Horse Health Care: A Veterinary Science Perspective

Horse Health Care: A Veterinary Science Perspective

Edited by Eliza Melton

MURPHY & MOORE
www.murphy-moorepublishing.com

Published by Murphy & Moore Publishing,
1 Rockefeller Plaza,
New York City, NY 10020, USA
www.murphy-moorepublishing.com

Horse Health Care: A Veterinary Science Perspective
Edited by Eliza Melton

International Standard Book Number: 978-1-63987-309-8 (Hardback)

Cataloging-in-Publication Data

Horse health care : a veterinary science perspective / edited by Eliza Melton.
p. cm.
Includes bibliographical references and index.
ISBN 978-1-63987-309-8
1. Horses--Health. 2. Horses. 3. Veterinary medicine. I. Melton, Eliza.
SF285.3 .H67 2022
636.1--dc23

TABLE OF CONTENTS

PREFACE

Horses are a common breed of domestic pets. They are also used for recreation purpose for humans such as for horse riding, racing events, polo, etc. They require a high degree of health care to prevent infections and disease outbreak. Some of the most prominent diseases in horses are colic, equine encephalomyelitis, azoturia, west nile virus, etc. Colic refers to a series of conditions characterized by variable degrees of abdominal pain. It is the most common digestive disorder in horses. Equine encephalomyelitis is caused by mosquitoes which carry viruses. The symptoms include lack of coordination, depression, fever, poor reflexes and a drooping lower lip. Vaccination can help in prevention of equine encephalomyelitis. Azoturial is a medical condition that affects the muscles of horses. It can result in cramping, stiffness, elevated temperature and sweat. West nile virus is caused by the bite of an infected mosquito. It can result in brain inflammation and meningitis. The symptoms include impaired vision, weakness of hind limbs, convulsions and difficulty in swallowing. This book is a valuable compilation of topics, ranging from the basic to the most complex advancements in the field of horse health care. It aims to shed light on some of the unexplored aspects of this discipline. This book will help the readers in keeping pace with the rapid changes in this field.

The researches compiled throughout the book are authentic and of high quality, combining several disciplines and from very diverse regions from around the world. Drawing on the contributions of many researchers from diverse countries, the book's objective is to provide the readers with the latest achievements in the area of research. This book will surely be a source of knowledge to all interested and researching the field.

In the end, I would like to express my deep sense of gratitude to all the authors for meeting the set deadlines in completing and submitting their research chapters. I would also like to thank the publisher for the support offered to us throughout the course of the book. Finally, I extend my sincere thanks to my family for being a constant source of inspiration and encouragement.

Editor

1

Capillaria hepatica (Calodium hepaticum) infection in a horse

Akihiro Ochi[1], Tatsuro Hifumi[2], Takanori Ueno[1*] and Yoshinari Katayama[1]

Abstract

Background: *Capillaria hepatica* is a zoonotic parasite in humans and animals and has a worldwide distribution. However, infections in mammals apart from rodents, which are natural hosts of the parasite, have rarely been reported. This report describes the first known case of *C. hepatica* infection in a horse in Japan.

Case presentation: A 3-year-old filly without clinical signs was presented at a slaughterhouse in Japan. Gross examination revealed white to tan nodules 0.5 to 1.5 cm in diameter in the parenchyma of the liver. Histologically, the nodules had mature fibrous capsules and consisted of multifocal to coalescing granulomatous inflammations with numerous nematode eggs. The eggs were barrel shaped with an opercular plug on each end and double-layered shells; these findings are consistent with the features of *C. hepatica* eggs.

Conclusions: To our knowledge, this is the first case of *C. hepatica* infection in a horse in Japan. The pathological findings confirmed the presence of this pathogen in this part of the world, and they highlight the importance of this nematode in the differential diagnosis of hepatic granulomatous lesions in horses.

Keywords: *Capillaria hepatica*, Hepatic capillariasis, Horse

Background

Capillaria hepatica (now called *Calodium hepaticum*) is a nematode in the family Capillariidae and a zoonotic parasite with a worldwide distribution. The usual hosts for the parasite are rodents, especially wild rats and mice [1], but the parasites uncommonly infect various other mammals including humans [2]. In a review of *C. hepatica* infections in humans, 163 cases, including 72 genuine infections have been reported in Europe, North and South America, Asia and Oceania, especially in tropical and temperate zone [1]. In veterinary medicine, this parasite was found in at least 69 species in 25 mammalian families including Insectivora, Chiroptera, Lagomorpha, Artiodactyla, Perissodactyla, Hyracoidea, Marsupialia, Carnivora, and Primates [2]. The life cycle of *C. hepatica* is direct [3]. After the animal ingests embryonated eggs, larvae hatch in the intestine and migrate to the liver, where they mature, breed, and lay unembryonated eggs. These eggs are not passed in the feces of the host but remain in the liver until the animal dies and decomposes or the host is eaten by scavengers or predators. After the death of the host, the unembryonated eggs are released into the environment and become infective and embryonated. In contrast, ingestion of unembryonated eggs leads to spurious infection, and the non-infective eggs are shed into the environment with the feces.

Capillaria hepatica is a zoonotic nematode that inhabits the liver of the host during the adult stage of the life cycle. The presence of worms and eggs can provoke focal necrosis, fibrosis, and inflammatory reaction in the liver [4] and result in hepatic capillariasis in a variety of animals [1]. However, *C. hepatica* infection in horses is relatively rare and only two cases have been reported, in the United Kingdom and Canada [5, 6]. This case report describes the first known case of *C. hepatica* infection in a horse in Japan.

Case presentation

The subject was a 3-year-old female Thoroughbred presented at a municipal slaughter plant in Japan. It was in good body condition, showed no signs of illness, and passed ante-mortem inspection. On gross examination, within the liver there were multifocal, firm, homogenous white to tan nodules 0.5 to 1.5 cm in diameter scattered

* Correspondence: ueno@equinst.go.jp
[1]Equine Research Institute, Japan Racing Association, 1400-4 Shiba, Shimotsuke, Tochigi 329-0412, Japan
Full list of author information is available at the end of the article

in the parenchyma. On the cut surface, the nodules were rich in fibrous tissue with partial calcification. The nodules were harvested from the horse, fixed in 20% neutral buffered formalin, and sent to the Equine Research Institute of the Japan Racing Association for histological examination. After fixation, the nodules were decalcified in Morse's solution. All samples were embedded in paraffin wax, cut at 4 μm, and stained with hematoxylin and eosin.

Histological examination revealed multifocal to coalescing, partially calcified granulomatous lesions in the hepatic parenchyma. Each lesion measured up to about 1.5 cm and contained nematode eggs surrounded by a fibrous capsule (Fig. 1). The eggs were barrel shaped with an opercular plug at each end and a double-layered shell with a spoke-like pattern (Fig. 2); they measured about 50 by 20 μm. Lymphocytes, macrophages, and a few eosinophils were infiltrated around the lesions. Although there were no adult worms in the tissues, the eggs were identified as those of *C. hepatica* on the basis of their morphological characteristics.

Discussion and conclusions

Capillaria hepatica is a parasitic nematode with a worldwide distribution [3]. Rodents are considered the main reservoirs, but the parasite rarely infects other animals. In Japan, the prevalence of *C. hepatica* in rodents is unknown, but the eggs or adult worms, or both, have been reported in mice and rats [7, 8]. Moreover, hepatic capillariasis has been observed in 2.25% of 400 cattle, although the nematode was not classified as *C. hepatica* [9]. Sekikawa et al. [10] reported the first human case of *C. hepatica* in Japan. However, to our knowledge, *C. hepatica* in horses has not been reported in this country. In horses, hepatic capillariasis is rare and only two cases have been reported—in the United Kingdom and Canada

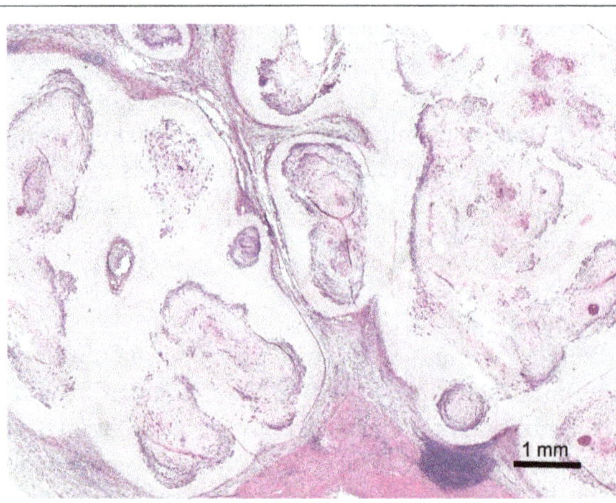

Fig. 1 Histology of the hepatic nodules. Multifocal to coalescing granulomatous lesions, with mild calcification, are present in the hepatic parenchyma. There are infiltrations of inflammatory cells, and edema is apparent at the periphery of the nodules. Hematoxylin and eosin stain

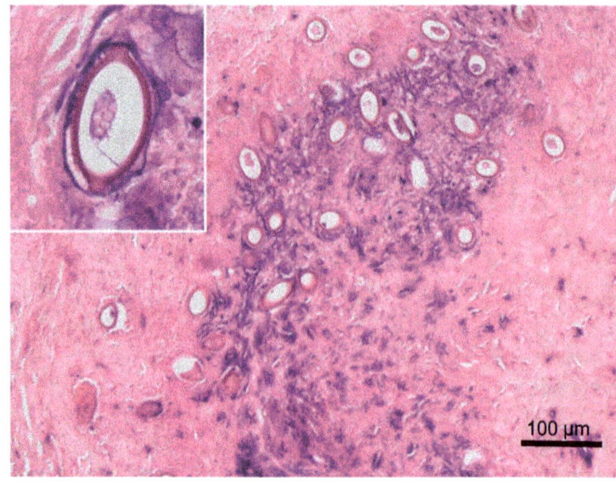

Fig. 2 *Capillaria hepatica* eggs. Most of the eggs are surrounded by fibrous tissue. Inset: The eggs are barrel-shaped and have a thick, two-layered wall with a reticulated surface. Hematoxylin and eosin stain

[5, 6]. The lesions consisted of fibrous connective tissue around eggs, as was seen in the present case.

Infection with *C. hepatica* occurs via the ingestion of embryonated eggs in the environment. In human cases, unsanitary practices, poor hygienic conditions, and the presence of dense rodent populations are thought to be predisposing factors of infection. [1]. In addition, the infections are usually found in children from 1 to 5 years old [11]. This higher incidence in children may be due to their more frequent soil-hand-mouth contact [12]. Children or adults with the habit of eating soil (geophagia or pica) are especially at risk of infection [13]. The habit of geophagia has been observed in horses and is considered to indicate nutritional deficiency or boredom [14]. Therefore, infection in horses is most likely due to accidental ingestion of the embryonated eggs with food, water, or soil, although the exact route in the present case was unknown.

Liver biopsy remains the gold standard method for the diagnosis of hepatic capillariasis [15], although other diagnostic methods are available in human medicine [1]. Imaging modalities such as ultrasound and computed tomography are helpful [16]. In addition, serologic methods such as indirect immunofluorescence can be used for screening purposes. However, these methods have not been widely used for diagnosis in veterinary medicine. A definitive diagnosis is commonly achieved by finding the adults or eggs, or both, in the liver.

This paper provides the first report of hepatic capillariasis in a horse in Japan. Although further investigations are needed to determine the prevalence of the nematode in horses, our findings indicate that *C. hepatica* infection should be considered in the differential diagnosis of hepatic granulomas in horses.

Acknowledgments
We thank Ms. Sayoko Shibata of the Equine Research Institute of Japan Racing Association for her technical help.

Funding
This study was supported by the Japan Racing Association.

Authors' contribution
AO conducted the pathological examination and drafted the manuscript. TH performed the gross examination and wrote the clinical report. TU and YK reviewed the manuscript. All authors read and approved the final manuscript.

Consent for publication
Not applicable.

Competing interests
The authors declare that they have no competing interests.

Author details
[1]Equine Research Institute, Japan Racing Association, 1400-4 Shiba, Shimotsuke, Tochigi 329-0412, Japan. [2]Laboratory of Veterinary Histopathology, Joint Faculty of Veterinary Medicine, Kagoshima University, Kagoshima 890-0065, Japan.

References
1. Fuehrer HP, Igel P, Auer H. *Capillaria hepatica* in man—an overview of hepatic capillariosis and spurious infections. Parasitol Res. 2011;109(4):969–79.
2. Fuehrer HP. An overview of the host spectrum and distribution of *Calodium hepaticum* (syn. *Capillaria hepatica*): part 2—Mammalia (excluding Muroidea). Parasitol Res. 2014;113(2):641–51.
3. Spratt DM, Singleton GR. Hepatic capillariasis. In: Samuel MW, Pybus JM, Kocan AA, editors. Parasitic diseases of wild mammals. USA: Wiley-Blackwell; 2008. p. 365–79.
4. Stalker M, Hayes M. Liver and biliary system. In: Maxie G, editor. Jubb, Kennedy, and Palmer's pathology of domestic animals, vol. 2. Elsevier: St. Louis; 2016. p. 258–352.
5. Munroe G. Pyloric stenosis in a yearling with an incidental finding of *Capillaria hepatica* in the liver. Equine Vet J. 1984;16(3):221–2.
6. Nation P, Dies K. Case report: *Capillaria hepatica* in a horse. Can Vet J. 1978; 19(11):315–6.
7. Momma K. Notes on modes of rat infestation with *Hepaticola hepatica*. Ann Trop Med Parasitol. 1930;24(1):109–13.
8. Iwaki T, Hatakeyama S, Nonaka N, Miyaji S, Yokohata Y, Okamoto M, et al. Survey on larval *Echinococcus multilocularis* and other hepatic helminths in rodents and insectivores in Hokkaido, Japan, from 1985 to 1992. Jpn J Parasitol. 1993;42:502–6.
9. Nakamura N. Parasitic lesions of bovine liver attributed to capillaria species. J Comp Pathol. 2005;132(2):228–31.
10. Sekikawa H, Hasegawa H, Otsuru M, Igarashi T, Kaneko H, Wada K, et al. First human case of *Capillaria hepatica* infection in Japan. Kiseichugaku Zasshi. 1991;40(6):528–32.
11. Juncker-Voss M, Prosl H, Lussy H, Enzenberg U, Auer H, Nowotny N. Serological detection of *Capillaria hepatica* by indirect immunofluorescence assay. J Clin Microbiol. 2000;38(1):431–3.
12. Wang Z, Cui J, Wang Y. Persistent febrile hepatomegaly with eosinophilia due to hepatic capillariasis in Central China. Ann Trop Med Parasitol. 2011; 105(6):469–72.
13. Ewing GM, Tilden I. *Capillaria hepatica*: report of fourth case of true human infestation. J Pediatr. 1956;48(3):341–8.
14. McGreevy P, Hawson L, Habermann T, Cattle S. Geophagia in horses: a short note on 13 cases. Appl Anim Behav Sci. 2001;71(2):119–25.
15. Li CD, Yang HL, Wang Y. Capillaria hepatica in China. World J Gastroenterol. 2010;16(6):698–702.
16. Sharma R, Dey AK, Mittal K, Kumar P, Hira P. *Capillaria hepatica* infection: a rare differential for peripheral eosinophilia and an imaging dilemma for abdominal lymphadenopathy. Ann Parasitol. 2015;61(1):61–4.

2

Metalloproteinases and their inhibitors are influenced by inhalative glucocorticoid therapy in combination with environmental dust reduction in equine recurrent airway obstruction

Ann Kristin Barton[1*], Tarek Shety[1,2], Angelika Bondzio[3], Ralf Einspanier[3] and Heidrun Gehlen[1]

Abstract

Background: Overexpression of matrix-metalloproteinases (MMPs) has been shown to lead to tissue damage in equine recurrent airway obstruction (RAO), as a misbalance with their natural inhibitors, the tissue inhibitors of metalloproteinases (TIMPs), occurs. This favors irreversible pulmonary fibrosis formation. Increased levels of MMPs, TIMPs or altered ratios between them can be used as biomarkers of respiratory disease. We hypothesized that levels of MMPs, TIMPs and their ratios correlate with improvement in clinical findings and bronchoalveolar lavage fluid (BALF) cytology after 10 days of inhalative glucocorticoid therapy and environmental dust reduction (EDR) and may be used to monitor treatment success.

Ten horses with a history of RAO participated in a prospective clinical study. Clinical and cytological scoring was performed before and after inhalative therapy using budesonide (1500 μg BID over 10 days) and EDR (bedding of wood shavings and wet hay as roughage). Gelatin zymography was performed for qualitative and semi-quantitative evaluation of MMP-2 and MMP-9 in BALF supernatant, while fluorimetry was used to evaluate MMP-8 activity. Additionally, specific equine ELISA assays were used for quantitative assessment of MMP-2, MMP-9, TIMP-1 and TIMP-2.

Results: A significant reduction in the total and several single parameters of the clinical score were found after 10 days of inhalative therapy and EDR. The concentrations of MMP-2, MMP-9, TIMP-1 and TIMP-2 (ELISA) as well as their activities (MMP-2 and MMP-9 zymography and MMP-8 fluorimetry) were significantly decreased after therapy. Significant improvements in MMP-8/TIMP-1 and MMP-8/TIMP-2 ratios were also found, differences between other ratios before and after therapy were insignificant.

Conclusions: Metalloproteinases and their inhibitors, in particular MMP-9 and TIMP-2, are valuable markers for clinical improvement in RAO.

Keywords: Horse, Lung, Inflammatory marker, Recurrent airway obstruction, Metalloproteinases, Tissue inhibitors of metalloproteinases

* Correspondence: Ann-Kristin.Barton@fu-berlin.de
[1]Equine Clinic, Freie Universitaet Berlin, Oertzenweg 19b, Berlin 10163, Germany
Full list of author information is available at the end of the article

Background

Severe equine asthma, commonly known as recurrent airway obstruction (RAO), is a very common pneumopathy in middle-aged to older horses with a prevalence of about 14% in the general horse population [1]. Older studies even found an incidence over 50% of this respiratory disease [2]. Thus, RAO is considered an important problem requiring veterinary attention as it leads to decreased performance capacity and major economic losses [3].

Equine RAO resembles human asthma and COPD in many ways. In all of them, so called remodeling of the pulmonary tissue occurs, which includes reduction of bronchial luminal caliber, smooth muscle hypertrophy, peribronchiolar fibrosis formation and airway epithelial cell hyperplasia, all impeding gas exchange [4, 5]. Control of remodeling may be the key to effective therapy and long-term success of managing these patients [6].

The extracellular matrix (ECM) stabilizes the inner structures of the lung, for which collagen is the most important ECM component. Therefore, the ECM is essential to insure the efficacy of gas exchange. To allow for growth and physiologic tissue repair, it underlies a continuous turnover, but a physiologic balance between synthesis and degradation needs to be maintained. Cleavage of ECM components takes place by zinc-depentant endopeptidases, so called matrix-metalloproteinases (MMPs) and is controlled by their natural inhibitors, the tissue inhibitors of matrix metalloproteinases (TIMPs) [6, 7]. Overwhelming proteolytic degradation in consequence of a dysbalance of MMP and TIMP activity leads to an inflammatory response and ultimately fibrosis formation [8, 9].

Several studies have been published focusing on MMP levels in equine RAO. Increased collagenolytic activity, as indicated by MMP-8 concentrations, was found in tracheal epithelium lining fluid (TELF) [10]. Levels of MMP-8 and MMP-13 were positively correlated with type-I collagen degradation [11].

Markedly increased elastinolytic activity in TELF, indicated by MMP-2 and –9, was also found in RAO [12, 13], but other authors found no disease-associated increase of MMP-2 levels and concluded that its major role may be the physiologic ECM turnover [14]. MMP-9 on the other hand shows very low levels in health, but increases dramatically during exacerbations of asthma and RAO as well as in idiopathic pulmonary fibrosis [15].

While levels of MMPs have been studied intensively in RAO, not much is known about their natural inhibitors, in particular TIMP-1 and TIMP-2, as well as the course of MMPs and TIMPs under different forms of therapy. The inhibitory effect of different tetracyclines, flunixin meglumine and pentoxifylline on elastinolytic activity after intravenous infusion of lipopolysaccharide (LPS) was evaluated [16]. All MMP inhibitors significantly decreased MMP activities, but pentoxifylline and oxytetracycline appeared to be the most effective. Collagenase activity also could be reduced by doxycycline inhibition in tracheal aspirates [10]. These authors concluded that MMP inhibitors might be a valuable new treatment approach to equine RAO. A similar effect was found in a clinical trial in human medicine, in which COPD patients with stable symptoms showed significant improvement in lung function after 4-weeks of doxycycline treatment [17].

Before testing MMP inhibitors in a clinical setting, we were interested in the course of MMPs and TIMPs under the cornerstone of RAO therapy, namely environmental dust reduction in combination with anti-inflammatory glucocorticoids, which were given in an inhalative approach to achieve high local concentrations in the lung. The focus of this study was the evaluation of possible correlations between clinical and cytological parameters with MMP-2, –8 and –9 as well as TIMP1- and –2 activities and concentrations before and after 10 days of inhalative budesonide therapy and environmental dust reduction (EDR).

Methods

Preparticipation examination

10 horses (4 geldings, 6 mares, age 16.5 ± 4.3 years, BDW 481 ± 80.4 kg) with a history of RAO were examined to evaluate the current disease status using a validated clinical score system, recommended by an international workshop [18, 19] and modified by including cytology of BALF instead of tracheal aspirates [20], the previous diagnosis was confirmed (Table 1). Horses in remission, not meeting the inclusion criteria for RAO exacerbation, but still showing parameters above reference values, were included into the study, as these patients account for a large part of our hospital population and often show further improvement under therapy.

BALF collection and processing

Under local anesthesia using 20 ml of 2% lidocaine[1] applied to the main bronchi, bronchoalveolar lavage was performed using a silicone catheter.[2] Five hundred milliliters of pre-warmed phosphate buffered saline[3] were infused and immediately aspirated. BALF was divided into 2 aliquots for cytological and biochemical examination. After centrifugation[4] (250 g, 10 min at 4 °C) the BALF supernatant was kept at –80 °C until further analysis. Cytology was performed using Wright-Giemsa staining and counting 500 cells at 500x magnification.

Gelatine zymography of elastases

Zymography was performed[5,6] following the manufacturer's instructions. Human MMP-2 and MMP-9 controls were used together with a multicolor broad protein range

Table 1 Clinical scoring system, modified from Ohnesorge et al. (1998): The highest score given in each subcategory counts as maximum points for this subcategory, maximum points of subcategories are summed up to gain the total score number

		Score	Max. Points
1. Coughing	No cough after manual compression of larynx	0	1
	from history, spontaneously or induced	1	
2. Dyspnoea at rest	moderately increased abdominal effort	1	3
	Nostril flare	3	
	Hypertrophy of abdominal muscles	3	
3. Percussion lung field	>1 hand increase	1	2
	>2 hands increase	2	
4. Lung auscultation	Wheezes and crackles	2	2
5. Endoscopy	Significantly increased secretions with moderate viscosity	1	2
	Highly increased secretions with high viscosity	2	
	Marked thickening of tracheal bifurcation [52]	1	
6. BALF cytology	Neutrophils <8%	0	3
	Neutrophils 8–15%	1	
	Neutrophils 15–25%	2	
	Neutrophils >25%	3	
7. Blood gas analysis	PAO_2-PaO_2: 0–7 mmHg	0	2
	PAO_2-PaO_2: 7–14 mmHg	1	
	PAO_2-PaO_2: >14 mmHg	2	

protein ladder as a control on each gel. Also, a sample of a healthy control horse (samples of a previous study) was applied to each gel to compare the signals to affected horses. Gels were scanned for digital analysis by densitometry using digital image analyzing software[7] to quantify the bands objectively as described previously [21].

ELISA of MMPs and TIMPs

Commercially available ELISA systems were used for quantification of MMP-2, MMP-9, TIMP-1 and TIMP-2 concentrations.[891011] Duplicate standards and samples were measured following the manufacturer's instructions and absorbance measured with an ELISA microplate reader[12] at 450 nm.

Fluorimetry MMP-8 assay

For the MMP-8 assay[13] the manufacturer's instructions were followed. Negative controls containing assay buffer and positive controls using recombinant human purified MMP-8 were included.

Inhalation therapy

Inhalation therapy was performed twice daily at a dosage of 1500 μg budesonide (Pulmicort™ suspension)[14] using an automatic inhalation device[15]. Although the study participants had been under environmental dust reduction (wood shavings as bedding and wet hay as roughage) at their home stables prior to the study, they were stabled in the clinic for overall 16 days to ensure the same conditions concerning stabling and application of inhalation therapy for all animals. During the phase of inhalation therapy a daily clinical examination ensured that no horse was suffering from complications or showed clinical signs of respiratory infection.

Check-up examination

After 10 days of inhalation therapy, the horses were examined following the same protocol as for the prepartticipation examination exclusive of thoracic radiography. Afterwards, they were discharged from the clinic with instructions to the owners concerning further management and therapy.

Statistical analysis

Statistical analysis was performed using SPSS Statistics[16] and results were expressed as mean ± standard deviation (SD). As parts of data were not found to be normally distributed using the Shapiro Wilks Test, non-parametric tests were used for the entire analysis. The level of significance was set at $P < 0.05$.

Spearman rank correlation coefficients were calculated between clinical and cytological parameters, MMP and TIMP concentrations or activities, respectively. The level of significance was set at $P < 0.05$.

The Wilcoxon signed ranks test was used to analyze differences before and after budesonide inhalation in combination with environmental dust reduction Again, the level of significance was set at $P < 0.05$.

Results

Clinical scoring

The anamnestic diagnosis of RAO was confirmed for all 10 horses. 7 horses were classified RAO in exacerbation, 3 in partial remission. All were subjected to treatment. The total examination score before and after therapy showed a significant difference before and after therapy ($P = 0.005$) with the endoscopy score being the single parameter of highest significance ($P = 0.007$).

Inhalation therapy and environmental dust reduction resulted in significantly decreased neutrophil ratio after therapy (25.7 ± 19.4%) compared to before therapy (42.92 ± 27%). As neutrophils decreased ($P = 0.013$), the relative percentage of macrophages increased ($P = 0.022$) from 32.77 ± 18.7% before therapy to 45 ± 16.57% after therapy.

Results of clinical scoring are shown in Table 2.

MMP-2 ELISA

The concentration of MMP-2 was significantly decreased after therapy (3.54 pg/ml ± 0.71 pg/ml) compared to before therapy (4.93 pg/ml ± 0.91 pg/ml, $P = 0.005$). MMP-2 activity in BALF detected by gelatin zymography was significantly decreased after therapy (5827.45 ± 5250.42) compared to that before therapy (12570.98 ± 9164.32, $P = 0.028$).

MMP-9 ELISA

MMP-9 concentration in BAL was significantly decreased after therapy (282.29 ng/ml ± 101.19 ng/ml) compared to before therapy (414.59 ng/ml ± 119.6 ng/ml, $P = 0.005$). The MMP-9 activity in gelatin zymography was significantly decreased after therapy (2942.95 ± 2440.24) compared to before therapy (11176.68 ± 11255.3, $P = 0.022$).

Table 2 Mean results ± standard deviation (Min-Max) of clinical scoring before and after therapy in 10 RAO horses

Parameter	Before therapy	After therapy	P
Coughing	0.5 ± 0.53 (0–1)	0.3 ± 0.48 (0–1)	0.157
Dyspnea at rest	1.1 ± 1.1 (0–3)	0.7 ± 0.82 (0–2)	0.046*
Percussion of the lung field	0 ± 0 (0–0)	0 ± 0 (0–0)	1
Lung auscultation	0 ± 0 (0–0)	0 ± 0 (0–0)	1
Endoscopy	1.5 ± 0.53 (1–2)	0.6 ± 0.52 (0–1)	0.007*
BALF cytology	2.4 ± 1.1 (0–3)	2 ± 1.25 (0–3)	0.157
Blood gas analysis	0.4 ± 0.7 (0–2)	0 ± 0 (0–0)	0.102
Total clinical score	6 ± 2.6 (2–10)	$3.1 \pm 2^{*\downarrow}$ (0–5)	0.005*

* marks significance at $P < 0.05$

Examples of MMP-2 and MMP-9 zymography before and after therapy are shown in Figs. 1a and b.

TIMP-1 ELISA

TIMP-1 concentration was significantly decreased after therapy (249.78 ± 59.56 pg/ml) compared to before therapy (308.80 ± 7.44 pg/ml, $P = 0.005$).

TIMP-2 ELISA

TIMP-2 concentration was also significantly decreased after therapy (18.76 ± 2.79 ng/ml) compared to before therapy (26.20 ± 1.49 ng/ml, $P = 0.002$).

MMP-8 fluorimetry

The activity of MMP-8 was significantly decreased after therapy (0.10 RFU ± 0.11 RFU) compared to before therapy (0.57 RFU ± 0.85 RFU, $P = 0.005$).

Results of MMP- and TIMP-measurements are presented in Table 3.

Correlation of clinical score and MMPs/TIMPs

Strong positive correlations were found between the total clinical scoring and concentrations of MMP-2 ($r = 0.66$), MMP-9 ($r = 0.83$), TIMP-1 ($r = 0.65$), TIMP-2 ($r = 0.72$) concentrations, MMP-8 activity ($r = 0.75$) and weakly for MMP-2 ($r = 0.47$) activity measured by gelatin zymography. All these correlations had a level of significance of $P < 0.01$, except MMP-2 zymography ($P = 0.036$). No significant correlation was found between the clinical examination score and MMP-9 zymography ($r = 0.30$).

Correlations of BALF cytology and MMPs/TIMPs

BAL neutrophil percentages showed no correlation with the concentrations of MMP-2 ($r = 0.39$), but significant correlations with MMP-9 ($r = 0.59$), TIMP-1 ($r = 0.65$), TIMP-2 ($r = 0.72$) concentrations and MMP-8 activity ($r = 0.78$) with $P < 0.01$. MMP-2 activity measured by gelatin zymography was also weakly correlated ($r = 0.45$), while MMP-9 ($r = 0.25$) activity was not ($P < 0.05$).

MMP/TIMP ratios

Significant differences were found for MMP-8 / TIMP-1 ($P = 0.002$) and MMP-8 / TIMP-2 ($P = 0.038$) ratios before and after therapy as shown in Table 4.

Discussion

Pathogenesis of airway remodeling – In human asthma, activation of fibroblasts leads to increases of ECM mass by overwhelming fibrosis formation, a process similar to bronchial remodeling in equine RAO. This is suspected to be the consequence of a pathologic dysbalance between proteolytic degradation of ECM components by MMPs, and excessive tissue repair primarily mediated by TIMP-1, which can be upregulated very effectively and

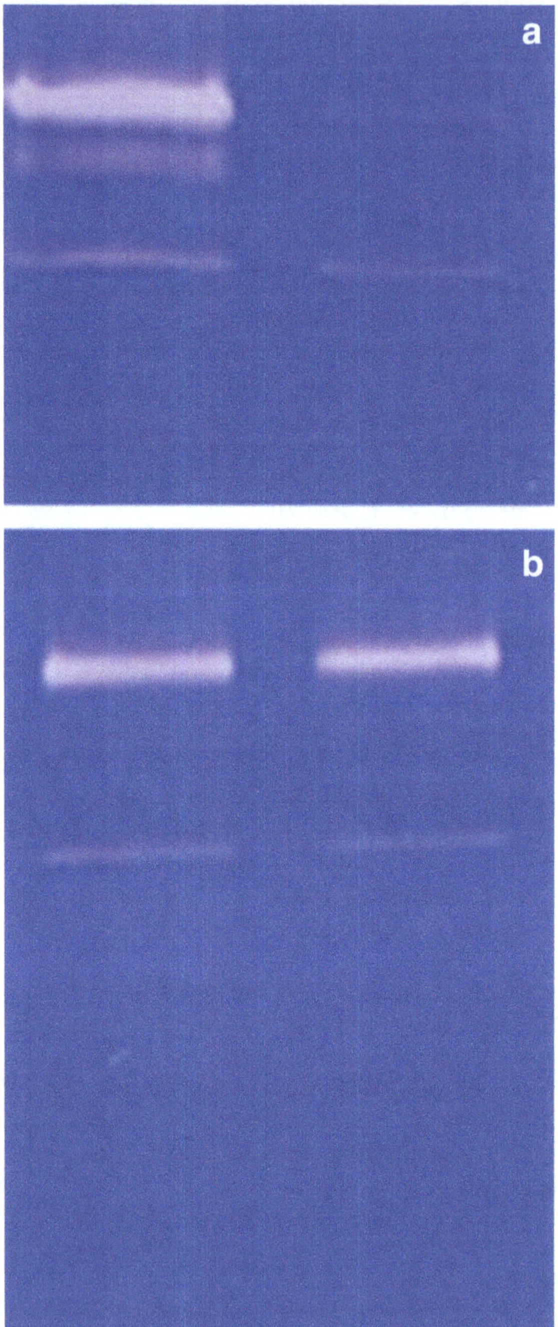

Fig. 1 Zymography of MMP-2 (*lower band*) and MMP-9 (*upper band*) before (*left*) and after (*right*) inhalation therapy in a horse showing clear improvement in clinical and cytologic data (**a**) versus a horse, in which therapy did not lead to significant improvement (**b**)

is capable of cleaving all active MMPs. Elastinolytic and collagenolytic activity was found in several studies on human asthma, in particular increased levels of MMP-9 [22, 23], but also MMP-2 [24, 25]. Former studies of our group showed that this is also true for several equine pneumopathies including RAO, inflammatory airway disease (IAD) and chronic interstitial pneumopathy compared to healthy controls [26, 27]. Compared to these controls, all horses of the presented study showed increased levels of MMP 2, 8 and 9 prior to therapy. Increased TIMP levels have also been found in humans suffering from asthma [23, 24, 28, 29] and the same was found for equine RAO in this study and previous [26, 27]. This may allow the suspicion that fibrosis formation as a long-term consequence of human asthma and equine RAO may be the ultimate result of continuous activation of tissue repair mechanisms or over-repair processes [30]. The most important source of MMP-8, MMP-9 and TIMP-1 are neutrophils, which are typically increased in RAO, accounting for more than 25% of BALF cytology by definition [1]. Therefore, decreases of these enzymes in accordance with decreasing percentages of neutrophils can be expected.

Effects of corticosteroids on MMPs and TIMPs - According to the GINA (global initiative for asthma) guidelines, inhalative therapy using various corticosteroids including budesonide is the key factor of asthma therapy after the control of acute disease exacerbation and is commonly used for persistent long-term management [31]. Reduced pulmonary function and increased inflammatory mediators are also found in equine RAO during phases of clinical remission [32] and corticosteroid treatment in combination with $ß_2$-mimetic bronchodilatators and secretolytic therapy is accepted as the most successful therapy after consequent environmental dust-control [1]. Inhalative treatment is becoming more and more popular in equine medicine and results may be more comparable to what is known in asthmatic patients, so we chose this route of application for our study. Glucocorticoids were shown to slow down the process of bronchial remodeling by downregulation of elastinolytic activity and TIMP upregulation at the same time [33], but other authors could not confirm this observation. Data of the presented study shows indeed the most significant decrease in MMP-9 compared to MMP-2 and 8, but there were also significant decreases in TIMP-1 and TIMP-2. Ex vivo studies demonstrated the ability of corticosteroids to decrease MMP-9 and TIMP-1 levels [34]. In human lung fibrosis, MMP-9 expression could be inhibited with steroids and immunosuppressants [35]. Fibrosis formation is also a long-term effect of equine RAO [36, 37] and it might be suspected that TIMPs decrease in reaction to decreasing MMPs. Nevertheless, ratios of elastases and TIMPs did not differ before and after inhalative therapy in combination with environmental dust control in the presented study.

Todorova et al. [30] studied the effect of inhaled budesonide combined with the bronchodilator formoterol on the metalloproteolytic balance between MMPs and TIMPs. This combination therapy inhibited upregulation

Table 3 MMP-2, MMP-9, TIMP-1 and TIMP-2 ELISA and MMP-8 fluorimetry measurements, the results are expressed as mean ± SD

	n	Before therapy	After therapy	*P*-value
MMP-2 ELISA [pg/ml]	10	4.93 ± 0.91	3.54 ± 0.71	0.005
MMP-9 ELISA [ng/ml]	10	414.59 ± 119.6	282.29 ± 101.19	0.005
TIMP-1 ELISA [pg/ml]	10	308.80 ± 7.44	249.78 ± 59.56	0.005
TIMP-2 ELISA [ng/ml]	10	26.20 ± 1.49	18.76 ± 2.79	0.002
MMP-8 Fluorimetry [RFU]	10	0.57 ± 0.85	0.1 ± 0.11	0.005
MMP-2 zymography	10	12570.98 ± 9164.32	5827.45 ± 5250.42	0.028
MMP-9 zymography	10	11176.68 ± 11255.3	2942.95 ± 2440.24	0.022

of prostaglandine and TIMP-1 production, MMP-9 levels and the MMP-9 / TIMP-1 ratio in human lung fibroblasts, whereas MMP-2 was not affected. Budesonide monotherapy required higher concentrations and formoterol alone had no effects. Therefore, the synergistic effect of budesonide and formoterol was considered the best option to reduce enhanced metalloproteolytic activity and may inhibit or at least reduce pulmonary fibrosis formation in asthma. We might have enhanced the effect of our therapy on MMPs in horses, if the budesonide had been combined with a $ß_2$-agonist like clenbuterol, which is commonly used in horses. This should be the subject of further studies. In asthmatic rats sensitized by ovalbumin and challenged with mist inhalation, steroid treatment not only reduced MMP-9 and TIMP-1 levels, but also improved hyperplasia of airway smooth muscle and basement membrane [38]. Inhalation of budesonide only influences MMP-9 and TIMP-1 levels in moderate to severe disease though, no effect of inhaled budesonide was found in subjects suffering from mild asthma [25].

Obase et al. [39] studied the effects of inhaled budesonide in children with mild and moderate symptoms of asthma on MMP-8 and TIMP-1 levels in induced sputum. Before the beginning of inhalation, MMP-8 was higher in asthma of moderate severity, TIMP-1 was lower and the MMP-8/TIMP-1 ratio was higher in mild and moderate asthma in comparison to healthy childeren. TIMP-1 levels increased in consequence of budesonide inhalation leading to normalization of the the MMP-8 / TIMP-1 ratio. Nevertheless, the excessive MMP-8 levels remained in the airways of children with moderate symptoms. Therefore, corticosteroids may be capable of controlling asthma symptoms, but may be insufficient in preventing the occurrence of airway remodeling involving MMP-8. Results of the presented study, however, show a significant reduction in MMP-8 activity after corticosteroid therapy, although most horses were in disease exacerbation before starting the inhalation protocol. There were also significant reductions in both TIMP concentrations as well as in the MMP-8 / TIMP-1 and the MMP-8 / TIMP-2 ratios. This shows that the MMP-8 / TIMP ratios in the horse do not normalize by upregulation of TIMP, but by downregulation of MMP-8. This seems pleasing and would improve prognosis in equine disease compared to human asthma, but further studies should be performed on the role of MMP-8, as airway remodeling is definitely a long-term effect of equine RAO leading to irreversible exercise insufficiency, but fibrosis formation might not be a direct consequence of TIMP overexpression in the horse.

New therapeutic approaches - MMPs themselves have been discussed as an ideal target for new therapeutic approaches as they play an active role in disease pathophysiology [40]. Inhibition of MMP activity has been studied in human cancer. Although this was not successful [41], new data suggests that selective inhibitors might find a role in acute and chronic anti-inflammatory therapy after all [42]. This includes asthma, where reduced airway inflammation and hyperresponsiveness was reported after local bronchial application of synthetic TIMP-2 [43]. TIMP-2 downregulated MMP-2 activity [44]. In addition to their antibiotic acitivity, tetracyclines act as effective MMP inhibitors. Doxycycline was studied in asthma models including different species [10, 45, 46]. After oral administration in mice, it reduced airway inflammation and hyperresponsiveness as well as MMP-9 expression. Further studies have shown that MMP-inhibition also decreases goblet cell hyperplasia, another component of airway remodeling in asthma [47], whichh is also known for equine RAO. In the horse, in-vitro studies showed reductions of proteolytic activity using acetylcysteine, pentamidine and diminazene [14, 48]. The clinical application of synthetic TIMPs in

Table 4 MMP/TIMP ratios before and after therapy ($n = 10$)

	MMP-2/ TIMP-1	MMP-2/ TIMP 2	MMP-9/ TIMP-1	MMP-9/ TIMP-2	MMP-8/ TIMP-1	MMP-8/ TIMP-2
Before therapy	0.016	0.188	1.343	15.824	0.002	0.022
After therapy	0.014	0.188	1.130	15.047	0.000*	0.005*

The (*) shows significance at $P < 0.05$

RAO horses is currently under consideration by our group.

Limitations - To our knowledge, this is the first study on the course of MMPs in RAO affected horses and a clinical trial, but we were faced with several limitations, so unintentional bias may have occurred at several points. Due to the fact that privately owned horses were included to the study, it was doubtful if stabling of all horses at their home stables was actually in a low-dust environment, as most horses were still in exacerbation and had increased MMPs at the beginning of therapy. The effect of therapy may therefore be based on the combined effect of inhalative glucocorticoid therapy and environmental dust reduction under clinic conditions, with the effect of the latter being quite variable. Even if horses had been stabled on wood shavings and fed wet hay, they may have come from a very dusty environment apart from these two conditions for enrolment in the study. A second group subjected to a low-dust-environment in the clinic only would have been preferable to control this effect and was planned to be included in the study, but unfortunately, not enough owners agreed to this protocol. Therefore, the actual bias caused by this is hard to assess. Another time-point of sampling after a few days of low-dust-environment before starting inhalation therapy would have been helpful as well, but again, owners wished for hospitalization as short as possible. On the other hand, it was not the aim of this study to prove the therapeutic effect of neither environmental dust reduction, which is commonly acceptected [1] nor inhaled budesonide, which has also already been published [49], but to study the course of MMPs and TIMPs under clinical improvement to evaluate their usefulness as biomarkers and correlation with clinical and cytological findings. Clinical scoring and even the quantitative tests may have been subject to bias as well. The clinical scoring was done by two independent observers, but these were not blinded to horses'enrolment in the study and the time-point as before or after therapy, which was due to the fact that subjects enrolled were clinic patients. Endoscopy and cytology was done by one observer and images scored by another later on randomly and blinded. ELISAs and zymography were performed, when all samples had been collected and stored, also randomly and blinded.

Conclusion

Despite the difficulties discussed above, the results of the presented study suggest that developing new therapeutic approaches to correct the misbalance between MMPs and TIMPs might be promising for treatment of asthma and equine RAO, which shares many features with human asthma disease. Due to their various effects in different organ systems, it seems safer to target MMPs actually relevant in this disease specifically and to use an inhalative approach to reach high local levels of the drug, while the remaining organism remains unaffected. In chronic pneumopathies, targeting MMP-2 and MMP-8, but in particular MMP-9 might be of therapeutic value [50]. First attempts in this direction have been taken in treating cancer, but less data is available on inhibition of MMP activity in chronic pneumopathies [51].

To our knowledge, TIMP-1 or TIMP-2 expression in equine RAO has not been studied so far. Studies in horses on the effect of inhaled glucocorticoids on MMPs or TIMPs have not been published either. Therefore, this is the first clinical study to show a correlation of MMP and TIMP levels to clinical findings and cytology. Parallels to results presented in papers on humans and laboratory animals allow the suspicion that the same mechanisms might apply in the horse regarding the effects of glucocorticoids, but further studies including a control group have to be performed to differentiate a possible therapeutic effect between glucocorticoid inhalation and envirnonmental dust reduction in horses affected by RAO.

Endnotes

[1]Lidocaine, bela-Pharm GmbH, Vechta, Germany

[2]Silicone Bronchoalveolar Lavage Catheter 300 cm, Smiths Medical ASD, Inc, USA

[3]Phosphate buffered saline, Lonza, Verviers, Belgium;[d-] Table Top Refrigerated Centrifuge Hermle Z326K, Hermle Labortechnik GmbH, Germany

[4]Gelatin zymogram gels, Life technologies, USA

[5]electrophoresis device XCell, Novex Experimental Technology, Japan

[6]ImageJ v1.47, Wayne Rasband, NIH, USA

[7]equine MMP-2 kit, USCN Life Science Inc., China

[8]equine MMP-2 kit, USCN Life Science Inc., China

[9]equine MMP-9 kit, USCN Life Science Inc., China

[10]equine TIMP-1 kit, USCN Life Science Inc., China

[11]equine TIMP-2 kit, USCN Life Science Inc., China

[12]ELISA microplate reader, BioRad Laboratories, USA

[13]Sensolyte™ 520 MMP-8 Assay Kit, Anaspec, Inc. Fermont, USA

[14]Pulmicort™ suspension, Astra Zeneca, Germany

[15]SaHoMa II mobile ultrasonic nebulizer, NEBU-TEC International, Germany

[16]SPSS Statistics, Version 17.0 released 2008, SPSS Inc., USA

Abbreviations

$AaDo_2$: Arterio-alveolar pressure difference; BALF: Bronchoalveolar lavage fluid; BDW: Body weight; BGA: Blood gas analysis; BID: Bis in die, twice daily; CIP: Chronic interstitial pneumopathy; COPD: Chronic obstructive pulmonary disease; ECM: Extracellular matrix; EDR: Environmental dust reduction; ELISA: Enzyme-linked immunosorbent assay; GINA: Global initiative for asthma; IAD: Inflammatory airway disease; LaGeSo: State Office of Health and Social Affairs Berlin; LPS: Lipopolysaccharide; MMP: Matrix metalloproteinase; PaO_2: Partial oxygen pressure; RAO: Recurrent airway obstruction;

Rpm: Rounds per minute; SD: Standard deviation; TELF: Tracheal epithelium lining fluid; TIMP: Tissue inhibitor of metalloproteinases

Acknowledgements
We thank the owners of the horses for participation in this study.

Funding
This study was funded by a research grant of the Freie Universitaet Berlin.

Authors contributions
AKB carried out the clinical examinations, participated in the conceivement, design and coordination of the study and drafted the manuscript. TS carried out the laboratory assays and performed the statistical analysis. AB participated in the coordination of the study and participated in the laboratory assays, RE participated in the coordination of the study and laboratory assays, HG conceived of the study, participated in its design and coordination. All authors read and approved the final manuscript.

Competing interests
The authors declare that they have no competing interests.

Consent for publication
Not applicable.

Author details
[1]Equine Clinic, Freie Universitaet Berlin, Oertzenweg 19b, Berlin 10163, Germany. [2]Animal Medicine Department, Faculty of Veterinary Medicine, Zagazig University, Zagazig, Egypt. [3]Institute of Veterinary Biochemistry, Freie Universitaet Berlin, Oertzenweg 19b, Berlin 10163, Germany.

References

1. Pirie RS. Recurrent airway obstruction: a review. Equine Vet J. 2014;46:276–88.
2. Bracher V, von Fellenberg R, Winder CN, et al. An investigation of the incidence of chronic obstructive pulmonary disease (COPD) in random populations of Swiss horses. Equine Vet J. 1991;23:136–41.
3. Roy MF, Lavoie JP. Tools for the diagnosis of equine respiratory disorders. Vet Clin North Am Equine Pract. 2003;19:1–17.
4. Lavoie JP. Recurrent Airway Obstruction (Heaves) and Summer-pasture-associated Obstructive Pulmonary Disease. In: McGorum BC, Dixon PM, Robinson NE, Schumacher J, editors. Equine Respiratory Medicine and Surgery. Edinburgh: W.B. Saunders; 2007. p. 565–90.
5. Lugo J, Harkema JR, deFeijter-Rupp H, et al. Airway inflammation is associated with mucous cell metaplasia and increased intraepithelial stored mucosubstances in horses. Vet J. 2006;172:293–301.
6. Lu P, Takai K, Weaver VM et al. Extracellular matrix degradation and remodeling in development and disease. Cold Spring Harb Perspect Biol. 2011; 3: doi: 10.1101/cshperspect.a005058.
7. Clutterbuck AL, Harris P, Allaway D, et al. Matrix metalloproteinases in inflammatory pathologies of the horse. Vet J. 2010;183:27–38.
8. Frantz C, Stewart KM, Weaver VM. The extracellular matrix at a glance. J Cell Sci. 2010;123:4195–200.
9. Chapman HA. Disorders of lung matrix remodeling. J Clin Invest. 2004;113:148–57.
10. Koivunen AL, Maisi P, Konttinen YT, et al. Collagenolytic activity and its sensitivity to doxycycline inhibition in tracheal aspirates of horses with chronic obstructive pulmonary disease. Acta Vet Scand. 1997;38:9–16.
11. Raulo SM, Sorsa TA, Kiili MT, et al. Evaluation of collagenase activity, matrix metalloproteinase-8, and matrix metalloproteinase-13 in horses with chronic obstructive pulmonary disease. Am J Vet Res. 2001;62:1142–8.
12. Raulo SM, Sorsa TA, Tervahartiala T, et al. MMP-9 as a marker of inflammation in tracheal epithelial lining fluid (TELF) and in bronchoalveolar fluid (BALF) of COPD horses. Equine Vet J. 2001;33:128–36.
13. Raulo SM, Sorsa TA, Maisi PS. Concentrations of elastinolytic metalloproteinases in respiratory tract secretions of healthy horses and horses with chronic obstructive pulmonary disease. Am J Vet Res. 2000;61:1067–73.
14. Koivunen AL, Maisi P, Konttinen YT, et al. Gelatinolytic activity in tracheal aspirates of horses with chronic obstructive pulmonary disease. Acta Vet Scand. 1997;38:17–27.
15. Atkinson JJ, Senior RM. Matrix metalloproteinase-9 in lung remodeling. Am J Respir Cell Mol Biol. 2003;28:12–24.
16. Fugler LA, Eades SC, Moore RM, et al. Plasma matrix metalloproteinase activity in horses after intravenous infusion of lipopolysaccharide and treatment with matrix metalloproteinase inhibitors. Am J Vet Res. 2013;74:473–80.
17. Dalvi PS, Singh A, Trivedi HR, et al. Effect of doxycycline in patients of moderate to severe chronic obstructive pulmonary disease with stable symptoms. Ann Thorac Med. 2011;6:221–6.
18. Ohnesorge B, Trötschel C and Deegen E. Diagnostic value of capnography in horses with RAO. Proceedings 5th World Equine Vet Assoc Congress 1998, p. 65–69.
19. Robinson NE. International workshop on equine chronic airway disease, Michigan State University 16–18 June 2000. Equine Vet J. 2001;33:5–19.
20. Dieckmann M, Deegen E. Clinical aspect of tracheobronchial aspirates cytology. Pferdeheilkunde. 1990;6:101–10.
21. Chung MK. Correlation Coefficient. In: Salkind J, editor. Encyclopedia of Measurement and Statistics. London: Sage; 2007.
22. Ohbayashi H, Shimokata K. Matrix metalloproteinase-9 and airway remodeling in asthma. Curr Drug Targets Inflamm Allergy. 2005;4:177–81.
23. Mattos W, Lim S, Russell R, et al. Matrix metalloproteinase-9 expression in asthma: effect of asthma severity, allergen challenge, and inhaled corticosteroids. Chest. 2002;122:1543–52.
24. Cataldo D, Munaut C, Noel A, et al. MMP-2-and MMP-9-linked gelatinolytic activity in the sputum from patients with asthma and chronic obstructive pulmonary disease. Int Arch Allergy Immunol. 2000;123:259–67.
25. Suzuki R, Kato T, Miyazaki Y, et al. Matrix metalloproteinases and tissue inhibitors of matrix metalloproteinases in sputum from patients with bronchial asthma. J Asthma. 2001;38:477–84.
26. Barton A, Shety T, Pelli A, et al. Evaluation of inflammatory markers and treatment success in inflammatory airway disease under the course of inhalation therapy and environmental dust reduction. Cabourg: Proceedings 2nd Havemeyer Workshop on IAD; 2014.
27. Barton A, Shety T, Bondzio A, et al. Metalloproteinases and their tissue inhibitors in comparison between different chronic pneumopathies in the horse, Med Inflamm. 2015, http://dx.doi.org/10.1155/2015/569512
28. Vignola AM, Riccobono L, Mirabella A, et al. Sputum metalloproteinase-9/ tissue inhibitor of metalloproteinase-1 ratio correlates with airflow obstruction in asthma and chronic bronchitis. Am J Respir Crit Care Med. 1998;158:1945–50.
29. Mautino G, Henriquet C, Jaffuel D, et al. Tissue inhibitor of metalloproteinase-1 levels in bronchoalveolar lavage fluid from asthmatic subjects. Am J Respir Crit Care Med. 1999;160:324–30.
30. Todorova L, Gürcan E, Westergren-Thorsson G, et al. Budesonide/ formoterol effects on metalloproteolytic balance in TGFb-activated human lung fibroblasts. Respir Med. 2009;103:1755–63.
31. Global Initiative for Asthma (GINA). Global strategy for asthma managementand prevention. NIH Publication 02–3659 issued January 1995 (updated 2004).
32. Lavoie-Lamoureux A, Leclere M, Lemos K, et al. Markers of systemic inflammation in horses with heaves. J Vet Intern Med. 2012;26:1419–26.
33. Hoshino M, Takahashi M, Takai Y, et al. Inhaled corticosteroids decrease subepithelial collagen deposition by modulation of the balance between matrix metalloproteinase-9 and tissue inhibitor of metalloproteinase-1 expression in asthma. J Allergy Clin Immunol. 1999;104:356–63.
34. Profita M, Gagliardo R, Di Giorgi R, et al. In vitro effects of flunisolide on MMP-9, TIMP-1, fibronectin, TGF-beta1 release and apoptosis in sputum cells freshly isolated from mild to moderate asthmatics. Allergy. 2004;59:927–32.
35. Gueders MM, Foidart JM, Noel A, et al. Matrix metalloproteinases (MMPs) and tissue inhibitors of MMPs in the respiratory tract: potential implications in asthma and other lung diseases. Eur J Pharmacol. 2006;533:133–44.
36. Kaup FJ, Drommer W, Deegen E. Ultrastructural findings in horses with chronic obstructive pulmonary-disease (COPD). 1. Alterations of the larger conducting airways. Equine Vet J. 1990;22:343–8.

37. Kaup FJ, Drommer W, Damsch S, et al. Ultrastructural findings in horses with chronic obstructive pulmonary disease (COPD) II: Pathomorphological changes of the terminal airways and the alveolar region. Equine Vet J. 1990;22:349–55.
38. Qiao HM, Lu JR, Cheng HJ, et al. Regulatory effects of inhaled steroids on expression of matrix metalloproteinase-9 and its inhibitor in asthmatic rats. Zhonghua Er Ke Za Zhi. 2005;43:591–4.
39. Obase Y, Rytilä P, Metso T, et al. Effects of Inhaled Corticosteroids on Metalloproteinase-8 and Tissue Inhibitor of Metalloproteinase-1 in the Airways of Asthmatic Children. Int Arch Allergy Immunol. 2010;151:247–54.
40. Fingleton B. MMPs as therapeutic targets–still a viable option? Semin Cell Dev Biol. 2008;19:61–8.
41. Vihinen P, Ala-aho R, Kahari VM. Matrix metalloproteinases as therapeutic targets in cancer. Curr Cancer Drug Targets. 2005;5:203–20.
42. Hu J, Van den Steen PE, Sang QXA, et al. Matrix metalloproteinase inhibitors as therapy for inflammatory and vascular diseases. Nat Rev Drug Discov. 2007;6:480–98.
43. Kumagai K, Ohno I, Okada S, et al. Inhibition of matrix metalloproteinases prevents allergen-induced airway inflammation in a murine model of asthma. Am J Respir Crit Care Med. 1999;159:325.
44. Kumagai K, Ohno I, Imai K, et al. The involvement of matrix metalloproteinases in basement membrane injury in a murine model of acute allergic airway inflammation. Clin Exp Allergy. 2002;32:1527–34.
45. Lee YC, Lee HB, Rhee YK, et al. The involvement of matrix metalloproteinase-9 in airway inflammation of patients with acute asthma. Clin Exp Allergy. 2001;31:1623–30.
46. Lee KS, Jin SM, Kim SS, et al. Doxycycline reduces airway inflammation and hyperresponsiveness in a murine model of toluene diisocyanate-induced asthma. J Allergy Clin Immunol. 2004;113:902–9.
47. Yoshisue H, Hasegawa K. Effect of MMP/ADAM inhibitors in goblet cell hyperplasia in cultured human bronchial epithelial cells. Biosci Biotechnol Biochem. 2004;68:2024–31.
48. Koivunen AL, Maisi P, Fang W, et al. Inhibition of the protease activity in tracheobronchial aspirates of horses with chronic obstructive pulmonary disease. Am J Vet Res. 1996;57:603–7.
49. Kampmann C, Ohnesorge B, Venner M, et al. Effects of inhaled budesonide on pulmonary mechanics and gas exchange for treatment of COPD. Equine Medicine. 2001;17:155–60.
50. Kupai K, Szucs G, Cseh S. Matrix metalloproteinase activity assays: Importance of zymography. J Pharmacol Toxicol Methods. 2010;61:205–9.
51. Ohbayashi H. Matrix metalloproteinases in lung diseases. Curr Protein Pept Sci. 2002;3:409–21.
52. Gerber V, Straub R, Marti E, et al. Endoscopic scoring of mucus quantity and quality: observer and horse variance and relationship to inflammation, mucus viscoelasticity and volume. Equine Vet J. 2004;36:576–82.

3

In vitro effects of platelet-rich gel supernatants on histology and chondrocyte apoptosis scores, hyaluronan release and gene expression of equine cartilage explants challenged with lipopolysaccharide

Jorge U. Carmona[1*], Diana L. Ríos[1], Catalina López[1], María E. Álvarez[1,2], Jorge E. Pérez[2] and Mabel E. Bohórquez[3]

Abstract

Background: Platelet-rich plasma (PRP) preparations are a common treatment in equine osteoarthritis (OA). However, there are controversies regarding the ideal concentration of platelets and leukocytes in these biological substances necessary to induce an adequate anti-inflammatory and anabolic response in articular cartilage. The aims were to study the influence of leukocyte- and platelet-rich gel (L-PRG) and pure platelet-rich gel (P-PRG) supernatants on the histological changes of cartilage, the degree of chondrocyte apoptosis, the production of hyaluronan (HA) and the gene expression of nuclear factor kappa beta (NFkβ), matrix metalloproteinase 13 (MMP-13), a disintegrin and metalloproteinase with thrombospondin motifs 4 (ADAMTS-4), collagen type I alpha 1 (COL1A1), collagen type II alpha 1 (COL2A1) and cartilage oligomeric matrix protein (COMP) in normal cartilage explants (CEs) challenged with lipopolysaccharide (LPS).

Results: Overall, 25 % L-PRG supernatant (followed in order of importance by, 50 % P-PRG, 25 % P-PRG and 50 % L-PRG) represented the substance with the most important anti-inflammatory and anabolic effect. 25 % P-PRG supernatant presented important anabolic effects, but it induced a more severe chondrocyte apoptosis than the other evaluated substances.

Conclusions: 25 % L-PRG supernatant presented the best therapeutic profile. Our results demonstrate that the biological variability of PRP preparations makes their application rather challenging. Additional in vivo research is necessary to know the effect of PRP preparations at different concentrations.

Keywords: Platelet-rich plasma, Cartilage explants, Chondrocyte apoptosis, Catabolic/anabolic gene expression, Growth factors

* Correspondence: carmona@ucaldas.edu.co
[1]Grupo de Investigación Terapia Regenerativa, Departamento de Salud Animal, Universidad de Caldas, Manizales, Colombia
Full list of author information is available at the end of the article

Background

Osteoarthritis (OA) is a chronic inflammatory disease that affects middle aged and older people worldwide [1]. This disease also affects horses and other animal species, which causes economic losses by diminishing the athletic potential of the affected animals and through the chronic use of anti-inflammatory drugs and nutraceuticals [2–4]. Thus, the horse is an important animal model to study both the pathophysiological mechanisms and the experimental treatments of OA [5, 6].

There are several extrinsic factors associated with OA development such as joint repetitive trauma, obesity, joint infection and osteochondrosis, amongst others [4]. During the OA developmental process, there are structural (histological) changes indicating the severity or degree of affectation of the articular cartilage [7]. This includes increased chondrocyte necrosis, cluster (complex chondrone) formation, fibrillation/fissuring, focal cell loss and diminished uptake of safranin-O fast green (SOFG) stain [8]. Furthermore, another important histological change associated with OA is chondrocyte apoptosis, which leads to loss of resident cells in the articular cartilage and results in severe alterations such as impaired extracellular matrix (ECM) remodelling [9]. This phenomenon has been described in both human and animal models of OA [10, 11]. Chondrocyte apoptosis could be detected by caspase-3 expression or terminal deoxynucleotidyl transferase dUTP nick end labelling (TUNEL) staining [12].

Together with the OA histological changes are several joint molecular alterations characterized by nuclear factor kappa beta (NFkβ) upregulation [13] that subsequently upregulates several catabolic and proinflammatory cytokines for cartilage such as interleukin-1 (IL-1) and tumour necrosis factor alpha (TNF-α), matrix metalloproteinases (MMPs - e.g. MMP-13), aggrecanases (i.e. a disintegrin and metalloproteinase with thrombospondin motifs 4 - ADAMTS-4), inducible synthases of nitric oxide and cyclooxygenase type 2 [14]. Consequently, a proinflammatory molecular milieu produces histological alterations in cartilage and induces molecular changes with clinical accompanying indicators such as pain and synovial effusion [4].

In the initial OA stages, joint tissues (e.g. cartilage) act by upregulating anabolic gene expression to induce cartilage ECM anabolism and to increase the synthesis of collagen type II alpha 1 (COL2A1), cartilage oligomeric matrix protein (COMP) and hyaluronan (HA) amongst other anabolic ECM components. However, as the OA progresses, the local expression and production of collagen type I alpha 1 (COL1A1) appears as a poor anabolic response by the osteoarthritic cartilage [15, 16].

Platelet-rich plasma (PRP) has been used as a therapy for OA in humans [17–19] and animals [20–23]. The rationale for the therapeutic use of PRP stems from the fact that platelets (PLTs) (but also white blood cells – WBC-) contained in PRP represent an important autologous source of some growth factors (GFs), which include transforming growth factor beta 1 (TGF-β_1), platelet derived growth factor isoform BB (PDGF-BB) [24, 25], and other anti-inflammatory cytokines such as interleukin 4 (IL-4) and the receptor antagonist of IL-1 (IL-1ra) [26, 27], which are implicated in the anabolic characteristics of OA [4, 28]. Furthermore, in vitro studies have revealed that PDGF-BB downregulates NFkβ [29, 30] and increases the proliferation of chondrocytes [29, 31], whereas TGF-β_1 increases the cartilage extracellular matrix (ECM) synthesis and promotes the differentiation of stem cells in chondrocytes [32].

Currently, there is controversy about which PRP preparation is ideal for the intra-articular treatment of patients with OA [33, 34]. Some in vitro [35–37] and clinical studies have suggested that leukoreduced PRP (also known as pure PRP [P-PRP]) preparations have better anabolic and anti-inflammatory effects for OA treatment than leukoconcentrate PRP (L-PRP) preparations, whereas other studies have described similar positive effects for both preparations [32, 38, 39].

Recently, we demonstrated in an in vitro system of cartilage inflammation that 50 % L-PRP releasate produced a more sustained temporal concentration of growth factors and anti-inflammatory cytokines than both 25 % L-PRP and P-PRP releasates and 50 % P-PRP releasate in relation to the concentration in culture media [40]. However, there is no information regarding the effects of these substances on the histology or ECM cartilage gene expression.

The study presented here shows complementary and novel information for the anabolic, anti-inflammatory effect of two supernatant concentrations (25 and 50 %) from both P-PRP and L-PRP preparations on equine cartilage explants (CEs) challenged with lipopolysaccharide (LPS). This research evaluates and compares the influence of both platelet-rich gel (PRG) supernatants on the histological changes of cartilage, the degree of chondrocyte apoptosis, the production of HA and the gene expression of NFkB, MMP-13, ADAMTS-4, COL1A1, COL2A1 and COMP in an in vitro system of cartilage inflammation and degeneration.

The hypothesis of this study is that L-PRG supernatants at a lower concentration (25 %) have better anti-inflammatory and anabolic effects than both PRG supernatants at the higher 50 % concentration and P-PRG supernatant at 25 % concentration in CEs challenged with LPS.

Methods

This study was approved by the committee on animal experimentation of the Universidad de Caldas, Manizales, Colombia.

Samples

Cartilage samples from the metacarpophalangeal joints from six horses, aged 4 to 9 years, were included in this study. The samples were taken from horses that were free from musculoskeletal disease and euthanised by a pentobarbital intravenous overdose for other medical reasons. All metacarpophalangeal joints were radiographed and macroscopically evaluated to exclude horses with OA-associated joint changes.

L-PRP and P-PRP preparation

Venous blood from one clinically healthy mare was used in order to avoid the great variability in the GF and cytokine concentrations in the PRG supernatants used in the experiments. Platelet concentrates were obtained through a manual double centrifugation tube method [41] that was previously validated and used clinically in horses with OA [21]. Blood was drawn from jugular venipuncture and immediately deposited in 4.5 mL tubes with sodium citrate solution (BD Vacutainer®, Becton Drive, Franklin Lakes, NJ, USA). After centrifugation at 120 × *g* for five minutes, the first 50 % of the top supernatant plasma fraction, adjacent to the buffy coat, was collected. This fraction was centrifuged at 240 × *g* for five minutes, and then the bottom quarter of the fraction was collected [41]. This fraction was considered as L-PRP. The upper plasma fraction was considered as P-PRP (Fig. 1). Whole blood and both PRP preparations were analysed for PLT and WBC counts using an impedance-based haematology device (Celltac-α MEK 6450, Nihon Kodhen, Japan).

Both PRP preparations were activated with calcium gluconate (Ropsohn Therapeutics Ltda®, Bogotá, Colombia) (ratio 1:10) and incubated at 37 °C for 1 h until clot retraction occurred. Fresh L-PRG and P-PRG supernatants were used to add to the culture media at two concentrations (25 % and 50 %). Aliquots of both PRG supernatants obtained were frozen at -86 °C for later quantification of PDGF-BB, TGF-β_1 and HA.

Cartilage explants culture and LPS challenge

Cartilage samples were obtained aseptically, and circular 4 mm diameter explants were obtained using a disposable biopsy punch (KAI Medical, Solingen, Germany). CEs were dissected from the articular surface without calcified cartilage layers and washed in phosphate-buffered saline.

CEs were stabilised in Dulbecco's Modified Eagle Medium (DMEM) (high glucose, 4500 mg/L) with L-glutamine and sodium bicarbonate and free of sodium pyruvate (DMEM, Lonza Group Ltd, Basel, Switzerland) and supplemented with streptomycin (100 μg/mL) and penicillin (100 μg/mL) without the addition of serum. Cultures were incubated in a 5 % CO_2 and water saturated atmosphere for 24 h and then replaced with fresh

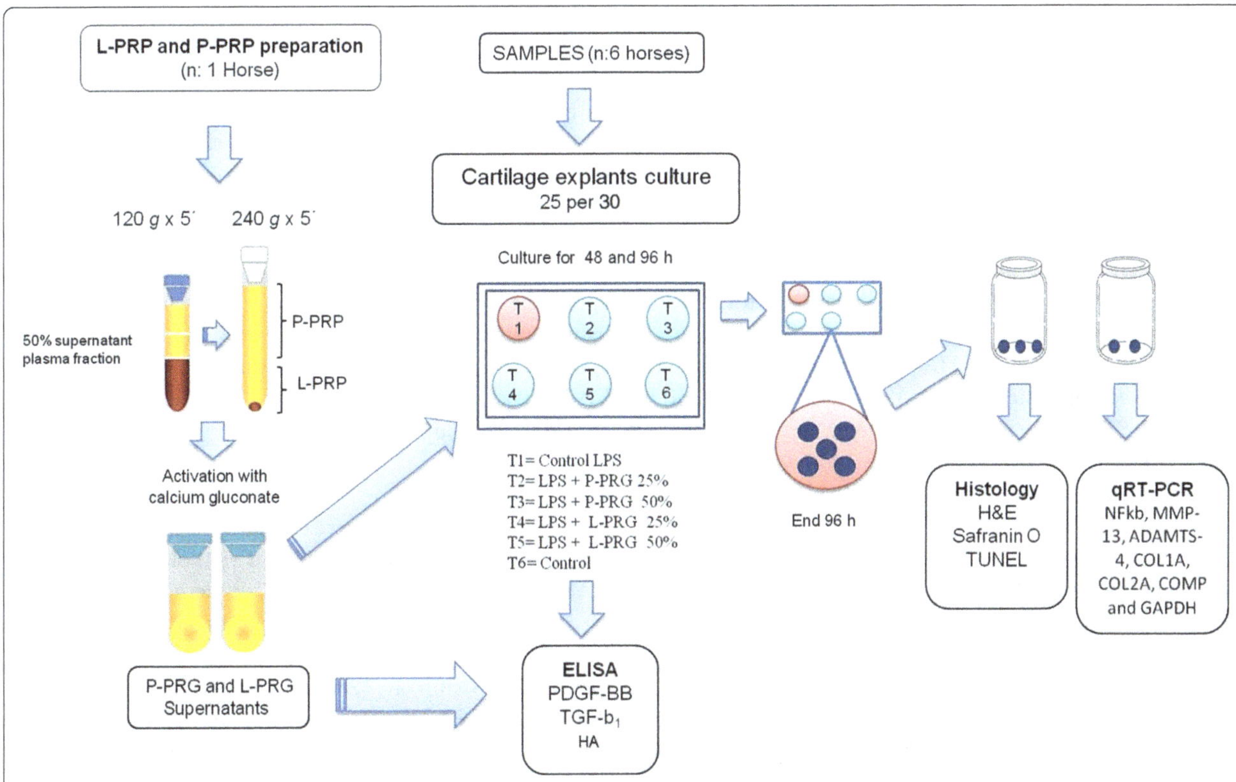

Fig. 1 Schematic workflow of the experiments of the study

culture media. At this time point (24 h), the CEs were challenged with 100 ng/mL of LPS (Sigma-Aldrich, St Louis, MO, USA) to induce inflammatory/catabolic damage of the cartilage [42, 43].

Study design

A total of 30 CEs were obtained from each horse. The study design included the evaluation of six experimental groups using five CEs per group from each horse as follows: one CE healthy control group without LPS and without addition of any PRG supernatant, one CE control group challenged with LPS and without addition of any PRG supernatant, and four CE groups cultured with L-PRG and P-PRG supernatants at two different concentrations (25 % and 50 %). After 1 h of incubation, L-PRG and P-PRG supernatants were added in order to obtain concentrations at 25 and 50 %. All CE groups were cultured at 96 h, after which the culture media were frozen in aliquots at -86 °C for later determination of HA concentration by ELISA. Furthermore, the CEs were deposited in buffered formaldehyde for histological analysis or in an RNA conserving solution (RNAlater, Life Technologies, Carlsbad, CA, USA) for quantitative gene expression of NFkB, MMP-13, ADAMTS-4, COL1A1, COL2A1 and COMP. The schematic diagram (Fig. 1) summarises the study design and methodology.

ELISA analysis

L-PRG and P-PRG supernatants and culture media at 96 h were used to determine the concentration of PDGF-BB, TGF-β_1 and HA via ELISA in duplicate. All proteins were assayed using commercial ELISA development kits from R&D Systems (Minneapolis, MN, USA). PDGF-BB (Human PDGF-BB DuoSet, DY220) and TGF-β_1 (Human TGF-β1 DuoSet, DY240E) were determined using human antibodies because there is a high sequence homology between these proteins in humans and horses [44, 45]. Furthermore, these kits have been used for the same purposes in other equine PRP studies [24, 25]. HA (Hyaluronan, DuoSet, DY3614) was determined using a multispecies detection ELISA kit. Standards provided for each ELISA kit were used to prepare each standard curve following the manufacturers' instructions. Absorbance readings were performed at 450 nm.

H&E histology evaluation

CEs were dehydrated in serial alcohol concentrations, fixed in wax blocks, cut into 3 μm slices and stained with either haematoxylin and eosin (H&E) or safranin O stains. The outcome parameters evaluated were: (1) chondrocyte necrosis, (2) cluster (complex chondrone) formation, (3) fibrillation/fissuring, (4) focal cell loss and (5) safranin-O stain uptake. All preparations were analysed using a light microscope in a 40× magnification following the OARSI histopathology initiative for histological assessments of osteoarthritis in the horse [8] (Table 1).

These variables were quantified using a 0–4 scale, with 0 being normal and 4 being abnormal (Table 1). Thus, a totally normal CE would score 0 and a maximally abnormal CE would score 15 [8]. Three sections randomly selected from each sample were evaluated blindly and the average score was used for comparison.

TUNEL assay for chondrocyte apoptosis

TUNEL staining was performed to detect DNA strand breakage using a commercial kit for cell and tissues (TACS TdT-Blue Label In situ Apoptosis Detection Kit, Trevigen, Inc., Gaitherburg, MD, USA). Briefly, the CEs were washed and dehydrated in serial alcohol concentrations, fixed in wax blocks and cut into 3 μm slices. The tissue sections were deparaffinised with xylene and ethanol and washed with PBS. The samples were covered with 50 μl of proteinase K solution and incubated for 15 min at 37 °C in a humidity chamber. The samples were washed with PBS and covered with 50 μl of labelling reaction mix. After this, the samples were immersed in a stop buffer solution for 5 min at room temperature to stop labelling reaction and once more washed twice with PBS for 2 min at room temperature. The samples were covered with 50 μl of antibody solution and incubated for 30 min at 37 °C then washed with PBS and covered with 50 μl of TACS Blue Label™ (Trevigen, Inc., Gaitherburg, MD, USA). These samples were washed with deionised water and counterstained with nuclear fast red. The controls were treated similarly except that terminal deoxynucleotidyl transferase was substituted by distilled water [46].

After the reaction, stained chondrocytes (grey-black) were analysed under a light microscope. Chondrocyte apoptosis was scored by a semiquantitative approach using a 0-4 scale, where 1 = 6–25 % of chondrocyte apoptosis; 2 = 26–50 % of chondrocyte apoptosis; 3 = 51–75 % of chondrocyte apoptosis and 4 = 76–100 % of chondrocyte apoptosis [47].

Molecular evaluation

CE samples were pulverised in liquid nitrogen and mixed with TRIzol reagent (Life Technologies, Carlsbad, CA, USA) for 5 min. The samples were centrifuged for 10 min at 10,000 × g, and the supernatant was mixed with 20 % chloroform (volume/volume) and then centrifuged for 15 min at 12,000 × g. The aqueous phase of the samples was removed and transferred to special columns (PureLink RNA Mini Kit, Life Technologies, Carlsbad, CA) for RNA extraction according to the manufacturer's instructions. RNA concentrations were

Table 1 Microscopic grading system for articular cartilage histology [8]

Articular cartilage		
Outcome parameter	Score	Description
Chondrocyte necrosis*	0	Normal section without necrosis
	1	No more than one necrotic cell located near the articular surface per 20x objective
	2	1e2 necrotic cells located near the articular surface per 20x objective
	3	2e3 necrotic cells located near the articular surface per 20x objective
	4	3e4 necrotic cells located near the articular surface per 20x objective
Cluster (complex chondrone) formation	0	No cluster formation throughout section
	1	Two chondrocytes (doublets) within same lacunae along superficial aspect of the articular cartilage section
	2	2e3 chondrocytes (doublets & triplets) within same lacunae along superficial aspect of the articular cartilage section
	3	3e4 chondrocytes within same lacunae along superficial aspect of the articular cartilage section
	4	Greater than four chondrocytes within same lacunae along superficial aspect of the articular cartilage section
Fibrillation/fissuring	0	No fibrillation/fissuring of the articular cartilage surface
	1	Fibrillation/fissuring of the articular cartilage restricted to surface and superficial zone
	2	Fissuring that extends into the middle zone
	3	Fissuring that extends to the level of the deep zone
	4	Fissuring that extends into the deep zone
Focal cell loss*	0	Normal cell population throughout the section
	1	A 10e20% area of acellularity per 20x field
	2	A 20e30% area of acellularity per 20x field
	3	A 40e50% area of acellularity per 20x field
	4	A greater than 50 % area of acellularity per 20x field
Safranin-O stain uptake	0	Normal staining
	1	Less than 25 % loss of staining characteristics
	2	25e50% loss of staining characteristics
	3	50e75% loss of staining characteristics
	4	Greater than 75 % loss of staining characteristics

*Chondrocyte necrosis is used to grade presence of lacunae with necrotic nuclei still present compared to focal cell loss which is most likely an extension of the pathologic change but lacunae or nuclei are no longer present

measured using a spectrophotometer (Nanodrop 2000, Thermo Scientific, Wilmington, DE, USA). Samples were diluted to a concentration of 5 ng/μL of RNA.

The samples were assayed for quantitative gene expression levels in a qRT-PCR device (StepOnePlus Real-Time PCR System, Life Technologies, Carlsbad, CA, USA) using a SuperScript III platinum SYBR Green One-Step qRT-PCR kit (Life Technologies, Carlsbad, CA, USA). Primers for NFkB, MMP-13, ADAMTS-4, COL1A1, COL2A1, COMP and GAPDH (glyceraldehyde 3-phosphate dehydrogenase) were designed and validated in the Colombian Centre for Bioinformatics and Computational Biology (BIOS) (Table 2).

The relative change in gene expression was determined via the comparative $2^{-\Delta\Delta CT}$ method [48]. GAPDH was used as the internal control (housekeeping gene), and cartilage samples from all horses that were not incubated with any treatment were used as reference samples.

Statistical and data analysis

The statistical analysis was performed with SPSS 19.0 software (IBM, Chicago, IL, USA). The Shapiro–Wilk test was used to assess the fit of the data set to a normal distribution (goodness of fit). All the parameters evaluated, except CE histology and apoptosis scores, demonstrated a normal distribution ($p > 0.05$). However, these data were normalised by using a transformation log (Y).

Platelet and WBC counts in whole blood and both PRP preparations were evaluated through a one-way analysis of variance (ANOVA), followed by a Tukey test. PDGF-BB, TGF-β_1 and HA concentrations from both PRG supernatants were compared using a t-non-paired test. A generalised lineal model (GLM), followed (when necessary) by a Tukey test, was used for comparing HA concentrations in culture media and gene expression at 96 h. The HA concentrations in fresh culture media with PRG supernatants at 1 h and 96 h were compared using a t-paired test. A $p < 0.05$ was accepted as statistically significant for all tests. Data are presented as mean ± mean standard error (m.s.e).

Results

Cell, growth factor and HA in L-PRP/L-PRG and P-PRP/P-PRG

PLT counts were significantly ($p < 0.05$) different between whole blood, L-PRP and P-PRP, with the lowest

Table 2 Genes and sequence of primers evaluated in the study

Targeted genes	Primer sequences (5'- > 3')	Product size (bps)
GAPDH, glyceraldehyde-3-phosphate dehydrogenase 6	Forward TCCCTGCTTCTACTGGTGCT Reverse TGACAAAGTGGTCGTTGAGG	306
NFkβ, nuclear factor of kappa light polypeptide gene enhancer in B-cells-like 1	Forward CGATTTCGATATGGCTGTGA Reverse CACCTTCTTCAGCTCCTTGG	399
MMP 13, matrix metallopeptidase 13 (collagenase 3) 7	Forward GCATTCAAAAAGGCCTTCAA Reverse GGAAGCACAAAGTGGCTTTT	356
ADAMTS 4, metallopeptidase with thrombospondin type 1 motif 4	Forward TGTCAGCTTGGTGGTGACTC Reverse GTTGAAGACATGGCCCAGTT	322
COL1A1, collagen, type I, alpha 1 11	Forward AGCCAGCAGATCGAGAACAT Reverse CTGGCCACCATACTCGAACT	309
COL2A1, collagen, type II, alpha 1 6	Forward primer ACGTCCAGATGACCTTCCTG Reverse primer GTCCACACCAAATTCCTGCT	326
COMP, cartilage oligomeric matrix protein 21	Forward CCACGTGAATACGGTCACAG Reverse TAGGAACCAGCGGTAGGATG	301

concentration for P-PRP (98.7 00 ± 4.600 PLT/μL), followed by whole blood (125.900 ± 3.400 PLT/μL) and L-PRP (312.800 ± 19.600 PLT/μL). WBC counts were also significantly different between the evaluated groups, with a higher concentration for L-PRP (35.100 ± 3.500 WBC/μL), followed by whole blood (8.300 ± 3.700 WBC/μL) and P-PRP (110 ± 40 WBC/μL). TGF-β_1 concentration was similar between L-PRG (1676.3 ± 312.4 pg/mL) and P-PRG (1356.9 ± 20.8 pg/mL). PDGF-BB had a significantly ($p < 0.05$) higher concentration in L-PRG (3053. 8 ± 956.7 pg/mL) when compared to P-PRG (372.7 ± 79.6 pg/mL). HA concentration was significantly ($p < 0.05$) higher in L-PRG supernatant (4.3 ± 1.7 pg/mL) in comparison to P-PRG supernatant (1.1 ± 0.21 pg/mL).

H&E histology evaluation

Chondrocyte necrosis scores were significantly ($p <$ 0.05) worse (higher) for CEs from the control group with LPS and those treated with 25 % L-PRG and 50 % P-PRG supernatants when compared to CEs of the control group and those treated with 50 % LPRG and 25 % P-PRG supernatants (Fig. 2a). Cluster formation was significantly higher for CEs from the control group plus LPS when compared to the rest of the CE groups evaluated. This histology parameter was similar among CEs from the healthy control group and those treated with both L-PRG supernatants and 25 % P-PRG supernatant, whereas CEs treated with 50 % P-PRG supernatant presented a significantly worse score than the aforementioned CE groups (Fig. 2b).

Fibrillation/fissuring scores were significantly ($p < 0.05$) higher in both control groups, although there was a statistical trend ($p = 0.10$) showing CEs of the healthy control group with lower score in comparison to CEs of the control group treated with LPS. In general, CEs treated with all PRG supernatants presented significantly ($p < 0.05$) lower scores. However, CEs treated with 50 % L-PRG and 25 % P-PRG supernatants were significantly lower than CEs of healthy control group (Fig. 2c).

Focal cell loss scores were significantly ($p < 0.05$) worse for the CEs of control group treated with LPS and those treated with 50 % P-PRG supernatant. CEs from the healthy control group and those treated with both 25 % PRG supernatants presented significantly ($p < 0.05$) lower scores than the rest of the CE groups (Fig. 2d). SOFG stain uptake score were significantly ($p < 0.05$) worse for CEs treated with 50 % L-PRG supernatant, followed by CEs of the control group challenged with LPS and both 25 % PRG supernatants. The best score for this histology parameter was found in CEs of the healthy control group and those treated with 50 % P-PRG supernatant (Fig. 2e).

The general histology total score was significantly ($p <$ 0.05) higher in CEs of the control group challenged with LPS when compared to CEs of the healthy control group and those treated with both L-PRG and 25 % P-PRG supernatant. In general, CEs treated with both 25 % PRG supernatants showed significantly ($p < 0.05$) better general histology score than the rest of the groups evaluated (Fig. 2f).

TUNEL assay for chondrocyte apoptosis

No chondrocyte apoptosis was detected in CEs of the healthy control group and those treated with both 50 % PRG supernatants. However, this cellular phenomenon was detected (and it was significantly higher [$p < 0.05$]) in CEs of the control group challenged with LPS and those treated with both 25 % PRG supernatants; although, the score for this parameter was apparently lower for those CEs treated with 25 % L-PRG supernatant (Fig. 2g).

Concentration of HA in culture media at 1 h and 96 h

At 1 h, HA concentrations varied significantly ($p < 0.05$) between all PRG supernatant groups evaluated. At 96 h, HA was released by all CE groups. However,

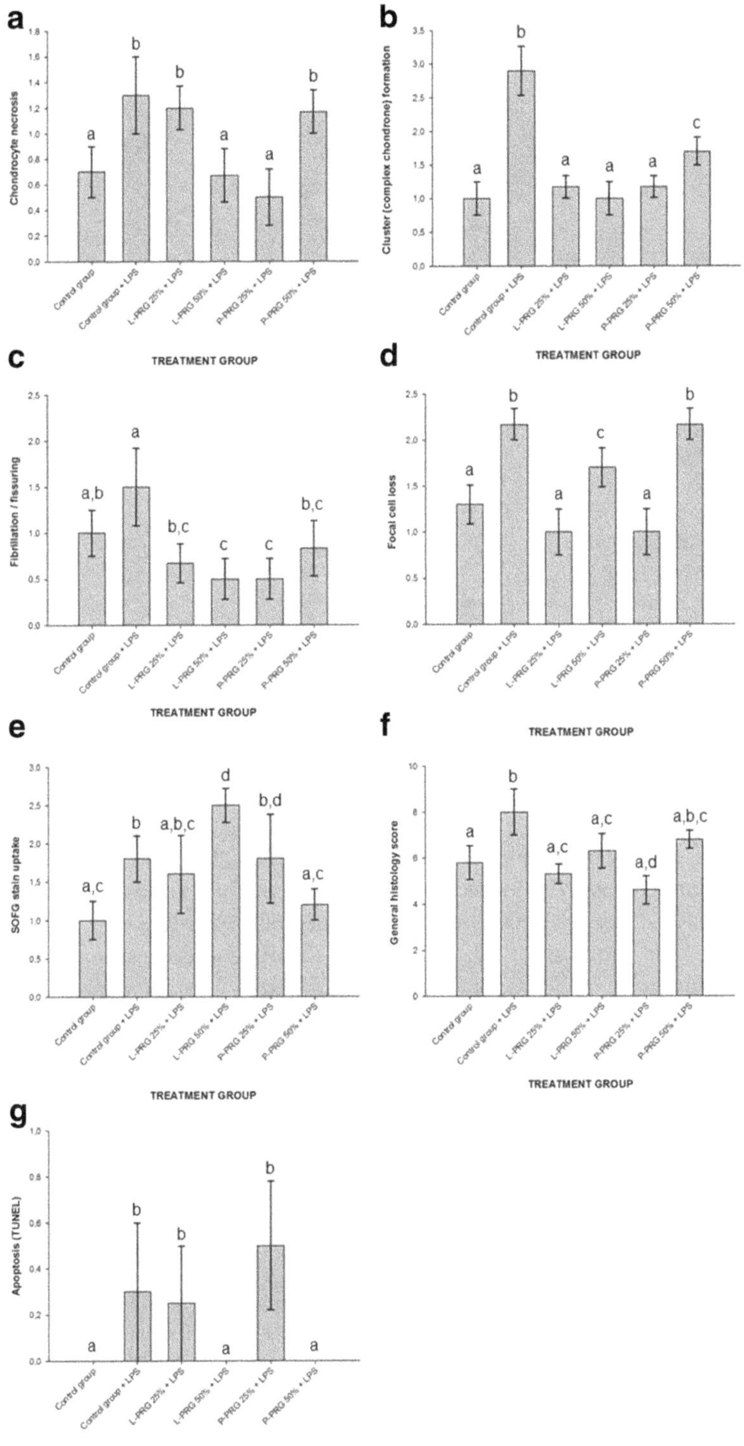

Fig. 2 Means (±standard error of the mean [s.e.m]) of the cartilage histology and chondrocyte apoptosis scores. **a** Chondrocyte necrosis. **b** Cluster formation. **c** Fibrillation/fissuring. **d** Focal cell loss. **e** SOFG stain uptake. **f** Total histology score. **g** Chondrocyte apoptosis. [a-b]Different lowercase letters denote significant ($p < 0.05$) differences between the groups evaluated by the Tukey test

the CE group cultured with 25 % P-PRG supernatant presented the highest significant ($p < 0.05$) HA release in comparison with the CE control group and the other CE PRG-treated groups. Notably, HA concentrations were different between CE PRG treated groups at 1 h and 96 h (Fig. 3).

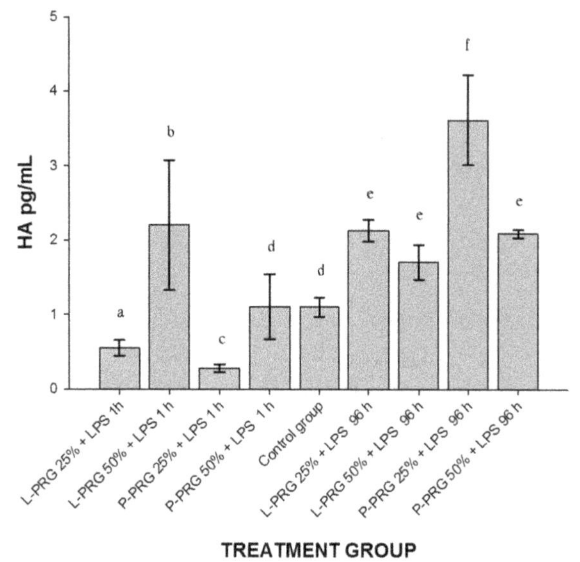

Fig. 3 Means (± s.e.m) of HA concentration in culture media from cartilage explant (CE) groups at 1 h and 96 h. [a-b] Different lowercase letters denote significant ($p < 0.05$) differences between the groups evaluated by the Tukey test over the same period of time. * Denotes significant differences between the same variable at different time periods by the t-paired test

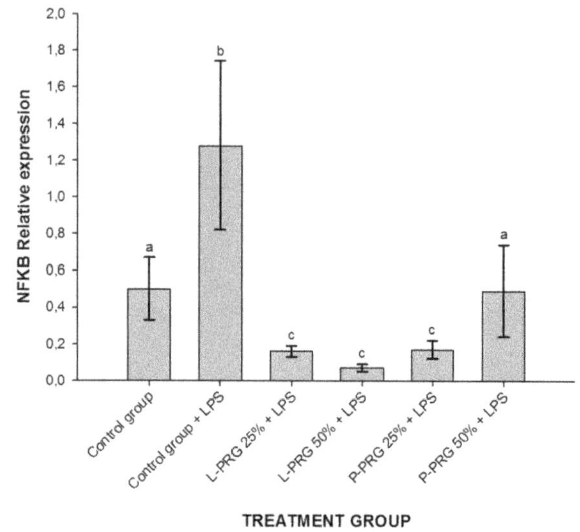

Fig. 4 Means (± s.e.m) of NFkB gene expression in CE groups at 96 h. [a-b] Different lowercase letters denote significant ($p < 0.05$) differences between the groups evaluated by the Tukey test

Gene expression

NFkB gene expression was significantly ($p < 0.05$) increased in CEs from the control group challenged with LPS in comparison to the rest of the CE groups evaluated. NFkB gene expression was significantly ($p < 0.05$) diminished in CEs treated with both 25 % PRG supernatants and 50 % P-PRG supernatant in comparison to the CEs from the healthy control group and those treated with 50 % P-PRG (Fig. 4).

CEs from the healthy control group and all PRG supernatant treatments presented a significant ($p < 0.05$) decrease of MMP-13 expression (Fig. 5). However, 25 % L-PRG supernatant induced a lesser expression of this gene in CEs when compared to CEs treated with 50 % P-PRG supernatant ($p < 0.05$). No significant differences were noticed for the expression of this catabolic gene in the CEs from the healthy control group and those treated with 50 % L-PRG, and 25 and 50 % P-PRG supernatants (Fig. 5).

All PRG supernatant treatments significantly ($p < 0.05$) decreased ADAMTS-4 gene expression in CEs when compared to CEs of both control groups (Fig. 6). Furthermore, CEs from the healthy control group and all PRG supernatant treatments showed significant ($p < 0.05$) COL1A1 gene downregulation when compared to CEs of the control group challenged with LPS (Fig. 7). L-PRG supernatants at different concentrations significantly ($p < 0.05$) diminished the COL2A1 gene expression in CEs in comparison to CEs treated with both P-PRG supernatant concentrations and the control group. Notably, there were not significant differences between these last three groups and CEs from the healthy control group for COL2A1 gene expression (Fig. 8). However, although this gene expression was statistically ($p = 0.09$) similar among CEs from both control groups, COL2A1gene expression was apparently higher in CEs from the healthy control group than in CEs challenged only with LPS (Fig. 8).

COMP gene expression was significantly ($p < 0.05$) diminished in CEs from the control group challenged with LPS and those treated with the 50 % L-PRG supernatant

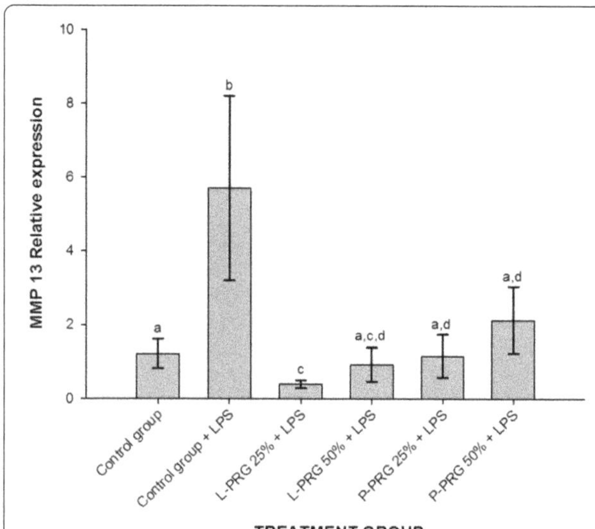

Fig. 5 Means (± s.e.m) of MMP-13 gene expression in CE groups at 96 h [a-b] Different lowercase letters denote significant ($p < 0.05$) differences between the groups evaluated by the Tukey test

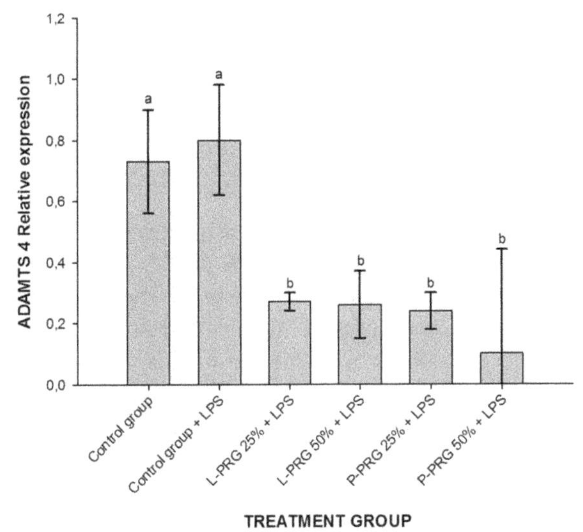

Fig. 6 Means (± s.e.m) of ADAMTS-4 gene expression in CE groups at 96 h. [a-b] Different lowercase letters denote significant ($p < 0.05$) differences between the groups evaluated by the Tukey test

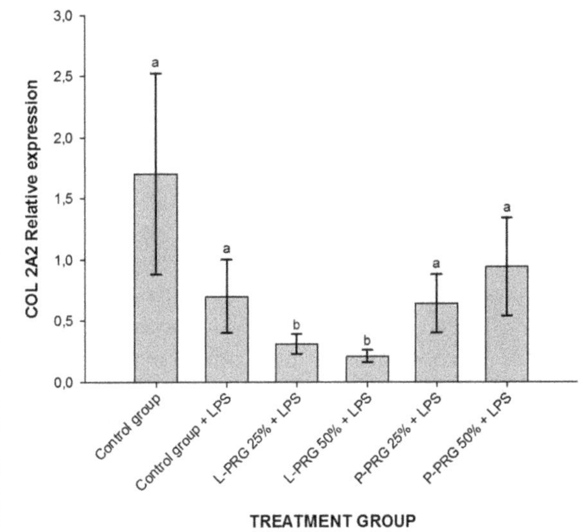

Fig. 8 Means (± s.e.m) of COL2A1 gene expression in CE groups at 96 h. [a-b] Different lowercase letters denote significant ($p < 0.05$) differences between the groups evaluated by the Tukey test

in comparison to CEs treated with both the 25 % PRG supernatants and the 50 % P-PRG supernatant. CEs from the healthy control group and those treated with both 25 % PRG supernatants presented similar increased COMP gene expression. However, CEs treated with both 25 % PRG supernatants demonstrated a significantly higher CE gene expression when compared to CEs treated with 50 % P-PRG supernatant (Fig. 9).

Discussion

Diverse PRP effects on cells and tissues are well recognised as depending on their varying preparations [38]. Thus, the molecular profile of a PRG supernatant is associated with the type and quantity of WBCs and PLTs initially present in PRP [25, 28]. However, after PRP is activated in a joint, it becomes a fibrin mesh or PRG that releases growth factors and cytokines and acts as an immune node inside the joint [49]. We currently believe that the cell ratio (PLT:WBC) in PRP is not as critical as the GF:GF or GF:cytokine ratios and concentrations

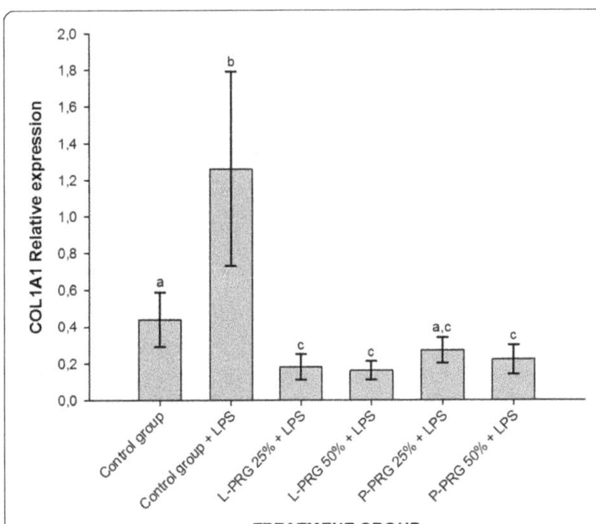

Fig. 7 Means (± s.e.m) of COL1A1 gene expression in CE groups at 96 h. [a-b] Different lowercase letters denote significant ($p < 0.05$) differences between the groups evaluated by the Tukey test

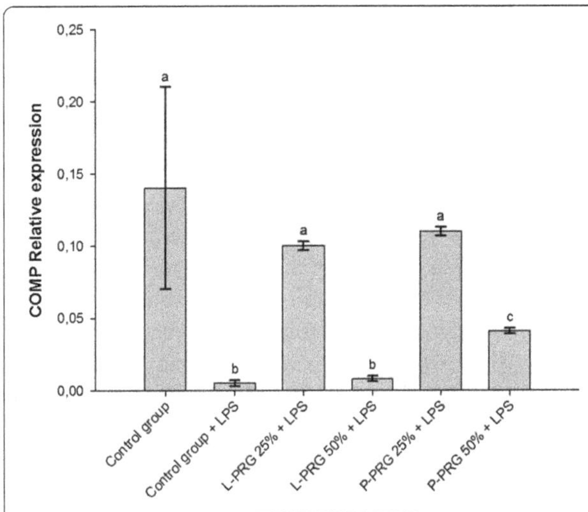

Fig. 9 Means (± s.e.m) of COMP gene expression in CE groups at 96 h. [a-b] Different lowercase letters denote significant ($p < 0.05$) differences between the blood component groups obtained with the same anticoagulant by the Tukey test

released into the joint fluid [50]. However, we also wish to clarify that this assumption could possibly be valid for the use of PRP in joints and not for the infiltrative use of this substance in tendons, ligaments or muscles, where not only is the growth factor concentration important, but also the fibrin mesh to allow growth factor storage, cell migration and cell proliferation [51].

Strong debates continue about the ideal PLT:WBC ratio and concentration in PRP [51]. Currently, there are several studies indicating that plasma with a poor quantity of PLTs and negligible WBs could be the best "PRP" preparations to treat OA and other musculoskeletal pathologies [35, 36, 52]. However, a recent in vitro study described molecular positive effects for several commercial kits which have concentrates at different PLT:WBC ratios and are used for OA treatment [39].

Thus, we decided to conduct an independent study to evaluate the effect of two different PRP preparations (obtained by a homemade lab method) at different concentrations on cartilage histology, chondrocyte apoptotic scores, HA release and catabolic and anabolic gene expression of CEs challenged with LPS. Exposure of CEs to LPS resulted in marked changes in the expression of genes involved in matrix formation and degradation as well as inflammation of which many were reduced by the addition of both PRG supernatants at different concentrations.

The use of LPS for inducing cartilage inflammation/degeneration is a classical methodological approach to perform diverse in vitro studies by simulating a system of inflammatory/degenerative arthropaty [42, 43, 53]; although, the use of recombinant IL-1β to induce in vitro articular cartilage degradation could be more suitable [54, 55]. However, it is important to clarify that the cellular receptors for LPS and IL-1β are closely interlinked and described as the TLR-IL-1 receptor (IL-1R) superfamily of receptors. When activated they induce a series of intercellular signalling pathways that converge on the activation of the transcription NFkB resulting in pro-inflammatory cytokine expression [55, 56].

It is important to mention that the evaluation of the anti-inflammatory effect of PRG supernatants by measuring the relative expression of the NFkB gene in the present study represents a very limited approach to understanding the activity signalling of this important inflammatory process [57]. However, an in vitro study in human chondrocytes revealed that activated PRP induced the expression and production of inhibitor-κBα (IκBα) (directly mediated by hepatocyte growth factor), which is responsible for the inhibition of the transcription of NFkB [58]. This finding has also been consistent for gingival fibroblasts and alveolar osteoblasts challenged with LPS and cultured with PRP preparations [59].

Notably, LPS challenge induced important structural (degenerative) changes accompanied with chondrocyte apoptosis in CEs, which were reverted or ameliorated in diverse degrees by PRG supernatants. However, the general histology score was significantly lower (better) for CEs treated with PRG supernatants, and some individual outcome parameters, such as chondrocyte necrosis, focal cell loss and SOFG uptake, were affected by some of these substances.

Chondrocyte necrosis was mostly observed in CEs treated with 25 % L-PRG and 50 % P-PRG supernatants. This finding could indicate that these substances at these specific concentrations were not able to reverse the catabolic effect mediated by endotoxin in CEs. Furthermore, it is also important to consider that both 25 % PRG supernatants presented chondrocyte apoptosis reaction similar to those observed in CEs from the control group challenged with LPS; although, CEs treated with 25 % P-PRG supernatant presented the highest score for this parameter. This last finding could possibly indicate that this substance at lower concentration is not able to reverse the cartilage catabolic effects of LPS and can induce additional chondrocyte apoptosis.

Focal cell loss was more evident for both 50 % PRG supernatants, possibly due to that chondrocytes being able to migrate inside the CEs towards the periphery through a chemotactic attractive stimulus in the culture media [60], such as the milieu of growth factors released from PRP [61–63]. In contrast, another explanation to demonstrate the cause of focal cell loss in the groups of CEs treated with higher concentrations of PRG supernatants could be attributed to chondrocyte necrosis or even chondrocyte apoptosis [64]. However, this lack of significant increase of these parameters occurred only for CEs treated with 50 % P-PRG supernatant, which could indicate that P-PRG preparations were not chondroprotective.

The SOFG uptake score was higher in CEs treated with 50 % L-PRG and 25 % P-PRG supernatants, and apparently this parameter was worst for CEs treated with 50 % L-PRG supernatant. This parameter is associated with the structural content of proteoglycans in the cartilage ECM [8], which indicate the quality and integrity of this structure. It is important to consider that 50 % L-PRG supernatant also induced downregulation of anabolic ECM genes, such as COL2A1 and COMP. Taken together, these histology and molecular findings indicate that higher concentrations of L-PRP preparations could be deleterious for osteoarthritic cartilage. One pitfall of the present research was that the release or accumulation of proteoglycans was not measured in the culture media of CEs. However, we consider that the combination of histology parameters and gene expression could be valid indicators for the degree of affection of ECM of the CEs of this study.

The combination of the general histology score, chondrocyte apoptosis findings, HA release to the culture media and the catabolic and anabolic cartilage ECM gene expression demonstrated that all PRG supernatants are "biosubstances" with mixed biological effects. In general, all PRG supernatants presented a potential anti-inflammatory effect and decreased the catabolic effects of LPS on CEs at the cellular and molecular level. However, the overall analysis of our results indicates that 25 % L-PRG supernatant (followed in order of importance by 50 % P-PRG, 25 % P-PRG and 50 % L-PRG) represented the substance with the most important anti-inflammatory and anabolic effect with lower affection of CEs at the histology level. Furthermore, 25 % P-PRG supernatant presented important anabolic effects, but it induced a more severe chondrocyte apoptosis than the other of the evaluated substances. This detrimental cell effect limits the potential clinical use of this substance at this concentration.

The present results can be complemented with the previous findings obtained by us in two in vitro studies, in which the production of anti-inflammatory and catabolic cytokines was measured in the culture media of synovial membrane explants (SME) [27] and CEs [40] challenged with LPS over 48 h and 96 h. In general, 25 % L-PRG and 50 % L-PRG supernatants presented the best anabolic and anti-inflammatory profile. However, in both studies, 25 % L-PRG supernatant produced a most significant reduction of TNF-α production and a total higher production of IL-1ra over time than 50 % L-PRG [27, 40].

Currently, we use 3-5 mL doses of PRP to treat fetlock osteoarthritis in horses with a body weight of 300-450 kg. This PRP volume has also been used for other researches with good results [22]. Notably, the complete volume capacity for an equine fetlock joint has been calculated at 12.5 ± 1.0 mL [65]. Thus, if the PRP volume used is adjusted in relation to the volume capacity of this specific joint [65], the effective concentration of PRP in clinical conditions could be near to 40 %, without considering the additional volume of synovial fluid (2-2.5 mL), which could represent a final PRP/synovial fluid concentration of 40-60 %. In line with this, the PRP dose for this joint could possibly be adjusted at 25 % using between 1.5-2.0 mL. However, this hypothesis should be probed in patients with osteoarthritis or experimentally induced synovitis.

Our findings are in line with the results of Cavallo et al. [39] and Kreuz et al.[38], who found diverse and positive effects for L- and P-PRP preparations in human osteoarthritic chondrocytes and subchondral mesenchymal progenitor cells. Conversely, our results are different from other in vitro studies [34–36], which have concluded that only P-PRP preparations induce an anabolic effect in cartilage and L-PRP preparations only induce an opposite (catabolic) joint state.

This study had several limitations. First, this is an in vitro study, which does not reflect the exact biological phenomena occurring in the osteoarthritic joint. However, this in vitro system of cartilage inflammation and degeneration could be useful to demonstrate that L- and P-PRG supernatants could act in function of their concentration and could have different mechanisms of action to induce cartilage joint anabolism and, potentially, diminish pain and inflammation. Another limitation of this study was that blood of only one animal was used to produce the PRG supernatants evaluated to avoid the great variability in the CE responses to several PRP preparations. This situation is not practical in clinical conditions because autologous PRP should be used. However, the response of each patient in particular will depend in some measure on the concentration of the cells' proteins in PRP.

Conclusions

This study demonstrates that both L- and P-PRP preparations at different concentrations can induce different anti-inflammatory, anti-catabolic, anabolic and even catabolic responses in an in vitro system of cartilage inflammation and degeneration.

Apparently, 25 % L-PRG supernatant presented the best therapeutic profile when compared to the other PRP preparations examined, because it presented anti-inflammatory and anabolic effects with minimal cellular and structural changes in CEs. Our results once more demonstrate that the biological variability of PRP preparations makes their application rather challenging. Additional studies in animal models and in patients with OA should be performed to know the in vivo effect of PRP preparations at different concentrations.

Abbreviations

ADMTS-4, A disintegrin and metalloproteinase with thrombospondin motifs 4; ANOVA, analysis of variance; CEs, cartilage explants; COL1A1, collagen type I alpha 1; COL2A1, collagen type II alpha 1; COMP, cartilage oligomeric matrix protein; DMEM, Dulbecco's modified Eagle medium; ECM, extracellular matrix; ELISA, enzyme-linked immunosorbent assay; GF, growth factor; HA, hyaluronan; IL-1, interleukin 1; L-PRG, leukoconcentrated platelet-rich gel; L-PRP, leukoconcentrated platelet-rich plasma; LPS, lipopolysaccharide; MMP-13, matrix metalloproteinase 13; NFkβ, nuclear factor kappa beta; OA, osteoarthritis; PDGF-BB, platelet derived growth factor isoform BB; PLT, platelet; P-PRG, pure platelet-rich gel; P-PRP, pure platelet-rich plasma; PRG, platelet-rich gel; PRP, platelet-rich plasma; RBC, red blood cell; TGF-β_1, transforming growth factor beta-1; TNF-α, tumor necrosis factor alpha; WBC, leukocyte.

Acknowledgments

The authors thank Wilson Gómez and Fabio Robayo for their assistance and thank Policía Nacional de Colombia.

Funding

This project was supported by grant No.397-2011 of the National Program of Biotechnology from COLCIENCIAS, Bogotá D.C and by grant No 0250911 of the Vicerrectoría de Investigaciones y Postgrados of the Universidad de Caldas, Manizales, Colombia. D.L.R´s PhD scholarship was funded by COLCIENCIAS.

Authors' contributions
JUC had full access to all of the data in the study and takes responsibility for the decision to submit this work for publication. JUC designed the study and participated in data analysis and interpretation, manuscript drafting and critical revision. CL, DLR, MEA, JEP and MEB performed laboratory work and contributed to data collection, data analysis and interpretation and critical revision of the manuscript. All of the authors read and approved the final version of the manuscript to be published.

Competing interests
The authors declare that they have no competing interests.

Consent for publication
Not applicable.

Author details
[1]Grupo de Investigación Terapia Regenerativa, Departamento de Salud Animal, Universidad de Caldas, Manizales, Colombia. [2]Grupo de investigación Biosalud, Departamento de Ciencias Básicas para la Salud, Universidad de Caldas, Manizales, Colombia. [3]Grupo de Investigación en Citogenética, Filogenia y Evolución de Poblaciones, Universidad del Tolima, Ibagué, Colombia.

References
1. Marshall DA, Vanderby S, Barnabe C, MacDonald KV, Maxwell C, Mosher D, Wasylak T, Lix L, Stat P, Enns E, et al. Estimating the burden of osteoarthritis to plan for the future. Arthritis Care Res. 2015;4(10):22612.
2. Aragon CL, Hofmeister EH, Budsberg SC. Systematic review of clinical trials of treatments for osteoarthritis in dogs. J Am Vet Med Assoc. 2007;230(4):514–21.
3. Vandeweerd JM, Coisnon C, Clegg P, Cambier C, Pierson A, Hontoir F, Saegerman C, Gustin P, Buczinski S.Systematic review of efficacy of nutraceuticals to alleviate clinical signs of osteoarthritis. J Vet Intern Med. 2012;26(3):448–56.
4. Carmona JU, Prades M. Pathophisiology of osteoarthritis. Comp Equine. 2009;4(1):28–40.
5. McIlwraith CW, Fortier LA, Frisbie DD, Nixon AJ. Equine models of articular cartilage repair. Cartilage. 2011;2(4):317–26.
6. McCoy AM. Animal models of osteoarthritis: comparisons and key considerations. Vet Pathol. 2015;10:0300985815588611.
7. Neundorf RH, Lowerison MB, Cruz AM, Thomason JJ, McEwen BJ, Hurtig MB. Determination of the prevalence and severity of metacarpophalangeal joint osteoarthritis in Thoroughbred racehorses via quantitative macroscopic evaluation. Am J Vet Res. 2010;71(11):1284–93.
8. McIlwraith CW, Frisbie DD, Kawcak CE, Fuller CJ, Hurtig M, Cruz A. The OARSI histopathology initiative - recommendations for histological assessments of osteoarthritis in the horse. Osteoarthritis Cartilage. 2010;18 Suppl 3:S93–105.
9. Zamli Z, Sharif M. Chondrocyte apoptosis: a cause or consequence of osteoarthritis? Int J Rheum Dis. 2011;14(2):159–66.
10. Chang CH, Hsu YM, Chen YC, Lin FH, Sadhasivam S, Loo ST, Savitha S. Anti-inflammatory effects of hydrophilic and lipophilic statins with hyaluronic acid against LPS-induced inflammation in porcine articular chondrocytes. J Orthop Res. 2014;32(4):557–65.
11. Franciozi CE, Tarini VA, Reginato RD, Goncalves PR, Medeiros VP, Ferretti M, Dreyfuss JL, Nader HB, Faloppa F. Gradual strenuous running regimen predisposes to osteoarthritis due to cartilage cell death and altered levels of glycosaminoglycans. Osteoarthritis Cartilage. 2013;21(7):965–72.
12. Otsuki Y, Li Z, Shibata MA. Apoptotic detection methods–from morphology to gene. Prog Histochem Cytochem. 2003;38(3):275–339.
13. Marcu KB, Otero M, Olivotto E, Borzi RM, Goldring MB. NF-kappaB signaling: multiple angles to target OA. Curr Drug Targets. 2010;11(5):599–613.
14. Ownby SL, Fortuno LV, Au AY, Grzanna MW, Rashmir-Raven AM, Frondoza CG. Expression of pro-inflammatory mediators is inhibited by an avocado/ soybean unsaponifiables and epigallocatechin gallate combination. J Inflamm (Lond). 2014;11(1):8. doi:10.1186/1476-9255-1111-1188.
15. Ishijima M, Kaneko H, Kaneko K. The evolving role of biomarkers for osteoarthritis. Ther Adv Musculoskelet Dis. 2014;6(4):144–53.
16. Aigner T, Bartnik E, Zien A, Zimmer R. Functional genomics of osteoarthritis. Pharmacogenomics. 2002;3(5):635–50.
17. Campbell KA, Saltzman BM, Mascarenhas R, Khair MM, Verma NN, Bach Jr BR, Cole BJ. Does intra-articular platelet-rich plasma injection provide clinically superior outcomes compared with other therapies in the treatment of knee osteoarthritis? A systematic review of overlapping meta-analyses. Arthroscopy. 2015;29(15):00353–9.
18. Say F, Gurler D, Yener K, Bulbul M, Malkoc M. Platelet-rich plasma injection is more effective than hyaluronic acid in the treatment of knee osteoarthritis. Acta Chir Orthop Traumatol Cech. 2013;80(4):278–83.
19. Jang SJ, Kim JD, Cha SS. Platelet-rich plasma (PRP) injections as an effective treatment for early osteoarthritis. Eur J Orthop Surg Traumatol. 2013;23(5): 573–80.
20. Brossi PM, Moreira JJ, Machado TS, Baccarin RY. Platelet-rich plasma in orthopedic therapy: a comparative systematic review of clinical and experimental data in equine and human musculoskeletal lesions. BMC Vet Res. 2015;11:98.
21. Carmona JU, Argüelles D, Climent F, Prades M. Autologous platelet concentrates as a treatment of horses with osteoarthritis: a preliminary pilot clinical study. J Equine Vet Sci. 2007;27(4):167–70.
22. Pichereau F, Décory M, Cuevas Ramos G. Autologous platelet concentrate as a treatment for horses with refractory fetlock osteoarthritis. J Equine Vet Sci. 2014;34(4):489–93.
23. Silva RF, Carmona JU, Rezende CM. Intra-articular injections of autologous platelet concentrates in dogs with surgical reparation of cranial cruciate ligament rupture: a pilot study. Vet Comp Orthop Traumatol. 2013;26(4):285–90.
24. Giraldo CE, Alvarez ME, Carmona JU. Effects of sodium citrate and acid citrate dextrose solutions on cell counts and growth factor release from equine pure-platelet rich plasma and pure-platelet rich gel. BMC Vet Res. 2015;11:60.
25. Giraldo CE, Lopez C, Alvarez ME, Samudio IJ, Prades M, Carmona JU. Effects of the breed, sex and age on cellular content and growth factor release from equine pure-platelet rich plasma and pure-platelet rich gel. BMC Vet Res. 2013;9:29.
26. Rios DL, Lopez C, Carmona JU. Platelet-rich gel supernatants stimulate the release of anti-inflammatory proteins on culture media of normal equine synovial membrane explants. Vet Med Int. 2015;2015:547052.
27. Rios DL, López C, Álvarez ME, Samudio I, Carmona JU. Effects over time of two platelet gel supernatants on growth factor, cytokine and hyaluronan concentrations in normal synovial membrane explants challenged with lipopolysaccharide. BMC Musculoskelet Disord. 2015;16:153.
28. Andia I, Maffulli N. Platelet-rich plasma for managing pain and inflammation in osteoarthritis. Nat Rev Rheumatol. 2013;9(12):721–30. doi:10.1038/nrrheum.2013.1141. Epub 2013 Oct 1031.
29. Stewart K, Pabbruwe M, Dickinson S, Sims T, Hollander AP, Chaudhuri JB. The effect of growth factor treatment on meniscal chondrocyte proliferation and differentiation on polyglycolic acid scaffolds. Tissue Eng. 2007;13(2):271–80.
30. Montaseri A, Busch F, Mobasheri A, Buhrmann C, Aldinger C, Rad JS, Shakibaei M. IGF-1 and PDGF-bb suppress IL-1beta-induced cartilage degradation through down-regulation of NF-kappaB signaling: involvement of Src/PI-3 K/AKT pathway. PLoS One. 2011;6(12):e28663.
31. Brandl A, Angele P, Roll C, Prantl L, Kujat R, Kinner B. Influence of the growth factors PDGF-BB, TGF-beta1 and bFGF on the replicative aging of human articular chondrocytes during in vitro expansion. J Orthop Res. 2010;28(3):354–60.
32. Zhai G, Dore J, Rahman P. TGF-beta signal transduction pathways and osteoarthritis. Rheumatol Int. 2015;15:15.
33. Russell RP, Apostolakos J, Hirose T, Cote MP, Mazzocca AD. Variability of platelet-rich plasma preparations. Sports Med Arthrosc. 2013;21(4):186–90.
34. Sundman EA, Cole BJ, Fortier LA. Growth factor and catabolic cytokine concentrations are influenced by the cellular composition of platelet-rich plasma. Am J Sports Med. 2011;39(10):2135–40.
35. Kisiday JD, McIlwraith CW, Rodkey WG, Frisbie DD, Steadman JR. Effects of platelet-rich plasma composition on anabolic and catabolic activities in equine cartilage and meniscal explants. Cartilage. 2012;3(3):245–54.
36. Sundman EA, Cole BJ, Karas V, Della Valle C, Tetreault MW, Mohammed HO, Fortier LA. The anti-inflammatory and matrix restorative mechanisms of platelet-rich plasma in osteoarthritis. Am J Sports Med. 2014;42(1):35–41.
37. Braun HJ, Kim HJ, Chu CR, Dragoo JL. The effect of platelet-rich plasma formulations and blood products on human synoviocytes: implications for intra-articular injury and therapy. Am J Sports Med. 2014;42(5):1204–10.

38. Kreuz PC, Kruger JP, Metzlaff S, Freymann U, Endres M, Pruss A, Petersen W, Kaps C. Platelet-rich plasma preparation types show impact on chondrogenic differentiation, migration, and proliferation of human subchondral mesenchymal progenitor cells. Arthroscopy. 2015;13(15):00260-1.
39. Cavallo C, Filardo G, Mariani E, Kon E, Marcacci M, Pereira Ruiz MT, Facchini A, Grigolo B:. Comparison of platelet-rich plasma formulations for cartilage healing: an in vitro study. J Bone Joint Surg Am. 2014;96(5): 423–9.
40. Ríos DL, López C, Carmona JU. Evaluation of the anti-inflammatory effects of two platelet-rich gel supernatants in an in vitro system of cartilage inflammation. Cytokine. 2015;76(2):505–13.
41. Arguelles D, Carmona JU, Pastor J, Iborra A, Vinals L, Martinez P, Bach E, Prades M. Evaluation of single and double centrifugation tube methods for concentrating equine platelets. Res Vet Sci. 2006;81(2):237–45.
42. Bolt DM, Ishihara A, Weisbrode SE, Bertone AL. Effects of triamcinolone acetonide, sodium hyaluronate, amikacin sulfate, and mepivacaine hydrochloride, alone and in combination, on morphology and matrix composition of lipopolysaccharide-challenged and unchallenged equine articular cartilage explants. Am J Vet Res. 2008;69(7):861–7.
43. Byron CR, Orth MW, Venta PJ, Lloyd JW, Caron JP. Influence of glucosamine on matrix metalloproteinase expression and activity in lipopolysaccharide-stimulated equine chondrocytes. Am J Vet Res. 2003;64(6):666–71.
44. Penha-Goncalves MN, Onions DE, Nicolson L. Cloning and sequencing of equine transforming growth factor-beta 1 (TGF beta-1) cDNA. DNA Seq. 1997;7(6):375–8.
45. Donnelly BP, Nixon AJ, Haupt JL, Dahlgren LA. Nucleotide structure of equine platelet-derived growth factor-A and -B and expression in horses with induced acute tendinitis. Am J Vet Res. 2006;67(7):1218–25.
46. Furuta N, Yoshioka I, Fukuizumi T, Tominaga K, Nishihara T, Fukuda J. Morphological features of cartilage observed during mandibular distraction in rabbits. Int J Oral Maxillofac Surg. 2007;36(3):243–9.
47. Fraser A, Fearon U, Reece R, Emery P, Veale DJ. Matrix metalloproteinase 9, apoptosis, and vascular morphology in early arthritis. Arthritis Rheum. 2001; 44(9):2024–8.
48. Livak KJ, Schmittgen TD. Analysis of relative gene expression data using real-time quantitative PCR and the 2(-Delta Delta C(T)) Method. Methods. 2001;25(4):402–8.
49. Dohan DM, Choukroun J, Diss A, Dohan SL, Dohan AJ, Mouhyi J, Gogly B. Platelet-rich fibrin (PRF): a second-generation platelet concentrate. Part III: leucocyte activation: a new feature for platelet concentrates? Oral Surg Oral Med Oral Pathol Oral Radiol Endod. 2006;101(3):e51–55.
50. Giusti I, D'Ascenzo S, Manco A, Di Stefano G, Di Francesco M, Rughetti A, Dal Mas A, Properzi G, Calvisi V, Dolo V. Platelet concentration in platelet-rich plasma affects tenocyte behavior in vitro. Biomed Res Int. 2014;2014: 630870. doi:10.1155/2014/630870. Epub 632014 Jul 630823.
51. Dohan Ehrenfest DM, Bielecki T, Mishra A, Borzini P, Inchingolo F, Sammartino G, Rasmusson L, Evert PA. In search of a consensus terminology in the field of platelet concentrates for surgical use: platelet-rich plasma (PRP), platelet-rich fibrin (PRF), fibrin gel polymerization and leukocytes. Curr Pharm Biotechnol. 2012;13(7):1131–7.
52. McCarrel TM, Minas T, Fortier LA. Optimization of leukocyte concentration in platelet-rich plasma for the treatment of tendinopathy. J Bone Joint Surg Am. 2012, 94(19):e143(141-148).
53. Pearson W, Fletcher RS, Kott LS, Hurtig MB. Protection against LPS-induced cartilage inflammation and degradation provided by a biological extract of Mentha spicata. BMC Complement Altern Med. 2010;10(19):1472–6882.
54. Santoro A, Conde J, Scotece M, Abella V, Lopez V, Pino J, Gomez R, Gomez-Reino JJ, Gualillo O. Choosing the right chondrocyte cell line: Focus on nitric oxide. J Orthop Res. 2015;27(10):22954.
55. Bougault C, Gosset M, Houard X, Salvat C, Godmann L, Pap T, Jacques C, Berenbaum F. Stress-induced cartilage degradation does not depend on the NLRP3 inflammasome in human osteoarthritis and mouse models. Arthritis Rheum. 2012;64(12):3972–81.
56. Vezina Audette R, Lavoie-Lamoureux A, Lavoie JP, Laverty S. Inflammatory stimuli differentially modulate the transcription of paracrine signaling molecules of equine bone marrow multipotent mesenchymal stromal cells. Osteoarthritis Cartilage. 2013;21(8):1116–24.
57. Brenner D, Blaser H, Mak TW. Regulation of tumour necrosis factor signalling: live or let die. Nat Rev Immunol. 2015;15(6):362–74.
58. Bendinelli P, Matteucci E, Dogliotti G, Corsi MM, Banfi G, Maroni P, Desiderio MA. Molecular basis of anti-inflammatory action of platelet-rich plasma on human chondrocytes: mechanisms of NF-kappaB inhibition via HGF. J Cell Physiol. 2010;225(3):757–66.
59. Anitua E, Zalduendo M, Troya M, Padilla S, Orive G. Leukocyte inclusion within a platelet rich plasma-derived fibrin scaffold stimulates a more pro-inflammatory environment and alters fibrin properties. PLoS One. 2015;10(3):e0121713.
60. Morales TI. Chondrocyte moves: clever strategies? Osteoarthritis Cartilage. 2007;15(8):861–71.
61. O'Connell GD, Tan AR, Cui V, Bulinski JC, Cook JL, Attur M, Abramson SB, Ateshian GA, Hung CT. Human chondrocyte migration behaviour to guide the development of engineered cartilage. J Tissue Eng Regen Med. 2015, 28(10). doi:10.1002/term.1988.
62. Kruger JP, Hondke S, Endres M, Pruss A, Siclari A, Kaps C. Human platelet-rich plasma stimulates migration and chondrogenic differentiation of human subchondral progenitor cells. J Orthop Res. 2012;30(6):845–52.
63. Schar MO, Diaz-Romero J, Kohl S, Zumstein MA, Nesic D. Platelet-rich concentrates differentially release growth factors and induce cell migration in vitro. Clin Orthop Relat Res. 2015;473(5):1635–43.
64. Thomas CM, Fuller CJ, Whittles CE, Sharif M. Chondrocyte death by apoptosis is associated with the initiation and severity of articular cartilage degradation. Int J Rheum Dis. 2011;14(2):191–8.
65. Ekman L, Nilsson G, Persson L, Lumsden JH. Volume of the synovia in certain joint cavities in the horse. Acta Vet Scand. 1981;22(1):23–31.

4

Relationships between body dimensions, body weight, age, gender, breed and echocardiographic dimensions in young endurance horses

D. S. Trachsel[1,2*], A. Giraudet[2], D. Maso[2], G. Hervé[2], D. D. Hauri[3], E. Barrey[4] and C. Robert[2,4]

Abstract

Background: The heart's physiological adaptation to aerobic training leads to an increase in heart chamber size, and is referred to as the Athlete's heart. However, heart dimensions are also related to body weight (BWT), body size, growth and (in some species) breed. There are few published data on the relationships between heart dimensions and growth or aerobic training in Arabian and Arabian-related endurance horses. Therefore the objective of the present study was to describe the influence of body dimensions (body length (BL), thoracic circumference (TC), withers height (WH)), BWT, age, gender, breed (*purebred Arabians, part-bred Arabians, Anglo-Arabians, and Others*) and the initiation of endurance training on echocardiographic measurements in competition-fit endurance horses aged 4 to 6 years.

Results: Most left atrial (LA) and left ventricular (LV) dimensions increased with age, whereas LA and LV functional indices did not. Although there was no gender difference for LV dimensions, females had larger LA dimensions. In terms of breed, *Anglo-Arabians* had the largest LV dimensions. Regression models indicated that the included explanatory factors had a weak influence on heart dimensions. Age, body dimensions, breed and gender showed the most consistent influence on LA dimensions, whereas BWT, breed and kilometres covered in competition showed the most consistent influence on LV dimensions.

Conclusion: The increase in echocardiographic dimensions with age indicates on-going growth in our population of 4 to 6 year-old horses. We also observed small changes associated with the initiation of endurance training. Morphometric dimensions had a greater influence on LA dimensions, whereas LV dimensions were also influenced (albeit weakly) by parameters associated with exercise intensity. These results may therefore reflect early adaptations linked to the initiation of endurance training.

Keywords: (3-10): equine, Echocardiography, Cardiovascular, Non-invasive cardiac assessment, Endurance, Body weight, Body dimensions, Gender, Age, Breed

Background

The Athlete's heart is a physiological adaptation to aerobic training and athletes (especially endurance athletes) have larger hearts and thus a larger stroke volume than non-endurance trained or sedentary humans [1, 2]. The Athlete's heart has also been described in various types of racehorse and endurance horses [3–7] and has been linked to the appearance of heart murmurs albeit with little impact on performance [6, 8–10]. Furthermore, a high VO_{2max} (an index of exercise capacity) in horses has been related to larger left ventricular (LV) dimensions and LV mass [11, 12]. Larger hearts have been associated with better performance in some studies, [4, 5, 13] but not in others [14] and the discrepancy between these studies can certainly be explained by varying parameters used to assess performance. It is nevertheless the case that in most equestrian sport

* Correspondence: dagmart@sund.ku.dk
[1]CIRALE-Hippolia, Médecine Sportive, RD 674, F-14430 Goustranville, France
[2]Université Paris-Est, Ecole Nationale Vétérinaire d'Alfort, 7 avenue du Général de Gaulle, F-94704 Maisons-Alfort, France
Full list of author information is available at the end of the article

disciplines, horses that train more, race more, earn more or participate in elite competitions have larger hearts than their peers [4, 5, 7, 13].

However, other factors (such as body dimensions, body weight (BWT) [5, 6, 15], breed [16, 17] and gender [5, 6, 13]) might influence the heart's dimensions. Some of the studies in this field included non-fully mature horses [3, 5, 13], whereas others also included adult horses [6, 7]. Especially in young individuals, growth is an important matter, and age at maturity differs from one breed to another [18–21]. Furthermore, training methods and the physical demands of competition differ from one discipline to another. Thus, conclusions based on data from one breed and/or discipline cannot necessarily be fully extrapolated to another breed and/or discipline. Hence, the primary objective of the present study was to describe the development of the heart in young Arabian-type horses aged between four and six years, an age at which endurance training is usually initiated. The second objective was to assess a possible association between external factors and the echocardiographic dimensions of the heart's chambers and great vessels in these horses.

Methods

Population

Between 2011 and 2014, echocardiographic measurements were recorded during field exercise tests and at the annual finals of the French National Championships for young endurance horses. The field tests were organised by the research group for all interested endurance horses owners four times a year. Only horses aged between 4 and 6 years at the time of presentation and with at least one purebred Arabian parent were included in the study. All horses were examined by the official veterinarians on site and had thus been authorised to race prior to enrolment in the study. Each horse was identified by its French national identification number and was included only once in our subsequent analyses. The study design was approved by the local institutional Ethical Committee (ComEthANSES/ENVA/UPEC, Maisons-Alfort, France; approval number: 12/07/11-1). All owners provided their written, informed consent to participation before the horses underwent any study procedures and were told that they could withdraw their horse from the study at any time.

For each horse, body length (BL, in cm: the distance between the shoulder at the palpable portion of the greater tubercle and the palpable portion of the ischial tuberosity), thoracic circumference (TC, in cm: circumference measured at girth placement), withers height (WH, in cm: height at the highest point of the withers) were measured with a tape measure. The BWT (in kg) was measured using a portable horse-weighing platform (Horse weigh® Tokyo model, Horse Weigh Ltd, Llandrindod Wells, UK, http://www.horseweigh.com). The body surface area (BSA, in m^2) [22] was calculated using the following equation: $BSW = 0.101 \times BWT^{2/3}$. Horses were divided into age groups: *Group 4y* included all 4-year old horses, *Group 5y* included all 5-year old horses, and *Group 6y* included all 6-year old horses. Each horse's gender and breed were also recorded. Although all the horses necessarily had a least one purebred Arabian parent (given the study's inclusion criterion), they were divided into four breed groups for further analysis: *Group purebred Arabians* comprised all the purebred Arabians and the Shagya Arabians, *Group part-bred Arabians* comprised crossbreeds between Arabians and Warmbloods, *Group Anglo-Arabians* comprised Anglo-Arabians or Anglo-Arabian crossbreed, and lastly, *Group Others* comprised all other Arabian crossbreeds.

Given that the owners of the included horses applied a very broad variety of training programmes, it was not possible to objectively quantify the horses' training history. However, a rough estimation of each horse's activity prior to echocardiography was derived by noting the total number of kilometres covered in competition since the first registered competition (Km-career) and the numbers of days since the first registered competition (d-career) from the records in the French Equestrian Federation's database (FFECompet https://ffecompet.ffe.com/cheval [23]).

Echocardiographic measurements

Transthoracic, two-dimensional echocardiography (2DE) was performed on resting horses before they participated in the endurance competitions or field exercise tests. The echocardiography was performed by two experienced clinicians (AG for the 68 examinations in 2011, and DST for the 272 examinations in 2012-2014) using a portable ultrasound system (Vivid I, General Electric Healthcare Europe GMBH, France) that enabled synchronous recording of the electrocardiogram (ECG). The field conditions and the limited time available for the examinations precluded the realisation of Doppler ultrasound examinations and allowed only recordings from the right parasternal long axis views, as described elsewhere in detail [24–27].

The measurements were made under supervision of the experienced clinicians by two well-trained persons independent of those who examined the horses (DM, GH). To summarise, the dimension of the aortic (sinus) diameter (AOD), and the maximal pulmonary artery diameter (PAD) were measured at end-diastole on the right parasternal long-axis 2 DE views of the left and right ventricular outflow tract, respectively. The atrial dimensions were assessed in a right parasternal long-axis 2 DE view centred on the LA by measuring the maximal LA diameter (LAD_{max}), and LA area (LAA_{max}) at end-systole prior to mitral valve opening, the LA diameter (LAD_a) and LA area (LAA_a) at the onset of the electrocardiographic P wave prior to active contraction, and the minimal LA diameter (LAD_{min}) and LA area (LAA_{min}) at the time of mitral valve closure. The LV dimensions were also assessed in a right parasternal long-axis 2DE view but centred to visualize the LV apex. From this view, the interventricular septal thickness (IVS), the LV internal diameter (LVID), and the LV free wall thickness (LVFW) were measured on a line midway between the papillary muscles and the mitral valve annulus, perpendicular to the IVS and LVFW and parallel to the mitral valve annulus at end-diastole (d) and peak systole (s). Using the same view LV internal area (LVIA) and LV internal length (LVIL) were measured at end-diastole (d) and at peak systole (s).

The LA areas were used to calculate functional indices of LA contraction including the active LA fractional area change [Active LA FAC = $(LAA_a - LAA_{min})/LAA_a \times 100$], the passive LA fractional area change [Passive LA FAC = $(LAA_{max} - LAA_a)/LAA_{max} \times 100$], the total LA fractional area change [Total LA FAC = $(LAA_{max} - LAA_{min})/LAA_{max} \times 100$], and the active-to-total LA area change [active:total LA AC = $(LAA_a - LAA_{min})/(LAA_{max} - LAA_{min})$] [25].

For measured LV dimensions, the relative wall thickness at end-diastole [RWT = $(IVS_d + LVFW_d)/LVID_d$], the mean wall thickness at end-diastole [MWT = $(IVS_d + LVFW_d)/2$] and the LV_{mass} [$1.04\times[(LVID_d + LVFW_d + IVS_d)^3 - LVID_d] - 13.6$] were calculated.[5, 11, 24]. Two functional indices for the LV were calculated: the LV fractional shortening [LV FS = $(LVID_d - LVID_s)/LVID_d \times 100$]) and the LV fractional area change [LV FAC = $(LVIA_d - LVIA_s)/LVIA_d \times 100$] [5, 11, 24, 27].

Further, the cardiac output [CO = SV × HR] and the stroke volume [SV = $LVIV_d - LVIV_s$], based on LV internal volume at end-diastole (LVIV_d) and at peak systole (LVIV_s), were calculated using the equation $5/6\times LVIA^2/LVIL$ (describes as the "4CAL equation" by McConachie et al. [28]).

In order to compare the relative proportions of the heart's chambers, the $LAA_{max}/LVIA_d$, and $LAD_{max}/LVID_d$ ratios were calculated. Further, the AOD/PAD ratio was established.

All measurements were made offline on the basis of digitally stored cine-loop recordings and were averaged over two or three non-consecutive cardiac cycles. The heart rate (HR) was determined and the rhythm was assessed on the ECGs recorded synchronously on the cine-loops.

Statistical analyses

Based on a visual assessment of histograms and of normal probability plots, normality of the data distribution was given and parametric methods were applied.

Influences of age category, gender and breed were tested using an analysis of variance (ANOVA) with Holm-Sidak post-hoc tests for multiple comparisons. Further, pooled males (geldings and intact males) were compared with females using a Student's *t*-test. Dichotomous variables were compared in a Chi^2 test. The threshold for statistical significance was set to $p < 0.05$.

Univariate regression models were established for LA and LV echocardiographic measurements and for explanatory factors with continuous data (BWT, BSA, WH, TC, BL, Km-career, d-career). Multivariate regression models were then developed for the most relevant LA and LV measurements. Based on an assessment of the residuals, log-linear regression models were used if necessary. The log transformation of the outcomes allowed reaching normality of the residuals. All explanatory factors were included in the initial model. Thereafter, quadratic and cubic terms were also included for the BWT in the initial models. Non-relevant explanatory factors were excluded by stepwise elimination based on the adjusted R^2 and the Akaike information criterion (AIC). However, models were not considered to be relevant if the final adjusted R^2 was below 10 %. No interactions between explanatory factors were considered in the models.

All statistical analyses were performed using commercially available software (GraphPad Prism®, version 6.05, GraphPad Software, San Diego, CA, USA, www.graphpad.com, SigmaStat®, version 3.5, Systat Software GmbH, Erkrath, Germany, R-software®, version 3.1.0, R Development Core Team, Vienna, Austria).

Results

Three hundred and forty horses were included in the study. The demographic characteristics of the study population are summarised in Table 1. Given that the field conditions limited the available time per horse, the number of missing data varied from one measurement to another. The numbers of available data per measurement are given in Additional files 1, 2, 3 and 4. Most horses were females or geldings, and intact males were significantly underrepresented (Chi^2 $p < 0.01$). Furthermore, most of the horses were *purebred* or *part-bred Arabians*, whereas *Anglo-Arabians* and *Others* were significantly underrepresented (Chi^2 $p = 0.03$). There were slightly more horses in *Group 6y* than in the two other groups. The measured HR was slightly higher than the usual resting HR for horses, and no arrhythmias were observed on the reviewed cine-loops.

The p-values obtained in ANOVAs for age groups, genders and breed groups are presented in Additional files 5, 6 and 7. In summary, the BWT and the BSA were significantly greater in 5-year old horses than in 4-year

Table 1 Demographic characteristics of the study population

	4-year-olds	5-year-olds	6-year-olds	Total	$p^{\#}$
Number	101	109	130	340	n.s.
	Mean (± SD)	Mean (± SD)	Mean (± SD)	Mean (± SD)	
HR (bpm)	44 (±10)	44 (±9)	43 (±10)	43 (±9)	n.s.
BWT (kg)	405.9^{a} (±39.2)	422.9^{b} (±35.3)	411.1^{a} (±37.0)	413.4 (±37.6)	*
BSA (m^2)	3.9^{a} (±0.2)	4.0^{b} (±0.2)	3.9^{a} (±0.2)	3.9 (±0.2)	*
WH (cm)	152.9 (±3.8)	153.5 (±4.0)	152.5 (±4.3)	152.9 (±4.0)	n.s.
TC (cm)	173.5 (±7.6)	174.7 (±6.8)	173.1 (±5.8)	173.8 (±6.7)	n.s.
BL (cm)	154.2 (±7.3)	154.7 (±7.5)	152.9 (±7.4)	153.9 (±7.4)	n.s.
d-career (days)	109.7^{a} (±69.5)	302.5^{b} (±175.1)	576.3^{c} (±268.8)	351.5 (±276.5)	**
Km-career (km)	44.3^{a} (±49.7)	130.5^{b} (±82.8)	435.8^{c} (±323.6)	223.0 (±269.8)	**
Gender					
females	42	52	64	158	**
geldings	34	36	48	118	
intact males	25	21	18	64	
Breed					
Purebred Arabian	49	64	88	201	*
Part-bred Arabians	39	30	31	100	
Anglo-Arabians	5	11	8	24	
Others	8	4	3	15	

#, results from ANOVAs or Chi^2 tests, as appropriate; *, significant at $p < 0.05$; **, significant at $p < 0.01$; n.s., not significant; results marked with a different superscript letter differed significant from the other results in the row. For *p*-values, see Additional file 5

or 6-year old horses. The body dimensions in *Group 5y* were also slightly (but not significantly) higher than those in the other two age groups.

Further, the horses in *Group 6y* had significantly longer careers and had covered significantly more kilometres in competition than those in the other age groups. Likewise, values for Km-career and d-career were also significantly higher in *Group 5y* than in *Group 4y.*

The two-dimensional LA dimensions increased fairly steadily with age and significant differences were noted when comparing *Group 4y* with *Group 5y* or *Group 4y* with *Group 6y* (Additional file 6). However, the largest difference was observed when comparing *Group 4y* and *Group 6y*. LA area measurements also increased with age, although the differences between the age groups were not significant. The LA functional indexes did not differ significantly with age. *Group 5y* and *Group 6y* did not differ significantly in terms of any of the LA dimensions.

AOD and AOD/PAD increased constantly from *Group 4y* to *Group 6y*, whereas PAD was lower in *Group 4y* than in *Group 5y* (Additional file 6).

Most LV echocardiographic measurements (Additional file 7) also increased with age and the largest differences were observed when comparing *Group 4y* and *5y*. The differences between *Group 5y* and *6y* were less pronounced but were most marked for two-dimensional measurements. In contrast, increases in area measurements were more regular over the studied age range. *Group 5y* and *6y* did not differ significantly in terms of any of the LV measurements. We did not observe any age-related changes for IVS_s, IVS_d, $LVFW_s$, $LVFW_d$, MWR, RWT, LV FS, LV FAC and CO.

Overall, gender differences were small (Additional files 5, 6 and 7). The comparison between genders showed that females had a larger TC than intact males or pooled males. Geldings had slightly greater WH and BWT than the other groups, and intact males had the lowest values for all morphometric dimensions; however, the differences were not statistically significant. There were no gender differences in Km-career or d-career. Intact males had the smallest two-dimensional LA dimensions, whereas females had the largest LA area measurements (Additional file 6). These differences in dimensions led to a significant gender difference for one of the LA functional indices: the passive LA FAC was highest in intact males. There were no significant differences for other comparisons. With regard to the great vessels, the AOD was slightly (but not significantly) lower in females. The PAD was significantly greater in females when compared with geldings or with all males. Hence, the ratio AOD/PAD was also smaller in females than in geldings or in all males. There were no gender differences in the LV measurements (Additional file 7).

There were no differences for Km-career or d-career between the breed groups. In our population *purebred Arabians* were smallest and lightest, whereas *Anglo-Arabians* were tallest and heaviest (Additional file 5). Further, none of the differences in LA dimensions between breed groups were statistically significant (Additional file 6). However, two-dimensional LA measurements were highest in *Anglo-Arabians*, whereas in *part-bred Arabians* and *Others* these dimensions were slightly smaller than in *purebred Arabians*. The same difference was not apparent for area measurements, and *purebred Arabians* even showed a trend towards highest values. There were no obvious differences in AOD or in PAD between the breeds.

As seen for the LA, all LV measurements were highest in *Anglo-Arabians* and for most measurements lowest in *part-bred Arabians* and *Others* (Additional file 7). The largest differences were observed for measurements made at end-diastole, and were statistically significant for IVS_d, $LVID_d$, LV_{mass} and SV.

Univariate linear regression models revealed very weak influences of the explanatory variables on echocardiographic measurements (Additional files 1 and 2). Less than 14 % of the total variability in the LV dimensions ($LVIA_d$: $R^2 = 11.0$ %; LVIV_d: $R^2 = 12.4$ %; SV: $R^2 = 12.6$ %) and in the LV_{mass} ($R^2 = 13.7$ %) was explained by the BWT or BSA. Less than 11 % of the total variability of the LA measurements was explained by TC (LAD_a: $R^2 = 11.0$ %; LAA_{max}: $R^2 = 11.0$ %).

In the multivariate regression models, the values for the adjusted R^2 were also low and the chosen explanatory factors accounted for less than 18 % of the total variability in the echocardiographic measurements (Additional files 3 and 4). Furthermore, the analyses for LA and LV measurements showed different patterns. For LA measurements, the values for the adjusted R^2 were higher than those obtained for LV measurements, and most of the LA measurements were related to morphometric measurements.

In these multivariate regression models, BL showed a positive influence on LAD_{max}, BL and TP showed a positive influence on LAD_a and AOD. BL and WH had a positive influence on LAD_{min}. LAA_a and LAA_{min} increased with increasing WH, TP and BL, whereas LAA_{max} increased only with increasing TP and WH. BWT had positive influence only on LAD_{max}, AOD and PAD. BSA is not reported as results were identical to those for BWT.

For most LA measurements, age positively influenced the dimensions. Hence older horses displayed larger dimensions, except for the PAD, which decreased with age.

Although *Anglo-Arabians* showed a trend towards larger two-dimensional LA measurements, breed had a negative influence on LAD_{max}, LAA_a and LAA_{min} in the multivariate regression models and belonging to a breed other than *purebred Arabians* was associated with a decrease in the mentioned LA dimensions.

As seen in the ANOVAs, multivariate regressions showed that gender was variously associated with the magnitude of some LA measurements. Intact males and geldings showed lower LAD_a, LAD_{min}, LAA_a and LAA_{min} values than females did. Intact males and geldings had smaller PADs but higher AODs than females. The Km-career and d-career variables were not associated with the LA measurements. The PAD increased with Km-career and decreased very slightly with d-career.

For LV measurements (Additional file 4), most measurements were positively associated with BWT. This was especially true for LV_{mass}, $LVIA_d$, and derived values such as LVIV_d and SV. When considering other morphometric measurements, WH had positive influence on $LVIA_d$, LVIV_d and SV, and BL had a negative influence on $LVIA_d$, LVIV_d and SV. The results for BSA are not reported in detail because they were identical to those for BWT.

In comparison to *purebred Arabians*, LV_{mass} was higher in the *Anglo-Arabians* and lower in the *part-bred Arabians*. Gender and age had only a slight influence on LV measurements. However, Km-career was positively associated with LV_{mass}, $LVIA_d$ and LVIV_d.

Discussion

The present study reports changes in echocardiographic dimensions of the heart in young Arabian type horses at the end of their growth period and at the beginning of their endurance training for competitions. All external variables included in the analyses influenced to some extent several of the measured dimensions. Morphometric dimensions, age and breed showed most consistently an influence on LA measurements, whereas BWT, breed and Km-career had most consistently an influence on LV measurements.

All the horses in the study population had at least one purebred Arabian parent. Our study population was chosen to be representative of the horses participating in endurance competitions. This choice was in accordance with literature data indicating that purebred or mixed-breed Arabians are largely overrepresented in endurance competitions, although some other breeds do participate [29, 30]. In view of the inclusion criteria, the division into several breed groups may seem arbitrary. However, there were significant differences between these breed groups. *Purebred Arabians* were the smallest and lightest - giving them advantage over other breeds in endurance competitions [29, 30]. Body dimension and BWT were highest in *Anglo-Arabians* that in turn led also to larger LV_{mass}. Nevertheless, in the multivariate regression models, belonging to breeds other than *purebred Arabians* was associated with smaller LA measurements. This indicated that the smallest horses in our population did not necessarily have the smallest hearts and hence that other factors must be considered.

BWT and body dimensions were higher in *Group 5y* than in *Group 4y*, which was presumably due to on-going growth. In contrast, the smaller body dimensions in *Group 6y* (especially WH and BL, which are less influenced by body condition) might be due to the selection of smaller, lighter, more compact horses for more demanding competitions. Indeed, high BWT in endurance horses has been associated with failure to finish competitions, particularly due to lameness [29, 30]. Furthermore, horses in *Group 6y* had covered a greater distance in competition (Km-career) and thus were certainly subjected to harder training, which may have resulted in a lower BWT. Training reduces fat content and increases muscle mass. Therefore, it would have been interesting to measure lean body weight. BWT and especially fat-free mass were associated with better indices of performances in Standarbreds, [31, 32] and fat-free mass was also associated with a higher VO_{2max}. However, too low BWT or too low percentage of body fat is detrimental in human athletes [33, 34]. The optimal percentage of body fat has not yet been established for horses, although body fat was around 8 % in well-performing athletic horses [29, 32, 35]. As is the case for human athletes, the optimal percentage of body fat doubtless varies from one discipline to another [34, 36].

All heart dimensions increased with age. The difference between 4 and 5 years of age was greater than the difference between 5 and 6 years of age. In univariate and multivariate regression analyses, for most heart dimensions a weak relationship was observed with BWT or TC (especially for LA measurements). The higher values for the R^2 in regression models of LA measurements and of the dimensions of the great vessels, and their relationship with body dimensions (rather than BWT) might indicate that these dimensions are more strongly related to the horse's morphotype. Al-Haidir et al. also have reported that some echocardiographic measurements are somewhat more strongly associated with TC than they are with BWT [37]. However, due to the present study's inclusion criteria, the range of body dimensions and weights was narrower than in the work by Al-Haidir et al. [37]. Concomitant increases in all dimensions are seen with growth, and growth has to be taken into consideration when studying young individuals. Different breeds have differing growth rates. Thoroughbreds and Standardbreds are fast-growing breeds and reached 83 % of the adult BWT by the age of 2 years, whereas the growth rate is slower in other breeds and by the age of 2 years Warmbloods, Anglo-Arabians and Lusitanos reached 80 %, 75 % and 77 % of their adult BWT, respectively [20, 21]. Arabians have been classified as slow-growing horses [38]. Accordingly, they are still growing between the ages of 4 and 6 years. This contrasts with Standardbred horses, which are considered to reach maturity between the ages of 3.5 and 5 years [6]. Although growth certainly affects the LV dimensions, the latter are also greatly modulated by other factors. In particular, training is a strong stimulus for cardiac hypertrophy, and we detected a weak but significant association between Km-career and some of the LV measurements. This very weak association might be due to the poorly elaborated performance parameters (Km-career, d-career) and also due to the generally low level of endurance training seen at this age [39]. A training-related increase in LV dimensions has been observed in Thoroughbreds [3], Standardbreds [5, 6] and elite Arabians [7]. The absence of a change in RWT indicated that the heart's adaptation to exercise in our population is more similar to that seen in Standardbreds [5, 6] than to that seen in Thoroughbreds, [3] or elite Arabians [7]. Further, this finding might also illustrate differences in training practices among different breeds. We did not find any association between LA dimensions and Km-carrer. This is in contrast to studies in human athletes that showed also greater LA dimensions in presence of an Athlete's heart [40, 41]. However, the endurance training in our study population was probably not intensive enough to induce changes in LA dimensions.

The results of our regression analyses agree with another study reporting small values for the R^2 for LV measurements in young (2-year-old) Standardbreds [6]. However, values for the R^2 increased with age in this previous study, particularly for LV_{mass}. This comparison also suggests that our population's training was not yet hard enough to induce marked changes in heart dimensions.

In accordance with previous studies [42–44], there were no age-related differences in LA and LV functional indexes.

Females had the largest TC. Given that LA measurements were related to TC in our regression models, we were not surprised to find that females had also the largest LA measurements. On the contrary, intact males had the smallest LA dimensions. In contrast to other studies [5, 13, 44], gender did not appear to influence LV dimensions in our study population. One explanation could be that the intensity of the aerobic training in endurance horses at this age is not high enough to bring out the full potential for hypertrophy in intact males. Another explanation might be related to the custom of French endurance trainers/owners to breed females at the age of 5 years. Gestation may have induced changes in heart dimensions (as seen in humans and dogs), although these changes are usually reversible [45, 46].

The present study had a number of limitations. Due to field conditions and the limited time available per horse, not all echocardiographic views of heart chambers could be taken, and some views were of poor quality. Similarly, it was not possible to perform Doppler examinations and thus screen for possible regurgitations. Due to these technical issues there were several missing data. Nevertheless our analyses were based on a large body of data. Given that the measured heart chamber dimensions can be influenced by the transducer position and the views obtained [47, 48], not all of our measurements can be validly compared with the literature values. Our comparison with previous studies is therefore limited to the consideration of factors that influence heart dimensions. Second, the use of only longitudinal views meant that our LV measures could probably be underestimated [47]. Furthermore, the measured HRs were slightly over resting values, and the shorter filling time at these HRs might have affected ours results, especially for diastolic measurements. Nevertheless, the HRs measured in our studies were only slightly higher than those reported in the literature for endurance horses [7, 48]. Lastly, the fact that the recordings and measurements were made by several operators probably decreased the precision of our measurements [25, 49].

Differentiating the effects of growth from the effects of training would have required the use of a control group. In principle, a control group should comprise untrained, non-competing horses of the same age. Unfortunately, this type of population was not available in our research setting. Furthermore, follow-up measurements of our study population 3-4 years later or measurements from a control group of mature, elite endurance horses would have provided information on the effects of more intensive aerobic training. In accordance with results from Sleeper et al. [7] reporting greater LVID, LV_{mass} and SV in elite Arabians (mean age 21.1, age range 7-17) than in non-elite Arabians, data from our research group show that in a smaller group of endurance horses (n = 11; nine purebred Arabians and two others; four females, six geldings and one intact male; mean age ten, range 8-13 years) participating in races of least 120 km, the main differences relative to younger horses were seen for LVID, LVIA, LVIL and LVIV, with greater differences appearing in peak systolic measurements. Furthermore, in the older horses, LV_{mass} was higher and LV FAC and LV FS were lower. The greater LV dimensions and LV_{mass} agree with literature data on various breeds [4, 6, 7] and are certainly related to a greater aerobic training volume at this age. These considerations strengthen our hypothesis whereby the training load in younger horses was not intense enough to induce marked cardiac hypertrophy. Our findings with regard to LV FAC and LV FS are more difficult to explain, since the Athlete's heart does not feature any changes in LV function at rest [1, 41]. The results might be best explained by the fact that older horses were more used to being handled and therefore showed a narrower range of heart rates than younger horses. Indeed, the HRs for adult endurance horses reported in the literature were slightly lower than in the present study [7, 48].

Furthermore, the performance parameters used in the present study (Km-career, d-career) were very rough. In France, purebred Arabians are not trained intensively between the ages of 4 and 6 years and training is not as standardised as it is in Thoroughbreds or Standardbreds [39]. Furthermore, some horses were bred during this period, which decreased the training period. Therefore, it was not possible to analyse objective parameters, such as gains, speed at kilometre, or numbers of start [4, 5, 13, 14]. The most accessible parameters were Km-career and d-career, since this information was freely available in the FEE database. We hypothesised that a horse having participated in a greater number of competitions or longer competitions would have been trained harder. Even though we observed a weak relationship between Km-career and some LV measurements, better performance indicators are clearly needed. Long-term information on the endurance horses' competitive performance was not yet available at the time of the present study and will be addressed in the future.

Lastly, we had no possibility to record and therefore to compare echocardiographic measurements taken before and after exercise. This comparison would have provided valuable information on cardiac adaptation to effort in competition [50, 51] but was outside the scope of the present study. Hence this topic merits further research.

Conclusion

In a population of endurance horses aged four to six years, the main changes in cardiac dimensions were observed between age groups and are probably due to ongoing growth, even though the initiation of endurance training may also have had some effect. In particular, LV measurements were related (albeit weakly) to performance parameters, which might reflect the adaption to the initiation of aerobic training. Gender differences were not apparent in our young population, although there were significant differences between breeds. Despite being the smallest horses, *purebred Arabians* did not have the smallest hearts. Small body size might be an advantage in endurance competitions. However, other factors, such as the heart's dimensions relative to the body dimension, or the capacity of a rapid HR recovery after the race, appear to be important and should be studied in the future. Further longitudinal studies are needed, in particular to validate specific performance indicators for endurance horses.

Additional files

Additional file 1: Results of the univariate linear regression analyses, showing the weak influence (expressed as R^2) of the chosen explanatory parameters on left atrial (LA) and great vessel echocardiographic dimensions. (DOCX 16 kb)

Additional file 2: Results of the univariate linear regression analyses, showing the weak influence (expressed as R^2) of the chosen explanatory parameters on left ventricular (LV) echocardiographic dimensions. (DOCX 16 kb)

Additional file 3: Results of the multivariate regression analyses, showing the influence of external factors considered as independent variables on left atrial (LA) and great vessel echocardiographic dimensions. (DOCX 29 kb)

Additional file 4: Results of the multivariate regression analyses, showing the influence of external factors considered as independent variables on left ventricular (LV) echocardiographic dimensions. (DOCX 37 kb)

Additional file 5: Results of the ANOVAs and Student's t-tests reporting p-values for comparisons of morphometric measurements between age groups, genders and breeds groups. (DOCX 17 kb)

Additional file 6: Results of the ANOVAs and Student's t-tests reporting p-values for comparisons of left atrial (LA) and great vessels dimensions between age groups, genders and breeds groups. (DOCX 18 kb)

Additional file 7: Results of the ANOVAs and Student's t-tests reporting p-values for comparisons of left ventricular (LV) echocardiographic dimensions between age groups, genders and breeds groups. (DOCX 21 kb)

Abbreviations

2DE: Two-dimensional echocardiography; active LA FAC: Active left atrial fractional area change; active:total LA AC: Active-to-total left atrial area change; AIC: Akaike information criterion; ANOVA: Analyse of variance; AOD: The dimension of the aortic (sinus) diameter; BL: Body length; BSA: Body surface area; BWT: Bodyweight; CO: Cardiac output; d: At end-diastole; d-career: Numbers of days since the first recorded official competition; ECG: Electrocardiogram; HR: Heart rate; IVS: Interventricular septal thickness; Km-career: Number of km covered in completion since the first recorded official competition; LA: Left atrium; LAA_a: Left atrial area prior to active contraction, at the onset of the electrocardiographic P-wave; LAA_{max}: Maximum left atrial area at end-systole, prior to mitral valve opening; LAA_{min}: Minimum left atrial area at end-diastole, after mitral valve closure; LADa: Left atrial diameter prior to active contraction, at the onset of the electrocardiographic P-wave; LAD_{max}: Maximum left atrial diameter at end-systole, prior to mitral valve opening; LAD_{min}: Minimum left atrial diameter at end-diastole, after mitral valve closure; LV FAC: Left ventricular fractional area change; LV FS: Left ventricular fractional shortening; LV: Left ventricular; LVFW: Left ventricular free wall thickness; LVIA: Left ventricular internal area; LVID: Left ventricular internal diameter; LVIL: Left ventricular internal length; LVIV: Left ventricular internal volume; LV_{mass}: Left ventricular mass; MWT: Mean wall thickness; PAD: Maximal pulmonary artery diameter; passive LA FAC: Passive left atrial fractional area change; RWT: Relative wall thickness; s: At peak systole; SV: Stroke volume; TC: Thoracic circumference; total LA FAC: Total left atrial fractional area change; WH: Withers height

Acknowledgements

We would like to acknowledge all the horse owners, riders and trainers as well as collaborators of the project GenEndurance and the Société Hippique Française for making this study possible. Further, we thank Dr Neus Palau Barreda for her valuable assistance during data analysis.

Funding

The study was funded by the French National Studs (IFCE), the Eperon Funds, the French Arabian Horse Association (ACA), the Institut National de Recherche Agronomique (INRA) and the Ecole Nationale Vétérinaire d'Alfort (ENVA).

Authors' contributions

DST and AG recorded the echocardiographic views, DST, DM and GH performed echocardiographic measurements and some of the statistical analyses, DDH advised on and performed the statistical analyses, and DST, CR and EB conceived, designed and coordinated the study and drafted the manuscript. All authors read and approved the final manuscript.

Authors' information

The current address of the corresponding author (DST) is University of Copenhagen, Faculty of Health and Medical Sciences, Department of Veterinary Clinical and Animal Science, Dyrlægevej 100, 1870 Frederiksberg C, Denmark. The current address of GH is Selas Hunaudaye Vétérinaires, 5 PA Carrefour du Penthièvre, 22640 Plestan, France.
Parts of this study have been presented as posters at the 9th ICEPP in Chester (2014) and at the 7th ECEIM congress in Prague (2014).

Competing interest

The authors declare that they have no competing interests.

Consent for publication

Not applicable.

Author details

[1]CIRALE-Hippolia, Médecine Sportive, RD 674, F-14430 Goustranville, France. [2]Université Paris-Est, Ecole Nationale Vétérinaire d'Alfort, 7 avenue du Général de Gaulle, F-94704 Maisons-Alfort, France. [3]Office Fédéral de la Statistique, Espace de l'Europe 10, CH-2010 Neuchâtel, Switzerland. [4]INRA, GABI-UMR1313, 78350 Jouy-en-Josas, France.

References

1. Pluim BM, Zwinderman AH, van der Laarse A, van der Wall EE. The athlete's heart. A meta-analysis of cardiac structure and function. Circulation. 2000;101(3):336–44.
2. D'Andrea A, Limongelli G, Caso P, Sarubbi B, Della Pietra A, Brancaccio P, et al. Association between left ventricular structure and cardiac performance during effort in two morphological forms of athlete's heart. Int J Cardiol. 2002;86(2-3):177–84.
3. Young LE. Cardiac response to training in 2-year-old Thoroughbreds: an echocardiographic study. Equine Vet J Suppl. 1999;30:195–8.
4. Young LE, Rogers K, Wood JL. Left ventricular size and systolic function in Thoroughbred racehorses and their relationships to race performance. J Appl Physiol (1985). 2005;99(4):1278–85.
5. Buhl R, Ersboll AK, Eriksen L, Koch J. Changes over time in echocardiographic measurements in young Standardbred racehorses undergoing training and racing and association with racing performance. J Am Vet Med Assoc. 2005;226(11):1881–7.
6. Buhl R, Ersboll AK. Echocardiographic evaluation of changes in left ventricular size and valvular regurgitation associated with physical training during and after maturity in Standardbred trotters. J Am Vet Med Assoc. 2012;240(2):205–12.
7. Sleeper MM, Durando MM, Holbrook TC, Payton ME, Birks EK. Comparison of echocardiographic measurements in elite and nonelite Arabian endurance horses. Am J Vet Res. 2014;75(10):893–8.
8. Young LE, Rogers K, Wood JL. Heart murmurs and valvular regurgitation in thoroughbred racehorses: epidemiology and associations with athletic performance. J Vet Intern Med. 2008;22(2):418–26.
9. Young LE, Wood JL. Effect of age and training on murmurs of atrioventricular valvular regurgitation in young thoroughbreds. Equine Vet J. 2000;32(3):195–9.
10. Buhl R, Ersboll AK, Eriksen L, Koch J. Use of color Doppler echocardiography to assess the development of valvular regurgitation in Standardbred trotters. J Am Vet Med Assoc. 2005;227(10):1630–5.
11. Young LE, Marlin DJ, Deaton C, Brown-Feltner H, Roberts CA, Wood JL. Heart size estimated by echocardiography correlates with maximal oxygen uptake. Equine Vet J Suppl. 2002;34:467–71.

12. Sampson SN, Tucker RL, Bayly WM. Relationship between VO2max, heart score and echocardiographic measurements obtained at rest and immediately following maximal exercise in thoroughbred horses. Equine Vet J Suppl. 1999;30:190–4.
13. Seder JA, Vickery III CE, Miller PM. The relationship of selected two-dimensional echocardiographic measurements to the racing performance of 5431 yearlings and 2003 two-year-old Thoroughbred racehorses. J Equine Vet Sci. 2003;23(4):149–67.
14. Leadon D, McAllister H, Mullins E, Osborne M. Electrocardiographic and echocardiographic measurements and their relationships in Thoroughbred yearlings to subsequent performance. Equine Exp Physiol. 1991;3:22–9.
15. Zucca E, Ferrucci F, Croci C, Di Fabio V, Zaninelli M, Ferro E. Echocardiographic measurements of cardiac dimensions in normal Standardbred racehorses. J Vet Cardiol. 2008;10(1):45–51.
16. Al-Haidar A, Farnir F, Deleuze S, Sandersen CF, Leroux AA, Borde L, et al. Effect of breed, sex, age and body weight on echocardiographic measurements in the equine species. Res Vet Sci. 2013;95(1):255–60.
17. Gehlen H, Haubold A, Stadler P. Reference values for echocardiographic parameters of trained and untrained Icelandic horses. Dtsch Tierarztl Wochenschr. 2007;114(10):374–7.
18. Kocher A, Staniar WB. The pattern of thoroughbred growth is affected by a foal's birthdate. Livest Sci. 2013;154:204–14.
19. Valette JP, Robert C, Denoix JM. Use of linear and non-linear functions to describe the growth of young sport- and race-horses born in Normandy. Animal. 2008;2(4):560–5.
20. Fradinho MJ, Bessa RJB, Ferreira-Dias G, Caldeira RM. Growth and development of the Lusitano horse managed on grazing systems. Livest Sci. 2016;186:22–28.doi:10.1016/j.livsci.2015.06.006.
21. Heugebaert S, Garcia-Launay F, Trillaud-Gey C, Dubroeucq HH, Arnaud G, Bigot G, et al. Modélisation de la croissance des poulains : première étape vers de nouvelles recommandations alimentaires. In: 36ème Journee de la Recherche Equine. Saumur: Institut français du cheval et de l'équitation; 2010. p. 61-68.
22. Brown DJ, Rush JE, MacGregor J, Ross Jr JN, Brewer B, Rand WM. M-mode echocardiographic ratio indices in normal dogs, cats, and horses: a novel quantitative method. J Vet Intern Med. 2003;17(5):653–62.
23. FFE Compet [https://ffecompet.ffe.com/cheval]
24. Grenacher PA, Schwarzwald CC. Assessment of left ventricular size and function in horses using anatomical M-mode echocardiography. J Vet Cardiol. 2010;12(2):111–21.
25. Schwarzwald CC, Schober KE, Bonagura JD. Methods and reliability of echocardiographic assessment of left atrial size and mechanical function in horses. Am J Vet Res. 2007;68:735–47.
26. Reef VB. Cardiovascular ultrasonography. In: Reef VB, editor. Equine diagnostic ultrasound. Philadelphia: W.B. Saunders; 1998. p. 215–72.
27. Schefer KD, Bitschnau C, Weishaupt MA, Schwarzwald CC. Quantitative analysis of stress echocardiograms in healthy horses with 2-dimensional (2D) echocardiography, anatomical M-mode, tissue Doppler imaging, and 2D speckle tracking. J Vet Intern Med. 2010;24(4):918–31.
28. McConachie E, Barton MH, Rapoport G, Giguere S. Doppler and volumetric echocardiographic methods for cardiac output measurement in standing adult horses. J Vet Intern Med. 2013;27(2):324–30.
29. Lawrence L, Jackson S, Kline K, Moser L, Powell D, Biel M. Observations on body weight and condition of horses in a 150-mile endurance ride. J Equine Vet Sci. 1992;12(5):320–4.
30. Garlinghouse SE, Burrill MJ. Relationship of body condition score to completion rate during 160 km endurance races. Equine Vet J Suppl. 1999;30:591–5.
31. Leleu C, Cotrel C. Body composition in young standardbreds in training: relationships to body condition score, physiological and locomotor variables during exercise. Equine Vet J Suppl. 2006;36:98–101.
32. Kearns CF, McKeever KH, Kumagai K, Abe T. Fat-free mass is related to one-mile race performance in elite standardbred horses. Vet J. 2002;163(3):260–6.
33. Brownell KD, Steen SN, Wilmore JH. Weight regulation practices in athletes: analysis of metabolic and health effects. Med Sci Sports Exerc. 1987;19(6):546–56.
34. Rodriguez NR, Di Marco NM, Langley S. American College of Sports Medicine position stand. Nutrition and athletic performance. Med Sci Sports Exerc. 2009;41(3):709–31.
35. Kearns CF, McKeever KH, Abe T. Overview of horse body composition and muscle architecture: implications for performance. Vet J. 2002;164(3):224–34.
36. Fleck SJ. Body composition of elite American athletes. Am J Sports Med. 1983;11(6):398–403.
37. Al-Haidar A, Leroux AA, Borde L, Deleuze S, Cerri S, Sandersen CF, et al. Relationship between echocardiographic measurements and body size in horses. J Equine Vet Sci. 2013;33(2):107–14.
38. Martin-Rosset W. Growth and development in the equine. In: 2nd European workshop on Equine Nutrition: Dijon. France: Wageningen Academic Publishers; 2005. p. 15–50.
39. Robert C: Veterinary aspects of training and racing endurance horses. In: Hinchcliff KW, Kaneps AJ, Geor RJ, editors. Equine Sports Medicine and Surgery. 2nd edn. Philiadelphia: Saunders Elsevier; 2014. p. 1083-1106.
40. Maron BJ, Pelliccia A. The heart of trained athletes: cardiac remodeling and the risks of sports, including sudden death. Circulation. 2006;114(15):1633–44.
41. Utomi V, Oxborough D, Whyte GP, Somauroo J, Sharma S, Shave R, et al. Systematic review and meta-analysis of training mode, imaging modality and body size influences on the morphology and function of the male athlete's heart. Heart. 2013;99(23):1727–33.
42. Stewart JH, Rose RJ, Barko AM. Echocardiography in foals from birth to three months old. Equine Vet J. 1984;16(4):332–41.
43. Lombard CW, Evans M, Martin L, Tehrani J. Blood pressure, electrocardiogram and echocardiogram measurements in the growing pony foal. Equine Vet J. 1984;16(4):342–7.
44. Rovira S, Munoz A. Two-dimensional- and M-mode echocardiographic measurements and indices of cardiac function in Spanish colts and fillies of different age. J Vet Med Sci. 2009;71(7):957–64.
45. Hunter S, Robson SC. Adaptation of the maternal heart in pregnancy. Br Heart J. 1992;68(6):540–3.
46. Valensise H, Novelli GP, Vasapollo B, Borzi M, Arduini D, Galante A, et al. Maternal cardiac systolic and diastolic function: relationship with uteroplacental resistances. A Doppler and echocardiographic longitudinal study. Ultrasound Obstet Gynecol. 2000;15(6):487–97.
47. Al Haidar A, Farnir F, Deleuze S, Sandersen CF, Amory H. Comparison of the repeatability of echocardiographic measurements from different modes and views in horses of various breeds and sizes. J Equine Vet Sci. 2010;30(6):287–97.
48. dos Santos Michima LE, Latorre SM, de Andrade AFC, Fernandes WR. B-mode and M-mode echocardiography of endurance horses raised in São Paulo State Brazil. J Equine Vet Sci. 2004;24(10):451–7.
49. Sampson SN, Jacobson RL, Sande RD, Susumi CJ, Larntz KJ, Tucker RL, et al. Reproducibility and repeatability of M-mode echocardiographic measurements collected from 25 normal horses. J Equine Vet Sci. 1999;19(1):51–7.
50. Bertone JJ, Paull KS, Wingfield WE, Boon JA. M-mode echocardiographs of endurance horses in the recovery phase of long-distance competition. Am J Vet Res. 1987;48(12):1708–12.
51. Amory H, Votion DM, Fraipont A, Goachet AG, Robert C, Farnir F, et al. Altered systolic left ventricular function in horses completing a long distance endurance race. Equine Vet J Suppl. 2010;38:216–9.

5

Equine dendritic cells generated with horse serum have enhanced functionality in comparison to dendritic cells generated with fetal bovine serum

Anja Ziegler[1*], Helen Everett[2], Eman Hamza[1,6], Mattia Garbani[3], Vinzenz Gerber[4], Eliane Marti[1] and Falko Steinbach[5*]

Abstract

Background: Dendritic cells are professional antigen-presenting cells that play an essential role in the initiation and modulation of T cell responses. They have been studied widely for their potential clinical applications, but for clinical use to be successful, alternatives to xenogeneic substances like fetal bovine serum (FBS) in cell culture need to be found. Protocols for the generation of dendritic cells ex vivo from monocytes are well established for several species, including horses. Currently, the gold standard protocol for generating dendritic cells from monocytes across various species relies upon a combination of GM-CSF and IL-4 added to cell culture medium which is supplemented with FBS. The aim of this study was to substitute FBS with heterologous horse serum. For this purpose, equine monocyte-derived dendritic cells (eqMoDC) were generated in the presence of horse serum or FBS and analysed for the effect on morphology, phenotype and immunological properties. Changes in the expression of phenotypic markers (CD14, CD86, CD206) were assessed during dendritic cell maturation by flow cytometry. To obtain a more complete picture of the eqMoDC differentiation and assess possible differences between FBS- and horse serum-driven cultures, a transcriptomic microarray analysis was performed. Lastly, immature eqMoDC were primed with a primary antigen (ovalbumin) or a recall antigen (tetanus toxoid) and, after maturation, were co-cultured with freshly isolated autologous $CD5^+$ T lymphocytes to assess their T cell stimulatory capacity.

Results: The microarray analysis demonstrated that eqMoDC generated with horse serum were indistinguishable from those generated with FBS. However, eqMoDC incubated with horse serum-supplemented medium exhibited a more characteristic dendritic cell morphology during differentiation from monocytes. A significant increase in cell viability was also observed in eqMoDC cultured with horse serum. Furthermore, eqMoDC generated in the presence of horse serum were found to be superior in their functional T lymphocyte priming capacity and to elicit significantly less non-specific proliferation.

Conclusions: EqMoDC generated with horse serum-supplemented medium showed improved morphological characteristics, higher cell viability and exhibited a more robust performance in the functional T cell assays. Therefore, horse serum was found to be superior to FBS for generating equine monocyte-derived dendritic cells.

Keywords: Dendritic cell, Horse, Fetal bovine serum

* Correspondence: anja.ziegler@vetsuisse.unibe.ch; f.steinbach@surrey.ac.uk
[1]Department of Clinical Research and Veterinary Public Health, Vetsuisse Faculty, University of Bern, Länggassstrasse 124, 3001 Bern, Switzerland
[5]Faculty of Health and Medical Sciences, School of Veterinary Medicine, University of Surrey, Daphne Jackson Road, Guildford GU2 7AL, UK
Full list of author information is available at the end of the article

Background

Dendritic cells are antigen-presenting cells specialized in uptake and presentation of antigens to T cells [1]. They are the only antigen-presenting cells capable of inducing primary immune responses in naïve T cells and are thus pivotal for the development of T cell responses [2, 3]. The function of dendritic cells is reflected in a number of specific properties. Their distinct shape with many cellular processes offers a large surface area for antigen recognition and uptake [4]. Furthermore, the high surface expression of MHC class II in connection with high levels of costimulatory molecules allows for optimal stimulation of T cells. Initially, studies using dendritic cells have been hindered by difficulties in obtaining sufficient numbers of these cells, as their frequency is very low (<1%). The discovery that granulocyte-macrophage colony stimulating factor (GM-CSF) was the key cytokine needed to differentiate viable dendritic cells from murine blood [5] allowed the development of standardized methods to generate large numbers of dendritic cells ex vivo from hematopoietic progenitors. In humans, dendritic cells can be generated from peripheral blood $CD14^+$ monocytes by using GM-CSF and Interleukin-4 (IL-4) [6, 7]. Due to the higher frequency of $CD14^+$ cells, this method has been widely used to generate dendritic cells for experimental purposes in the human field and for immunotherapy. Monocyte-derived dendritic cells (MoDC) were shown to be homogeneous and could be fully matured using autologous monocyte-conditioned medium [8, 9] or, alternatively, through a cocktail of inflammatory cytokines, namely IL-1β, Tumor necrosis factor-α (TNF-α), IL-6 and Prostaglandin E2 (PGE_2) [10]. The generation of MoDC has been described in a number of domestic animal species such as cattle [11], pigs [12], sheep [13] and horses [14–17].

Fetal bovine serum (FBS) represents an important source of nutrients for in vitro cell growth, metabolism and proliferation [18] and is widely used in cell culture media. Prior to the emergence of variant Creutzfeldt-Jakob disease as a result of the bovine spongiform encephalitis (BSE) crisis at the end of last century, FBS was considered reasonably safe for humans. In animals however, the safety of FBS was always more questionable with more animal diseases potentially being transmissible between species. The main advantage in using serum from unborn animals consists in the absence of interfering substances like inflammatory molecules, hormones or exogenous antigens, including feed-derived components. However, FBS batches are known to be heterogeneous in their performance and need to be batch-tested. Moreover, diluted and altered FBS has been sold recently in Europe, underlining the challenges to FBS selection [19]. Accordingly, FBS production is increasingly subject to regulations and restrictions, not least to protect animals under the 3R guidelines and reduce unnecessary pain, suffering, distress or lasting harm.

In recent years, the ex vivo generation of dendritic cells for the induction of anti-tumor responses has been a focus point for cancer immunotherapy research [20–23]. When generating dendritic cells for clinical applications, such as tumor vaccines, reproducibility and safety are of paramount importance. The use of FBS as a poorly defined cocktail of proteases and other active substances has always been less than ideal, and for both humans and animal species, the use of xenogeneic reagents needs to be avoided.

The utility of autologous serum or serum free media for the generation of MoDC has been questioned [24–26]. In horses, the use of homologous serum for cell culture has been described widely in systems other than DC generation or maintenance. Hamza et al. [27] used autologous serum in cell culture for functional assays involving equine peripheral blood mononuclear cells (PBMC). The use of horse serum for culture of primary equine bronchial fibroblasts [28] has also been described.

In the present study we examined the morphology, viability, phenotype and functional properties of eqMoDC generated under different serum conditions. For this purpose, three FBS batches from two different manufacturers were compared to horse serum produced in one of our laboratories. The data demonstrate that eqMoDC generated in the presence of heterologous horse serum perform equally well or better than dendritic cells generated with FBS.

Methods

Horses and blood samples

Blood samples were collected from the jugular vein of six healthy horses (4 geldings, 2 mares) using Sodium-Heparin containing vacutainers (Vacuette®; Greiner, St.Gallen, Switzerland). The horses were of diverse breeds (Warmblood, Freiberger, Icelandic horse) and spanned a large age range (4–25 years, mean age = 12.7 years). They had been vaccinated yearly against equine influenza and tetanus, and dewormed regularly. The horses belonged to the Swiss Institute of Equine Medicine, Vetsuisse Faculty, University of Bern.

Horse and fetal bovine sera

For preparation of horse serum (HS), blood was collected from a healthy horse into Serum Clot Activator containing vacutainers (Vacuette®; Greiner, St.Gallen, Switzerland). HS was separated by leaving the blood to clot for 2 h followed by centrifugation at 2684×g (Rotanta 46 RSC centrifuge, Hettich AG, Bäch, Switzerland) for 10 min at 4 °C and inactivation for 30 min at 56 °C in a water bath. Serum was then stored at -20 °C until used.

Three commercially available batches of fetal bovine serum were used: FBS (A15-101), Lot A10106-1060 (PAA Pasching, Austria); FBS (S0113), Lot 1107A (Biochrom GmbH, Berlin Germany); FBS Superior (S0613), Lot 0503B, (Biochrom).

In vitro generation of eqMoDC

PBMC were isolated by two sequential Ficoll density gradient centrifugations, using Biocoll 1.090 g/ml and 1.077 g/ml (Biochrom) as described by Mauel et al. [14]. The PBMC-containing fraction was then washed twice in PBS and re-suspended in PBS supplemented with 2 mM EDTA and 0.5% of FBS or HS. Monocytes were isolated by magnetic separation (MACS technology, Miltenyi Biotec GmbH, Bergisch-Gladbach, Germany) according to the manufacturer's standard protocols, using a monoclonal anti-equine CD14 antibody (clone 105) [29]. Briefly, PBMC were first incubated with anti-CD14 and, after a washing step, with secondary goat anti-mouse micro beads. The cells were then separated on a LS column (Miltenyi Biotec GmbH). 2×10^6 monocytes were incubated in a 12-well tissue culture plate (Falcon, BD Biosciences, San Jose CA, USA) in 2 ml RPMI 1640 medium with HEPES and L-glutamine (Gibco, Life Technologies Ltd, Paisley UK) supplemented with 1% penicillin and streptomycin (Gibco), 1% MEM vitamins, 1% Na pyruvate, 1% Non-essential amino acids (all Biochrom) and either 10% FBS (A15-101), FBS (S0113), FBS (S0613) or 5% HS.

Endotoxin contamination was assessed in all serum-supplemented media using a qualitative in vitro end-point endotoxin assay (ToxinSensor™, GenScript, Piscataway, NJ, USA). Lipopolysaccharide (LPS) levels were below 0.06 I.U./ml in all media. Differentiation into eqMoDC was induced by addition of 25 ng/ml recombinant (r.) equine GM-CSF and 10 ng/ml (r.) equine IL-4 (both Kingfisher Biotech Inc., St. Paul MN, USA) and cells were cultured for 3 days. Cells were monitored daily by light microscopy for changes in morphology.

Viability assessment

Viability of three day old immature eqMoDC was assessed using the Alexa Fluor 488 annexin V/Dead Cell Apoptosis Kit for Flow Cytometry (Invitrogen Life Technologies, Paisley, UK) according to the protocol provided by the manufacturer. Briefly, cells were harvested from the cell culture plates, washed and an aliquot of cells was suspended in 0.4% Trypan Blue for counting using a hemocytometer (Neubauer). The cells were resuspended in annexin-binding buffer, incubated with 5 μl AF488 annexin V and 1 μl of 100 μg/ml propidium iodide for 15 minutes at room temperature, then analysed immediately by flow cytometry.

Analysis of eqMoDC phenotype by flow cytometry

MoDC phenotypes were assessed by surface marker expression analysis using the following monoclonal antibodies: anti-equine CD14 mAb (clone 105) [29], anti-human CD206 clone 3.29B1.10 (Beckman Coulter, High Wycombe, UK) and anti-human CD86 clone IT2.2 (Becton Dickinson, Oxford, UK). Unlabelled antibodies were labelled using anti-mouse IgG1 zenon Kits (Invitrogen Life Technologies). Appropriate isotype controls were used. Analysis of cells was performed using a BD LSRII Flow Cytometer (BD Biosciences) and FlowJo software 6 (Tree Star Inc. Ashland OR, USA).

Transcriptome analysis of eqMoDC populations

RNA was extracted from cell pellets of 1×10^6 cells using the RNAqueous micro Kit (Life Technologies, Qiagen, Crawley, UK) and stored at -80 °C. RNA quality was assessed with the RNA 6000 Pico Labchip kit on the Agilent 2100 Bioanalyzer (Agilent Technologies, Berkshire, United Kingdom). The Ovation PicoSL WTA System v2 kit (NuGEN, Leek, The Netherlands) was used to amplify cDNA from 50 ng total RNA. The MinElute Reaction Cleanup Kit (Qiagen) option was used to purify cDNA, and 1 μg was then labelled using a one-color DNA labelling kit (NimbleGen, Madison, USA). For each sample, 4 μg labelled cDNA was hybridised to the NimbleGen 12 × 135 K custom equine arrays (Roche, Madison, USA). Three biological repeats were analysed for each data set. Hybridised arrays were scanned at 2 μm resolution with the Agilent High-resolution C Microarray Scanner (Agilent, Wokingham, UK). Microarray images were processed using DEVA v1.2.1 software (Roche, Madison, USA) to obtain a report containing the signal intensity values corresponding to each probe. The raw data was pre-processed using the DEVA v1.2.1 software by log2 transformation followed by RMA normalisation and summarisation to yield a signal intensity value for each probe set. The data set was then filtered by variance and Principal Component Analysis (PCA) was performed using Qlucore v2.0 software (Qlucore, Lund, Sweden). Variance levels were set using the δ/δ_{max} method.

EqMoDC maturation and functional T cell stimulation assays

For antigen-presentation assays, immature eqMoDC were re-suspended at 2×10^5 cells per 150ul of RPMI 1640 complete medium containing FBS or HS and incubated for 90 min at 37 °C either with 20 μg/ml tetanus toxoid (Schweizerisches Serum und Impfinstitut Bern, Switzerland) as a recall antigen, or 20 μg/ml of the primary antigen ovalbumin (OVA, kindly provided by the Swiss Institute for Allergy and Asthma Research, University of Zürich, Davos Switzerland), or with medium alone as a control. After antigen uptake, eqMoDC were washed and cultured in a 96-well round bottom tissue culture plate

(Sarstedt, Nümbrecht, Germany) at 2×10^4 eqMoDC per well in quadruplicates.

For maturation, antigen-primed eqMoDC were exposed overnight to a maturation cocktail comprising 1 μg/ml LPS (Sigma-Aldrich St. Louis MO, USA), 1 μg/ml PGE_2 (Enzo Life Sciences, Exeter, UK), 20 ng/ml equine TNF-α, 10 ng/ml equine IL-1β, 20 ng/ml equine IL-6 and 100 ng/ml equine IFN-γ (all R&D Systems, Abingdon, UK) according to Moyo et al. [17].

Fresh CD5$^+$ T lymphocytes were enriched by positive selection using MACS technology as above-mentioned, employing an anti-equine CD5 mAb (clone CVS5, Abd Serotec, Kidlington UK) and re-suspended in RPMI 1640 medium containing FBS or HS, respectively. Purity of CD5$^+$ lymphocytes after bead selection was assessed by flow cytometry and was shown to be > 94%. 10^5 autologous CD5$^+$ T lymphocytes were added to the MoDC in the 96-well plate and co-cultured for 5 days at 37 °C/5% CO_2. 5 μCi/well [^{3}H] thymidine (Perkin Elmer, Waltham MA, USA) was added for the last 18 h of culture. DNA was then harvested onto a glass fibre filter plate and thymidine incorporation was measured on a scintillation counter (Inotech, LabLogic Systems Inc., Brandon FL, USA).

A mixed leukocyte reaction (MLR) was performed in addition to the autologous co-cultures by incubating matured eqMoDC with CD5$^+$ T lymphocytes from another horse.

Statistical analysis

Statistical analyses were carried out using the software program NCSS 8 (NCSS, Kaysville, Utah 84037, USA). Descriptive statistics showed that the data were not normally distributed. Therefore, non-parametric tests were used. The proportion of non-viable immature MoDC (Fig. 2), as well as the yield of immature eqMoDC (Table 1), was compared between the four serum culture conditions by using a non-parametric paired sample Wilcoxon (signed rank) test. The same test was used to determine differences in surface marker expression between eqMoDC before and after maturation (Fig. 3). A one-way ANOVA with Tukey-Kramer test for multiple comparisons was used to assess significant differences between the individual serum conditions within one maturation state (Fig. 3).

Non-parametric paired sample Wilcoxon (signed rank) test was again used to assess differences in serum conditions with regard to induction of T cell proliferation by antigen-primed MoDC (Figs. 5 and 6). Overall, p-values ≤ 0.05 were considered significant.

Results

Morphology of differentiating eqMoDC differs between cells generated in the presence of HS or FBS

During differentiation from monocytes, MoDC undergo a distinct change in morphology. Equine CD14$^+$ monocytes

Table 1 Cell counts of immature eqMoDC generated after 3 days in vitro

Horse	HS	FBS (A15-101)	FBS (S0113)	FBS (S0613)
A	100	96	106.7	106.7
B	100	91.3	95.7	91.3
C	100	97.9	111.5	119.8
D	100	83.1	57.7	90
E	100	74.7	100.6	64.4
F	100	65.6	71.1	70.3
Mean (SD)	100 * (0)	84.8 * (12.75)	90.6 (21.37)	84.4 (21.02)

An identical number of monocytes from 6 horses (A-F) were differentiated in parallel and the resulting numbers of cells after three days counted. Results are shown as percentages with the number of cells generated with HS set as 100%. Using non-parametric paired Wilcoxon signed-rank test, only the comparison of HS vs. A15-101 was statistically significant (p ≤ 0.05), as indicated by the asterisks

presented themselves as round cells that adhere quickly to cell culture plates. After 24 hours of stimulation, a formation of tight cell clusters could be seen. These became larger and denser as differentiation progressed (Fig. 1). Also, cellular dendrites could be seen by that time protruding from the clusters. After another 24 to 48 hours, the differentiated eqMoDC detached from the clusters and could be identified as large, heterogeneously formed cells with distinctive long dendrites. Marked differences in the morphology of the differentiating eqMoDC between serum conditions were observed. Cluster formation seemed to be impaired in all cells cultured with FBS in comparison to cells cultured in the presence of HS, where the vast majority of cells had formed into very distinct dense clusters (Fig. 1a). Cluster formation was less clear with both FBS from Biochrom (Fig. 1b, c) and almost non-observable with FBS batch A15-101 (Fig. 1d). Also, in the clusters that were present in FBS treated cells, fewer dendrites could be seen in comparison to HS. With FBS S0113 in particular, several long spindly cells were seen that could be an indicator of excess IL-4 in the culture [7]. However, identical concentrations of IL-4 were used for all serum conditions. When looking at individual cells in the 40× magnification (Fig. 1, small inlaid pictures), no significant differences could be determined between serum conditions. An intriguing finding with FBS A15-101 were large round objects enclosed by a clearly visible membrane, as indicated by the arrow in Fig. 1d.

Immature eqMoDC generated in the presence of HS exhibit a higher viability

It is essential for dendritic cells generated in vitro to maintain viability and thus be able to perform their functional tasks in downstream assays without becoming saturated with apoptotic material. Table 1 exhibits relative cell counts of differentiated eqMoDC following 3 days of incubation, starting with an identical number of

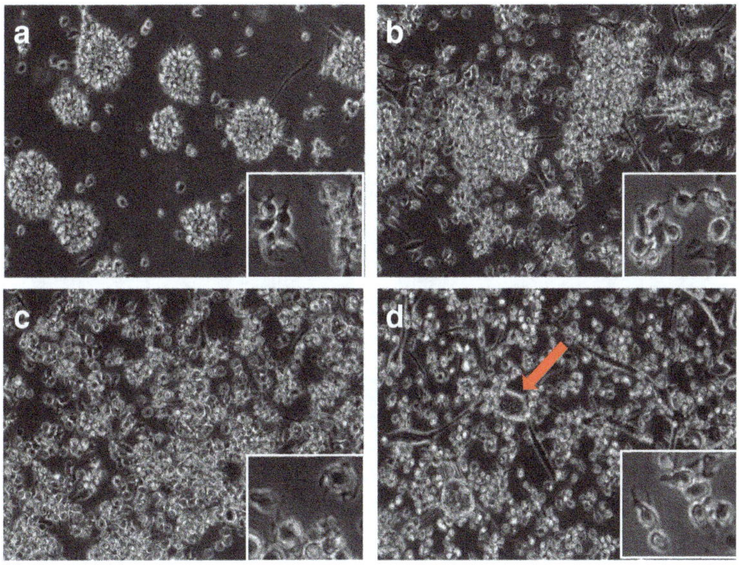

Fig. 1 Morphology of eqMoDC at day 2 at 10× (large pictures) and 40× magnification (small inlaid pictures). Cells were incubated in the presence of HS (**a**), FBS batch S0113 (**b**), FBS batch S0613 (**c**) and FBS batch A15-101 (**d**), respectively. Pictures are representative of cells from 6 tested horses. The arrow in (**d**) indicates giant cells, presumably after uptake of apoptotic material, only seen in the FBS A15-101 condition

cells for all serum conditions. Cell yield was significantly lower with A15-101 serum in comparison to HS. To assess differences in viability between the individual serum conditions, immature eqMoDC were tested using annexin V and propidium iodide staining and analysed by flow cytometry for the presence of apoptotic and/or dead cells. Figure 2 shows that cells cultured in the presence of any of the three FBS exhibited a significantly higher percentage of dead cells than cells cultured with HS. While differences between the individual FBS were non-significant, the highest proportion of dead cells could be observed in the cells incubated with the A15-101 serum.

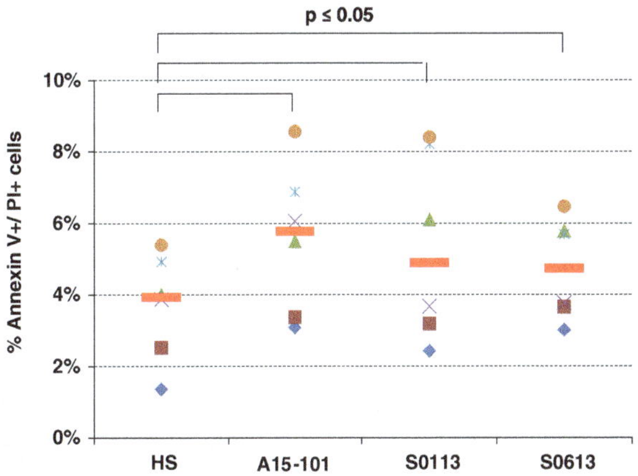

Fig. 2 Proportion of non-viable immature eqMoDC measured by flow cytometry. The AF488 annexin V/Dead Cell Apoptosis Kit (Invitrogen) was used for the analysis according to the protocol provided in the kit. Each symbol indicates a separate horse (n = 6), with red lines indicating the median value. A non-parametric paired sample Wilcoxon (signed rank) test was used to determine significant differences between HS and the respective FBS condition. P-values ≤ 0.05 were considered statistically significant

Surface marker expression of eqMoDC reflects maturation status and is comparable between serum conditions

Differentiation and maturation of eqMoDC in vitro is reflected by changes in the expression of surface markers. To compare our findings with previous results and established knowledge [17] CD14, CD86, and CD206 were selected for analysis by flow cytometry on eqMoDC before and after maturation and for comparison of eqMoDC generated under the different serum conditions. While CD14 is a monocyte marker that should be markedly down-regulated during the differentiation process from monocytes to MoDC, CD206 is a particular marker for immature MoDC to be down-regulated upon activation. CD86 was expected to be up-regulated during maturation/activation of MoDC. As expected, no significant difference could be observed in CD14 expression between immature and mature eqMoDC under any serum condition (Fig. 3a). Interestingly, CD14 remained significantly more highly expressed in immature eqMoDC obtained under the influence of the FBS batches (S0113) or (S0613) than in the presence of the A15-101 FBS batch. For CD86 expression, no significant difference between serum conditions could be observed (Fig. 3b). Nonetheless, eqMoDC incubated with the maturation cocktail showed an up-regulation of CD86 under all serum conditions. This up-regulation was statistically significant for FBS batches

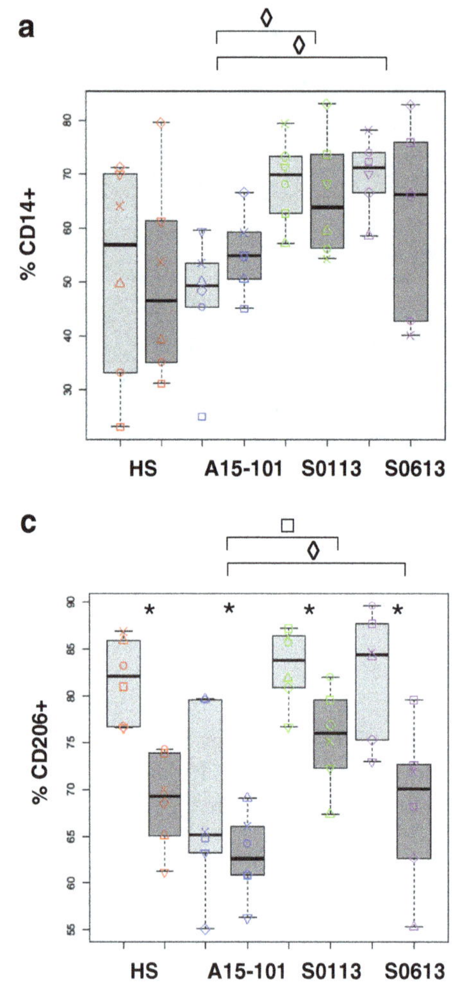

Fig. 3 Surface marker expression of eqMoDC generated under the different serum conditions. EqMoDC were analysed by flow cytometry for cell surface expression of CD14 (**a**), CD86 (**b**) or CD206 (**c**). Results are displayed as percentage of positive cells for the respective marker. EqMoDC were generated under the respective serum conditions and were incubated overnight with the maturation cocktail (mature eqMoDC; dark grey boxplots) or maintained as immature eqMoDC (light grey boxplots). A non-parametric paired sample Wilcoxon (signed rank) test was used to identify significant differences between the HS condition and the different FBS conditions, respectively, within the maturation state (◊ indicates differences between immature eqMoDC; □ indicates differences between mature eqMoDC). The same test was also applied to investigate significant differences between immature and mature eqMoDC within each serum condition (indicated by asterisks). P-values ≤ 0.05 were considered statistically significant

A15-101, S0113 and S0613. The difference in median values between immature versus mature eqMoDC was particularly low for HS. This was due to a considerable expression of CD86 already on immature eqMoDC. CD206 was clearly expressed upon differentiation of immature eqMoDC under all culture conditions, albeit at significantly lower levels in the presence of FBS A15-101 (median, range. 65.2%, 55.1–79.6%) compared to FBS batch S0113 (83.8%, 76.7–87.2%), or FBS batch S0613 (84.5%, 73–89.6) and also to HS (82.1%, 76.6–86.9%), although this difference was not statistically significant. A significant down-regulation of CD206 upon maturation could be observed in all four serum conditions (Fig. 3c).

Transcriptome comparison of eqMoDC preparations and populations

While the above results demonstrate that HS provided results similar to FBS for the differentiation of equine eqMoDC, there is a considerable lack of antibodies in the horse system to perform a more comprehensive analysis. Aiming to test for hidden features, we resorted to gene expression profiling using equine-specific microarray analysis. Expression profiles of all three cell types were analysed by 3D PCA, which demonstrated that while monocytes (Mo), immature eqMoDC (iMoDC) and mature eqMoDC (mMoDC) are distinct populations, there was no detectable effect of the serum conditions on the gene expression profile of the different cell types (Fig. 4).

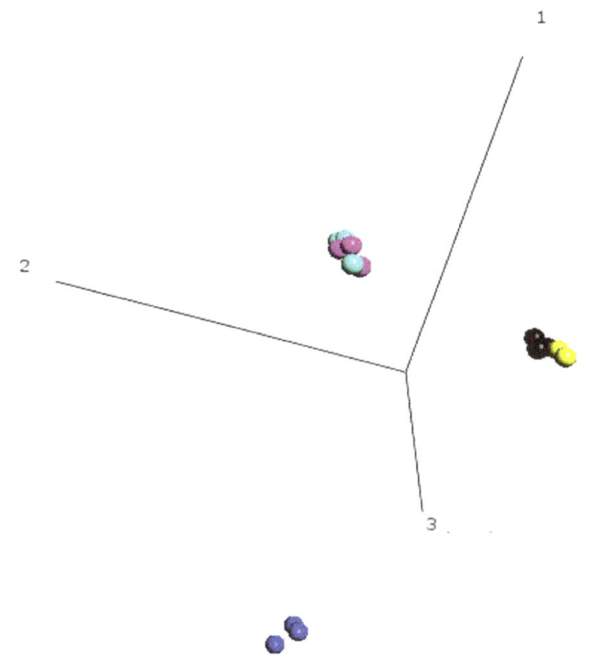

Fig. 4 Gene expression analysis of equine monocytes (Mo) and eqMoDC. Mo (dark blue), iMoDC (black, FBS batch S0113; yellow, HS) and mMoDC (light blue, FBS batch S0113; pink, HS) were generated in parallel from three horses each. Principal component analysis (PCA) was carried out on the differentially expressed genes (1331 variables) and demonstrated that while the gene expression profiles of the different MoDC stages are separate and different to Mo, the genetic profile of the different sera cannot be further separated. Three biological repeats (horses) were analyzed using Qlucore, one dataset (iMoDC, HS) was discarded due to a technical issue in the hybridization of the sub-arra

Induction of T cell proliferation by antigen-primed MoDC

We analysed the eqMoDC generated under the different serum conditions for their ability to induce proliferation of T cells following antigen presentation. After the uptake of either tetanus toxoid as recall antigen, or OVA as a primary antigen, MoDC were incubated with autologous or heterologous (MLR) CD5$^+$ T cells and proliferation of T cells was measured. While no proliferation could be observed in T cells incubated with medium only for the HS condition (median (range) 107 (67–170) cpm), T cells incubated with FBS showed a notable background proliferation (median (range) 4384 (300–20667) cpm with A15-101; 10709 (1935–36199) cpm with S0113; 5385 (1049–57954) cpm with S0613, respectively) (Fig. 5a). Similarly, non-specific proliferation of T cells co-incubated with non-primed MoDC was significantly higher in all FBS conditions (median (range) 15924 (5843–55404) cpm with A15-101; 12545 (5657–58043) cpm with S0113; 17719 (14952–72847) cpm with S0613, respectively) than in the HS condition (median (range) 6993 (2844–24414) cpm) (Fig. 5b). As expected, the strongest induction of T cell proliferation was observed with heterologous MoDC in the MLR control (Fig. 6a), followed by autologous tetanus toxoid-primed MoDC as a recall antigen presentation (Fig. 6b). T cell proliferation was least pronounced when using the primary antigen OVA (Fig. 6c). Serum culture conditions were compared for each antigen condition. The gradation between MLR, tetanus toxoid vs. OVA-elicited T cell responses was most evident in the HS condition, with horses exhibiting a median stimulation index for MLR of 5.14 (range 1.48–10.86) while for tetanus toxoid the SI was 2.75 (range 2.04–5.9). Three horses exhibited a stimulation index > 2 for OVA (median = 1.84; range 1.5–2.79). Use of HS in culture resulted in consistently higher stimulation indices when compared to the FBS conditions for MLR, tetanus and OVA, albeit not all differences were statistically significant.

Discussion

Dendritic cells are key players in the immune system, particularly competent in modulating the immune

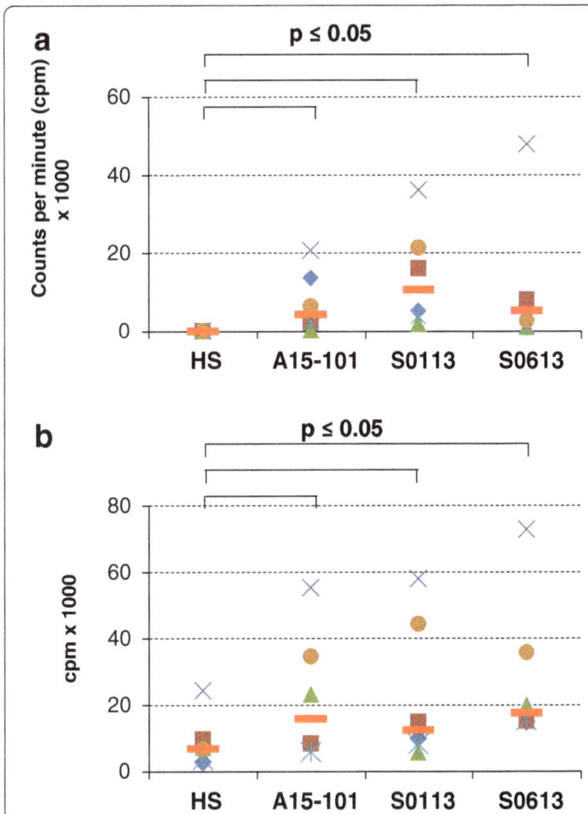

Fig. 5 Non-specific background proliferation induced by the different serum conditions. T cell proliferation was measured by [^{3}H] thymidine incorporation assay after a 5 day incubation of either CD5$^+$ T cells alone (**a**) or co-incubation of CD5$^+$ T cells with non antigen-primed eqMoDC (**b**). Each symbol indicates a separate horse (n = 6), with red lines indicating the median value. Non-parametric paired sample Wilcoxon (signed rank) tests were used to compare HS with each FBS and p-values ≤ 0.05 were considered statistically significant

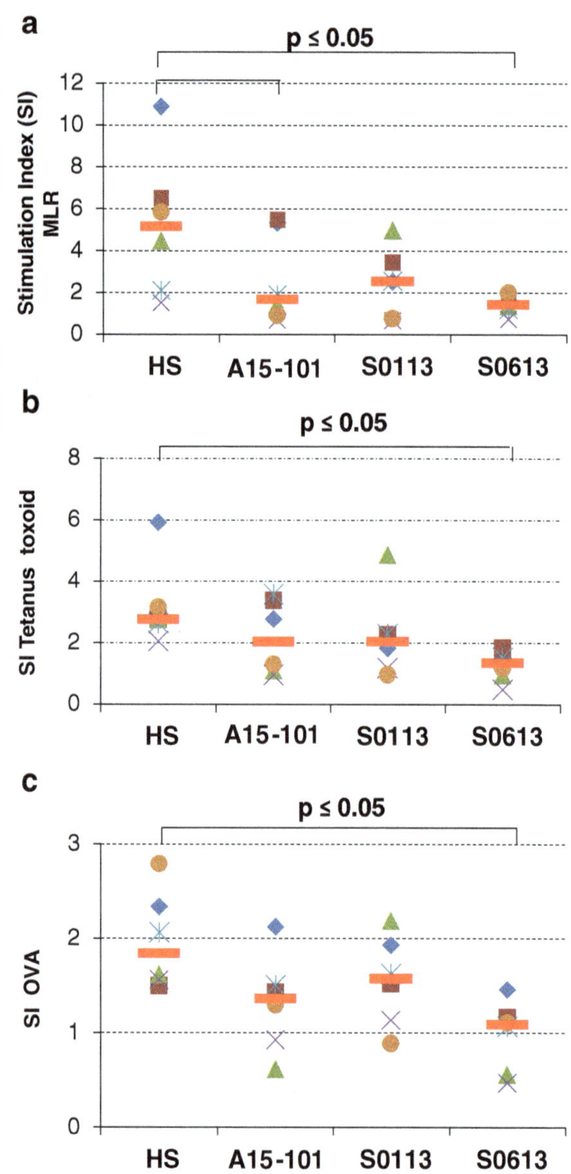

Fig. 6 T cell proliferation induced by eqMoDC. T cells were stimulated with heterologous eqMoDC (mixed leukocyte reaction [MLR]) (**a**), as well as autologous eqMoDC primed with tetanus toxoid (**b**) or OVA (**c**). Results are displayed as stimulation indices (cpm with stimulation/cpm without stimulation). Each symbol indicates a separate horse (n = 6), with red lines indicating the median value. Non-parametric paired sample Wilcoxon (signed rank) tests were used to determine significant differences between the HS and the three FBS, respectively. P-values ≤ 0.05 were considered statistically significant

responses [1]. Thus they are promising tools both for cancer immunotherapy and to limit immune responses to treat allergic reactions [30, 31]. The ability to generate these otherwise scarce immune cells in large quantities from progenitors and in particular monocytes, reinitiated research in this field around 20 years ago [6, 7, 32]. The identification of distinct DC populations in vivo, among them DC specialized in cross-presenting antigens to $CD8^+$ cytotoxic T cells [33] has widened the opportunities to study specialized subsets of DC. MoDC remain the first choice for personalized therapeutic approaches, such as loading DC ex vivo, as they were shown to substitute for all DC functions, including cross-presentation [34].

Fetal bovine serum (FBS) is widely used in cell culture media, but has come under more intense scrutiny in recent years: as well as being a possible source for disease transmission its use in therapeutic vaccines may lead to adverse immune reactions against FBS [35, 36]. The problem of batch variability, including the contamination with LPS (which is detrimental to MoDC differentiation), was immediately recognised as an issue for therapeutic use of DC [37].

Early work to replace the 5–10% FBS commonly used to generate human MoDC by an equal amount of human sera (either autologous or batch tested) has not been successful (Steinbach et al., unpublished; various personal communications). This was explained by the plasticity of monocytes as uncommitted myeloid cells during differentiation allowing them to acquire a macrophage rather than a DC phenotype [38]. It was accordingly suggested to replace the 10% FBS by 1% autologous plasma, but while the phenotypical and functional data were analogous to FBS-derived MoDC, the DC yield obtained was very low (around 20% compared to FBS based protocols) with a significantly reduced enrichment [9]. This was offset by larger scale production [39], which, however, does not address the issue of cell debris from dead cells in such cultures.

In horses, previous studies to generate MoDC under the influence of GM-CSF and IL-4 used FBS [14, 16, 17] and pilot studies have also shown the potential use of such ex vivo generated MoDC for treatment of tumors [40]. However, previous experience where FBS-specific IgE was induced through MoDC application [36], eliminated such equine MoDC for the purpose of allergen immunotherapy.

In a preliminary experiment, we compared the use of autologous and heterologous equine serum with FBS from PAA (A15-101), which was used in one of our laboratories for the maintenance of cells lines. Intriguingly, while both equine serum preparation delivered encouraging results, the A15-101 FBS led to morphologically more heterogeneous populations with giant cells that we presumed to be the result of cell death followed by phagocytosis, not matching previous descriptions [14, 17]. Since the results obtained with the two serum preparations from horses were very similar, we decided to generate a heterologous serum to achieve a better standardisation for subsequent experiments. In addition, it became necessary to expand our study to other FBS batches able to reproduce previous results

[17]. Thus, we decided to conduct a small study comparing three different FBS with HS during the generation of equine MoDC and their application in functional assays. The aim was to determine if equine MoDC could be successfully generated using horse serum that was freshly prepared rather than commercial serum that previously failed to deliver equine MoDC (Steinbach et al., unpublished).

The differentiation from monocytes to MoDC is characterised by the formation of tight cell clusters, where cells gradually become non-adherent and develop typical dendrites [6, 41]. It was notable that equine MoDC differentiated with HS developed larger clusters faster than monocytes incubated with FBS, which showed only limited clustering by day 2 (Fig. 1). It is not known whether the formation of cell clusters and thus close cell-to-cell contact is necessary for differentiating monocytes to become fully functional, but eqMoDC cultured in the presence of HS were also significantly more viable. It is thus likely that cell-cell signalling within clusters promotes viability of cells in culture. Not surprisingly and in line with the preliminary data, FBS batch A15-101 showed the highest proportion of non-viable cells. These results, however, do not explain whether HS contains additional viability factors which are lacking in FBS, or whether the changes and additions made to FBS batch A15-101 were detrimental to eqMoDC differentiation. Interestingly, there seems to be an inherent variation between individual horses in the proportion of non-viable cells that was independent of the serum used. Regardless of the serum condition, the same horse delivered the highest as well as the lowest proportion of dead cells. Thus, it is reasonable to propose that individual disposition (from genetics to an individual's current health status) likely affects the generation of eqMoDC ex vivo. This resonates an earlier study showing that monocytes from Lupus Erythematosus patients required more GM-CSF and IL-4 to obtain viable DC [42].

As with the morphology and viability, clear differences were observed for the phenotype between the four tested sera: again, eqMoDC incubated with the two FBS from Biochrom displayed very similar phenotypes and maturation patterns, which were likely due to a similar FBS composition that should be observed using high performance FBS batches. Slightly surprising though was the relatively high level of CD14 remaining on MoDC generated with the Biochrom FBS. Since we tested all media for LPS this can be excluded as the causative factor. MoDC generated with HS expressed slightly higher levels of CD86 already at the immature stage. Overall, though all cells displayed a phenotype in accordance with MoDC differentiation and maturation and only trends were observed that made cells treated with HS preferable, i.e. is more in line with the published gold standard, to those treated with FBS. Accordingly, it was not surprising that in a whole transcriptome analysis the three differentiation stages were clearly separable, whereas the different sera clustered strongly together similar to previous results [17]. This is not astonishing, since across a whole population of cells of the same lineage, only minute shifts in gene expression will suffice to induce the changes in protein expression and morphology such as observed by flow cytometry. This emphasises that all four sera delivered equine MoDC of some quality.

It is important to consider that ultimately, DC are not defined by the presence or absence of certain markers, but by their functional ability to stimulate T cells. Here, HS clearly demonstrated an advantage through not inducing non-specific proliferation. This result, observed with all batches of FBS, may reflect their xenogenous and antigenetic nature, with T cells in adult horses reacting against foreign serum components or exogenous agents. To exclude the latter we tested the FBS batches for the presence of pestivirus RNA (a common contaminant of FBS) and can exclude this as a factor. However, as all horses in this study were regularly vaccinated, a sensitisation to foreign proteins present in these vaccines may well have occurred and has been described for equine vaccines before [43]. The strongest proliferation was induced in the heterologous mixed leukocyte reaction (MLR) followed by an antigen-specific recall response against tetanus toxoid. This was to be expected compared to a primary antigen like OVA, where the response relies on the activation of naïve rather than memory T cells. Using the stimulation index to determine the specific reaction above the background, the best performance was observed with HS.

Conclusion

It can be concluded that eqMoDC generated in the presence of HS showed improved morphological characteristics, higher cell viability and were superior with a more robust performance in the functional T cell assays. While HS did not perform significantly better in all assays, it is the mixture of results that favours HS for the generation of eqMoDC. While PAA's FBS (A15-101) did not perform worst in all experiments, its inferior performance in morphology and viability assays and the lack of clarity surrounding its composition and thereby functional reproducibility exclude this product completely from use [19]. While FBS can in general be considered further for in vitro research, the results here re-emphasize the need for batch testing. These results are very encouraging for the clinical application of equine MoDC and confirm a most recent report using cells generated with horse serum for recall responses [44]. However, the effect of autologous serum or different serum conditions on the phenotype and function of equine MoDC had not been systematically investigated previously. Prior to clinical application, though horse sera need to be tested extensively for extraneous agents, like the widespread equine hepaciviruses and or treated for inactivation of such. Thus, the serum free generation of MoDC would be desirable, but this has proven inefficient, resulting in very limited cell numbers [8, 45] and is still a matter of debate [24–26, 46, 47]. With the recent progress in defining serum free media for various purposes (discussed in [48]) this goal can be achieved in the near future, but requires further studies to ensure good compliance with MoDC functionality as well.

Acknowledgements
We would like to thank Dr. Andreas Zurbriggen, Department of Clinical Research and Veterinary Public Health, Vetsuisse Faculty, University of Bern for his continuous support, Dr. Bettina Wagner at the Department of Population Medicine and Diagnostic Sciences, College of Veterinary Medicine, Cornell University, Ithaca, 825 NY 14853, USA for providing the anti-equine CD14 antibody. We are also thankful to Biochrom GmbH for providing the FBS samples used in this study.

Funding
This work was supported by a grant of the Department of Clinical Research VPH, Vetsuisse Faculty, University of Bern, by the Swiss National Science Foundation grant no. 310030-160196/1 and by the APHA grant SCRD0092 'Systems Biology for Veterinary Species'.

Authors' contributions
AZ carried out the immunological experiments, assisted in the design of the study and drafted the manuscript. HE carried out the transcriptome analysis. EH participated in and supervised the immunological experiments. MG was responsible for production and purification of the ovalbumin used in this study. VG provided the horses used in this study and edited the manuscript. EM participated in the design and coordination of the study and assisted with statistical analysis and preparation of the manuscript and figures. FS conceived the study, participated in its design and edited the manuscript. All authors read and approved the final manuscript.

Competing interests
The authors declare that they have no competing interests.

Consent for publication
Not applicable.

Author details
[1]Department of Clinical Research and Veterinary Public Health, Vetsuisse Faculty, University of Bern, Länggassstrasse 124, 3001 Bern, Switzerland. [2]Virology Department, Animal and Plant Health Agency-Weybridge, Woodham Lane, Addlestone, Surrey KT15 3NB, UK. [3]Swiss Institute of Allergy and Asthma Research (SIAF), University of Zürich, Davos, Switzerland. [4]Swiss Institute of Equine Medicine, University of Bern, Bern, Switzerland. [5]Faculty of Health and Medical Sciences, School of Veterinary Medicine, University of Surrey, Daphne Jackson Road, Guildford GU2 7AL, UK. [6]Department of Zoonoses, Faculty of Veterinary Medicine, Cairo University, Cairo, Egypt.

References

1. Steinman RM. The dendritic cell system and its role in immunogenicity. Annu Rev Immunol. 1991;9:271–96. Review.
2. Croft M, Duncan DD, Swain SL. Response of naive antigen-specific CD4$^+$ T cells in vitro: characteristics and antigen-presenting cell requirements. J Exp Med. 1992;176(5):1431–7.
3. Cella M, Sallusto F, Lanzavecchia A. Origin, maturation and antigen presenting function of dendritic cells. Curr Opin Immunol. 1997;9(1):10–6.
4. Steinman RM, Nussenzweig MC. Dendritic cells: features and functions. Immunol Rev. 1980;53:127–47. Review.
5. Inaba K, Inaba M, Romani N, Aya H, Deguchi M, Ikehara S, Muramatsu S, Steinman RM. Generation of large numbers of dendritic cells from mouse bone marrow cultures supplemented with granulocyte/macrophage colony-stimulating factor. J Exp Med. 1992;176(6):1693–702.
6. Sallusto F, Lanzavecchia A. Efficient presentation of soluble antigen by cultured human dendritic cells is maintained by granulocyte/macrophage colony-stimulating factor plus interleukin 4 and downregulated by tumor necrosis factor alpha. J Exp Med. 1994;179(4):1109–18.
7. Peters JH, Gieseler R, Thiele B, Steinbach F. Dendritic cells: from ontogenic orphans to myelomonocytic descendants. Immunol Today. 1996;17:273–8.
8. Romani N, Reider D, Heuer M, Ebner S, Kämpgen E, Eibl B, Niederwieser D, Schuler G. Generation of mature dendritic cells from human blood. An improved method with special regard to clinical applicability. J Immunol Methods. 1996;196(2):137–51.
9. Bender A, Sapp M, Schuler G, Steinman RM, Bhardwaj N. Improved methods for the generation of dendritic cells from nonproliferating progenitors in human blood. J Immunol Methods. 1996;196(2):121–35.
10. Jonuleit H, Kühn U, Müller G, Steinbrink K, Paragnik L, Schmitt E, Knop J, Enk AH. Pro-inflammatory cytokines and prostaglandins induce maturation of potent immunostimulatory dendritic cells under fetal calf serum-free conditions. Eur J Immunol. 1997;27(12):3135–42.
11. Werling D, Hope JC, Chaplin P, Collins RA, Taylor G, Howard CJ. Involvement of caveolae in the uptake of respiratory syncytial virus antigen by dendritic cells. J Leukoc Biol. 1999;66(1):50–8.
12. Paillot R, Laval F, Audonnet JC, Andreoni C, Juillard V. Functional and phenotypic characterization of distinct porcine dendritic cells derived from peripheral blood monocytes. Immunology. 2001;102:396–404.
13. Chan SS, McConnell I, Blacklaws BA. Generation and characterization of ovine dendritic cells derived from peripheral blood monocytes. Immunology. 2002;107(3):366–72.
14. Mauel S, Steinbach F, Ludwig H. Monocyte-derived dendritic cells from horses differ from dendritic cells of humans and mice. Immunology. 2006; 117(4):463–73.
15. Dietze B, Cierpka E, Schäfer M, Schill W, Lutz MB. An improved method to generate equine dendritic cells from peripheral blood mononuclear cells: divergent maturation programs by IL-4 and LPS. Immunobiology. 2008; 213(9–10):751–8.
16. Cavatorta DJ, Erb HN, Flaminio MJ. Ex vivo generation of mature equine monocyte-derived dendritic cells. Vet Immunol Immunopathol. 2009;131(3–4):259–67.
17. Moyo NA, Marchi E, Steinbach F. Differentiation and activation of equine monocyte-derived dendritic cells are not correlated with CD206 or CD83 expression. Immunology. 2013;139(4):472–83.
18. Bettger WJ, McKeehan WL. Mechanisms of cellular nutrition. Physiol Rev. 1986;66(1):1–35. Review.
19. Köppele W. Unbekannte Zusätze. Laborjournal. 2013;9:67–69.
20. Tacken PJ, Jolanda I, de Vries M, Torensma R, Figdor CG. Dendritic-cell immunotherapy: from ex vivo loading to in vivo targeting. Nat Rev Immunol. 2007;7:790–802.
21. Palucka KA, Banchereau J. Cancer immunotherapy via dendritic cells. Nat Rev Cancer. 2012;12:265–77.
22. Apostolopoulos V, Pietersz GA, Tsibanis A, Tsikkinis A, Stojanovska L, McKenzie IF, Vassilaros S. Dendritic cell immunotherapy: clinical outcomes. Clin Transl Immunology. 2014;3(7), e21.
23. Anguille S, Smits EL, Bryant C, van Acker HH, Goossen H, Lion E, Fromm PD, Hart DN, van Tendeloo VF, Berneman ZN. Dendritic Cells as Pharmacological Tools for Cancer Immunotherapy. Pharmacol Rev. 2015;67(4):731–53.
24. Pietschmann P, Stöckl J, Draxler S, Majdic O, Knapp W. Functional and phenotypic characteristics of dendritic cells generated in human plasma supplemented medium. Scand J Immunol. 2000;51(4):377–83.

25. Loudovaris M, Hansen M, Suen Y, Lee SM, Casing P, Bender JG. Differential effects of autologous serum on CD34(+) or monocyte-derived dendritic cells. J Hematother Stem Cell Res. 2001;10(4):569–78.
26. Garderet L, Cao H, Salamero J, Vergé V, Tisserand E, Scholl S, Gorin NC, Lopez M. In vitro production of dendritic cells from human blood monocytes for therapeutic use. J Hematother Stem Cell Res. 2001;10(4):553–67. Review.
27. Hamza E, Doherr MG, Bertoni G, Jungi TW, Marti E. Modulation of allergy incidence in icelandic horses is associated with a change in IL-4-producing T cells. Int Arch Allergy Immunol. 2007;144(4):325–37.
28. Franke J, Abs V, Zizzadoro C, Abraham G. Comparative study of the effects of fetal bovine serum versus horse serum on growth and differentiation of primary equine bronchial fibroblasts. BMC Vet Res. 2014;10:119.
29. Kabithe E, Hillegas J, Stokol T, Moore J, Wagner B. Monoclonal antibodies to equine CD14. Vet Immunol Immunopathol. 2010;138(1–2):149–53.
30. Grabbe S, Beissert S, Schwarz T, Granstein RD. Dendritic cells as initiators of tumor immune responses: a possible strategy for tumor immunotherapy? Immunol Today. 1995;16(3):117–21. Review.
31. Steptoe RJ, Thomson AW. Dendritic cells and tolerance induction. Clin Exp Immunol. 1996;105(3):397–402. Review.
32. Porcelli S, Morita CT, Brenner MB. CD1b restricts the response of human CD4-8- T lymphocytes to a microbial antigen. Nature. 1992;360(6404):593–7.
33. Merad M, Sathe P, Helft J, Miller J, Mortha A. The dendritic cell lineage: ontogeny and function of dendritic cells and their subsets in the steady state and the inflamed setting. Annu Rev Immunol. 2013;31:563–604.
34. Cheong C, Matos I, Choi JH, Dandamudi DB, Shrestha E, Longhi MP, Jeffrey KL, Anthony RM, Kluger C, Nchinda G, Koh H, Rodriguez A, Idoyaga J, Pack M, Velinzon K, Park CG, Steinman RM. Microbial stimulation fully differentiates monocytes to DC-SIGN/CD209^{+} dendritic cells for immune T cell areas. Cell. 2010;143:416–29.
35. Selvaggi TA, Walker RE, Fleisher TA. Development of antibodies to fetal calf serum with arthus-like reactions in human immunodeficiency virus-infected patients given syngeneic lymphocyte infusions. Blood. 1997;89(3):776–9.
36. Mackensen A, Dräger R, Schlesier M, Mertelsmann R, Lindemann A. Presence of IgE antibodies to bovine serum albumin in a patient developing anaphylaxis after vaccination with human peptide-pulsed dendritic cells. Cancer Immunol Immunother. 2000;49(3):152–6.
37. Schuler G, Steinman RM. Dendritic cells as adjuvants for immune-mediated resistance to tumors. J Exp Med. 1997;186(8):1183–7.
38. Palucka KA, Taquet N, Sanchez-Chapuis F, Gluckman JC. Dendritic cells as the terminal stage of monocyte differentiation. J Immunol. 1998; 160(9):4587–95.
39. Berger TG, Feuerstein B, Strasser E, Hirsch U, Schreiner D, Schuler G, Schuler-Thurner B. Large-scale generation of mature monocyte-derived dendritic cells for clinical application in cell factories. J Immunol Methods. 2002; 268(2):131–40.
40. Steinbach F, Bischoff S, Freund H, Metzner-Flemisch S, Ibrahim S, Walter J, Wilke I, Mauel S. Clinical application of dendritic cells and interleukin-2 and tools to study activated T cells in horses - first results and implications for quality control. Vet Immunol Immunopathol. 2009;128(1–3):16–23.
41. Steinbach F, Krause B, Bläß S, Burmester GR, Hiepe F. Development of accessory phenotype and function during the differentiation of Monocyte-derived dendritic cells (MoDC). Res Immunol. 1998;149:627–32.
42. Steinbach F, Henke F, Krause B, Thiele B, Burmester GR, Hiepe F. Monocytes from SLE patients are severely altered in phenotype and lineage flexibility. Ann Rheum Dis. 2000;59:283–8.
43. Newton JR, Geraghty RJ, Castillo-Olivares J, Cardwell M, Mumford JA. Evidence that use of an inactivated equine herpesvirus vaccine induces serum cytotoxicity affecting the equine arteritis virus neutralisation test. Vaccine. 2004;22:4117–23.
44. Meulenbroeks C, van der Meide NM, Willemse T, Rutten VP, Tijhaar E. Recombinant Culicoides obsoletus complex allergens stimulate antigen-specific T cells of insect bite hypersensitive Shetland ponies in vitro. Vet Dermatol. 2015;26(6):467–109.
45. Toungouz M, Quinet C, Thille E, Fourez S, Pradier O, Delville JP, Velu T, Lambermont M. Generation of immature autologous clinical grade dendritic cells for vaccination of cancer patients. Cytotherapy. 1999; 1(6):447–53.
46. Lehner M, Morhart P, Stilper A, Holter W. Functional characterization of monocyte-derived dendritic cells generated under serum-free culture conditions. Immunol Lett. 2005;99(2):209–16.
47. da Silva SG, Saad ST, Gilli SC. An efficient protocol for the generation of monocyte derived dendritic cells using serum-free media for clinical applications in post remission AML patients. Ann Clin Lab Sci. 2014; 44(2):180–8.
48. van der Valk J, Brunner D, de Smet K, Fex Svenningsen A, Honegger P, Knudsen LE, Lindl T, Noraberg J, Price A, Scarino ML, Gstraunthaler G. Optimization of chemically defined cell culture media -replacing fetal bovine serum in mammalian in vitro methods. Toxicol In Vitro. 2010; 24(4):1053–63.

6

A randomised, double-blinded, placebo-controlled clinical study on intra-articular hyaluronan treatment in equine lameness originating from the metacarpophalangeal joint

Tytti M. Niemelä*, Riitta-Mari Tulamo and Anna K. Hielm-Björkman

Abstract

Background: Intra-articular inflammation resulting in lameness is a common health problem in horses. Exogenous intra-articular hyaluronic acid has been shown to provide an analgesic effect and reduce pain in equine and human osteoarthritis. High molecular weight non-animal stabilized hyaluronic acid (NASHA) has gained popularity in the treatment of human arthritic conditions due to its long-acting pain-relieving effects. The aim of this study was to compare the response to treatment of lameness localized in the equine metacarpophalangeal joint injected with non-animal stabilized hyaluronic acid (NASHA) and placebo (saline). Twenty-seven clinically lame horses with a positive response to diagnostic intra-articular anaesthesia of the metacarpophalangeal joint and with no, or at most mild, radiographic changes in this joint were included in the study. Horses in the treatment group ($n = 14$) received 3 mL of a NASHA product intra-articularly, and those in the placebo group ($n = 13$) received an equivalent volume of sterile 0.9 % saline solution.

Results: The change in the lameness score did not significantly differ between NASHA and placebo groups ($P = 0.94$). Scores in the flexion test improved more in the NASHA group compared with placebo ($P = 0.01$). The changes in effusion and pain in flexion were similar ($P = 0.94$ and $P = 0.27$, respectively) when NASHA and placebo groups were compared. A telephone interview follow-up of the owners three months post-treatment revealed that 14 of the 21 horses (67 %) were able to perform at their previous level of exercise.

Conclusions: In the present study, a single IA NASHA injection was not better than a single saline injection for reducing lameness in horses with synovitis or mild osteoarthritis. However, the results of this study indicate that IA NASHA may have some beneficial effects in modifying mild clinical signs but more research is needed to evaluate whether the positive effect documented ie. reduced response in the flexion test is a true treatment effect.

Keywords: Double-blinded, Clinical study, Lameness, Metacarpophalangeal joint, Non-animal stabilized hyaluronic acid (NASHA), Placebo-controlled

* Correspondence: tytti.niemela@helsinki.fi
Department of Equine and Small Animal Medicine, Faculty of Veterinary Medicine, University of Helsinki,, P.O. Box 5700014 Helsinki, Finland

Background

Over 70 % of racehorses suffer from lameness during their lifetime, and the cause of this is often intra-articular inflammation [1]. Acute or repetitive overload injuries of the metacarpo- or metatarsophalangeal joint can lead to synovitis or capsulitis of the joint [2]. Damage to the articular cartilage, subchondral bone, synovium, joint capsule or other soft tissues of the joint may lead to degeneration [3]. Inflammation of articular soft tissues can result in the synthesis of defective cartilage matrix components, leading to osteoarthritis [4]. This may remain clinically silent for a long period and only become clinically and radiographically evident when the disease has progressed to an irreversible state [5, 6]. Therefore, early detection and treatment of the disease, as well as prevention of further damage, is considered important.

Hyaluronan (HA) is a glycosaminoglycan that has an important role in the formation of proteoglycan aggregates in the cartilage. It is also a component of the synovial fluid. Synovial membrane type B cells and chondrocytes synthetize HA by disaccharide oligomerization [7]. Hyaluronan molecules restrict large plasma proteins from entering the synovial fluid, but facilitate the passage of small molecules for the maintenance of nutrition [8]. In osteoarthritis, the synthesis of HA is disrupted by increased levels of pro-inflammatory cytokines, free radicals and proteinases, resulting in HA with a significantly reduced molecular weight, more molecular polydisaccharides and a reduction in synovial fluid viscoelasticity [9].

Exogenous intra-articular (IA) HA has been shown to provide an analgesic effect and reduce pain in equine [10–15] and human osteoarthritis [16–24]. It is believed that exogenous HA stimulates the synthesis of HA by synoviocytes and promotes proteoglycan synthesis by chondrocytes [25]. HA can also indirectly contribute to the viscosity of the synovial fluid and lubricate unloaded joints. Furthermore, since the pain-relieving effect of IA HA within the injected joint often persists for considerably longer than the half-life of HA, it is likely that it provides not only symptom-modifying but also disease-modifying effects. The half-life of unmodified HA solutions can be less than 1 day [26, 27]. Recently, a high molecular weight non-animal stabilized hyaluronic acid (NASHA) product) has gained popularity in the treatment of human arthritic conditions due to its long-acting pain relieving effects [8, 17, 18, 20–24].

Currently, only one double-blinded placebo-controlled clinical equine study on IA HA treatment has been published [15]. That study reported a superior effect of HA and polysulphated glycosaminoglycan compared with placebo in reducing the lameness score. Overall, the efficacy of intra-articular HA in relieving inflammation and pain has only been examined in a few clinical and experimental equine studies [11–15, 28, 29]. In horses with medically induced synovitis, White et al. [28] found HA to relieve lameness compared with placebo. However, in a surgically induced equine osteoarthritis model, no changes in the lameness score were detected after HA treatment compared with a control treatment [29].

Some osteoarthritis models in animals have shown that high molecular weight HA preparations are superior to less polymerized HA forms [30, 31]. In a clinical equine trial comparing HA preparations differing in molecular weight, better clinical results were reported using HA of a higher molecular weight [32], but more research on the different preparations is needed. In this study, a NASHA product for human use (Durolane, Bioventus) was used. It has a long half-life (up to 32 days) [33] and remains in the synovial structures for a considerably longer period than other HA products [17, 18, 34].

We compared an IA injection of this NASHA product with an IA injection of placebo. The aim of the study was to examine whether the change in lameness originating from a metacarpophalangeal joint, from before the injection to after the injection, would differ between the two treatment groups. The IA injections were given on the day of the clinical baseline examination and after two weeks the horses returned for a second clinical examination. Our hypothesis was that the outcome measures would improve more in the horses treated with NASHA compared with those treated with placebo.

Methods

Design

The study was carried out as a randomised double-blind and placebo-controlled trial with a parallel group design and equal allocation ratio. It was planned and it is reported according the CONSORT statement (http://www.consort-statement.org/checklists/view/32-consort/). The study was approved by the Viikki Campus Research Ethics Committee of the University of Helsinki (31 March 2010). All horse owners signed a study consent sheet before the start of the study and owner was allowed to stop the study of the horse without giving any particular reason. Reasons for removing the horse from the study could have been side-effects caused by the NASHA or placebo products, additional orthopaedic or other health problems occurring after the first clinical examination and/or owners' lack of compliance or failure to follow the instructions given after the first clinical examination.

Population

Horses with lameness due to synovitis of the metacarpo- or metatarsophalangeal joint, with or without mild osteoarthritis, were recruited to the study. Synovitis of all durations was acceptable. Only adult, non-geriatric (i.e. age between 4–17 years), Finnhorse, Standardbred and Warmblood horses of all disciplines were eligible. In addition, large-sized ponies (withers 140–148 cm) were accepted (for convenience, referred to as horses in the text). Inclusion criteria were a positive response to diagnostic intra-articular anaesthesia of the affected metacarpo- or metatarsophalangeal joint and no radiographic signs of remodelling of the affected joint. This excluded horses with more severe chronic osteoarthritis. In addition, horses with intra-articular osteochondral or other fragments were excluded. Bilaterally lame horses and horses that had received intra-articular medications such as corticosteroids or HA within the previous three months, or per oral NSAIDs within 15 days, were not eligible. Furthermore, horses with concurrent pathologies, such as clinically significant ligament, tendon or other soft tissue injuries in the affected limb, were excluded.

Clinical exam and interventions

The study was advertised at stables, via the Internet page of the Faculty of the Veterinary Medicine [35], in equine clinics and in horse sport magazines. Horse owners contacted the University to have their horses included in the study and a telephone interview was conducted. An assistant not otherwise tied to the study enrolled the participants. Within a week after the horse owners had contacted the University to have their horses included, potential cases were presented to the Veterinary Teaching Hospital of the University of Helsinki for the first baseline clinical examination. This first examination was performed on the same day that each horse arrived at the hospital.

The horses were subjected to a complete lameness examination by the evaluating veterinarian (TMN). A standardized scale of 0–5 [36] was used to grade lameness. Effusion of the affected joint was recorded on a scale of 0–4 (0 = no effusion, 1 = mild, 2 = moderate, 3 = severe effusion, 4 = severe swelling of the joint region) [28, 37]. Other palpation findings, such as thickening of the joint capsule, were also recorded (yes/no thickening). A flexion test of the affected and the contralateral limb was performed and the lameness was recorded on a scale of 0–4 (0 = no increase, 1 = slight increase, 2 = moderate increase, 3 = considerable increase in the baseline lameness, 4 = non-weight-bearing lameness) [29]. To exclude confounding flexing reactions, for instance because of sensitiveness to handling, and thereby help the researchers to evaluate the reaction of the affected limb, the contralateral non-lame leg was always flexed first. The result of this contralateral flexion test was not recorded.

Pain when flexing the affected distal limb was also recorded on a scale of 0–3. This pain score was created by the authors and was recorded as follows: 0 = no pain on flexion, 1 = mild pain, i.e. the horse shows some reaction, such as moving the limb, 2 = moderate pain, i.e. the horse retracts the limb repeatedly during the 1 min flexion period, 3 = severe pain, i.e. the flexion test cannot be properly performed.

To localize the lesion and to decide if the horse was eligible for the study, a routine diagnostic aseptic arthrocentesis with an 18-gauge/3.8-cm needle was performed through the lateral sesamoidean ligament and 10 mL mepivacaine hydrochloride (Scandicain, Astra Zeneca) was injected into the joint. The response to the intra-articular anaesthesia was evaluated 10 min post-injection and was considered positive if a subjectively evaluated 80–100 % amelioration of lameness was evident. Radiographic examination of the joint with four standard views was performed (lateromedial, dorsopalmar, dorsolateral-palmaromedial and dorsomedial-palmarolateral), and all radiographs were evaluated by the same veterinarian (TMN).

Before starting the study, a non-blinded assisting technician created a computer generated randomization list using an Internet-based program [38]. The block size was 4 and no strata were used. Horses fulfilling the inclusion criteria were assigned to the treatment or control group according to the randomization list. The list and the NASHA and placebo products were kept in a locked locker at the university that only the non-blinded assisting veterinarian and his technician could access. Horses in the treatment group were injected with 3 mL NASHA into the affected joint, while horses in the control group received an equivalent volume of the sterile 0.9 % saline solution (Sodium chloride 9 mg/mL, B Braun) into the joint. Injections were administered on the same day that each horse arrived at the hospital, after confirming eligibility, the source of lameness and evaluating the radiographs.

Treatments were double-blinded so that the assisting veterinarian prepared the syringes according to the randomization list and performed the NASHA and saline injections, and neither the evaluating veterinarian (TMN) nor the owners were allowed in the treatment room during the procedure. Owners remained blinded until after the second clinical examination and the evaluating veterinarian (TMN) until after the statistical analyses were performed.

Second clinical examination and follow-up

Horses were allowed 30 min hand-walking per day and free access to a small paddock during the following two weeks, after which the second clinical examination was performed. Palpation findings and other outcome measures were re-evaluated and recorded (TMN). After the second clinical examination, the double-blinded trial part was concluded and the horses in the control group also received an IA NASHA injection to treat the lameness. To ensure that all treatment injections were performed by the same veterinarian, the assisting veterinarian also injected the placebo group with the NASHA. Follow-up information was collected two and a half to three months post-treatment by interviewing all owners by telephone.

The primary outcome measure was the change in the lameness score from baseline to the second clinical examination in the two intervention groups. The secondary outcome measures were the change in the effusion of the affected joint, in the lameness after the flexion test and in pain in flexion from baseline to the second clinical examination.

Statistical methods

A sample size calculator [39] was used with a 95 % confidence level and 80 % power, and the sample size was estimated at 11–14 horses per group based on 87 % of cases showing clinical improvement in an earlier study on HA for the treatment of naturally occurring arthritic conditions in horses [13]. In the placebo group, the proportion that would improve was estimated to be 20–30 %, where 20 % is 10 % lower than the percentage that has been used in the placebo groups in human studies [40, 41].

Data analysis was performed with a computer-based statistical program (SPSS Software, IBM). The final values for the outcome measures were subtracted from the baseline values to form variables of change, allowing positive and negative values. These variables of change were used in the comparison between groups with the independent-samples Mann–Whitney *U*-test (ranks). The demographic data and outcome measures at baseline were compared between the two treatment groups using the independent-samples Mann–Whitney *U*-test, or in the case of nominal categorical variables, Fisher's exact test or the likelihood ratio test. Furthermore, the outcome measures within groups were compared between the baseline examination and the second clinical examination using the Wilcoxon signed-rank test. All the above statistics were calculated for the population intended to treat ($n = 30$) and for the metacarpophalangeal patients only ($n = 27$). Value of $P < 0.05$ was considered significant.

Results

Sixty-eight horse owners were interviewed, which resulted in 36 horses being invited to the first clinical baseline examination. Altogether, 30 horses fulfilling the inclusion criteria were included in the study. However, as only three horses that concluded the study had lameness due to synovitis of the metatarsophalangeal joint, these were omitted from some of the analyses, leaving 27 horses with synovitis of the metacarpophalangeal joint as the primary study population (Table 1, Fig. 1). All the 27 horses completed the study. For the included horses, all examinations were performed between May 2010 and May 2012.

In 16 horses, lameness had previously been localised to the joint from which the lameness originated at baseline. Fifteen horses had received HA and/or corticosteroid treatment more than 3 months before entering the study in the same joint from which the lameness originated at baseline, while nine horses had not previously received any medications for musculoskeletal problems.

No significant differences in signalment, the use of the horse, outcome measures or the number of horses with findings in radiographs were found between the NASHA and placebo treatment groups at the first clinical (baseline) examination (Table 1). The baseline lameness score ranged from 1 to 3 (out of 0–5) and the most frequent lameness score was 2 ($n = 13$, 48 %). In 7 (26 %) horses, the lameness score was 1 and in 7 (26 %) cases 3.

When the change in the lameness score as the primary outcome measure was compared between the NASHA

Table 1 Demographic variables and outcome measures in the first clinical baseline examination of the placebo and NASHA groups ($n = 27$) and *P*-values for the comparison between treatment groups at the first clinical baseline examination

Variable	Placebo	NASHA	*P*-value
Number of horses	13	14	
Age (~years): Mean (range)	8.4 (4–17)	7.2 (4–12)	0.55
Gender: Mare/Stallion/Gelding %	46 %/15 %/39 %	43 %/21 %/36 %	0.09
Purpose: Harness race horse/Riding horse %	54 %/46 %	71 %/29 %	0.44
Breed: Standardbred/Finnhorse/Wamblood/Pony %	31 %/39 %/15 %/15 %	43 %/50 %/7 %/0 %	0.65
Affected limb: RF/LF %	46 %/54 %	71 %/29 %	0.25
Baseline lameness (AAEP)[a]: 0/1/2/3/4/5 %	0 %/15 %/39 %/46 %/0 %/0 %	0 %/36 %/57 %/7 %/0 %/0 %	0.05
Effusion[b]: 0/1/2/3/4 %	23 %/46 %/0 %/31 %/0 %	29 %/29 %/35 %/7 %/0 %	0.83
Lameness in the flexion test[c]: 0/1/2/3/4 %	0 %/0 %/8 %/61 %/31 %	0 %/0 %/29 %/50 %/21 %	0.33
Pain in flexion[d]: 0/1/2/3 %	0 %/31 %/23 %/46 %	7 %/29 %/36 %/28 %	0.46
Mild findings in radiographs: Yes/No %	54 %/46 %	50 %/50 %	1.00

[a] AAEP scale 0–5
[b] 0 = no effusion, 1 = mild, 2 = moderate, 3 = severe effusion, 4 = severe swelling of the metacarpal joint region
[c] 0 = no increase, 1 = slight increase, 2 = moderate increase, 3 = considerable increase in baseline lameness, 4 = non-weight-bearing lameness
[d] 0 = no pain at flexion, 1 = mild pain, 2 = moderate pain, 3 = severe pain

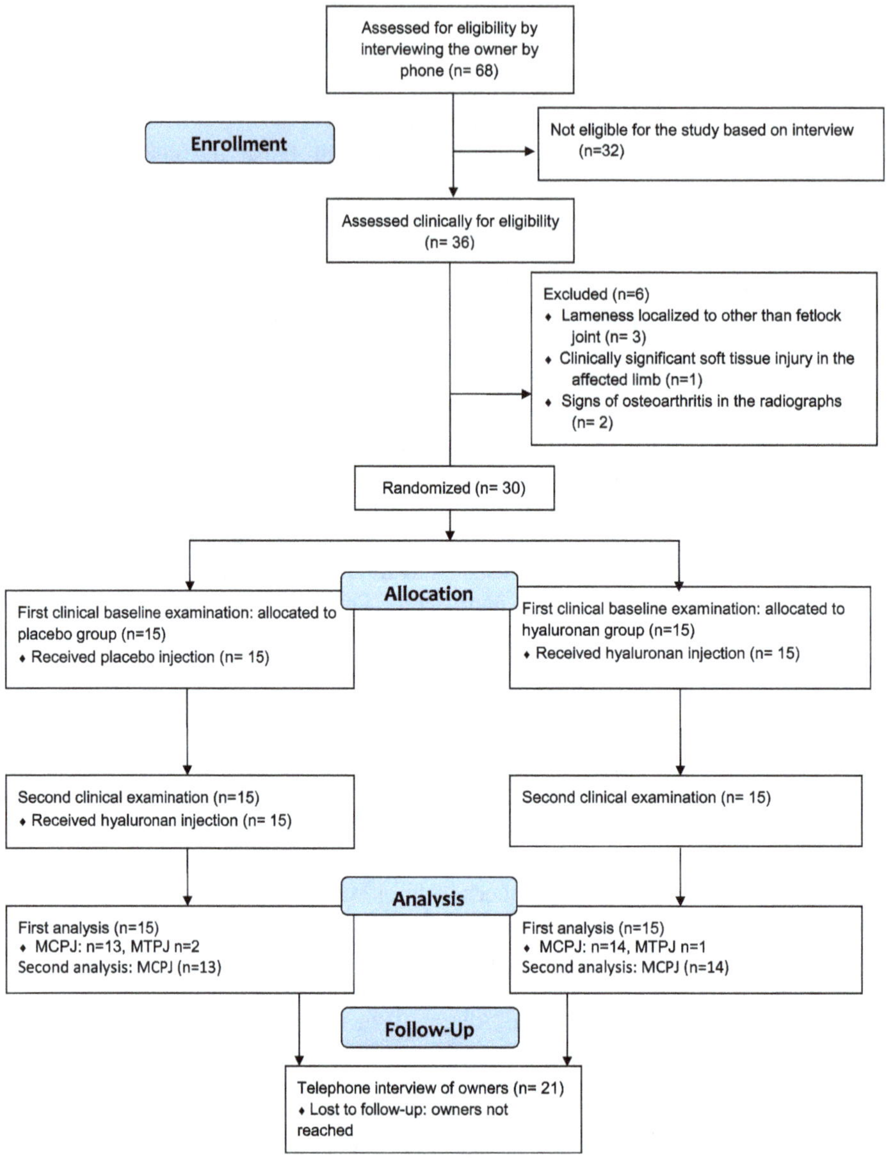

Fig. 1 Flow diagram showing the number of horses in different phases of the study. MCPJ = metacarpophalangeal joint; MTPJ = metatarsophalangeal joint

and the placebo groups, no significant difference was seen ($P = 0.94$, Table 2). When the changes in the secondary outcome measures were compared respectively, a significant difference was recorded for the change in the response to the flexion test ($P = 0.01$, Table 2). In contrast, the change in effusion and in the pain in flexion was similar in the placebo and NASHA groups ($P = 0.94$ and $P = 0.27$, respectively, Table 2). All results were similar when the three horses with metatarsophalangeal joint problems had been included.

No adverse effects of either intra-articular NASHA or saline injection could be seen in any of the horses. Based on the follow-up telephone interview at 2.5–3 months, 14 of the 21 horses (67 %) had been able to return to their previous level of use, but two of these had later developed other musculoskeletal problems. Six horse owners were not reached for the follow-up interview. Seven of the 21 horses (33 %) were no longer used in the same discipline or at the same performance level.

Discussion

In this study, the effect of intra-articular NASHA in relieving synovitis and lameness in clinical patients was evaluated. Apart from the study of Gaustad and Larsen [15], this is to our knowledge the only double-blinded placebo-controlled clinical equine study on intra-articular HA, and this study focused on a single joint. Although the difference in the baseline lameness score

Table 2 Medians (and ranges) of outcome measures in the placebo and NASHA groups, with *P*-values for the within-groups comparison of outcome measures between the first baseline and second clinical (end) examination, and *P*-values for the comparison between groups (*P* of change between interventions) of the change in outcome measures after the second clinical examination

Outcome measure	Placebo baseline	Placebo end	*P* within placebo	NASHA baseline	NASHA end	*P* within NASHA	*P* for change between interventions
Lameness[a]	2 (1–3)	2 (0–3)	0.005	2 (1–3)	0 (0–3)	0.02	0.94
Effusion[b]	1 (0–3)	1 (0–3)	0.48	1 (0–3)	1 (0–3)	0.56	0.94
Flexion test[c]	3 (2–4)	3 (1–4)	0.07	3 (2–4)	1 (0–3)	0.002	0.01
Pain[d]	2 (1–3)	1 (0–3)	0.04	2 (0–3)	0 (0–2)	0.01	0.27

[a] AAEP scale 0–5
[b] 0 = no effusion, 1 = mild, 2 = moderate, 3 = severe effusion, 4 = severe swelling of the metacarpal joint region
[c] 0 = no increase,1 = slight increase, 2 = moderate increase, 3 = considerable increase in baseline lameness, 4 = non-weight-bearing lameness
[d] 0 = no pain at flexion, 1 = mild pain, 2 = moderate pain, 3 = severe pain

was almost statistically significant, the groups of the present study were comparable (Table 1), as the baseline clinical and demographic variables did not significantly differ between them. This is important in a clinical study, since variables such as the level of physical activity of the horses cannot be fully controlled for. Gaustad and Larsen [15] also reported comparable treatment groups in their study (n = 77), but the HA treatment group (n = 28) was not separated from the PSGAG group (n = 27). Moreover, their study included horses with traumatic arthritis as well as other diagnoses in several high motion joints but the distribution of diagnoses between groups was not reported.

Most of the previous studies on IA HA treatment in horses are not comparable with the present study, since only two of them [15, 28] were blinded placebo-controlled studies and only one of the clinical studies [14] focused on a single joint. Furthermore, White et al. [28] used a prospective experimental study design with only 4 horses per group. Lameness was evaluated by measuring stride length, and not using the more subjective but, standardised, AAEP scale [36], which also takes into account the weight-bearing component of lameness. As in the present study, Gaustad and Larsen [15] found a significantly reduced lameness score in both the treatment and placebo groups. However, in contrast to their study, improvement in the lameness score of horses injected IA with NASHA in the present study, was not better than in the placebo group. The different result in the study of Gaustad and Larsen [15] might be explained by the more severe mean baseline lameness, the larger sample size, the multiple joints involved, or the presence of different joint diseases, compared with the present study. As in our study, Frisbie et al. [29] reported a lack of improvement in the lameness score with respect to treatment when HA was administered to horses with experimentally induced osteoarthritis. However, histologically, significantly less cartilage fibrillation was seen with HA treatment compared with controls [29].

A response to the flexion test was the only outcome measure which improved more in the NASHA group compared with the placebo group (Table 2). In addition to the lameness score, the flexion pain score improved both within the placebo and the NASHA groups (Table 2). It is possible that saline by itself might have had a positive effect, as also shown by Gaustad et al. [42]. They reported a significant improvement in horses with arthritis after repeated injections of a 2 mL NaCl solution. There was also a significant decrease in the lameness score when this NaCl-injected group was compared with the rest-only group. The synovial membrane has been shown to respond to IA injections of saline, and an increase in the synovial fluid HA concentration after an injection of saline into equine joints has been reported [43]. Furthermore, in both the study of Gaustad et al. [42] and the present study, the therapeutic effect of the local anaesthetic cannot be excluded. However, the improvement also seen in the placebo group might be explained by the two weeks of light exercise (half an hour of hand-walking per day) between clinical examinations, which may have been sufficient to improve relatively low-grade lameness, especially in harness racehorses undergoing heavy training. Furthermore, our study design was based on the assumption of a large difference in lameness improvement between groups based on an earlier study of HA for the treatment of naturally occurring arthritic condition in horses [13], so our originally calculated number of cases was probably too low to show smaller differences between groups.

Despite the lack of improvement in the other outcome measures of the present study, the greater improvement in the flexion test score in the NASHA group (Table 2) shows that IA NASHA may have some beneficial clinical sign modifying effects. Flexion tests are an integral part of a lameness examination. Although flexion tests may have some limitations, the distal limb flexion test has been shown to be very specific for the disease and the pain arising from the metacarpophalangeal joint [44].

Treatment with high molecular weight IA HA is of interest in human orthopaedics, and recent research has demonstrated it to be effective and long-acting in the treatment of human osteoarthritis [20–24]. Based on cross-linking, the NASHA has a prolonged residence time and results in a viscous HA gel in the joint [34]. Previously, exogenous HA has been shown to disappear from the joint within seven days [45], and synovitis also enhances the clearance of HA from the joint [46]. However, Altman et al. [18] found a prolonged reduction in pain after a NASHA treatment in human knee osteoarthritis patients with a maximum effect at 6 weeks post-treatment. Similarly, Gaustad and Larsen [15] reported that a significant number of horses became sound between 3 and 6 weeks post-injection. Exogenous HA has also been shown to increase the synthesis of HA by human synovial cell lines, which could explain the prolonged effect of exogenous HA [47]. Thus, the improvement in lameness in the NASHA group might have been greater if the period between the examinations in the present study had been longer than 2 weeks. However, since our study population consisted of clinical client-owned patients, it would have been unethical to delay the treatments of the horses receiving placebo for a longer period and all the first placebo-injected horses were therefore treated at the second examination. The third assessment was performed as a telephone interview to avoid long-distance travel for many of the patients. Most horses (14 of 21, i.e. 67 %) were able to perform at their previous level based on subjective assessment by owners or trainers.

A clinical study design sets limits on a placebo-control set-up. In addition, the lack of significant difference in the change of lameness score between the NASHA and placebo groups also reflects the difficulty in conducting clinical studies, as variation between intervention groups is always inevitably present, despite the lack of a statistically significant difference in demographic variables and in baseline outcome measures, as in the present study (Table 1). The severity of the disease can vary, despite a uniform lameness score or other clinical scores.

Selection bias was minimized by recruiting horses through several media and from a variety of riding and racehorse stables around southern Finland. On the other hand, this may also have caused a selection of horses which have been unresponsive to previous treatments or a selection of horse owners or trainers who overall train their horses differently compared with the general horse owner or trainer population. The population in the present study may also have been too heterogeneous, i.e. with variety of disciplines, training levels and training conditions may have caused excessive variation in the response to the NASHA injection and in the lack of a significant difference in most of the outcome measures.

No adverse effects of the intra-articular NASHA injection could be seen in any of the horses. A transient treatment related adverse effect of IA HA has been reported in up to 10.0 % of cases in an equine study [13] and 12.5 % in a human NASHA study [18].

Conclusions

In the present study, a single IA NASHA injection was not better than IA saline for reducing lameness in horses with synovitis or mild osteoarthritis in the metacarpophalangeal joint. However, this study shows indication that it may have some beneficial effects in modifying clinical signs. A single IA injection of NASHA might be useful in the treatment of acute synovitis, but more research is needed on the effects of NASHA in other equine joint disease states as well as on its mechanism of action.

Abbreviations

HA: hyaluronic acid; IA: Intra-articular; NASHA: non-animal stabilized hyaluronic acid.

Competing interests

The authors declare that they have no competing interests.

Authors' contributions

TMN carried out the clinical study of all horses, evaluation of radiographs, and drafted the manuscript. R-MT and AKH-B participated in the design of the study and helped to draft the manuscript. All authors read and approved the final manuscript.

Acknowledgements

Financial support from the Department of Equine and Small Animal Medicine and the Veterinary Teaching Hospital, University of Helsinki, is acknowledged. This study was partially supported by a grant from the Finnish Foundation of Veterinary Research, the Finnish Veterinary Foundation and the Erkki Rajakoski Foundation of the Finnish Trotting Association, which are acknowledged. We wish to thank Timo Paananen, DVM, for his assistance in treatments and adjunct professor Vesa Niskanen for the statistical advice.

References

1. Morris EA, Seeherman HJ. Clinical evaluation of poor performance in the racehorse: the results of 275 evaluations. Equine Vet J. 1991;23:169–74.
2. McIlwraith CW. Pathobiology of joints and their reaction to insult and injury. In: Stashak TS, editor. Adams' Lameness in Horses. 5th ed. Baltimore: Lippincott Williams & Wilkins; 2001. p. 469–79.
3. Buckwalter JA, Brown TD. Joint injury, repair, and remodelling: roles in post-traumatic osteoarthritis. Clin Orthop Rel Res. 2004;423:7–16.
4. Caron JP. Osteoarthritis. In: Ross MW, Dyson SJ, editors. Lameness in the Horse. 2nd ed. St Louis: Saunders; 2011. p. 655–68.
5. Frisbie DD. Synovial joint biology and pathobiology. In: Auer JA, Stick JA, editors. Equine Surgery. 3rd ed. St Louis: Saunders; 2006. p. 1036–55.
6. Rousseau JC, Delmas PD. Biological markers in osteoarthritis. Nat Clin Pract Rheumatol. 2007;3:346–56.
7. Gadher SJ, Woolley DE. Comparative studies on adherent rheumatoid synovial cells in primary culture: characterisation of the dendritic (stellate) cell. Rheumatol Int. 1987;7:13–22.
8. Goldberg VM, Buckwalter JA. Hyaluronans in the treatment of osteoarthritis of the knee: evidence for disease-modifying activity. Osteoarthr Cartilage. 2005;13:216–24.
9. Balazs EA, Denlinger J. Viscosupplementation: a new concept in the treatment of osteoarthritis. J Rheumatol. 1993;20 suppl 39:2–9.
10. Åsheim Å, Lindblad G. Intra-articular treatment of arthritis in racehorses with sodium hyaluronate. Acta Vet Scand. 1976;17:379–94.
11. Rose RJ. The intra-articular use of sodium hyaluronate for the treatment of osteoarthrosis in the horse. N Z Vet J. 1979;27:5–8.

12. Auer JA, Fackelman GE, Gingerich DA, Fetter AW. Effect of hyaluronic acid in naturally occurring and experimentally induced osteoarthritis. Am J Vet Res. 1980;41:568–74.
13. Ruth DT, Swites BJ. Comparison of the effectiveness of intra-articular hyaluronic acid and conventional therapy for the treatment of naturally occurring arthritic conditions in horses. Equine Pract. 1985;7:25–9.
14. Aviad AD, Arthur RM, Brencick VA, Ferguson HO, Teigland MB. Synacid vs. Hylartin V in equine joint disease. J Equine Vet Sci. 1988;8:112–6.
15. Gaustad G, Larsen S. Comparison of polysulphated glycosaminoglycan and sodium hyaluronate with placebo in treatment of traumatic arthritis in horses. Equine Vet J. 1995;27:356–62.
16. Dougados M, Nguyen M, Listrat V, Amor B. High Molecular weight sodium hyaluronate (Hyalectin) in osteoarthritis of the knee; a 1 year placebo-controlled trial. Osteoarthr Cartilage. 1993;1:97–103.
17. Åkermark C, Berg P, Björkman A, Malm P. Non-Animal Stabilised Hyaluronic Acid in the Treatment of Osteoarthritis of the Knee: A Tolerability Study. Clin Drug Inv. 2002;22:157–66.
18. Altman RD, Åkermark C, Beaulieu AD, Schnitzer T. Efficacy and safety of a single intra-articular injection of non-animal stabilized hyaluronic acid (NASHA) in patients with osteoarthritis of the knee. Osteoarthr Cartilage. 2004;12:642–9.
19. Balazs EA. Viscosupplementation for treatment of osteoarthritis: from initial discovery to current status and results. Surg Technol Int. 2004;12:278–89.
20. Raman R, Dutta A, Day N, Sharma HK, Shaw CJ, Johnson GV. Efficacy of Hylan G-F 20 and Sodium Hyaluronate in the treatment of osteoarthritis of the knee—A prospective randomized clinical trial. Knee. 2008;15:318–24.
21. Abate M, Pulcini D, Di Iorio A, Schivone C. Viscosupplementation with intra-articular hyaluronic acid for treatment of osteoarthritis in the elderly. Curr Pharm Des. 2010;16:631–40.
22. Chevalier X, Jerosch J, Goupille P, van Dijk N, Luyten FP, Scott DL, Bailleul F, Pavelka K. Single intra-articular treatment with 6 ml hylan G-F 20 in patients with symptomatic primary osteoarthritis of the knee: a randomised, multicentre, double-blind, placebo controlled trial. Ann Rheum Dis. 2010;69:113–9.
23. Arden NK, Åkermark C, Andersson M, Todman MG, Altman RD. A randomized saline-controlled trial of NASHA hyaluronic acid for knee osteoarthritis. Curr Med Res Opin. 2014;30:279–86.
24. Leighton R, Åkermark C, Therrien R, Richardson JB, Andersson M, Todman MG, Arden NK. NASHA hyaluronic acid vs methylprednisolone for knee osteoarthritis: a prospective, multicentre, randomized, non-inferiority trial. Osteoarthr Cartilage. 2014;22:17–25.
25. Frean SP, Abraham LA, Lees P. In vitro stimulation of equine articular cartilage proteoglycan synthesis by hyaluronan and and carprofen. Res Vet Sci. 1999;67:183–90.
26. Brown TJ, Laurent UB, Fraser JR. Turnover of hyaluronan in the synovial joints: elimination of labelled hyaluronan from the knee joint of the rabbit. Exp Physiol. 1991;76:125–34.
27. Lindehayn HH, Heilmann HH, Niederhausen HUW, Pohlenz K. Elimination of tritium-labelled hyaluronic acid from normal and osteoarthritic rabbit knee joints. Eur J Chem Clin Biochem. 1997;35:355–63.
28. White GW, Stites T, Hamm J, Pool R. Evaluation of the efficacy of various preparations of sodium hyaluronate in an induced equine carpitis model. J Equine Vet Sci. 1999;19:331–7.
29. Frisbie DD, Kawack CE, McIlwraith CW, Werpy NM. Evaluation of polysulfated glycosaminoglycan or sodium hyaluronan administered intra-articularly for treatment of horses with experimentally induced osteoarthritis. Am J Vet Res. 2009;70:203–9.
30. Kikuchi T, Yamada H, Shimmei M. Effect of high molecular weight hyaluronan on cartilage degradation in a rabbit model of osteoarthritis. Osteoarthr Cartilage. 1996;4:99–110.
31. Shimizu C, Kubo T, Hirasawa Y, Coutts R, Amiel D. Histomorphometric and biochemical effect of various hyaluronans on early osteoarthritis. J Rheumatol. 1998;25:1813–9.
32. Phillips MW. Clinical trial comparison of intra-articular sodium hyaluronate products in the horse. Equine Vet Sci. 1989;9:39–40.
33. Edsman K, Hjelm R, Lärkner H, Nord LI, Karlsson A, Wiebensjö Å, Höglund AU, Kenne AH, Näsström J. Intra-articular Duration of Durolane™ after Single Injection into the Rabbit Knee. Cartilage. 2011;2(4):384–8.
34. Lindqvist U, Tolmachev V, Kairemo K, Åström G, Jonsson E, Lundqvist H. Elimination of stabilised hyaluronan from the knee joint in healthy men. Clin Pharmacokinet. 2002;41(8):603–13.
35. University of Helsinki - Faculty of Veterinary Medicine. http://www.vetmed.helsinki.fi/english/research/(2010) Accessed 1 April 2010.
36. Anonymous. Definition and Classification of Lameness. In: Guide for Veterinary Service and Judging of Equestrian Events. Lexington: Amer Assoc Equine Pract; 1991. p. 19.
37. de Grauw JC, van de Lest CHA, Brama PAJ, Rambags BPB, van Weeren PR. In vivo effects of meloxicam on inflammatory mediators, MMP activity and cartlage biomarkers in equine joints with acute synovitis. Equine Vet J. 2009;41:693–9.
38. Research randomizer. https://www.randomizer.org/(2010). Accessed 1 Feb 2010
39. Working in Epidemiology. http://www.winepi.net/uk/index.htm (2010) Accessed 1 Feb 2010
40. Richette P, Ravaud P, Conrozier T, Euller_Ziegler L, Mazières B, Maugars Y, Mulleman D, Clerson P, Chevalier X. Effect of hyaluronic acid in symptomatic hip osteoarthritis: a multicenter, randomized, placebo-controlled trial. Arthritis Rheum. 2009;60:824–30.
41. Pham T, Le Henanff A, Ravaud P, Dieppe P, Paolozzi L, Dougados M. Evaluation of the symptomatic and structural efficacy of a new hyaluronic acid compound, NRD101, in comparison with diacerein and placebo in a 1 year randomised controlled study in symptomatic knee osteoarthritis. Ann Rheum Dis. 2004;63:1611–7.
42. Gaustad G, Dolvik NI, Larsen S. Comparison of intra-articular injection of 2 ml of 0.9 % NaCl solution with traumatic arthritis. Am J Vet Res. 1999;60:1117–21.
43. Tulamo R-M. 1991. Am J Vet Res. 1991;52:1940–4.
44. Kearney CM, van Weeren PR, Cornelissen BPM, den Boom P, Brama PAJ. Which anatomical region determines a positive flexion test of the distal aspect of a forelimb in a non-lame horse? Equine Vet J. 2010;42:547–51.
45. Antonas KN, Fraser JRE, Muirden KD. Distribution of biologically labelled radioactive hyaluronic acid injected into joints. Ann Rheum Dis. 1973;32:103–11.
46. Myers SL, Brandt KD, Eilam O. Even low-grade synovitis accelerates the clearance of protein from the canine knee: Implications for the measurement of synovial fluid "markers" of osteoarthritis. Arthr Rheum. 1995;38:1085–91.
47. Smith MM, Ghosh P. The synthesis of hyaluronic acid by human synovial fibroblasts is influenced by the nature of the hyaluronate in the extracellular environment. Rheumatol Int. 1987;7:113–22.

7

Pharmacokinetics and *in vitro* efficacy of salicylic acid after oral administration of acetylsalicylic acid in horses

Kathrin Buntenkötter[1], Maren Osmers[1], Ina Schenk[2], Wilhelm Schänzer[2], Marc Machnik[2], Michael Düe[3] and Manfred Kietzmann[1*]

Abstract

Background: Although acetylsalicylic acid (ASA) is not frequently used as a therapeutic agent in horses, its metabolite SA is of special interest in equestrianism since it is a natural component of many plants used as horse feed. This led to the establishment of thresholds by horse sport organizations for SA in urine and plasma. The aim of this study was to investigate plasma and urine concentrations of salicylic acid (SA) after oral administration of three different single dosages (12.5 mg/kg, 25 mg/kg and 50 mg/kg) of acetylsalicylic acid (ASA) to eight horses in a cross-over designed study.

Results: In the 12.5 mg/kg group, SA concentrations in urine peaked 2 h after oral administration (2675 μg/mL); plasma concentrations peaked at 1.5 h (17 μg/mL). In the 25 mg/kg group, maximum concentrations were detected after 2 h (urine, 2785 μg/mL) and 1.5 h (plasma, 23 μg/mL). In the 50 mg/kg group, maximum concentrations were observed after 5 h (urine, 3915 μg/mL) and 1.5 h (plasma, 45 μg/mL). The plasma half-life calculated for SA varied between 5.0 and 5.7 h. The urine concentration of SA fell below the threshold of 750 μg/mL (set by the International Equestrian Federation FEI and most of the horseracing authorities) between 7 and 26 h after administration of 12.5 and 25 mg/kg ASA and between 24 and 36 h after administration of 50 mg/kg ASA. For ASA, IC_{50} were 0.50 μg/mL (COX-1) and 5.14 μg/mL (COX-2). For salicylic acid, it was not possible to calculate an IC_{50} for either COX due to insufficient inhibition of both cyclooxygenases.

Conclusion: The established SA thresholds of 750 μg//mL urine and 6.5 μg/mL plasma appear too generous and are leaving space for misuse of the anti-inflammatory and analgetic compound ASA in horses.

Keywords: Acetylsalicylic acid, Salicylic acid, COX-inhibition, Pharmacokinetics, Horses

Background

Salicylic acid (SA) is one of the oldest nonsteroidal anti-inflammatory drugs (NSAIDs) and has been used as an antipyretic agent and in acute rheumatic events in humans for a long time [1]. Also in veterinary medicine, it has been administered in cases of joint disease in dogs and horses [2]. Acetylsalicylic acid (ASA) was synthesized to have the same effects as SA with an improved gastric and systemic tolerability profile [3]. After administration, ASA is rapidly converted to SA [4]. Additionally, ASA is sensitive to methanol, heat, change of pH and other factors. So, ASA itself cannot be detected with sufficient accuracy, because it is dissociated to SA and acetylic acid, even during sample storage and LC-MS analysis. Even though ASA is not frequently used as a therapeutic agent in horses, its metabolite SA is of special interest in equestrianism since it is a natural component of many plants used as horse feed, e.g. alfalfa hay or willow bark. Therefore, SA concentrations can be found in blood and urine samples of horses after consumption of any of these plants [5]. This led to the establishment of thresholds by horse sport organizations for SA in urine and plasma to avoid positive doping cases due to accidental feed intake, resulting in false positive. The International Equestrian Federation (FEI) and most of the

* Correspondence: manfred.kietzmann@tiho-hannover.de
[1]Institute of Pharmacology, Toxicology and Pharmacy, University of Veterinary Medicine Hannover Foundation, Hannover, Germany
Full list of author information is available at the end of the article

horseracing authorities (for example in Europe, U.S.A.) have set SA thresholds at 750 μg/mL in urine and 6.5 μg/mL in plasma [6]. These threshold levels were based on several studies [5, 7, 8], in which the average urine concentration of SA was dependent on the horse's diet and country of origin. However, the thresholds were established on a arbitrary statistical basis and not extrapolated from any irrelevant plasma or urine concentration as proposed by Toutain and Lassourd [9].

The study presented aimed to investigate average time intervals elapsed until plasma and urine concentrations fall below the threshold after oral administration of different dosages of ASA. Recommended ASA dosages for horses in literature vary between 5 and 100 mg/kg and from twice daily to every other day [10]. Main indications are inflammatory processes, pain and fever. In this cross-over designed study, eight horses received 12.5 mg/kg, 25 mg/kg, and 50 mg/kg ASA orally once daily. Blood and urine samples were analyzed via HPLC-MS/MS. Furthermore, to assess the efficacy of salicylates on COX-1 and COX-2 inhibition in horses, the IC_{50}, i.e. the drug concentration required to inhibit 50% of COX activity *in vitro*, was determined for ASA and SA in a whole blood assay.

Methods

Pharmacokinetic study

Animals

The animal study protocol was approved by the regional administration of the governmental body (LAVES; Lower Saxony, Germany; 33.9-42502-04-11/0512). Eight standardbred horses (4 mares, 4 geldings, 12.4 ± 3.2 years old; 656 ± 95 kg body weight) were used in this study. Horses were housed in stables of Serumwerk Memsen, WDT, Germany (owner of the horses) with straw bedding and daily turnout. They were fed a diet free from detectable SA contamination consisting of hay, grass, beets and water *ad libitum*. All horses were healthy on the basis of a clinical examination prior to the study.

Animal study

Three dosages of ASA were chosen: 12.5 mg/kg, 25 mg/kg, and 50 mg/kg bodyweight once daily. Horses received single oral doses of the ASA powder (Pyrinagil®, Veyx, Schwarzenborn, Germany) mixed with syrup in 100 mL syringes. The study was conducted in a 4-way, 3-treatment cross-over design with a washout period of at least 2 weeks. Blood samples were drawn in lithium heparin tubes at the following timepoints: −24, −21, −18 (blank samples), 0.25, 0.5, 0.75, 1, 1.5, 2, 3, 4, 6, 8, 12, 14, 16, 24, 36, 48, 72, 96, 120, 144 and 168 h after treatment. Plasma was separated after centrifugation (10 min at 1400 × g) immediately after withdrawal. Three blank urine samples (sampled during spontaneous emiction) were taken from each horse between 24 and 18 h before treatment. Urine samples were taken at 2, 5, 7, 12, 24, 36, 48, 72, 96, 120, 144, 168 and 192 h after treatment for each dosage tested; for 50 mg/kg ASA, an additional sample was taken after 216 h. Both, urine and plasma samples were stored at −20 °C until analysis (storage time about 4 weeks).

Quantification of SA in urine and plasma

Initially, it had been planned to measure ASA and SA in urine and plasma samples. However, this this was not feasible as ASA turned out to be sensitive to methanol, heat, change of pH and was continuously dissociated to SA, even during LC-MS analysis. ASA could therefore not be detected with sufficient accuracy so that it was decided to convert all ASA to SA and to measure total salicylates in plasma and urine by increasing the pH to 13–14. Since SA is the main metabolite of ASA, no other metabolites such as gentisic or salicyluric acid were quantified. Quantification of SA was partially based on methods described previously [11] and accomplished by an internal standard calibration. SA concentrations were determined using chromatographic peak area/concentration ratios and linear regression analysis to IS area ratios.

Materials and chemicals

Ammonium acetate, glacial acetic acid, potassium hydroxide, sodium dihydrogen phosphate-monohydrate, di-sodium hydrogen phosphate and methanol (analytical grade) were obtained from Merck (Darmstadt, Germany); acetonitrile (HPLC grade) was purchased from VWR (Darmstadt, Germany). Oasis ® HLB SPE cartridges (60 mg, 3 mL) were purchased from Roche (Mannheim, Germany). Deionised water was of MilliQ grade. SA and the internal standard D_4-SA were obtained from Sigma-Aldrich (Germany) and Toronto Research Chemicals (North York, Canada), respectively. For standard curves, pooled urine of horses with known SA concentrations as well as commercially available equine donor plasma (Sera Laboratories International, West Sussex, UK) were used.

Plasma sample preparation

For plasma samples, a direct injection method published by Thomas et al. [12] was modified. To 500 μL Milli-Q-water and 1 μg of the internal standard D4-SA 500 μl plasma were added. Samples taken up to 6 h (12.5 and 25 mg/kg) and up to 8 h after ASA administration were diluted 1:5 in Milli-Q-water before sample preparation. For protein precipitation, 1.5 mL acetonitrile were added and gently mixed. After centrifugation (10 min, 3000 U), 20 μL of KOH (5 mol/L) were added to the supernatant to alkalinize the sample to pH 13–14 for 20 min in order to hydrolyze all ASA to SA. To make the pH compatible with the HPLC column, the sample was adjusted to pH 1–2 by adding 20 μL HCl (6 mol/L) and centrifuged again (10 min, 1400 g). 200 μL aliquots were used for HPLC-MS/MS analysis.

Urine sample preparation

The sample preparation for the quantitative analysis of SA was performed following the method described by Schenk et al. [11] and included a solid phase extraction. Briefly, 2 μg of the internal standard D4-SA were added to 100 μL of urine and 900 μL of Milli-Q-water. Samples taken during the first 24 h after treatment were diluted 1:10 in Milli-Q-water (12.5 mg/kg and 25 mg/kg), whereas samples of the 50 mg/kg group were diluted 1:50. To enforce hydrolysis of any remaining ASA to SA, the pH was adjusted to 13–14 by addition of 40 μL KOH (1 mol/l). After 20 min an adjustment to pH 7 was achieved by addition of 0.2 mL phosphate buffer (Na_2HPO_4/NaH_2PO_4,0.8 mol/l). After centrifugation (5 min, 500 g), solid phase extraction was performed with conditioned Oasis® HLB 3 cc (60 mg) extraction cartridges (Waters corp., Milford, MA, USA). Samples were then evaporated to dryness in a rotary evaporator and dried residues dissolved in 200 μL ammonium acetate/acetonitrile (30:20, v/v) for HPLC-MS/MS injection.

Instrumentation-liquid chromatography

The liquid chromatography system comprised an Agilent Series 1100 LC (Agilent Technologies, Waldbronn, Germany). Analyte separation (plasma and urine samples) was achieved with a Nucleodur Pyramid column (70 × 4 mm, 5 μm particle size) from Macherey-Nagel (Düren, Germany). For plasma samples, a Gemini C_6 Phenyl (4 × 2 mm) guard column was added (Phenomenex, Aschaffenburg, Germany). The mobile phase comprised ammonium acetate buffer (5 mmol/l ammonium acetate, 0.1% glacial acid in MilliQ water, pH 3.5; solvent A) and acetonitrile (solvent B). The following programmed mobile phase gradient was used for analyte separation: gradient B 0–100% in 7 min, held for 1 min at 100% B, reequilibration time at 0% B for 3 min, run time 11 min. The mobile phase flow rate was 800 μL/min. The retention time was 5.2 min.

Instrumentation-mass spectrometry

Mass analysis was performed on an API 3200 triple-quadrupole mass spectrometer (AB Sciex, Darmstadt, Germany), equipped with an electrospray ionisation (ESI) interface. Samples were measured in the negative operation mode at an interface temperature 450 °C with an ion spray voltage of −4500 V. Collision-induced dissociation with nitrogen was performed at a collision gas pressure of 2.9×10^{-3} Pa. Diagnostic ions were detected in the multiple reaction monitoring mode (MRM). The transition ions monitored for SA were m/z 137 → −93; m/z 137 → −65; m/z 137 → −41; m/z 137 → −75; those for d_4-SA were m/z 141 → −97; and m/z 141 → −69. The quantifying ion for urine samples were m/z 137 → −75 (collision energy −38 eV) and m/z 137 → 65 (collision energy −40 eV) for plasma, respectively. Data acquisition and analysis were accomplished with Analyst® software (version 1.4.2, AB Sciex).

Method validation

The method was validated according to the guidelines of the European Horseracing Scientific Liaison Committee [13]. Validation parameters were selectivity, recovery, linearity, limit of quantification, limit of detection, analyte stability, precision, and accuracy. The calibration range was 5 to 250 μg/mL (urine samples) and 0.3 to 20 μg/mL (plasma samples).

Recovery was only calculated for urine, as plasma concentrations were determined by direct injection. To prove stability, quality control samples were stored under the same conditions as post administration samples for a minimum of 4 weeks.

Pharmacokinetic analysis

Pharmacokinetic parameters of SA in plasma were calculated with WinNonlin® 5.3 (Pharsight, Mountain View, USA), using a non-compartmental analysis. Because the SA concentration in plasma samples of untreated horses was below of the LLOQ (0.3 μg/ml), the absolute values were used for the PK calculation. The following information was obtained: C_{max}, T_{max}, clearance (Cl/F), MRT, elimination rate constant, half-life λ_z and AUC_{last}.

Pharmacodynamic study, COX-1 assay, COX-2 assay

Materials and chemicals

Compounds used for the pharmacodynamic study were ASA and SA (all Sigma Aldrich, Munich, Germany). Substances were diluted in dimethyl sulfoxide (DMSO; Merck, Darmstadt, Germany) in concentrations from 0.1 to 1000 mmol/L. LPS (*Escherichia coli* O111:B4) used for COX-2 assays was obtained from Sigma Aldrich, Munich, Germany. Samples were analyzed for thromboxane B_2 and prostaglandin E_2 concentrations using enzyme immunoassays (Cayman Chemicals, Ann Arbor, MI, USA).

Animals and study design

According to Brideau *et al.* [14] and McCann et al. [15], the COX-1 inhibition was quantified by each substance's ability to inhibit the formation of clot-induced Thromboxane B_2 (TXB_2) using blood from six clinically healthy warmblood horses (five mares and one gelding). To assess COX-2 inhibition, LPS-induced Prostaglandin E_2 (PGE_2) production was measured.

In vitro assay

For the COX-1 assay, blood was drawn by jugular venipuncture into vacuum tubes containing no anti-coagulant (Greiner bio-one, Frickenhausen, Germany). Immediately afterwards, blood aliquots (500 μL) were transferred into polypropylene tubes prepared with 5 μL of vehicle (DMSO), ASA or SA at final concentrations of 0.1, 1, 10, 100, or 1000 μmol/L. After mixing, tubes were incubated for 1 h at 37 °C to allow the blood to clot. Samples were then centrifuged at 4 °C and 2000 × g for 10 min. Supernatants were stored at −80 °C until analysis.

For the COX-2 assay, plasma was drawn in lithium heparin tubes (Vacutainer, BD, Heidelberg, Germany). Aliquots of 500 μL were transferred into polypropylene tubes and preincubated with 10 μL LPS dissolved in phosphate buffered saline (100 μg/mL). After 5 min of incubation at 37 °C, ASA or SA were added. A further incubation period of 24 h at 37 °C followed. One aliquot of blood was not incubated with LPS and used as control. Samples were centrifuged as described above and supernatants stored at −80 °C. A pre-incubation with a COX-1 inhibitor was not included in the performed COX-2 assay. After thawing, samples were diluted in EIA buffer (1:10) and used directly for the immunoassays without a preliminary extraction. The immunoassays were performed according to the manufacturer's instructions (Dynatech Microplate Reader, Dynatech Laboratories, Denkendorf, Germany).

Table 1 Precision and accuracy of the analytical method, summary results for plasma and urine

Concentration (μg/ml)	Intraday precision (%) ($n = 6$ per conc.)	Interday precision (%) ($n = 18$ per conc.)	Accuracy (%) ($n = 6$ per conc.)
Plasma			
1	4.6	10.3	2.3
5	4.8	1.1	4.8
10	3.1	3.4	1.6
Urine			
10	5.1	13.0	6.3
50	3.4	4.5	5.1
200	8.8	3.2	2.2

Statistical analysis

Data were analyzed with a commercially available software program (GraphPad Prism 5.03 software; GraphPad Software, Inc., La Jolla, CA, USA) by use of a one-way-repeated measures analysis of variance followed by the Bonferroni *post hoc* test. Values of $P < 0.05$ were considered statistically significant. The concentration leading to a 50% inhibition of COX activity (IC_{50}) was calculated with WinNonlin® Professional Edition, Version 5.3, Inhibitory Effect Sigmoid Imax Model (Pharsight, Mountain View, USA).). The vehicle control was used as baseline (0% inhibition).

Results

Validation of the analytical method

Identification of SA was ensured by its specific retention time and four characteristic ion transitions. As no SA free horse urine and plasma was available, traces of SA could be detected in each sample. Nevertheless, the SA

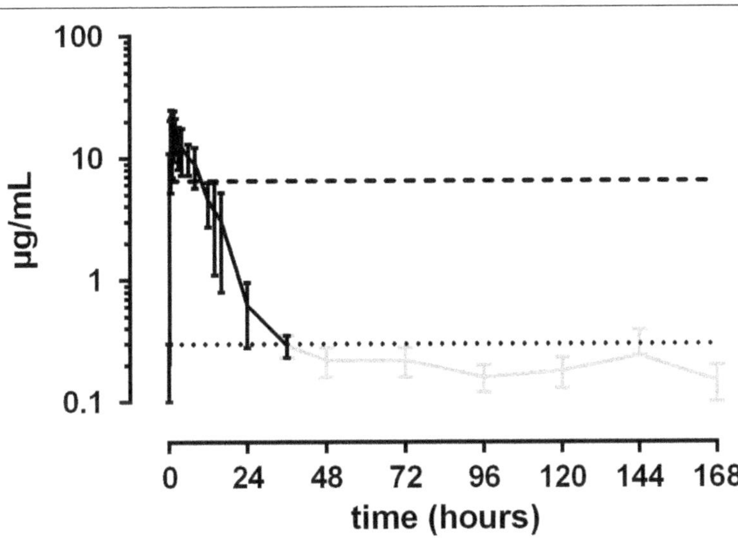

Fig. 1 Mean values (± S.D.) of SA concentrations in plasma of horses after a single oral dose of 12.5 mg/kg BW ($n = 8$). Black line = values > LLOQ. Grey line = values < LLOQ. Dotted line = LLOQ. Dashed line = threshold concentration (FEI)

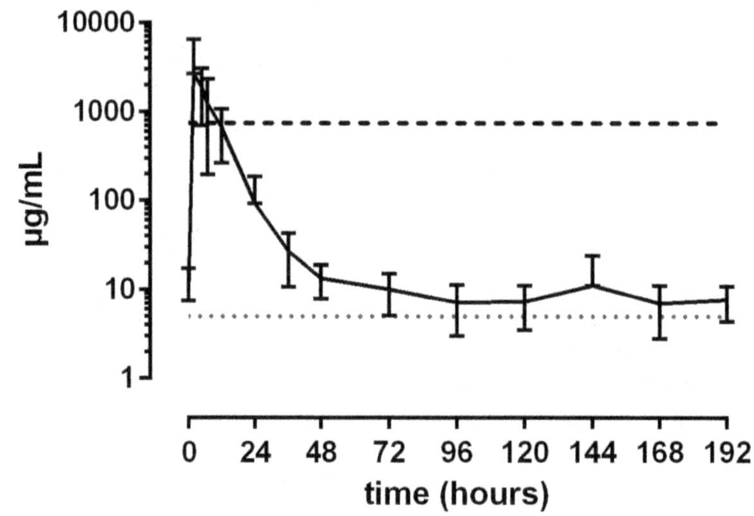

Fig. 2 Mean values (± S.D.) of SA concentrations in urine of horses after a single oral dose of 12.5 mg/kg BW ($n = 8$). Black line = values > LLOQ. Grey line = values < LLOQ. Dotted line = LLOQ. Dashed line = threshold concentration (FEI)

concentrations were mostly below the LLOQ and could easily be discriminated from the spiked samples. Plasma and urine samples spiked with SA that had been stored under the same conditions as the post administration samples, storage at −20 °C for four weeks did not show any significant difference in analyte degeneration (one-tailed *T*-test). Recovery was calculated to be 51% in urine.

Calibration curves were found linear in plasma and urine relating to the specified concentration ranges. The LLOD was estimated at 1 µg/mL for urine and 0.1 µg/mL for plasma. The LLOQ was determined at 5 µg/mL for urine and 0.3 µg/mL for plasma. Summary results for precision and accuracy are listed in Table 1.

Plasma and urine concentrations of SA after oral ASA administration

12.5 mg/kg ASA: Maximum plasma concentrations (C_{max})between 14.5 and 26.9 µg/mL were measured 0.5 h to 1.5 h after administration of ASA. Only in one horse C_{max} was reached eight hours after treatment. Plasma concentrations fell below the set threshold of 6.5 µg/mL between 6 and 16 h after treatment. Basal SA levels were measured 36 to 48 h after treatment (Fig. 1). In urine, maximum SA concentrations were achieved between 2 and 7 h after administration of ASA, with results varying between 699 and 10200 µg/mL. Values fell below the threshold of 750 µg/mL between 7 and 26 h after administration.

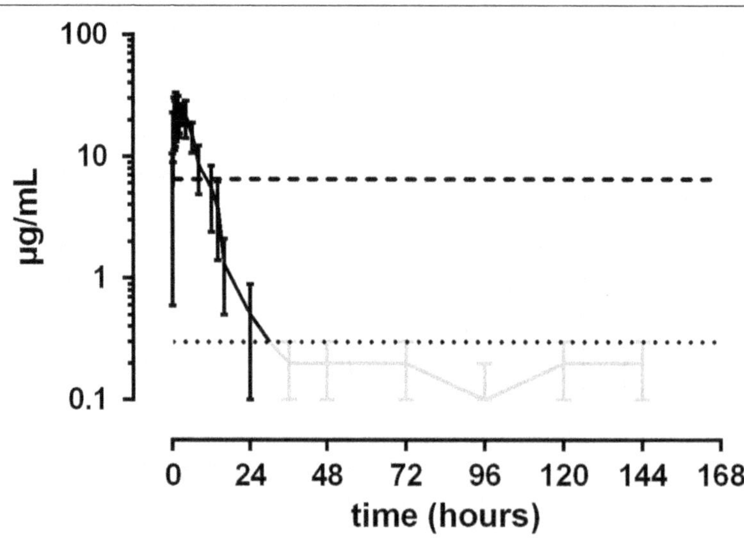

Fig. 3 Mean values (± S.D.) of SA concentrations in plasma of horses after a single oral Black line = values > LLOQ. Grey line = values < LLOQ. Dotted line = LLOQ. Dashed line = threshold concentration (FEI)dose of 25.0 mg/kg BW ($n = 8$)

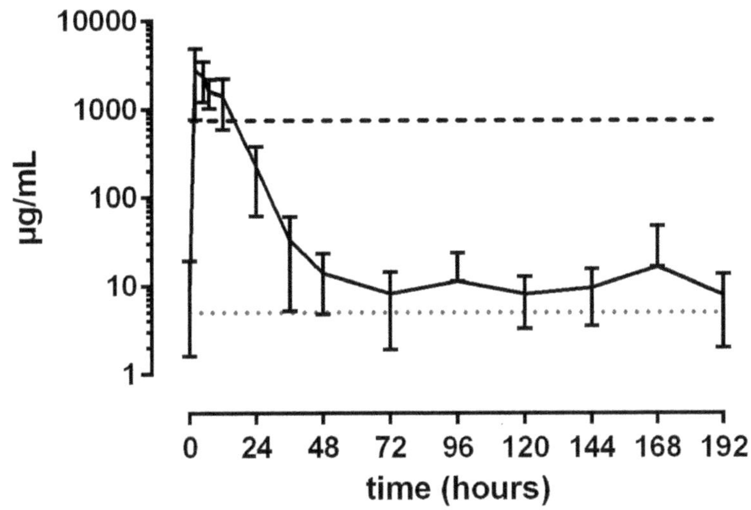

Fig. 4 Mean values (± S.D.) of SA concentrations in urine of horses after a single oral dose of 25.0 mg/kg BW ($n = 8$). Black line = values > LLOQ. Grey line = values < LLOQ. Dotted line = LLOQ. Dashed line = threshold concentration (FEI)

One horse did not exceed the urine threshold SA at all (Fig. 2).

25 mg/kg ASA: C_{max} was reached between 0.5 and 6 h after administrartion (19.1 to 37.8 µg/mL), while plasma concentrations dropped below the threshold of 6.5 µg/mL SA between 12 and 24 h. Between 36 and 48 h after treatment basal levels were reached in all horses (Fig. 3). All horses showed the highest urinary excretion of SA between 2 and 5 h after treatment, with values from 1550 to 7640 µg/mL SA. Between 7 and 24 h after administration, all horses featured urine SA levels below the threshold (Fig. 4).

50 mg/kg ASA: Plasma SA levels peaked between 1 and 6 h after administration (35.1 to 62.7 µg/mL). Plasma levels fell below the threshold at 12 h ($n = 2$), 14 h ($n = 1$), 24 h ($n = 3$) and 36 h ($n = 2$) after administration. Basal levels could be observed again between 36 and 48 h after administration (Fig. 5). Peak urine SA concentrations were measured between 2 and 7 h (2810 to 9640 µg/mL). Values fell below the threshold between 12 and 36 h (Fig. 6).

A plasma clearance (Cl/F) of 82.2 mL·h/kg, resulting in a calculated half-life of 5.2 h (12.5 mg/kg), 97.1 mL·h/kg with a half-life of 5.0 h (25 mg/kg), and 114.0 mL·h/

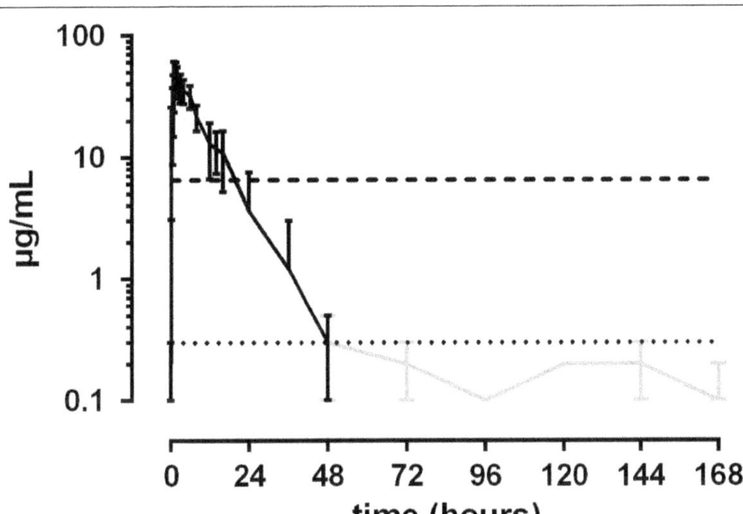

Fig. 5 Mean values (± S.D.) of SA concentrations in plasma of horses after a single oral dose of 50.0 mg/kg BW ($n = 8$). Black line = values > LLOQ. Grey line = values < LLOQ. Dotted line = LLOQ. Dashed line = threshold concentration (FEI)

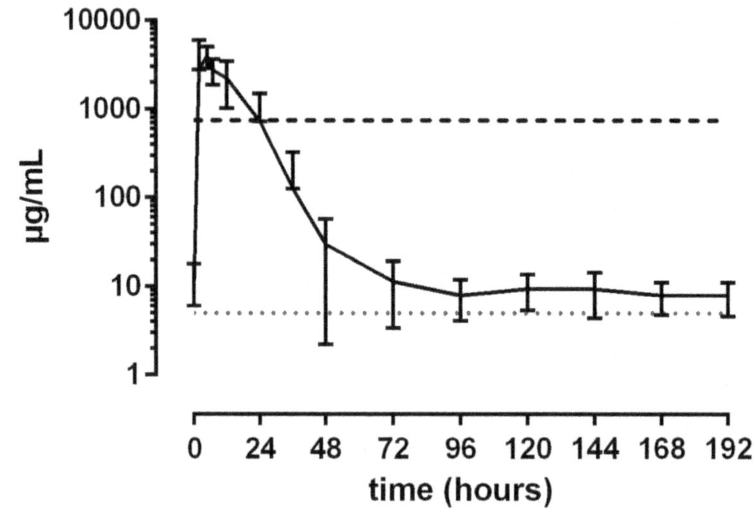

Fig. 6 Mean values (± S.D.) of SA concentrations in urine of horses after a single oral dose of 50.0 mg/kg BW (*n* = 8). Black line = values > LLOQ. Grey line = values < LLOQ. Dotted line = LLOQ. Dashed line = threshold concentration (FEI)

kg with a half-life of 5.7 h (50 mg/kg) were calculated (Table 2). The MRT varied between 7.26 and 8.39 h.

Pharmacodynamic study

In order to determine IC_{50} values, the inhibition of COX-1 and COX-2 activity was plotted against different concentrations of ASA (Table 3 and Fig. 7). The vehicle control was used as the baseline (0% inhibition). The IC_{50} of ASA was 1.68 μmol/L (0.50 μg/mL, COX-1) and 17.02 μmol/L (5.14 μg/mL, COX-2), respectively. No IC_{50} could be calculated for SA because of an insufficient COX-Inhibition (IC_{50} > 100 μmol/L (COX-1) and > 1000 μmol/L (Cox-2)).

Discussion

A method for the quantitative analysis of SA in horse urine and plasma has been developed and validated. Because of the distinctive instability of ASA during the whole process of sample storage, preparation and analysis, it was decided to convert ASA completely to SA.

Table 2 Plasma SA pharmacokinetics data after oral administration of ASA (12.5, 25.0, 50.0 mg/kg) to horses, mean ± S.D. of eight horses per treatment

Parameter	Units	12.5 mg/kg	25.0 mg/kg	50.0 mg/kg
Cmax	μg/ml	19.75 ± 5.22	30.06 ± 7.44	51.66 ± 11.27
Tmax	h	2.0 ± 2.5	2.5 ± 2.3	2.2 ± 1.7
Cl/F	ml/h/kg	82.2 ± 18.4	97.1 ± 19.9	114.0 ± 31.9
AUC*last*	h x μg/ml	154.9 ± 31.8	264.9 ± 63.2	457.1 ± 114.8
λZ	1/h	0.145 ± 0.040	0.148 ± 0.041	0.145 ± 0.061
λZ T½	h	5.1 ± 1.4	5.0 ± 1.3	5.7 ± 2.8
MRT	h	7.26 ± 2.13	7.81 ± 1.70	8.39 ± 3.67

Thus the origin of analysed SA values may be caused by a medication with SA or ASA which is metabolized to SA as well as by SA as a feeding component of plant origin (alfalfa hay, willow bark). With a LLOD (LLOQ) of 0.1 μg/mL (0.3 μg/mL) plasma the method is sensitive enough to detect an ASA administration, because mean population values of SA were reported to be about 0.23 μg/mL. The LLOD (LLOQ) for urine was determined to be 1 (5) μg/mL which is adequate considering the high mean population value of 27.3 μg/mL [11]. The SA concentration in plasma and urine samples (blanks) of the horses used in the described study was less than 0.3 μg/mL plasma and between <5 and 51 μg/mL urine.

According to our data, ASA inhibits COX-1 more potently than COX-2, with IC_{50} values of 1.68 μmol/L and 17.02 μmol/L, respectively. This finding is supported by the fact that ASA is known to only inhibit COX-1 irreversibly [16, 17]. The IC_{50} values calculated for ASA confirm results from other non-equine where ASA IC_{50} values from 1.67 to 4.45 μmol/L for COX-1 and from 5.34 to 15.9 μmol/L for COX-2 were described [18–21]. On the contrary, Vane and Botting [22] calculated an

Table 3 Inhibition of COX-1 and COX-2 activity (%) by ASA and SA; calculated based on in vitro assays (mean ± S.D. of experiments with equine blood samples of 6 horses)

Concentration (μmol/l)	ASA		SA	
	COX I	COX II	COX I	COX II
0.1	9.1 ± 3.6	9.8 ± 4.6	19.6 ± 9.5	4.7 ± 2.3
1.0	30.8 ± 16.0	12.6 ± 8.3	13.0 ± 5.7	15.3 ± 9.3
10.0	87.0 ± 11.5	37.9 ± 29.3	22.8 ± 10.0	10.3 ± 3.4
100.0	93.6 ± 10.3	60.9 ± 23.4	32.2 ± 21.1	−4.7 ± 3.2
1000.0	92.7 ± 12.9	75.7 ± 32.7	65.8 ± 28.4	26.8 ± 11.3

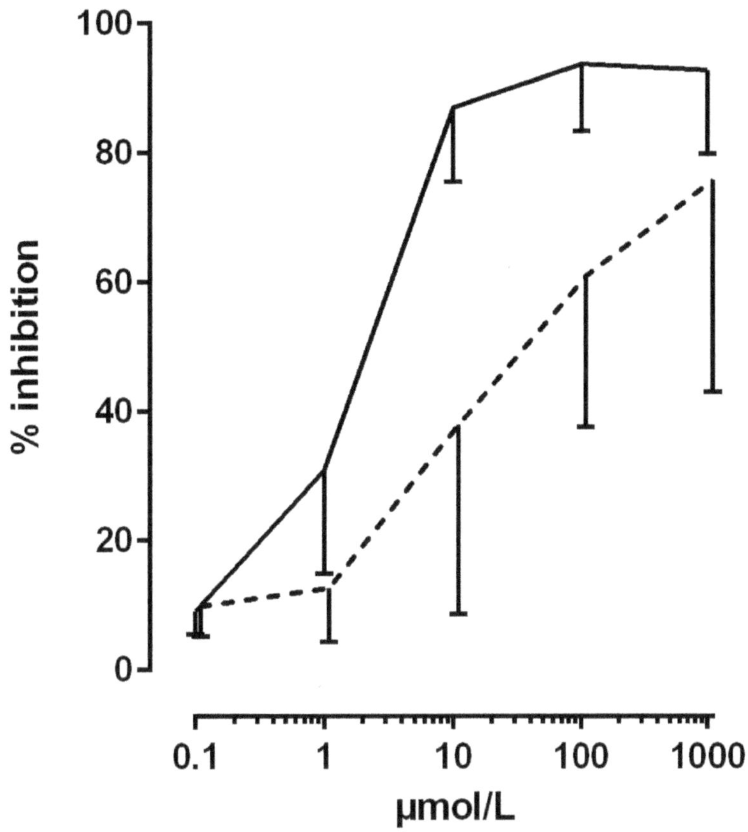

Fig. 7 Inhibition of COX-1 (black line) and COX-2 (dashed line) by ASA as a result of in vitro assays performed with equine blood; mean ± S.D. of 6 single experiments

ASA IC_{50} of 278 µmol/L for COX-2. SA did not inhibit either COX effectively enough to calculate an IC_{50} value for the concentrations used in this study (up to 1000 µmol/L). Similar findings have been reported in other studies [18, 19, 21]. However, since SA does have a clinically proven effect [23] there has to be another mode of action. An action trough NF-κB or gentisic acid is just mentioned, but no specific role of these factors has been proposed to explain the anti-inflammatory activity of SA [21, 24].

In doping control the international threshold for SA in plasma is 6.5 µg/mL. This means that a SA confirmation may only be reported as "positive" if the detected concentration is above this limit. A SA concentration above this threshold can not be explained by SA as a feeding component. Measuring SA concentrations below the threshold level, it remains unclear if the measured SA concentration is caused by an ASA or SA medication or by SA as a feeding component [5, 11]. The presented excretion study should give evidence in how far this threshold is exceeded after a therapeutic medication of ASA.

The threshold was exceeded by 30 min and eight 8 h following oral administration of 25 and 50 mg/kg ASA, respectively. Twenty-four hours after administration of 25 mg/kg and thirty-six hours after administration of 50 mg/kg plasma concentrations of all horses were below the threshold again. The lower dosage of 12.5 mg/kg which may be used because of the antithrombotic effects of ASA, led to "positive" concentrations for 12 h after administration. Thus the detection period of an ASA administration in a blood sample is rather short.

The detection of an ASA medication is even more difficult in urine samples when applying the urine threshold of 750 µg/mL. Concentrations higher than this level were only detected for 24 h after the 50 mg/kg and for 12 h after administration of the 25 or 12.5 mg/kg dose. After administration of 12.5 mg/kg one horse did not exceed the threshold at all.

As the detection period of an ASA medication (time of SA above the threshold) is less than one day in almost all horses of our study, it has to be discussed whether its therapeutic effect can be controlled adequately with the existing rules.

Broome et al. [4] described a rapid decline of the ASA concentration after intravenous administration of 20 mg/kg ASA to horses. The ASA concentration was below 0.1 µg/mL after four hours [4]. Comparing the ASA concentrations measured by Broome et al. (2003)

with the IC_{50} values calculated in the described study, it can be concluded that a COX-1 inhibitory effect may be reached for a period of about 3 to 4 h. A COX-2 inhibition should be expected for only 1.5 h. There are hints that salicylates accumulate in synovial fluid after systemic administration, as demonstrated *in vitro* by Friebe et al. [25] who simulated a systemic ASA treatment with 20 mg/kg I.V. in the isolated perfused equine distal limb. Extrapolated from synovial fluid concentrations measured in *vitro*, a COX-1 inhibitory effect can be expected in the joint for about 6 to 8 h (COX-1) and 2 h (COX-2). The results of the *in vitro* and *in vivo* studies [26] indicate that even if SA values in plasma and urine fall below the thresholds, one cannot exclude any therapeutic effect, especially since NSAIDs are generally known to accumulate in inflammatory exudate [27].

Conclusion

The established SA thresholds of 750 μg//mL urine and 6.5 μg/mL plasma appear too generous and are leaving space for misuse of the anti-inflammatory and analgetic compound ASA especially for countries where horse feed is not naturally rich in salicylates.

Abbreviations

ASA: Acetylsalicylic acid; COX: Cyclooxygenase; DMSO: Dimethyl sulfoxide; FEI: International Equestrian Federation; HPLC-MS/MS: High performance liquid chromatography–mass spectrometry; LLOQ: Lower limit of quantification; LPS: Lipopolysaccharide; PGE: Prostaglandin E; SA: Salicylic acid; TXB: Thromboxane B

Acknowledgements

The authors would like to thank the German Equestrian Federation (FN, Warendorf, Germany) for financial support.

Funding

German Equestrian Federation (FN, Warendorf, Germany).

Authors'contributions

Study design: MK, MD, KB. Pharmacokinetic study: KB, MF. In vitro study: KB, MF, MK. Analytics: KB, IS, MM. Preparation of the manuscript: KB, MF, IS, MK. Critical review of the manuscript: WS, MM, MD. All authors read and approved the final manuscript.

Competing interests

The authors declare that they have no competing interests.

Consent for publication

Not applicable.

Author details

[1]Institute of Pharmacology, Toxicology and Pharmacy, University of Veterinary Medicine Hannover Foundation, Hannover, Germany. [2]Institute for Biochemistry, German Sport University, Cologne, Germany. [3]Sassenberg, Germany.

References

1. Maclagan T. The treatment of rheumatism by salicin and salicylic acid. Br Med J. 1876;1:627.
2. Dun F. Veterinary medicines, their actions and uses. 9th ed. Edinburgh: David Douglas; 1895. p. 601–5.
3. Dreser H. Pharmakologisches über Aspirin (Acetylsalicylsäure). Pflügers Archiv Eur J Physiol. 1899;76:306–18.
4. Broome TA, Brown MP, Gronwall RR, Casey MF, Meritt KA. Pharmacokinetics and plasma concentrations of acetylsalicylic acid after intravenous, rectal, and intragastric administration to horses. Can J Vet Res. 2003;67:297–302.
5. Beaumier P, Fenwick J, Young L, Hazen S, Hama K, Laviolette B, Deocampo Z, Park H, Sio N, Timmings S, Todi F. Salicylic acid in the horse: Studies conducted for agriculture canada by the canadian race testing laboratories. In: The Canadian Section, Association of Official Racing Chemists, Can Test Limited, Mann Testing Laboratories Ltd. and Lynn & Johnston Laboratories Inc. 1983. p. 12–20.
6. Anonymus. Final version vet regs salicylic acid threshold. Fédération Equestre Internationale (FEI). 2010.
7. Moss MS, Blay P, Houghton E, Horner MW, Teale P, Smith RL, Sloan T. Normal and post-administration concentrations of salicylic acid in thoroughbred horses. In: Macmillan Publishers (HK) Limited, Hong Kong and The Royal Hong Kong Jockey Club, Hong Kong. 1985. p. 97–102.
8. Lakhani KH, Lambert M, Sluyter F, Devolz R, Maylin G, Higgins AJ. Estimation of the critical threshold value for presence of salicylic acid in the urine of thoroughbred horses. In: R & W Communications, Newmarket. 2004. p. 67–77.
9. Toutain PL, Lassourd V. Pharmacokinetic/pharmacodynamic approach to assess irrelevant plasma or urine drug concentrations in postcompetition samples for drug control in horses. Equine Vet J. 2002;34:242–9.
10. Robinson N. Table of drugs, approximate doses. In: Ed Robinson N, editor. Appendix 1: Table of drugs, approximate doses. Philadelphia: WB Saunders Company; 1997. p. 753–60.
11. Schenk I, Machnik M, Roettgen H, Flenker U, Guddat S, Schänzer W. Evaluation of salicylic acid concentrations in horse blood and urine with regard to the actual threshold, Proceedings 19th International Conference of Racing Analysts and Veterinarians. Philadelphia: ICRAV; 2012.
12. Thomas A, Guddat S, Kohler M, Krug O, Schänzer W, Petrou M, Thevis M. Comprehensive plasma-screening for known and unknown substances in doping controls. Rapid Commun Mass Spectrom. 2010;24:1124–32.
13. Anonymus. Guidelines for analysis of samples from pharmacokinetic studies, Guidelines of EHSLC, 03. London: The Jockey Club, Portman Square; 2002.
14. Brideau C, van Staden C, Chan CC. In vitro effects of cyclooxygenase inhibitors in whole blood of horses, dogs, and cats. Am J Vet Res. 2001;62:1755–60.
15. McCann ME, Andersen DR, Zhang D, Brideau C, Black WC, Hanson PD, Hickey GJ. In vitro effects and in vivo efficacy of a novel cyclooxygenase-2 inhibitor in dogs with experimentally induced synovitis. Am J Vet Res. 2004;65: 503–12.
16. Vane JR, Bakhle YS, Botting RM. Cyclooxygenases 1 and 2. Ann Rev Pharmacol Toxicol. 1998;38:97–120.
17. Vane JR, Botting RM. The mechanism of action of aspirin. Thromb Res. 2003; 110:255–8.
18. Cromlish WA, Kennedy BP. Selective inhibition of cyclooxygenase-1 and –2 using intact insect cell assays. Biochem Pharmacol. 1996;52:1777–85.
19. Cryer B, Feldman M. Cyclooxygenase-1 and cyclooxygenase-2 selectivity of widely used nonsteroidal anti-inflammatory drugs. Am J Med. 1998; 104:413–21.
20. Giuliano F, Warner TD. Ex vivo assay to determine the cyclooxygenase selectivity of non-steroidal anti-inflammatory drugs. Br J Pharmacol. 1999; 126:1824–30.
21. Hinz B, Kraus V, Pahl A, Brune K. Salicylate metabolites inhibit cyclooxygenase-2-dependent prostaglandin E(2) synthesis in murine macrophages. Biochem Biophys Res Commun. 2000;274:197–202.
22. Vane JR, Botting RM. New insights into the mode of action of anti-inflammatory drugs. Inflamm Res. 1995;44:1–10.
23. Preston SJ, Arnold MH, Beller EM, Brooks PM, Buchanan WW. Comparative analgesic and anti-inflammatory properties of sodium salicylate and acetylsalicylic acid (aspirin) in rheumatoid arthritis. Br J Clin Pharmacol. 1989; 27:607–11.

24. Kopp E, Ghosh S. Inhibition of NF-kappa B by sodium salicylate and aspirin. Science. 1994;265:956–9.
25. Friebe M, Schumacher S, Stahl J, Kietzmann M. Synovial distribution of "systemically" administered acetylsalicylic acid in the isolated perfused equine distal limb. BMC Vet Res. 2013;9:56.
26. Lehmann W, Wintzer HJ, Frey HH. Kinetics of Anti-Inflammatory Drugs in Serum and Synovia of Horses. Dtsch tierärztl Wschr. 1981;88:218–20.
27. Lees P, Taylor JBO, Higgins AJ, Sharma SC. Phenylbutazone and Oxyphenbutazone Distribution into Tissue Fluids in the Horse. J vet Pharmacol Therap. 1986;9:204–12.

Modulating effects of exercise training regimen on skeletal muscle properties in female polo ponies

Metha Chanda[1], Ratchakrit Srikuea[1], Worakij Cherdchutam[2], Arthit Chairoungdua[1] and Pawinee Piyachaturawat[1*]

Abstract

Background: The match play patterns in equestrian polo are unique and require specific training programs to ensure sport performance. The effect of commonly used exercise training regimens on the adaptation of skeletal muscle is unclear. The present study investigated the modulating effects of the classic training regimen, comprised of aerobic exercise training with increasing exercise intensities and varying duration combined with match play, on the properties of muscle in polo ponies. Nine healthy adult female polo ponies were subjected to four consecutive subsets of 1 year classic training regimen including basal activity (B), low intensity (L), low to moderate intensity (LM), and low to moderate intensity training plus match play during polo tournament (LMP), respectively. At the end of each training period, gluteus medius muscle samples were taken for determination of muscle fiber type distribution, muscle metabolic capacity, capillary density, and lipid and glycogen content. The expression profile of metabolic genes including succinate dehydrogenase (SDH), phosphofructokinase (PFK), glycogen phosphorylase (PYG), and glycogen synthase (GYS) were also measured.

Results: Among all exercise training subsets, only LMP exercise period caused an increase in the number of oxidative fibers (type IIa), along with increases in properties related to oxidative metabolism including high capillary density, intramuscular lipid content, and expression of SDH and PYG genes, with a corresponding decrease in the number of type IIx muscle fibers.

Conclusion: The combination of low to moderate and high intensity training in LMP are only sufficient to induce changes in oxidative characteristics. As the first scientific evidence providing such insight about the classic polo training regimen, the data forms a basis for further consideration in training program design.

Keywords: Exercise training, Horse, Match play, Polo pony, Skeletal muscle adaptation

Background

Achievement in competition of athletic horses depends on genetic contributions and the ability to improve muscle performance via exercise training. The effectiveness of the response to the training depends upon the extent of stimuli [1], training volume, as determined by frequency, intensity, and duration [2]. Adaptation of muscle properties to exercise training is well documented in several equestrian disciplines including racing [2, 3], endurance riding [4], and show jumping [5]. Aerobic exercise training is generally included in basic exercise training programs in all equestrian horses inducing adaptation of skeletal muscle towards oxidative characteristics [2, 6, 7]. Increases in the proportion of oxidative muscle fibers (type IIa), number of capillaries, and SDH activity have been demonstrated after aerobic exercise training in Thoroughbred horses [2]. Moreover, aerobic training reportedly increases activity of 3-hydoxyacyl-CoA dehydrogenase (HAD) and citrate synthase (CS) accompanied by decreased glycogen utilization in Standardbred horses [6]. At a cellular level, exercise training effects several genes responsible for oxidative energy metabolism and muscle structure. Training increases expression of cytochrome c oxidase subunit 4 (COX4), pyruvate dehydrogenase complex (PDC), and pyruvate dehydrogenase kinase (PDK) in Thoroughbred horse [8, 9]. In contrast, anaerobic exercise training

* Correspondence: pawinee.pia@mahidol.ac.th
[1]Department of Physiology, Faculty of Science, Mahidol University, Rama 6 Rd., Rachatewee, Bangkok 10400, Thailand
Full list of author information is available at the end of the article

promotes glycolytic capacity in some sport disciplines, i.e. Thoroughbred racehorses [10].

Although the majority of horses in equestrian sports undergo individual exercise training and competition, the difference in exercise regimen is notable in equestrian polo. Polo ponies are trained as a group during the preparation period before tournaments. In tournaments, two teams of four players play against each other on a grass field area of approximately ten acres [11]. A game is made up of 4–6 periods (chukkas) 7 min in duration each. The common training regimen in equestrian polo, consists of three phases of increasing intensity, starting with low to moderate intensity – walking and trotting – and progressing to high intensity — particular field training for specific activities and match play [12]. During polo games, the horses undergo intermittent high intensity exercise as well as swift changes in speed and direction. Hence, both muscle oxidative and glycolytic capacities are crucial factors for accomplishment during polo match play in seasonal tournaments. Unfortunately, there is no evidence of the effectiveness of the classic exercise training regimen commonly used in polo ponies on their skeletal muscle properties. Therefore, the present study investigated the effects of the polo training regimen on the skeletal muscle properties related to the muscular performance including fiber type composition, metabolic capacity, substrate utilization, and the expression of metabolic genes in polo ponies.

Methods

Horses

Nine healthy polo ponies (mares, age 11.9 ± 2 years, weight 452.6 ± 14.8 kg) from a Thai polo and equestrian club (Pattaya, Chonburi, Thailand) were recruited. All horses regularly participated in polo seasonal tournaments (5 months/year). They were housed in 3 × 3 m^2 separate stalls, fed with standard commercial pellet twice daily, and had free access to water and pangola hay.

Exercise training program and muscle sampling

All horses were subjected to a training program with progressive increases in exercise intensity. Horses were randomly assigned to participate in 0–14 goal match play during polo tournament. The exercise program consisted of four consecutive periods of different exercise intensities including basal activity (B); low intensity (L); low to moderate intensity exercise (LM); and low to moderate intensity plus match play (LMP). The LMP period was divided into low to moderate intensity exercise (LM), training match play (TM), and official match play (OM). The activities, mode, frequency, and duration of each training period are summarized in Table 1. Exercise intensity was determined by heart rate (HR), expressed as a percent of maximum heart rate (%HR_{max}) based on the regression analysis [13]. The duration of training period, speed, distance covered, and HR were recorded using Polar RC3 GPS sport watches connected to H3 heart rate sensors (Polar Electro, Kempele, Finland). Blood lactate concentrations were determined before and immediately after exercise sessions and match play using an Accutrend® Plus system autoanalyzer (Roche Diagnostics, Rotkreuz, Switzerland). During training match or official match play, all parameters were recorded from the horses ridden by the player at position number 2 (attack) for four chukkas.

Twenty-four hours after each training session, gluteus medius samples were taken by microbiopsy according to the modified method of Lindholm and Piehl [14]. Briefly, skin was subcutaneously injected with local anesthesia (1 ml of 2 % lidocaine) (L.B.S. Laboratory, Bangkok, Thailand). Then, muscle samples were taken at the middle of an imaginary line from tuber coxae to the greater trochanter of femoral bone at 50 mm depth using a 14 G semi-automated microbiopsy needle (SuperCore™, Argon Medical Devices, Texas, USA). The biopsy depth used has been employed in previous studies to collect mixed types of muscle fibers [15–17]. Muscle samples (wet weight approximately 60–70 mg) were divided into two portions. A piece of each sample was immediately embedded with optimal cutting temperature (O.C.T.) compound (Electron Microscopy Sciences, Pennsylvania, USA), then frozen in melting isopentane (Sigma-Aldrich, Missouri, USA), and stored at −80 °C for histochemical/immunohistochemical analyses. The other muscle portion was directly frozen in liquid nitrogen and stored at −80 °C for molecular analyses.

Histochemical and immunohistochemical analyses

Transverse cross-sections of O.C.T. preserved samples were obtained using cryostat (Leica Biosystems, Nussloch, Germany) at −20 °C. Five μm thickness serial sections were stained for succinate dehydrogenase (SDH) level, fiber type composition, and capillary density evaluations. The intramuscular lipid and glycogen contents were also stained using ten μm thickness serial sections. All protocols were performed at room temperature unless noted.

Fiber type composition

Muscle fiber types were determined according to the modified method of Kawai et al. [18]. Sections were air dried for 10 min and pre-incubated in 1 % normal goat serum (Sigma-Aldrich, Missouri, USA) for 10 min. Thereafter, three different primary monoclonal antibodies were applied separately including: 1) fast myosin (Sigma-Aldrich, Missouri, USA) (1:4000) that specifically binds with myosin heavy chain (MHC) IIa and IIx; 2) SC-71 (Developmental Studies Hybridoma Bank, Iowa, USA) (1:1000) that specifically binds with MHC-IIa;

Table 1 Practical classic exercise training regimen for one year

Training phase	Training period	Exercise mode	Exercise frequency	Exercise duration (estimated min)	Exercise intensity
1. Basal activity (B)	1st -22nd wk	Resting in stable and pasturing in paddock during off-season	Graze in the paddock 2–3 h a day	-	-
2. Low intensity exercise training (L)	23th-26th wk	Walking only	Twice a day, 6 days/week	~60	Very low
3. Low to moderate intensity exercise training (LM)	27th-30th wk	Walking (25 min) → Trotting (15min) → Walking (20 min)	Twice a day, 6 days/week	~60	Low to Moderate
4. Low to moderate intensity exercise training plus match play (LMP)	31st-53rd wk	Walking (25 min) → Trotting (15min) → Walking (20 min) (LM session)	Twice a day or once a day on the day with competition. 6 days/week	~60	Low to Moderate
		Training (TM) or official (OM) match play sessions	A horse plays 2–4 chukkas a day, 3–4 days/week	~7	Moderate to Very hard

On competition days in LMP period (polo tournaments), horses trained at low to moderate intensity exercise (LM session) in the morning and participated in polo match play in the evening 3–4 day/week

and 3) BF-35 (Developmental Studies Hybridoma Bank, Iowa, USA) (1:1000) that reacts with all MHCs except MHC-IIx. The serial sections were then incubated overnight in a moist chamber. After washing with PBS, the sections were incubated with goat anti-mouse IgG conjugated with horseradish peroxidase (HRP) secondary antibody (Merck Millipore, Massachusetts, USA) (1:500) for 2 h and washed with PBS. Subsequently, sections were incubated with diaminobenzidine tetrahydrochloride (DAB) (Sigma-Aldrich, Missouri, USA) in a dark environment for 3 min and mounted with temporary mounting medium (Vectors Lab, California, USA).

Muscle oxidative capacity

Oxidative fibers were determined by SDH staining according to the method previously described [19]. Briefly, muscle sections were incubated at 37 °C in solution containing 0.2 M PBS, succinic acid disodium, and nitroblue tetrazolium (Sigma-Aldrich, Missouri, USA) in a dark environment for 1 h. Thereafter, the sections were rinsed with series of acetone (30, 60, and 30 % concentrations) followed by distilled water prior to mounting with temporary mounting medium (Vectors Lab, California, USA).

Intramuscular lipid and glycogen content

Lipid content was determined using Oil Red O staining according to the method of Lillie and Ashburn [20]. Glycogen content was evaluated by using Periodic Acid Schiff (PAS) staining according to the modified method of Kocsis et al. [21].

Capillary density

The number of capillaries were analyzed using double labeling of anti-endothelial cell (CD31) and dystrophin protein to visualize muscle fiber. Briefly, the sections were pre-fixed with ice-cold acetone at 4 °C for 10 min, then rehydrated with PBS. After blocking with 10 % normal goat serum (Sigma-Aldrich, Missouri, USA) for 1 h, the sections were simultaneously incubated with polyclonal rabbit anti-CD31 primary antibody (Abcam, Cambridge, UK) (1:100) and monoclonal mouse anti-dystrophin primary antibody (Sigma-Aldrich, Missouri, USA) (1:100) for 1 h, and then washed with PBS. Thereafter, Alexa Fluor 568 conjugated-goat anti-mouse secondary antibody (Invitrogen, California, USA) (1:500) and Alexa Fluor 488 conjugated-goat anti-rabbit secondary antibody (Invitrogen, California, USA) (1:500) were applied simultaneously for 1 h. After washing with PBS, the sections were post-fixed with 4 % paraformaldehyde for 10 min and counterstained with DAPI (Invitrogen, California, USA) (1:10,000) for 5 min. The stained sections were mounted with fluoroshield mounting medium (Sigma-Aldrich, Missouri, USA).

Image analysis

All stained sections were visualized under a microscope (Olympus BX53) connected with a digital camera (Olympus DP73) (Olympus, Tokyo, Japan) and captured at 200× magnification, except fiber type composition determination that were captured at 100× magnification. All histological images were quantified using ImageJ software version 1.47v. Histological images of SDH, Oil Red O, and PAS stained sections were analyzed as the area of expression according to the modified method of Rinnankoski-Tuikka et al. [22]. A minimum of four captured images were analyzed for each staining. The color images were converted to 8-bit gray-scale (range of grey levels 0–255) images before processing. The threshold of staining was manually adjusted and kept constant between samples. The oxidative capacity, intramuscular lipid, and glycogen contents were expressed as percentage of the measured area. Muscle fiber types were classified according to the specific reaction with antibodies as type I, IIa, IIa/x, and IIx. The percentage of fiber distribution and cross-sectional area were measured and calculated from between 300–500 muscle fibers. The capillary density was quantified as capillary per fiber ratio from 150 to 250 muscle fibers.

Quantitative real-time PCR for mRNA expression

Total RNAs were extracted from muscle samples using a Trizol® Reagent (Ambion, Texas, USA) and enhancing precipitation with Rnase-free glycogen (Ambion, Texas, USA) according to the manufacturer's instructions. The purity and yield of total RNA were determined by measuring the absorbance at 260 and 280 nm using a NanoDrop 2000c UV–vis spectrophotometer. cDNAs were synthesized by using iScript™ cDNA synthesis kit (Bio-Rad, California, USA) and stored at −20 °C until analysis. The cDNA products were analyzed by real-time PCR using KAPA SYBR® FAST quantitative PCR kit (Kapa Biosystems, Massachusetts, USA) in StepOne Real Time PCR system (Applied Biosystems, Massachusetts, USA). The followings are sequences of the target gene primers: SDH (NM_001163823), 5'-GGCTCTACGAGTGCATC CTC-3' and 5'-GCCCAAATACTTGTCCCCGT-3'; PFK (NM_001081922), 5'-TCCAGCCAGCTTCCTCAATTCT G-3' and 5'-CATCCAGGGCAACCGAGTG-3'; GYS (NM_001126125), 5'-GCTTTGGGACACCTGCAACA-3' and 5'-GCCAGGAACTCACCCAGGAAC-3'; PYG (NM_001145253), 5'-TCGACAGATCATCGAGCAGC-3' and 5'-CTTTAAACCGGTCGTGGTGC-3'; β-actin (NM_00 1081838), 5'-GCACCAGGGCGTGATGG-3' and 5'-TCG ATGGGGTACTTGAGGGT-3'. The mRNA level of each gene was normalized to mRNA level of β-actin.

Statistical analysis

The data from histological analysis and metabolic enzyme mRNA expression were analyzed using one-way ANOVA with repeated measurement followed by Tukey's post hoc. Normal distribution and homogeneity of variance were analyzed by Kolmogorov Smirnov test and Levene's test, respectively. Paired Student's t-test was used where applicable. The statistical analysis was performed using SPSS version 18.0.0. All data are expressed as means ± SD. Significant differences were considered at $p < 0.05$.

Results

Heart rate and blood lactate concentration

Heart rate and blood lactate concentration in relation to distance covered and speed during each exercise training period of the classic polo training regimen are shown in Table 2. The maximum heart rate during exercise in B period was 37.1 ± 1 bpm (17 ± 1.1 % HR_{max}) and 41.7 ± 2.9 bpm (19 ± 1.3 % HR_{max}) during exercise in L period. The maximum heart rate increased substantially during LM period (HR = 144.3 ± 20.5 bpm, 65.6 ± 6.2 % HR_{max}) ($p < 0.01$). When horses participated in a polo match play, maximum heart rate increased substantially to approximately 175.0 ± 5.2 bpm (80 ± 1.7 % HR_{max}) in TM sessions and 195.3 ± 13.1 bpm (88.8 ± 6.7 % HR_{max}) with a maximum heart rate of 208 bpm during OM sessions. Of note, exercise in both L and LM periods produced blood lactate below threshold (<4 mmol/L); while, exercise in both kinds of match play (TM and OM) sessions produced blood lactate above threshold (>4 mmol/L). Furthermore, lactate concentration during OM was considerably higher than during TM (OM; 8.9 ± 0.6 mmol/L vs. TM; 4.2 ± 0.8 mmol/L). Maximum heart rate variation corresponded to exercise intensity – low, moderate, and moderate to very hard for L, LM, and LMP, respectively.

Muscle fiber type composition and fiber size

As shown in Fig. 1, muscle fiber types were differentially stained for specific expression of myosin heavy chain (MHC) isoforms. In the basal period (B), gluteus medius muscle consisted of type I, type IIa, type IIa/x, and type IIx at approximately 25.1 ± 8.0, 44.9 ± 6.0, 5.8 ± 2.4, and 24.8 ± 6.3 %, respectively. The percentage of muscle fiber type IIx significantly decreased in LMP compared to B and L periods ($p < 0.01$) (Fig. 2a). The decrease in the number of type IIx was accompanied by an increase in the number of type IIa and I muscle fibers, but this finding was not statistically significant ($p > 0.05$). Analysis of changes of fiber type in individual animals revealed 8 out of 9 animals experienced increases in type IIa fibers, and 7 out of 9 animals experienced increases in type I fibers after the LMP period compared to after the L period. Additional details are provided in the Additional file 1. The cross-sectional area (CSA) (μm^2) for muscle fiber types I, IIa, IIa/x, and IIx, were 2971 ± 549.5, 3176 ± 822.7, 3177 ± 578.9, and 4100 ± 434.2 μm^2 respectively. No statistically significant differences in CSA of individual muscle fiber types were found throughout the course of the study (Fig. 2b).

Oxidative capacity, substrate contents, and capillary density

Histological images of SDH staining, as well as intramuscular lipid and glycogen contents are shown in Fig. 3. The number of SDH-positive fibers significantly increased after the polo tournament period (LMP) compared to B and L periods (B; 35.9 ± 11.2 % vs. LMP; 74.4 ± 4.7 %, $p < 0.01$ and L; 36.9 ± 8.6 % vs. LMP; 74.4 ± 4.7 %, $p < 0.01$). Intramuscular lipid content also increased significantly after LMP period (B; 4.0 ± 0.8 % vs. LMP; 7.8 ± 2.0 %, $p < 0.01$ and L; 4.2 ± 0.2 % vs. LMP; 7.8 ± 2.0 %, $p < 0.01$); whereas, glycogen content was not altered throughout the study (Table 3). The capillary density expressed as capillary per fiber ratio significantly increased after LMP period (B; 1.0 ± 0.1 % vs. LMP; 1.4 ± 0.2 %, $p < 0.01$ and L; 1.0 ± 0.2 % vs. LMP; 1.4 ± 0.2 %, $p < 0.01$) (Fig. 4).

Table 2 Heart rate, blood lactate, speed, distance, and duration of a single bout of exercise in each exercise training period

Parameters		Consecutive exercise training periods for 1 year					
		B (22 weeks)	L (4 weeks)	LM (4 weeks)	LMP (22 weeks)		
					LM session	M	
						TM session	OM session
Distance covered (km)		-	6.6 ± 0.2	7.3 ± 0.1	7.3 ± 0.3	2.8 ± 0.1	1.4 ± 0.01
Duration (min)		-	58.3 ± 1.2	60.3 ± 0.6	60.1 ± 0.5	11.3 ± 0.8	7.9 ± 0.3
Speed (km/h)	Maximum speed	-	-	16.9 ± 1.1	17.0 ± 0.7	37.1 ± 5.2	47.4 ± 2.9
	Average speed	-	6.7 ± 0.1	6.7 ± 0.7	6.7 ± 0.8	14.7 ± 1.2[£†]	10.4 ± 0.4[£† ¶]
HR (bpm)	Resting HR	37.1 ± 1	37.3 ± 1.3	36.0 ± 2.5	36.7 ± 1.6	38.0 ± 2.0	42.3 ± 3.5
	Maximum HR	-	41.7 ± 2.9	144.3 ± 20.5	147.3 ± 13.3	175.0 ± 5.2	195.3 ± 13.1
	Average HR	-	38.0 ± 4	72.0 ± 4*	68.3 ± 4.4	132.3 ± 4.5[£ †]	137.0 ± 5.0[£ †]
	% HR_{max}	17 ± 1.1	19 ± 1.3	65.6 ± 6.2	66.8 ± 4.1	80 ± 1.7[£ †]	88.8 ± 6.7[£ †]
Blood lactate (mmol/L)	Before exercise	-	<0.9	1.4 ± 0.3	1.3 ± 0.2	1.9 ± 0.1	1.2 ± 0.1
	Immediately after exercise	<0.9	<0.9	1.1 ± 0.1	1.1 ± 0.1	4.2 ± 0.8[†]	8.9 ± 0.6[† ¶]

The activities in each period are different in the exercise intensity (means ± SD) ($n = 4$)
B basal activity, *L* low intensity exercise, *LM* low to moderate intensity exercise, *LMP* low to moderate intensity exercise plus match play, *M* match play, *TM* training match, *OM* official match, *HR* Heart rate
[£] $p < 0.01$; significantly different from L period
[†] $p < 0.01$; significantly different from LM
[¶] $p < 0.01$; significantly different from TM
[*] $p < 0.01$; significantly different from L period

Expression of metabolic genes

As the exercise intensity and the histological results of basal activity (B) and low intensity exercise training (L) period were similar, mRNA expression analysis at B period was omitted. After the polo tournaments (LMP period), expression of SDH and PYG genes increased significantly (~3.5 fold, $p < 0.01$, and ~3 fold, $p < 0.05$, respectively); whereas, there was a tendency to increase expression of PFK and GYS genes (~1.6 fold, $p = 0.076$, and ~2.3 fold, $p = 0.072$, respectively) (Fig. 5).

Discussion

According to the unique pattern of competition in equestrian polo, the properties of skeletal muscle are crucial factors determining performance in official match play. Surprisingly, little is known about the effects of the classic exercise regimen in equestrian polo on the adaptation of skeletal muscle properties and their relationship to the specific physiological demands of the sport. Interestingly, the major finding in the present study showed the exercise training regimen, particularly in LPM period of equestrian polo involving high intensity activity, evoked adaptation towards oxidative characteristics rather than glycolytic properties. Additionally, the training volume of the other training phases (L and LM) in the classic training regimen were not sufficient to induce changes in muscle properties. The oxidative adaptation of muscle fibers in the present study was evident in both biochemical and histological alterations. Muscle fiber types transitioned from fast to slow MHC phenotypes together with increased capillary density, oxidative enzymes, and associated substrates. The findings represent the first report on muscle adaptation in response to the classic exercise regimen in polo ponies.

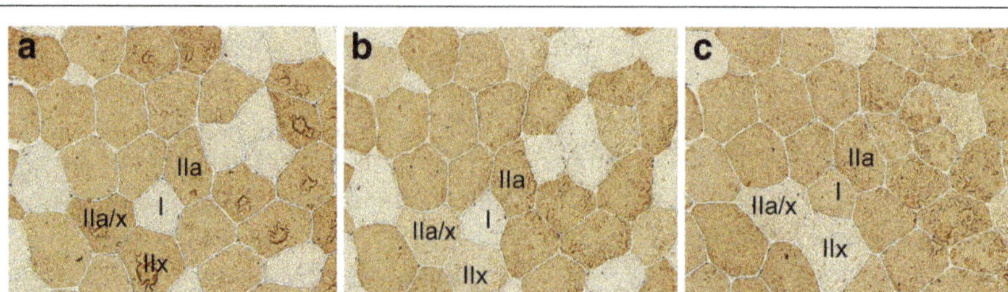

Fig. 1 Immunohistochemical staining of transverse sections of gluteus medius muscle from polo ponies at L period with monoclonal antibody against (**a**) MHC IIa, and IIx (fast myosin), (**b**) MHC IIa (SC-71), and (**c**) MHC all but IIx (BF-35). Muscle fibers are identified as type I (*unstained* in **a** and **b**), type IIa (*dark brown* stain in **b**) type IIa/x (*light stain* in **b** and **c**), and type IIx (*unstained* in **c**). Scale bars = 50 μm

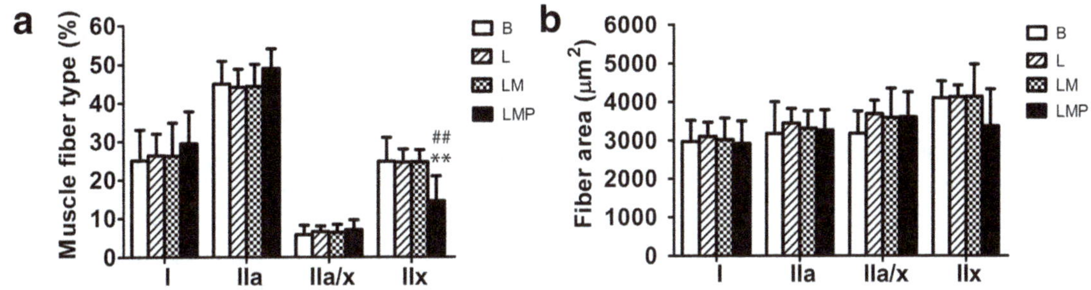

Fig. 2 Fiber type distribution and cross sectional area (CSA) (μm^2) of fibers in response to different exercise periods in polo ponies. **a** Changes in percentage of each muscle fiber type after basal activity (B), low intensity exercise training (L), low to moderate intensity exercise training (LM), and low to moderate intensity exercise training plus match play (LMP) periods. **b** Muscle CSA in response to the exercise regimen after B, L, LM, LMP periods. ** $p < 0.01$, significantly different from B value; $^{\#\#}p < 0.01$, significantly different from L value

Percent of maximal heart rate (%HR_{max}) has been used as an alternative to percent of VO_{2max} to indicate exercise intensity [13, 23, 24]. In the present study, exercise intensity was estimated from %HR_{max} and was classified as follows: very low (<50 % HR_{max}), low (50–63 % HR_{max}), moderate (64–76 % HR_{max}), hard (77–93 % HR_{max}), and very hard (≥94 % HR_{max}) as previously described [23]. Exercise intensity in L and LM were considered very light (L: 17 %%HR_{max}; LM: 33%HR_{max}), with a higher average heart rate during exercise in LM period reflecting the slightly higher intensity of exercise compared to L period. When horses participated in polo match play ,~7 min/chukka, they spent ~1 min ridden above 90 % HR_{max} (HR ≈ 195–208 bpm), followed by ~3 min ridden within ~68–89 % HR_{max} (HR ≈ 150–195 bpm), and another ~3 min ridden within ~41–68 % HR_{max} (HR ≈ 90–150 bpm). Thus, the majority of exercise period during match play in LMP period was considered moderate to very hard. The classical exercise pattern in equestrian polo utilizes both aerobic and anaerobic energy [24]. The latter is commonly indicated by blood lactate accumulation [25, 26]. In the present study, after low intensity (L) and low to moderated intensity (LM) exercise periods, blood lactate concentrations were far below the anaerobic threshold (<4 mmol/L), indicating these training regimens rely mainly on aerobic energy metabolism. However, it is worth noting that both intermittent high intensity exercise training match play (TM) and official match play (MO) in the LMP produced blood lactate concentrations above the anaerobic threshold (>4 mmol/L), indicating the anaerobic energy pathway becomes involved during polo match play. Accordingly, muscle glycolytic capacity is also crucial for this sport; however, classic exercise training regimens promotes the muscle oxidative capacity in all polo ponies rather than anaerobic properties found in only a few horses (Fig. 5c). The disparity between high glycolytic capacity required in match play and a training program promoting oxidative capacity only does not promote the sport capability of polo ponies. As glycolytic capacity is enhanced by anaerobic exercise training, the question arises as to whether additional anaerobic exercise –such as sprint exercise training – could increase glycolytic capacity, in turn, improving sport performance.

The effect of aerobic exercise training on muscle fiber type composition in horses has been reported [27, 28]. Transitions of MHC from type IIx to IIa during early training phases at approximately 3 months were observed [28]. As training duration increased up to 8 months, further muscle fiber transitions from MHC IIa to I were noted [20]. The changes reflected a dose–response relationship between exercise duration and magnitude of muscle property changes [21]. In the present study, type IIx fibers decreased along with marginal

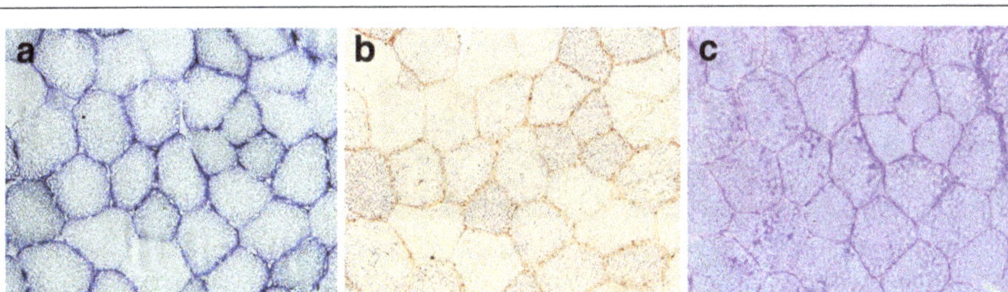

Fig. 3 Histochemical staining of gluteus medius muscle from polo ponies at L period. **a** SDH staining shows the *dark-purple* color that marks oxidative enzyme activity. **b** *Oil red* O staining shows the lipid droplet (*red color*) within the muscle fiber. **c** PAS Schiff reagent staining shows the *red-purple* color of the glycogen rich fiber. Scale bars = 50 μm

Table 3 Oxidative (SDH) capacity, intramuscular lipid content, and glycogen content (% area of expression) after basal activity (B), low intensity exercise training (L), low to moderate intensity exercise training (LM), and low to moderate intensity exercise training plus match play (LMP) periods

Metabolic properties	Consecutive exercise training activities			
	B	L	LM	LMP
Oxidative (SDH) capacity	35.9 ± 11.2	36.9 ± 8.6	46.1 ± 6.0	74.4 ± 4.7**,##
Lipid content	4.0 ± 0.8	4.1 ± 0.2	4.5 ± 0.9	7.8 ± 2.0**,##
Glycogen content	30.7 ± 4.7	30.2 ± 1.7	30.5 ± 2.8	29.9 ± 3.2

Each values were expressed as Mean ± SD ($n = 9$)
**$p < 0.01$, significantly different from B value
##$p < 0.01$, significantly different from L value

increases in type IIa muscle fibers in the post-LMP period. Analysis of fiber type changes in individual animals revealed eight out of nine animals showed increases in type IIa fibers, and seven out of nine animals showed increases in type I fibers after LMP compared to after L period. Thus, exercise intensity, duration, and the time course for sample collection are the primary variables accounting for the present results. As muscle samples were obtained at 1 month (L period), 2 months (LM period), and 7 months (LMP period) post-exercise onset (B period); it is possible insufficient exercise volume after 1 and 2 months of exercise training explains the lack of observable changes in fiber composition. Samples to represent LMP period were collected after 7 months of training; therefore, muscle fiber transitions from MHC IIa to I may be partially attributed to training duration instead of mode or phase; however, there was only a marginal increase in MHC IIa and a very slight increase in MHC I at the end of LMP period (Fig. 2a).

Increased oxidative capacity, as evidenced by SDH-positive staining, was concomitant with increased capillary density in polo ponies as has been reported in studies of angiogenesis [29]. Increased blood flow to muscle leads to splitting of capillaries as well as extensive endothelial cell proliferation and the formation of microtubes [30]. Thus, the classic exercise training regimen promotes oxidative properties in skeletal muscle of polo ponies.

In addition, expression of metabolic gene mRNA was consistent with phenotypic adaptation to training in polo ponies. At the end of polo tournaments, increased expression of oxidative marker (SDH) gene was closely correlated with increased numbers of SDH positive-stained fibers, indicating the classic exercise regimen induced oxidative capacity adaptation at a cellular level. Also, as anaerobic glycolysis exclusively uses carbohydrates in the absence of oxygen, increases in PYG along with marginal elevations of GYS and PFK mRNA expression were consistent with the increase in anaerobic glycolysis during polo tournaments. The classic exercise training regimen could increase, to a lesser extent than oxidative characteristics, glycolytic properties in muscle of polo ponies.

Since there were no changes to muscle properties after LM training period in the classic exercise regimen, polo ponies may start participating in polo tournaments with insufficient sport-specific performance. As a result, polo

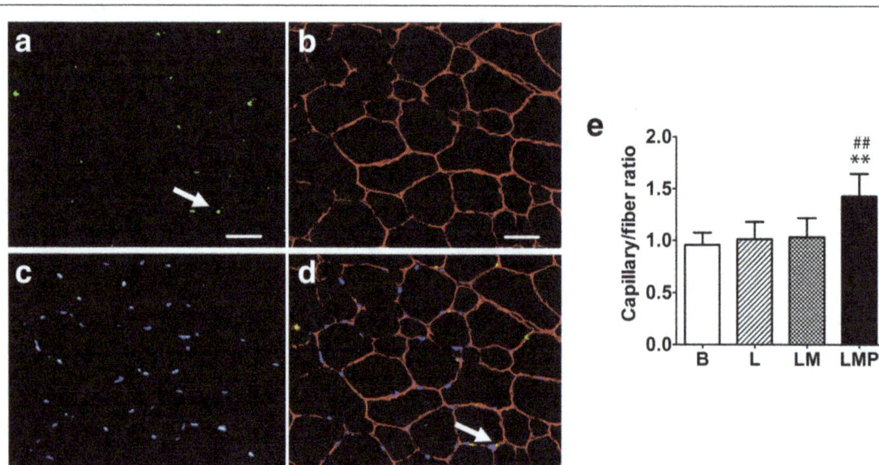

Fig. 4 Number of capillary density in response to different exercise regimens in polo pony including basal activity (B), low intensity exercise training (L), low to moderate intensity exercise training (LM), and low to moderate intensity exercise training plus match play (LMP) periods. **a** Immunostaining of CD31 to illustrate number of capillaries, (**b**) dystrophin protein visualization of muscle fiber membrane structure, (**c**) counterstaining with DAPI for nuclear localization and (**d**) merged image. *White arrows* indicate the capillary (*green spot*) within the muscle fiber. Scale bars = 50 μm. **e** Capillary density expressed as capillary per fiber ratio. Scale bars = 50 μm. ** $p < 0.01$, significantly different from B value; ##$p < 0.01$, significantly different from L value

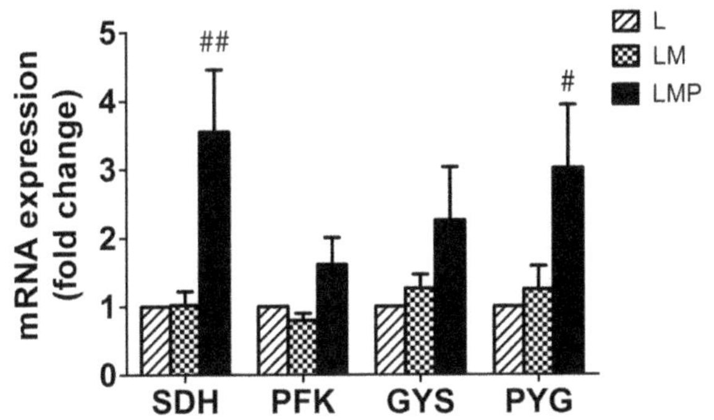

Fig. 5 Alterations in gene expression related to different exercise periods in polo ponies. Fold changes of metabolic enzyme mRNA expression including succinate dehydrogenase (SDH), phosphofructokinase (PFK), glycogen synthase (GYS), and glycogen phosphorylase (PYG) after basal activity (B), low intensity exercise training (L), low to moderate intensity exercise training (LM), and low to moderate intensity exercise training plus match play (LMP)periods. $^{\#\#}p < 0.01$, significantly different from L value; $^{\#}p < 0.05$, significantly different from L value

ponies are at potential risk of physical injury and metabolic disorders – such as exertional rhabdomyolysis – during and after polo match play. To improve muscle performance and minimize injury risk, starting exercise training further in advance of competition, as well as incorporating more intensity and longer duration sessions may be useful for the improvement of muscle performance.

Conclusion

The classic exercise regimen in polo ponies profoundly enhances oxidative capacity of muscle. To a lesser extent, it had a tendency to elevate glycolytic capacity. These results provide beneficial information for future research on the development of training programs to improve specific muscle performance in equestrian polo and associated equestrian sports.

Section

Clinical pathology, physiology and immunology.

Abbreviations

B: Basal activity; CSA: Cross-sectional area; DAB: Diaminobenzidine tetrahydrochloride; DAPI: 4',6-diamidino-2-phenylindole; GYS: Glycogen synthase; L: Low intensity exercise; LM: Low to moderate intensity exercise; LMP: Low to moderate intensity exercise plus match play; MHC: Myosin heavy chain; O.C.T.: Optimal cutting temperature; OM: Official match play; P: Phosphate buffer saline; PAS: Periodic acid–Schiff; PFK: Phosphofructokinase; PYG: Glycogen phosphorylase; SD: Standard deviation; SDH: Succinate dehydrogenase; SPSS: Statistical package for the social sciences; TM: Training match play

Acknowledgements

Our sincere thanks go to Mr. Harald Link, the President of the Thailand Equestrian Federation and the Thai Polo and Equestrian Club; and Ms. Nunthinee Tanner for the allocation of horses participating in this study. We also thank Dr. Santiago Bachmann and Dr. Teerapol Sathaporn for their animal arrangement, restraint, and care throughout the experiment. We are grateful to Professor Dr. Chumpol Pholpramool for critical reading of the manuscript and comments.

Funding

This work was financially supported by Kasetsart Veterinary Development Funds, Kasetsart University, Faculty of Veterinary Medicine. Bangkok, Thailand.

Authors' contributions

MC, RS and PP designed the experiment, collection of samples, immunohistochemical analysis, data analysis and write up manuscript. WC and AC performed functional analysis and biochemical analysis, respectively. PP adviser for the study and corresponding author. All authors read and approved the final manuscript.

Competing interests

The authors declare that they have no competing interests.

Consent for publication

Not applicable.

Author details

[1]Department of Physiology, Faculty of Science, Mahidol University, Rama 6 Rd., Rachatewee, Bangkok 10400, Thailand. [2]Department of Large Animal and Wildlife Clinical Science, Faculty of Veterinary Medicine, Kasetsart University Kamphaeng Saen Campus, Nakornpathom 73140, Thailand.

References

1. Tyler CM, Golland LC, Evans DL, Hodgson DR, Rose RJ. Skeletal muscle adaptations to prolonged training, overtraining and detraining in horses. Pflugers Arch. 1998;436(3):391–7.
2. Rivero JL, Ruz A, Marti-Korff S, Estepa JC, Aguilera-Tejero E, Werkman J, Sobotta M, Lindner A. Effects of intensity and duration of exercise on muscular responses to training of thoroughbred racehorses. J Appl Physiol (1985). 2007;102(5):1871–82.
3. Miyata H, Sugiura T, Kai M, Hiraga A, Tokuriki M. Muscle adaptation of Thoroughbred racehorses trained on a flat or sloped track. Am J Vet Res. 1999;60(12):1536–9.
4. Rivero J, Ruz MC, Serrano A, Diz A. Effects of a 3 month endurance training programme on skeletal muscle histochemistry in Andalusian, Arabian and Anglo-Arabian horses. Equine Vet J. 1995;27(1):51–9.
5. Rietbroek NJ, Dingboom EG, Joosten BJ, Eizema K, Everts ME. Effect of show jumping training on the development of locomotory muscle in young horses. Am J Vet Res. 2007;68(11):1232–8.
6. Hodgson DR, Rose RJ, DiMauro J, Allen JR. Effects of a submaximal treadmill training programme on histochemical properties, enzyme activities and glycogen utilisation of skeletal muscle in the horse. Equine Vet J. 1985;17(4):300–5.
7. Eaton MD, Hodgson DR, Evans DL, Rose RJ. Effects of low- and moderate-intensity training on metabolic responses to exercise in thoroughbreds. Equine Vet J Suppl. 1999;30:521–7.
8. Eivers SS, McGivney BA, Fonseca RG, MacHugh DE, Menson K, Park SD, Rivero J-LL, Taylor CT, Katz LM, Hill EW. Alterations in oxidative gene expression in equine skeletal muscle following exercise and training. Physiol Genomics. 2010;40(2):83–93.

9. McGivney BA, McGettigan PA, Browne JA, Evans AC, Fonseca RG, Loftus BJ, Lohan A, MacHugh DE, Murphy BA, Katz LM, et al. Characterization of the equine skeletal muscle transcriptome identifies novel functional responses to exercise training. BMC Genomics. 2010;11:398.
10. Eto D, Yamano S, Mukai K, Sugiura T, Nasu T, Tokuriki M, Miyata H. Effect of high intensity training on anaerobic capacity of middle gluteal muscle in Thoroughbred horses. Res Vet Sci. 2004;76(2):139–44.
11. Ferraz GC, Soares OA, Foz NS, Pereira MC, Queiroz-Neto A. The workload and plasma ion concentration in a training match session of high-goal (elite) polo ponies. Equine Vet J Suppl. 2010;38:191–5.
12. Giraudet A. Veterinary aspects of training and competing polo ponies. In: Hinchcliff KW, Kaneps AJ, Geor RJ, Bayly W, editors. Equine sports medicine and surgery. 2nd ed. Philadelphia: Saunders Ltd; 2014. p. 1107–12.
13. Marlin DJ, Allen JC. Cardiovascular demands of competition on low-goal (non-elite) polo ponies. Equine Vet J. 1999;31(5):378–82.
14. Lindholm A, Piehl K. Fibre composition, enzyme activity and concentrations of metabolites and electrolytes in muscles of standardbred horses. Acta Vet Scand. 1974;15(3):287–309.
15. Galisteo AM, Agiüera E, Monterde JG, Miró F. Gluteus medius muscle fiber type composition in young Andalusian and Arabian horses. J Equine Vet Sci. 1992;12(4):254–8.
16. Lopez-Rivero JL, Serrano AL, Diz AM, Galisteo AM. Variability of muscle fibre composition and fibre size in the horse gluteus medius: an enzyme-histochemical and morphometric study. J Anat. 1992;181(Pt 1):1-10.
17. Ginneken MME. Adaptation of signal transduction and muscle proteome in trained horses. 2006.
18. Kawai M, Aida H, Hiraga A, Miyata H. Muscle satellite cells are activated after exercise to exhaustion in Thoroughbred horses. Equine Vet J. 2013;45(4):512–7.
19. Srikuea R, Symons TB, Long DE, Lee JD, Shang Y, Chomentowski PJ, Yu G, Crofford LJ, Peterson CA. Association of fibromyalgia with altered skeletal muscle characteristics which may contribute to postexertional fatigue in postmenopausal women. Arthritis Rheum. 2013;65(2):519–28.
20. Lillie RD, Ashburn LL. Supersaturated solutions of fat stains in dilute isopropanol for demonstration of acute fatty degeneration not shown by Herxheimer's technique. Arch Pathol. 1943;36:432–40.
21. Kocsis T, Baan J, Muller G, Mendler L, Dux L, Keller-Pinter A. Skeletal muscle cellularity and glycogen distribution in the hypermuscular Compact mice. Eur J Histochem. 2014;58(3):2353.
22. Rinnankoski-Tuikka R, Silvennoinen M, Torvinen S, Hulmi JJ, Lehti M, Kivela R, Reunanen H, Kainulainen H. Effects of high-fat diet and physical activity on pyruvate dehydrogenase kinase-4 in mouse skeletal muscle. Nutr Metab (Lond). 2012;9(1):53.
23. Medicine ACS. Benefit and risks associated with physical activity. In: Thompson WR, Gordon NF, Pescatello LS, editors. ACSM's guidelines for exercise testing and prescription. 8th ed. Philadelphia: Wolters Kluwer Health; 2010. p. 3–6.
24. Zobba R, Ardu M, Niccolini S, Cubeddu F, Dimauro C, Bonelli P, Dedola C, Visco S, Parpaglia MLP. Physical, hematological, and biochemical responses to acute intense exercise in polo horses. J Equine Vet Sci. 2011;31(9):542–8.
25. Spurway NC. Aerobic exercise, anaerobic exercise and the lactate threshold. Br Med Bull. 1992;48(3):569–91.
26. Murphy M, O'Connor L, Walsh D, Condon S. Oxygen dependent lactate utilization by Lactobacillus plantarum. Arch Microbiol. 1985;141(1):75–9.
27. Guy PS, Snow DH. The effect of training and detraining on muscle composition in the horse. J Physiol. 1977;269(1):33–51.
28. Serrano A, Quiroz-Rothe E, Rivero J-L. Early and long-term changes of equine skeletal muscle in response to endurance training and detraining. Pflugers Arch. 2000;441(2–3):263–74.
29. Brown MD, Hudlická O. Angiogenesis in Skeletal and Cardiac Muscle. In: Fan T-PD, Kohn EC, editors. The New Angiotherapy. Totowa, NJ: Humana Press; 2002. p. 213-48.
30. Prior BM, Yang H, Terjung RL. What makes vessels grow with exercise training? J Appl Physiol. 2004;97(3):1119–28.

9

A serosurvey of selected cystogenic coccidia in Spanish equids: first detection of anti-*Besnoitia* spp. specific antibodies in Europe

Daniel Gutiérrez-Expósito[1], Ignacio García-Bocanegra[2], Daniel K. Howe[3], Antonio Arenas-Montes[2], Michelle R. Yeargan[3], SallyAnne L. Ness[4], Luis M. Ortega-Mora[1] and G. Álvarez-García[1*]

Abstract

Background: Equine besnoitiosis, caused by *Besnoitia bennetti,* and equine protozoal myeloencephalitis (EPM), caused by *Sarcocystis neurona* and *Neospora hughesi* are relevant equine diseases in the Americas that have been scarcely studied in Europe. Thus, a serosurvey of these cystogenic coccidia was carried out in Southern Spain. A cross-sectional study was performed and serum samples from horses (n = 553), donkeys (n = 85) and mules (n = 83) were included. An *in-house* enzyme-linked immunosorbent assay (ELISA) was employed to identify a *Besnoitia* spp. infection and positive results were confirmed by an a posteriori western blot. For *Neospora* spp. and *Sarcocystis* spp., infections were detected using *in-house* ELISAs based on the parasite surface antigens *N. hughesi* rNhSAG1 and *S. neurona* rSnSAG2/3/4. Risk factors associated with these protozoan infections were also investigated.

Results: Antibodies against *Besnoitia* spp., *Neospora* spp. and *Sarcocystis* spp. infections were detected in 51 (7.1%), 46 (6.4%) and 20 (2.8%) of 721 equids, respectively. The principal risk factors associated with a higher seroprevalence of *Besnoitia* spp. were the host species (mule or donkey), the absence of shelter and the absence of a rodent control programme. The presence of rodents was the only risk factor for *Neospora* spp. infection.

Conclusions: This study was the first extensive serosurvey of *Besnoitia* spp. infection in European equids accomplished by two complementary tests and gives evidence of the presence of specific antibodies in these populations. However, the origin of the infection is still unclear. Further parasite detection and molecular genotyping are needed to identify the causative *Besnoitia* and *Neospora* species. Finally, cross-reactions with antibodies directed against other species of *Sarcocystis* might explain the positive reactions against the *S. neurona* antigens.

Keywords: *Besnoitia* spp., *Sarcocystis* spp., *Neospora* spp., Spain, Serosurvey, Horse, Donkey, Mule, Risk factors

Background

Cystogenic coccidia such as *Sarcocystis* spp., *Neospora* spp., and *Besnoitia* spp. have been reported to affect equids. *Sarcocystis neurona* and *Neospora hughesi* are the causative agents of equine protozoal myeloencephalitis (EPM), a serious neurological disease of horses in the Americas [1]. Moreover, besnoitiosis in donkeys caused by *Besnoitia bennetti* in donkeys is an emerging disease in the United States [2].

Several serosurveys of *Sarcocystis* spp. and/or *Neospora* spp. infections have been carried out in horses and donkeys in Europe (France, Italy, Czech Republic, Sweden and Spain) [3, 4]. However, *Besnoitia* spp. infection has not been studied in depth in European equids apart from only two reports of equine besnoitiosis. The first case of besnoitiosis in a horse was reported in Northern France [5]. Recently, the disease was suspected in seven donkeys from Southern Spain since tissue cysts were detected by histopathology [6]. Apart from *B. bennetti,* two additional

* Correspondence: gemaga@vet.ucm.es; gemaga@ucm.es
[1]SALUVET, Animal Health Department, Faculty of Veterinary Sciences, Complutense University of Madrid, Ciudad Universitaria s/n, 28040 Madrid, Spain
Full list of author information is available at the end of the article

Besnoitia species (*B. besnoiti* and *B. tarandi*) also affect ungulates (i.e., bovines and cervidae) causing similar clinical signs and have been reported in Europe [7]. Besnoitiosis caused by *B. tarandi* has been documented in reindeer in the Artic regions [8], whereas besnoitiosis caused by *B. besnoiti* is a re-emergent cattle disease in western and Central Europe and has also been recently reported in roe deer and red deer in Spain [9–11].

Diagnostic tools that provide an accurate serological diagnosis of cystogenic coccidia infections must overcome cross-reactions. Particularly in equids, *N. hughesi* cross-reacts with *N. caninum* [12]. In addition, cross-reactions between anti-*B. bennetti* antibodies and *B. besnoiti* antigens have also been observed [13]. Thus, highly sensitive and specific tests are mandatory in order to confirm an infection. Enzyme-linked immunosorbent assays (ELISAs)-based on recombinant proteins provide an accurate diagnosis of *S. neurona* and *N. hughesi* infection [14, 15]. A *B. besnoiti* tachyzoite extract-based ELISA is a routinely employed screening technique for *Besnoitia* spp. infection and a western blot is used as a confirmatory test in various ungulate species [2, 16]. In addition, a novel ELISA based on the enrichment of specific antigens has been demonstrated to be highly specific for the diagnosis of bovine besnoitiosis [17].

The goal of the present work was to determine the presence of specific antibodies against *Besnoitia* spp., *Neospora* spp. and *Sarcocystis* spp. in horses, donkeys and mules from southern Spain (Andalusia). This was the first serosurvey of *Besnoitia* spp. infection in European equids. Moreover, the first results of anti-*Neospora* spp. antibodies detection in Spanish equids are presented.

Methods

Sampled areas and experimental design

A cross-sectional study was carried out between January and March of 2010 in equine herds from Andalusia (southern Spain; 36° N - 38° 60′ N, 1° 75′ W - 7° 25′ W), which is the Spanish region with the largest number of equines (see the discussion section).

A total of 721 samples from horses (n = 553), donkeys (n = 85) and mules (n = 83) were included. Specifically, samples from 616 horses were collected in a survey stratified by census tract. We used a convenience sampling technique to select the remaining samples. Horse samples were distributed across all provinces of Andalusia, whereas the donkey and mule samples were restricted to Cádiz Province (Fig. 1). ELISAs based on *S. neurona* and *N. hughesi* recombinant proteins were employed for the detection of anti-*Sarcocystis* spp. and anti-*Neospora* spp. antibodies. To detect anti-*Besnoitia* spp. antibodies, all serum samples were initially screened by a soluble extract-based ELISA, and positive results were confirmed by western blot. Animals seropositive according to the western blot were included in the data analysis.

Samples and data collection

Blood samples were collected by puncturing of the jugular vein using a sterile collection system (Vacutainer®, Becton, Dickinson and Company, USA). Next, the blood samples were centrifuged at 400 *g* for 15 min at 4 °C and the sera were separated and stored at −20 °C until further analysis.

Epidemiological data were collected by an on-farm interview with the owners (Additional file 1), who were informed of the goals of the study. The questionnaires were especially designed to collect information using "close-ended" questions to avoid ambiguous or lengthy answers. In total, 18 explanatory variables were included in the analysis: species (horse, mule and donkey), age classes (young: < 5 years, adult: 5–16 years and geriatric: > 16 years), gender (male and female), colour (dark and light), breed (Spanish, Arabian, Spanish-Arabian, other purebred and crossbred), province, activity (farming, leisure and work), type of housing (outside and individual or collective shelter), direct contact with other horses, mules or donkeys, presence of other animal species (domestic and wild birds, domestic and wild ruminants), presence of rodents, insecticide treatment, cleaning and disinfection methods and protocols, pest control programmes (insects and rodents) and water sources. The sero-status of any animals that shared the same habitat as the sampled equids was unknown.

Antigen production for serological tests

Culture-derived tachyzoites of *B. besnoiti* isolate -Bb-Spain 1 [18] were propagated and purified [19] to prepare antigens for the ELISA and western blot tests. Foetal bovine serum was previously checked for the absence of anti-*Besnoitia*, anti-*N. caninum* and anti-*T. gondii* antibodies by an immunofluoresce antibody test (IFAT) [18]. Soluble *B. besnoiti* tachyzoite antigens used in the ELISA were prepared and quantified as previously described [20] and maintained at −80 °C until use. *Besnoitia besnoiti* tachyzoites were pelleted and frozen at −80 °C for western blot.

Sarcocystis neurona and *N. hughesi* recombinant proteins were purified as described previously [14, 15] and maintained at 4 °C until use.

Serology

ELISAs *Besnoitia besnoiti* tachyzoite soluble extract was used as antigens because strong cross-reactions were present between *B. besnoiti* antigens and anti-*B. bennetti* specific antibodies as indicated by IFAT and western blot [13]. Serum samples were analysed in duplicate, as

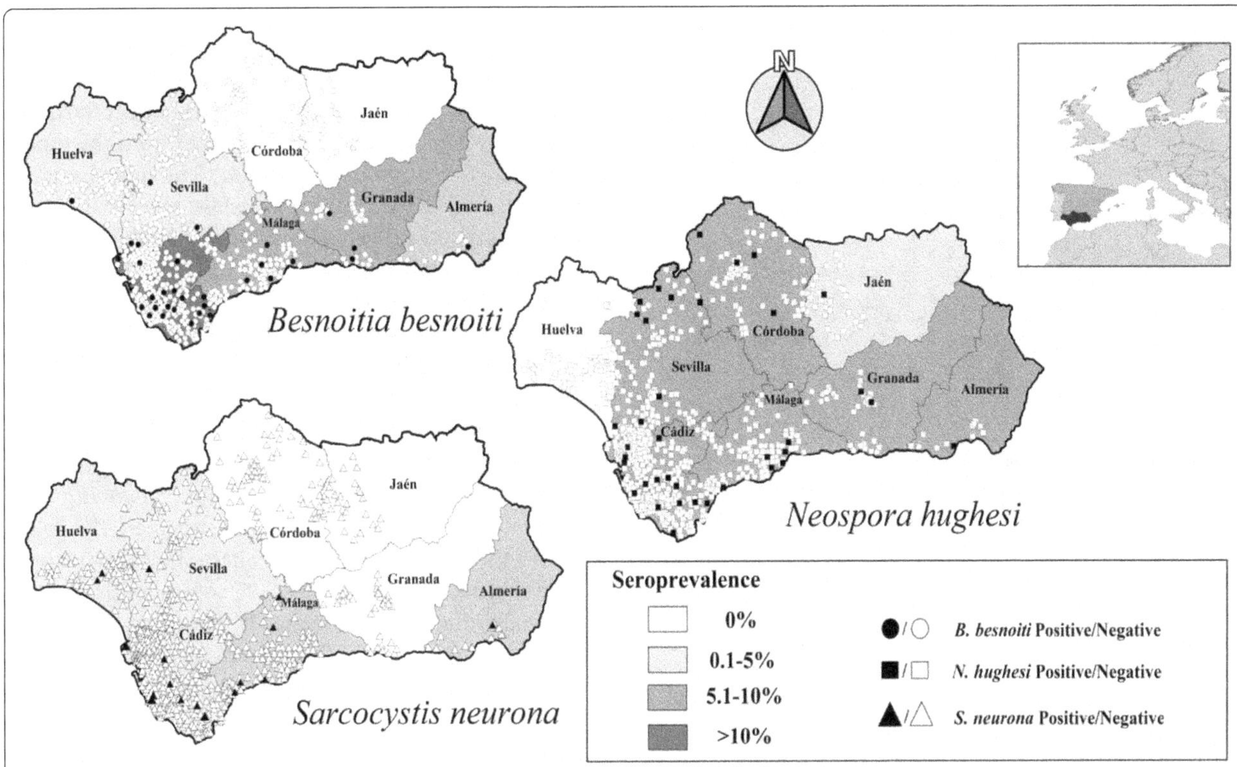

Fig. 1 Geographical distribution of equids sampled in Andalusia and seropositive results to *B. besnoiti*, *N. hughesi* and *S. neurona* infections. Positive results are marked in *black* and negative results are marked in *white*. Prevalence of infection by province is represented in *grey*

previously described [21], with a few modifications: (i) a blocking solution of phosphate buffered saline (PBS) containing 0.05% Tween 20 and 3% bovine serum albumin (Roche®) was used, and (ii) a rabbit peroxidase-labelled anti-horse IgG (H + L) antibody conjugate (INGENASA®) diluted at 1:5000 was used. The cut-off value was selected on the basis of three standard deviations of optical density (OD) values obtained with a panel of seronegative horse samples (n = 20). Positive and negative control sera tested by western blot consisted of chronically infected donkeys [13] and non-infected horses from USA and Spain, respectively. A cut-off at OD values higher than 0.40 was established and ELISA-positive results were confirmed by a western blot (Fig. 2).

Anti-*Neospora* spp. and anti-*Sarcocystis* spp. antibodies were detected using the recombinant *N. hughesi* surface antigen rNhSAG1 and *S. neurona* trivalent protein rSnSAG2/4/3 by means of previously described ELISAs [14, 15]. Percent positivity (PP) values of 20 and 15 were used as cut-offs for *N. hughesi* and *S. neurona* antigen-based ELISAs, respectively. The horse positive control serum employed in the *Neospora* spp.-based ELISA came from a mare that was experimentally infected during pregnancy with *N. hughesi*. The horse positive control serum for the *Sarcocystis* spp.-based ELISA was collected from two clinically affected horses with confirmed EPM by histopathology. The negative control serum for both ELISAs consisted of a serum collected from a weanling prior to infection with *S. neurona* [22]. This serum was negative by *S. neurona*-, *T. gondii*-, *N. caninum*-, and *N. hughesi*- based western blots.

SDS-PAGE and western blot

A total of 4 × 10^7 tachyzoites under non-reducing conditions were employed for the electrophoresis of *B. besnoiti* [23]. Tachyzoite antigens were transferred to a nitrocellulose membrane and, incubated with sera from either horses, donkeys or mules at a 1:20 dilution, followed by a peroxidase-conjugated anti-horse IgG (H + L) antibody diluted at 1:500 (INGENASA®, Madrid, Spain). Control sera were the same as used for the ELISA. The presence of at least three bands in at least two of the three principal antigenic areas (area I: 72.5, 58.9 and 51.4 kDa; area II: 38.7, 31.8 and 28.5 kDa; area III: 23.6, 19.1, 17.4, 14.5 kDa) was considered as a positive result for a *Besnoitia* spp. infection (Fig. 2) [23].

Statistical analysis

The prevalence of antibodies against *Besnoitia* spp., *Neospora* spp. and *Sarcocystis* spp. infections was

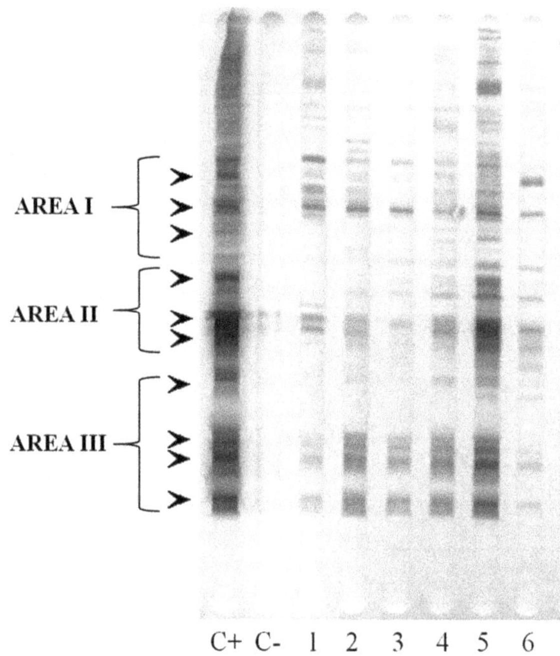

Fig. 2 Recognition of *Besnoitia* spp. tachyzoite antigens by western blot. Lines 1–6: samples from *Besnoitia* spp. ELISA seropositive equids. *Arrows* indicate recognition of antigenic bands in each of the three principal antigenic areas

estimated with the exact binomial confidence intervals of 95% [24].

To detect non-linear relationships and to homogenize the scales of the explanatory variables, all quantitative variables were transformed to qualitative variables using three categories of the 33rd and 66th percentiles as cut-off values. Tests of association were performed in three steps. First, a general linear univariate analysis was performed. The herd was the experimental unit, and the individual seroprevalence against *B. besnoiti* and *N. hughesi* was the dependent variable. Second, factors showing a *P-value* < 0.15 were further scrutinized for associations using Spearman's rank correlation coefficient (r) to avoid colinearity problems. When colinearity ($P < 0.05$ and $r > 0.4$) was present, only the variable more clearly linked to *Besnoitia* spp. and *Neospora* spp. seropositivity was retained. The third step involved a generalized estimating equations model (GEE) [25]. The number of seropositive animals was assumed to follow a binomial distribution and the herd was included as a random effect. A Poisson error distribution and a logit link function were considered.

An initial model was obtained using all of the potential explanatory variables and variables with a non-significant *P*-value were sequentially deleted. The quasi-likelihood under an independence model criterion was used to determine the best model in terms of its potential for explaining the results. Biologically plausible confounding factors were assessed using a Mantel-Haenszel analysis and confounding was considered to be potentially significant if the odds ratios (ORs) were shifted appreciably. Variables that altered the coefficients of the independent variables of interest by 30% or more when removed from the model were classified as confounding factors. The model was re-run until all of the remaining variables were statistically significant (i.e., the likelihood-ratio via Wald's test had $P < 0.05$), and a potential causal relationship with the response variable existed. SPSS 22.0 software (SPSS Inc., Chicago, IL, USA) was used for statistical analysis.

The association between *Besnoitia* spp. ELISA false-positive results and the presence of anti-*Neospora* spp. and anti-*Sarcocystis* spp. antibodies was estimated by using the chi-square test. A Mann–Whitney U test was used to compare differences in the anti-*Besnoitia* spp. antibody levels estimated by ELISA between the false-positive and true-positive results. These statistical analyses were performed with the InStat 3.05 software (GraphPad). Additionally, the test agreement expressed as the kappa-values (k) between the ELISA and the western blot tests was calculated using WinEpiscope 2.0 [26].

Results

Seroprevalence

Antibodies against *Besnoitia* spp., *Neospora* spp. and *Sarcocystis* spp. were detected in 51 (7.1%; $CI_{95\%}$: 5.2–8.9), 46 (6.4%; $CI_{95\%}$: 4.6–8.2) and 20 (2.8%; $CI_{95\%}$: 1.6–4.0) of 721 equids tested, respectively. Seropositivity against both *Besnoitia* spp. and *Neospora* spp. were confirmed in 0.8% (6/721), against both *Besnoitia* spp. and *Sarcocystis* spp. in 0.6% (4/721) and against both *Neospora* spp. and *Sarcocystis* spp. in 0.4% (3/721) equids (Table 1). A good agreement between the ELISA and the western blot tests was obtained (k = 0.6).

Cross-reactions between anti-Besnoitia spp. antibodies and other cystogenic coccidia

Antibodies against *Neospora* spp. and/or *Sarcocystis* spp. were detected in 8.7% (63/721) of the sampled animals (Table 2). Interestingly, true *Besnoitia*-seropositive animals that were also positive against *Neospora* spp. and/or *Sarcocystis* spp. had OD values higher than 0.8, whereas OD values of false *Besnoitia*-seropositive animals varied from 0.40 to 0.56 (Table 2) ($P < 0.001$, Mann–Whitney U test). However, the existence of *Besnoitia* spp. false-positive results was not significantly associated with seropositivity against *Neospora* spp. or *Sarcocystis* spp. ($P = 0.55$).

Risk factors

Due to the low number of *Sarcocystis* spp. seropositive animals, risk factors were only analysed using *Besnoitia*

Table 1 Variables identified as significant ($P < 0.15$ in the univariate analysis) and included in the multivariate analysis

			Besnoitia besnoiti		*Neospora hughesi*	
Variables	Categories	No. analyzed [a]	Positive (%)	*P*-value	Positive (%)	*P*-value
Species	Horse	553	16 (2.9)	<0.001		
	Donkey	85	13 (15.3)			
	Mule	83	22 (26.5)			
Breed	Pure	370	18 (4.9)	0.005	30 (8.1)	0.021
	Crossbred	298	31 (10.4)		12 (4.0)	
Sex	Female	306	26 (8.5)	0.129		
	Male	415	25 (6.0)			
Province	Almeria	14	1 (7.1)	<0.001		
	Cadiz	320	40 (12.5)			
	Córdoba	60	0 (0.0)			
	Granada	38	3 (7.9)			
	Huelva	60	1 (1.7)			
	Jaen	30	0 (0.0)			
	Malaga	98	5 (5.1)			
	Seville	101	1 (1.0)			
Presence of shelters	Yes	407	15 (3.7)	<0.001	23 (5.7)	0.122
	No	280	35 (12.5)		23 (8.2)	
Presence of wild birds	Yes	403	40 (9.9)	0.001		
	No	275	9 (3.3)			
Presence of cattle	Yes	145	19 (13.1)	0.020	17 (11.7)	0.017
	No	417	29 (7.0)		24 (5.8)	
Presence of wild ruminants	Yes	41			8 (19.5)	0.006
	No	521			33 (6.3)	
Presence of rodents	Yes	388	35 (9.0)	0.001	34 (8.8)	0.002
	No	261	8 (3.1)		15 (5.7)	
Rodent control program	Yes	434	24 (5.5)	0.009		
	No	226	25 (11.1)			
Cleaning protocol	Yes	581	38 (6.5)	0.018	32 (5.5)	0.068
	No	86	12 (14.0)		9 (10.5)	
Disinfection protocol	Yes	536	32 (6.0)	0.006		
	No	127	17 (13.4)			

[a] Missing values were omitted

spp. and *Neospora* spp. seropositive animals as the dependent variables.

Eleven explanatory variables were selected from the univariate analysis for *Besnoitia* spp. infection ($P < 0.15$) (Table 2). The seroprevalence was significantly higher in mules (26.5%) and donkeys (13.3%) compared to that in horses (2.9%) (Table 2). The seroprevalence values differed among provinces for horses (Fig. 1) and the seroprevalence was lower in the presence of shelters, whereas it was higher in the presence of rodents (Table 2).

The principal risk factors associated with a *Besnoitia* spp. infection were species (mule and donkey) (OR = 12.06 and OR = 2.06, respectively), the absence of shelters (OR = 2.45) and the absence of rodent a control programme (OR = 5.34) (Table 3). The presence of rodents (OR = 4.83) was the only risk factor for a *Neospora* spp. infection (Table 3).

Discussion

In the present study, we investigated three cystogenic coccidial infections that have been little studied in European equids. In fact, clinical cases of EPM have not been diagnosed in the Old World. Regarding other epidemiological gaps, the definitive hosts of *N. hughesi* and *Besnoitia* spp. that affect ungulates are still unknown [7, 27]. In contrast, the definitive host of *S. neurona* (*Didelphis* spp.) appears to

Table 2 Detection of anti-*Besnoitia* spp., anti-*Sarcocystis* spp. and anti-*Neospora* spp. antibodies by ELISA

	n	Seropositive to *Sarcocystis* spp. (%)	Seropositive to *Neospora* spp. (%)	Seropositive to *Sarcocystis* spp. and *Neospora* spp. (%)	Seronegative to *Sarcocystis* spp. and *Neospora* spp. (%)
Besnoitia spp. seropositive[a]	51	4 (7.84%)	6 (11.76%)	0 (0.0%)	41 (80.39%)
Besnoitia spp. seronegative	641	11 (1.71%)	36 (5.61%)	1 (0.15%)	593 (92.51%)
Besnoitia spp. seronegative with a false-positive ELISA result	29	2 (6.89%)	1 (3.44%)	2 (6.89%)	24 (82.75%)
Total	721	17 (2.35%)	43 (5.96%)	3 (0.41%)	658 (91.26%)

[a]True *Besnoitia*-seropositive animals confirmed by western blot

be restricted to the New World, but other species of *Sarcocystis* are known to infect equids in the Old World [4].

This serosurvey was focused on Andalusia, which has the highest number of equid herds in Spain (44.3%) [28]. In addition, *Besnoitia* spp. infections have been reported in cattle and suspected in donkeys from Andalusia [6, 29]. In contrast, no data exist for *Neospora* spp. and *Sarcocystis* spp. infections in equids from this region. Thus, the impact of EPM is unknown.

The most relevant finding of this work was the first detection of specific antibodies against *Besnoitia* spp. in European equids. The diagnostic approach (i.e., an initial screening by ELISA followed by a confirmatory western blot) was previously used in serosurveys conducted in the absence of a panel of reference sera and a gold standard test [11, 16] using sera from clinically *Besnoitia* spp.-infected donkeys as a positive control [13, 23]. Additionally, serological cross-reactions with antibodies against *Neospora* spp. and *Sarcocystis* spp. were ruled out, probably due to the low antibody levels detected against *Neospora* spp. and *Sarcocystis* spp. in this study and the use of highly specific recombinant proteins. Since the *Besnoitia* ELISA can yield ambiguous results, a western blot or a more specific ELISA are mandatory in order to confirm the infection [17].

Outside of Europe, a few cases of *Besnoitia* spp. infections in various equid species (horse, donkey, mule and zebra) were attributed to *B. bennetti* infection in the mid-twentieth century in different sub-Saharan countries such as South Africa and Sudan [30–32]. It has been suggested that besnoitiosis may be an emerging disease in donkeys in the United States [2]. Furthermore, equine besnoitiosis in Europe was first reported in 1922 [5] in a horse in Northern France. The disease has not been diagnosed since, but in a recent outbreak of donkeys from Southern Spain besnoitiosis was suspected [6]. Seroprevalence rates of *Besnoitia* spp. infection in other ungulate species of Spain of 1% (2/2608) and 0% (0/2285) have been reported in wild and small domestic ruminants, respectively, in areas where bovine besnoitiosis is highly endemic [11, 33]. However, whether equids may be reservoirs or intermediate hosts of *B. besnoiti* should be further elucidated through molecular genotyping [34].

Interestingly, the highest seroprevalence of *Besnoitia* spp. infection was observed in donkeys and mules. However, a higher susceptibility to *Besnoitia* spp. infection in donkeys and mules compared to that in horses has not been demonstrated. Most of the clinical cases of equine besnoitiosis have been reported in donkeys [2, 35, 36]. Although less frequently, the disease has also been diagnosed in horses [30, 32, 37]. The differences in the

Table 3 Generalized estimating equations model of potential risk factors associated with *Besnoitia* spp. and *Neospora* spp. seropositivity

Variable	Category	β	Sig.	OR	95% CI	
Besnoitia spp.						
Species	Horse	*	*	*	*	*
	Donkey	0.723	0.116	2.060	0.836	5.075
	Mule	2.490	<0.001	12.061	3.907	37.235
Presence of shelters	Yes	*	*	*	*	*
	No	0.898	0.038	2.455	1.053	5.725
Rodent control program	Yes	*	*	*	*	*
	No	1.676	0.001	5.342	1.952	14.623
Neospora spp.						
Presence of rodents	Yes	1.575	0.003	4.831	1.680	13.890
	No	*	*	*	*	*

* Reference category; OR, Odds ratio; 95% CI, 95% Confidence interval

management and biosecurity measures between donkeys/mules and horse herds could be a feasible explanation for this finding. Similar to bovine besnoitiosis, parasite transmission might occur through direct contact during natural mating or from bites of blood-sucking arthropods, and animal movement might favour the spread of the disease [29]. Indeed, it was suggested that the use of repellents indoors may help to reduce mechanical transmission by blood-sucking insects [29]. In this study, data on treatment with ectoparasiticides were only recorded in 229 animals and 190 were treated (156 of the treated animals were horses; data not shown). In addition, the absence of shelters would also lead to a higher exposure to blood-sucking arthropods. Finally, whether rodents may act as intermediate hosts of *B. bennetti* as they do for other *Besnoitia* species (*B. akodoni, B. jellisoni, B. neotomofelis* and *B. wallacei*) has not been clarified yet [7, 9]. The *Besnoitia* species that parasitize equids must be elucidated. Because *B. besnoiti* and *B. bennetti* infections are serologically indistinguishable, further molecular analyses and parasite isolations are necessary in order to determine which *Besnoitia* species might be present in Spanish equids.

Antibodies against the aetiological agents of EPM (*N. hughesi* and *S. neurona*) were also researched in this study. However, the simple detection of a specific antibody does not confirm the diagnosis of the disease since EPM occurs in a small proportion of infected horses [1]. This initial serosurvey of *Neospora* spp. infection carried out in Spanish equids showed a low seroprevalence (6.4%) and that the presence of rodents was a risk factor for a *Neospora* spp. infection. These results agreed with other studies carried out in different European countries such as France, Sweden and Italy that revealed a seroprevalence of approximately 10% [3, 38, 39]. Little it is known about the role of rodents in the epidemiology of equine neosporosis. Rodents could be considered as a putative intermediate host of equine neosporosis, similarly to bovine neosporosis. In fact, *N. caninum* DNA could be detected in mice and rats in cattle herds with a previous history of neosporosis [40–42]. Equids likely become infected with *Neospora* spp. via the ingestion of oocysts shed by the definitive host, or possibly through vertical transmission [43, 44].

The *Neospora* species present in these equids remain to be elucidated, since cross-reactions between both existing *Neospora* species are widely known [12]. Indeed, the rNhSAG1-based ELISA clearly detects antibodies to the *N. caninum* orthologue [14]. In this study, *Neospora* spp. seropositive sera were demonstrated to be seropositive by *N. caninum*-based western blot, supporting this assumption (see Additional file 2).

Finally, anti-*Sarcocystis* spp. antibodies were detected in 2.8% equids and this level is similar to previous reports in France and northern Spain [45, 46]. Spanish horses are unlikely to be exposed to *S. neurona* due to the absence of the definitive host in Europe but cross-reactions with other species of *Sarcocystis* might explain positive reactions. In fact, the trivalent rSnSAG surface antigen chimaera-based ELISA was not validated with sera from European equids. Additionally, other latent *Sarcocystis* spp. cysts are present in equids and are often benign.

Conclusions

This is the first serosurvey of *Besnoitia* spp. and *Neospora* spp. infections carried out in Spain. This study found specific antibodies against *Besnoitia* spp. infection in European equids. Anti-*Neospora* spp. and *Sarcocystis* spp. antibodies were also found in a few animals. However, neither parasitic disease had been not previously diagnosed in Europe. Further parasite detection and molecular genotyping are needed to clarify the presence and identity of these three parasite species [11].

Endnotes

[1]See: http://www.mapama.gob.es/es/ganaderia/temas/sanidad-animal-higiene-ganadera/sanidad-animal/enfermedades/fiebre-nilo-occidental/F_O_Nilo.aspx#para4 (Accessed 25th of April 2017)

Abbreviations

B: Besnoitia; ELISA: Enzyme-linked immunosorbent assay; EPM: Equine protozoal myeloencephalitis; GEE: Generalized estimating equation; IFAT: Immunofluorescence antibody test; Ig: Immunoglobulin; k: Kappa value; kDa: Kilodalton; N: *Neospora*; OD: Optical density; OR: Odd ratio; S: *Sarcocystis*; SPSS: Statistical package for the social sciences

Acknowledgments

We would like to thank the Epidemiological Monitoring Program of the Regional Government of Andalusia and farmers for providing the samples. Finally, we also acknowledge Paula García-Lunar, Alejandro Jiménez-Meléndez and Carlos Diezma-Díaz for their excellent technical assistance.

Funding

This study was supported by several research projects (AGL 2010–20,561, CYTED Thematic Network 113RT0469 Protozoovac and by PLATESA S20137ABI-2906). Daniel Gutiérrez Expósito has been financially supported by the Ministry of Science and Innovation (grant no. BES-2011-043753).

Authors' contributions

DGE performed serological tests against *Besnoitia* spp. infection, analysed the data and drafted the manuscript; IGB and AAM provided serum samples, carried out the statistical analyses and drafted the manuscript; DKH and MRY performed the ELISA tests against *Neospora* spp. and *Sarcocystis* spp. infections; SLN provided positive control sera against a *Besnoitia* spp. infection; LMO and GAG contributed to the conception and design of the study. GAG analysed the data and drafted the manuscript. All authors critically reviewed the manuscript and agreed to the final version.

Competing interests
All authors declare that they or their institutions have no financial and personal relationship with other people or organizations that could inappropriately influence their work.

Consent for publication
The manuscript contains no individual person's data and does not require consent for publication.

Author details
[1]SALUVET, Animal Health Department, Faculty of Veterinary Sciences, Complutense University of Madrid, Ciudad Universitaria s/n, 28040 Madrid, Spain. [2]Animal Health Department, Faculty of Veterinary Sciences, University of Cordoba-Agrifood Excellence International Campus (ceiA3), Cordoba, Spain. [3]Department of Veterinary Science, M.H. Gluck Equine Research Center, University of Kentucky, Lexington, KY 40546-0099, USA. [4]Department of Clinical Sciences, College of Veterinary Medicine, Box 52, Cornell University, Ithaca, NY 14853, USA.

References

1. Howe DK, MacKay RJ, Reed SM. Equine protozoal myeloencephalitis. Vet Clin North Am Equine Pract. 2014;30:659–75.
2. Ness SL, Schares G, Peters-Kennedy J, Mittel LD, Dubey JP, Bowman DD, Mohammed HO, Divers TJ. Serological diagnosis of *Besnoitia bennetti* infection in donkeys (*Equus asinus*). J Vet Diagn Investig. 2014;26:778–82.
3. Bártová E, Machacova T, Sedlák K, Budíková M, Mariani U, Veneziano V. Seroprevalence of antibodies of Neospora spp. and Toxoplasma gondii in horses from southern Italy. Folia Parasitol. 2015;62:43.
4. Dubey JP, Howe DK, Furr M, Saville WJ, Marsh AE, Reed SM, Grigg ME. An update on *Sarcocystis neurona* infections in animals and equine protozoal myeloencephalitis (EPM). Vet Parasitol. 2015;209:1–42.
5. Henry A, Masson G. Globidiose cutanée du cheval. In: Traite de protozoologie médicale et vétérinare. París: Vigot Freres; 1922. p. 386–7.
6. Zafra R, Soria-López N, de Castro ED, Jaber J, Mozos E, Pérez J. Outbreak of besnoitiosis in donkeys (*Equus asinus*) in the south of Spain. J Comp Pathol. 2013;1:81.
7. Olias P, Schade B, Mehlhorn H. Molecular pathology, taxonomy and epidemiology of *Besnoitia* species (protozoa: Sarcocystidae). Infect Genet Evol. 2011;11:1564–76.
8. Dubey JP, Sreekumar C, Rosenthal BM, Vianna MC, Nylund M, Nikander S, Oksanen A. Redescription of *Besnoitia tarandi* (protozoa: Apicomplexa) from the reindeer (*Rangifer tarandus*). Int J Parasitol. 2004;34:1273–87.
9. EFSA. European food safety authority - bovine Besnoitiosis: an emerging disease in Europe. EFSA J. 2010;8:1499.
10. Arnal M, Gutiérrez-Expósito D, Martínez-Durán D, Regidor-Cerrillo J, Revilla M, Fernández de Luco D, Jiménez-Meléndez A, Ortega-Mora LM, Álvarez-García G. Systemic besnoitiosis in a juvenile roe deer (*Capreolus capreolus*). Transbound Emerg Dis. 2016; doi: 10.1111/tbed.12514.
11. Gutiérrez-Expósito D, Arnal MC, Martínez-Durán D, Regidor-Cerrillo J, Revilla M, Fernández de Luco D, Jiménez-Meléndez A, Calero-Bernal R, Habela Martínez-Estéllez MA, García-Bocanegra I, Arenas-Montes A, Álvarez-García G. The role of wild ruminants as reservoirs of Besnoitia besnoiti infection in cattle. Vet Parasitol. 2016;223:7–13.
12. Gondim LF, Lindsay DS, McAllister MM. Canine and bovine *Neospora caninum* control sera examined for cross-reactivity using *Neospora caninum* and *Neospora hughesi* indirect fluorescent antibody tests. J Parasitol. 2009;95:86–8.
13. Ness SL, Peters-Kennedy J, Schares G, Dubey JP, Mittel LD, Mohammed HO, Bowman DD, Felippe MJ, Wade SE, Shultz N, Divers TJ. Investigation of an outbreak of besnoitiosis in donkeys in northeastern Pennsylvania. J Am Vet Med Assoc. 2012;240:1329–37.
14. Hoane JS, Yeargan MR, Stamper S, Saville WJ, Morrow JK, Lindsay DS, Howe DK. Recombinant NhSAG1 ELISA: a sensitive and specific assay for detecting antibodies against *Neospora hughesi* in equine serum. J Parasitol. 2005;91:446–52.
15. Yeargan M, de Assis RI, Morrow J, Graves A, Reed SM, Howe DK. A new trivalent SnSAG surface antigen chimera for efficient detection of antibodies against *Sarcocystis neurona* and diagnosis of equine protozoal myeloencephalitis. J Vet Diagn Investig. 2015;27:377–81.
16. Gutiérrez-Expósito D, Ortega-Mora LM, Marco I, Boadella M, Gortázar C, San Miguel-Ayanz JM, García-Lunar P, Lavin S, Álvarez-García G. First serosurvey of *Besnoitia* spp. infection in wild European ruminants in Spain. Vet Parasitol. 2013;197:557–64.
17. Schares G, Langenmayer MC, Scharr JC, Minke L, Maksimov P, Maksimov A, Schares S, Barwald A, Basso W, Dubey JP, Conraths FJ, Gollnick NS. Novel tools for the diagnosis and differentiation of acute and chronic bovine besnoitiosis. Int J Parasitol. 2013;43:143–54.
18. Fernández-García A, Risco-Castillo V, Pedraza-Díaz S, Aguado-Martínez A, Álvarez-García G, Gómez-Bautista M, Collantes-Fernández E, Ortega-Mora LM. First isolation of *Besnoitia besnoiti* from a chronically infected cow in Spain. J Parasitol. 2009;95:474–6.
19. Pérez-Zaballos FJ, Ortega-Mora LM, Álvarez-García G, Collantes-Fernández E, Navarro-Lozano V, García-Villada L, Costas E. Adaptation of *Neospora caninum* isolates to cell-culture changes: an argument in favor of its clonal population structure. J Parasitol. 2005;91:507–10.
20. Álvarez-García G, Pereira-Bueno J, Gómez-Bautista M, Ortega-Mora LM. Pattern of recognition of *Neospora caninum* tachyzoite antigens by naturally infected pregnant cattle and aborted foetuses. Vet Parasitol. 2002;107:15–27.
21. Fernández-García A, Álvarez-García G, Risco-Castillo V, Aguado-Martínez A, Marcén JM, Rojo-Montejo S, Castillo JA, Ortega-Mora LM. Development and use of an indirect ELISA in an outbreak of bovine besnoitiosis in Spain. Vet Rec. 2010;166:818–22.
22. Fenger CK, Granstrom DE, Gajadhar AA, Williams NM, McCrillis SA, Stamper S, Langemeier JL, Dubey JP. Experimental induction of equine protozoal myeloencephalitis in horses using Sarcocystis sp. Sporocysts from the oposum (*Didelphis virginiana*). Vet Parasitol. 1997;68:199–213.
23. García-Lunar P, Ortega-Mora LM, Schares G, Gollnick NS, Jacquiet P, Grisez C, Prevot F, Frey CF, Gottstein B, Álvarez-García G. An inter-laboratory comparative study of serological tools employed in the diagnosis of *Besnoitia besnoiti* infection in bovines. Transbound Emerg Dis. 2013;60:59–68.
24. Thrusfield M, Ortega C, de Blas I, Noordhuizen JP, Frankena K. WIN EPISCOPE 2.0: improved epidemiological software for veterinary medicine. Vet Record. 2001;148:567–72.
25. Hanley JA, Negassa A, Edwardes MD, Forrester JE. Statistical analysis of correlated data using generalized estimating equations: an orientation. Am J Epidemiol. 2003;157:364–75.
26. Altman DG. Statistics in medical journals: developments in the 1980s. Stat Med. 1991;10:1897–913.
27. Dubey J, Liddell S, Mattson D, Speer C, Howe D, Jenkins M. Characterization of the Oregon isolate of *Neospora hughesi* from a horse. J Parasitol. 2001;87:345–53.
28. El sector equino en cifras. http://www.mapama.gob.es/es/ganaderia/temas/produccion-y-mercados-ganaderos/indicadoreseconomicossectorequino2015_tcm7-386080.pdf. Accessed 1 Feb 2017.
29. Alvarez-García G, Frey CF, Ortega-Mora LM, Schares G. A century of bovine besnoitiosis: an unknown disease re-emerging in Europe. Trends Parasitol. 2013;29:407–15.
30. Bennet SC. A peculiar equine sarcosporidium in the Anglo-Egyptian Sudan. Vet J. 1927;83:297–304.
31. Bigalke RD. New concepts on the epidemiological features of bovine besnoitiosis as determined by laboratory and field investigations. Onderstepoort J Vet Res. 1968;35:3–137.
32. Bigalke RD. Studies on equine besnoitiosis. J Parasitol. 1970;56:29.
33. Gutiérrez-Expósito D, Ortega-Mora LM, Ara V, Marco I, Lavín S, Carvajal-Valilla J, Morales A, Alvarez-García G. Absence of antibodies specific to *Besnoitia* spp. in European sheep and goats from areas in Spain where bovine besnoitiosis is endemic. Parasitol Res. 2017;116:445–8.
34. Madubata C, Dunams-Morel DB, Elkin B, Oksanen A, Rosenthal BM. Evidence for a recent population bottleneck in an Apicomplexan parasite of caribou and reindeer, *Besnoitia tarandi*. Infect Genet Evol. 2012;12:1605–13.
35. Dubey JP, Sreekumar C, Donovan T, Rozmanec M, Rosenthal BM, Vianna MC, Davis WP, Belden JS. Redescription of *Besnoitia bennetti* (protozoa: Apicomplexa) from the donkey (*Equus asinus*). Int J Parasitol. 2005;35:659–72.

36. Elsheikha HM, Mansfield LS, Morsy GH. Studies on besnoitiosis bennetti in miniature donkeys. J Egypt Soc Parasitol. 2008;38:171–84.
37. Van Heerden J, Els HJ, Raubenheimer EJ, Williams JH. Besnoitiosis in a horse. J S Afr Vet Assoc. 1993;64:92–5.
38. Pitel P, Lindsay D, Caure S, Romand S, Pronost S, Gargala G, Mitchell S, Hary C, Thulliez P, Fortier G. Reactivity against *Sarcocystis neurona* and *Neospora* by serum antibodies in healthy French horses from two farms with previous equine protozoal myeloencephalitis-like cases. Vet Parasitol. 2003;111:1–7.
39. Jakubek E, Lundén A, Uggla A. Seroprevalences of *Toxoplasma gondii* and *Neospora* sp. infections in Swedish horses. Vet Parasitol. 2006;138:194–9.
40. Machačová T, Ajzenberg D, Žákovská A, Sedlák K, Bártová E. *Toxoplasma gondii* and *Neospora caninum* in wild small mammals: seroprevalence, DNA detection and genotyping. Vet Parasitol. 2016;223:88–90.
41. Ferroglio E, Pasino M, Romano A, Grande D, Pregel P, Trisciuoglio A. Evidence of *Neospora caninum* DNA in wild rodents. Vet Parasitol. 2007;148:346–9.
42. Medina-Esparza L, Macías L, Ramos-Parra M, Morales-Salinas E, Quezada T, Cruz-Vázquez C. Frequency of infection by *Neospora caninum* in wild rodents associated with dairy farms in Aguascalientes, Mexico. Vet Parasitol. 2013;191:11–4.
43. Antonello AM, Pivoto FL, Camillo G, Braunig P, Sangioni LA, Pompermayer E, Vogel FSF. The importance of vertical transmission of *Neospora* spp. in naturally infected horses. Vet Parasitol. 2012;187:367–70.
44. Pusterla N, Mackie S, Packham A, Conrad PA. Serological investigation of transplacental infection with *Neospora hughesi* and *Sarcocystis neurona* in broodmares. Vet J. 2014;202:649–50.
45. Pitel P, Pronost S, Gargala G, Anrioud D, Toquet M, Foucher N, Collobert-Laugier C, Fortier G, Ballet J. Detection of *Sarcocystis neurona* antibodies in French horses with neurological signs. Int J Parasitol. 2002;32:481–5.
46. Arias M, Yeargan M, Francisco I, Dangoudoubiyam S, Becerra P, Francisco R, Sánchez-Andrade R, Paz-Silva A, Howe DK. Exposure to *Sarcocystis* spp. in horses from Spain determined by western blot analysis using *Sarcocystis neurona* merozoites as heterologous antigen. Vet Parasitol. 2012;185:301–4.
47. Dubey JP, Hattel AL, Lindsay DS, Topper MJ. Neonatal *Neospora caninum* infection in dogs: isolation of the causative agent and experimental transmission. J Am Vet Med Assoc. 1988;193:1259–63.

10

Isolation and molecular characterization of Mycobacterium bovis causing pulmonary tuberculosis and epistaxis in a Thoroughbred horse

Tiny Motlatso Hlokwe[1,4*], David Sutton[2,3], Patrick Page[2] and Anita Luise Michel[4]

Abstract

Background: Tuberculosis caused by *Mycobacterium bovis* (*M. bovis*) is very uncommon in horses worldwide.

Case presentation: In the current study, an eight-year-old male Thoroughbred in good body condition was admitted to the Equine Clinic at the Onderstepoort Veterinary Academic Hospital in 2005 due to bilateral epistaxis accompanied by coughing. Routine examinations were conducted to determine the cause of the condition. Endoscopic examination revealed the major source of the epistaxis as the trachea, whereas thoracic radiography indicated the presence of a primary pulmonary mass. *M. bovis* was isolated from a broncho-alveolar lavage (BAL) sample collected. The pulmonary mass reduced in size three months later following an oral administration of enrofloxacin (7.5 mg/kg PO SID). Genetic fingerprinting by spoligotyping identified the *M. bovis* isolate as spoligotype SB0868 strain. This *M. bovis* strain type was never described previously in South Africa (SA). This is the first case of *M. bovis* infection in a horse in SA which has been fully documented including clinical findings, isolation and genetic characterisation of the causative pathogen.

Conclusions: This report indicates that horses may contract and harbour *M. bovis* despite their lower susceptibility compared to other domestic animals. It also suggests that the infection may be more easily contained and eliminated from the host.

Keywords: Equine, Respiratory, Epistaxis, Zoonosis

Background

Mycobacterium bovis is the causative agent of bovine tuberculosis (BTB) in a variety of mammalian hosts. The worldwide status of BTB as a zoonosis is of great concern [1]. Horses are suggested to be more resistant to mycobacterial infections as compared to other livestock animals [2] and tuberculosis incidence in horses is extremely low, especially in countries implementing BTB control programs [3]. Currently, the most common causes of mycobacterial infections in horses are members of the *Mycobacterium avium* complex (MAC) species [4], but under conditions of high infection pressure from co-grazing cattle, *M. bovis* may cause clinical pulmonary infection in horses [5].

Amongst members of the *Mycobacterium tuberculosis* complex (MTBC), *M. bovis* has been more commonly isolated from horses than *M. tuberculosis* [3]. Isolation of *M. bovis* was reported from a cheek lesion of a 9-year-old horse from Nigeria [6]. Acid-fast bacilli were detected on a splenic aspirate from a 10-year-old mare with weight loss in Spain. This mare was euthanized and *M. bovis* infection confirmed by polymerase chain reaction (PCR) and culture of tissue samples. In the cited case, a rapid diagnosis was obtained by use of PCR following antemortem detection of acid-fast bacteria [7]. In another report, *M. bovis* was isolated from lymph nodes of a 4-year-old horse in France that had been in close contact with infected cattle, supporting that horses may be more easily

* Correspondence: HlokweT@arc.agric.za
[1]Zoonotic Diseases Section, ARC-Onderstepoort Veterinary Institute, Soutpan Rd., Onderstepoort 0110, South Africa
[4]Department of Veterinary Tropical Diseases, Faculty of Veterinary Science, University of Pretoria, Soutpan Rd., Onderstepoort 0110, South Africa
Full list of author information is available at the end of the article

infected under conditions of high *M. bovis* infection pressure [5]. Most recently, *M. bovis* infection was confirmed by PCR of tissue samples collected post mortem from a 2-year-old horse with diarrhea and weight loss associated with granulomatous enterocolitis [8]. An antibody response to *M. tuberculosis* antigens was detected in blood samples obtained ante-mortem from a 20-year-old horse with signs of cardiac insufficiency and ventral edema in Switzerland [9]. *M. tuberculosis* pulmonary infection was subsequently confirmed by PCR amplification of DNA extracts from formalin fixed paraffin embedded tissue samples. Generally serological diagnosis of tuberculosis is of limited value in animals and humans and humoral immune responsiveness to MTBC is indicative of progressive tuberculous lesion development [10].

In this report, we describe for the first time, the isolation and molecular characterization of *M. bovis* in a horse in South Africa.

Case presentation

An 8-year-old, 563-kg Thoroughbred gelding was admitted to the Equine Clinic, Onderstepoort Veterinary Academic Hospital with a primary complaint of bilateral epistaxis, first noted 6 days prior to admission. The epistaxis had increased in severity and frequency, and was accompanied by coughing. The gelding had been purchased for show jumping 1 month previously and transported approximately 1600 km to a new stable yard. No exercise intolerance was reported since purchase.

On presentation the gelding was in good body condition, bright, alert and responsive with good appetite. Body temperature was mildly elevated (38.6 °C; reference range (RR) 37.5–38.5), pulse rate was mildly elevated (46 beats per minute; RR: 28–40) and respiratory rate was normal (16 breaths per minute; RR: <20/min). Mucous membranes were pink and moist with no petechiae. Intermittent, mild epistaxis was evident at both nares. No crackles or wheezes were detected on thoracic auscultation and no spontaneous coughing or coughing on rebreathing examination was recorded. Moderate hypoalbuminemia (22 g/L; RR: 66–83) was present. Serological testing for *Aspergillus* antibodies was negative.

Respiratory endoscopy[1] revealed petechiae in the medial compartment of the left guttural pouch but no blood. Frank blood was observed in the trachea with hemorrhage originating from a tertiary bronchiole in the left dorsal lung lobe. Trans-endoscopic broncho-alveolar lavage was performed in the region of the hemorrhage and samples submitted for cytology, bacterial and fungal culture. Cytology of the BAL fluid was consistent with pulmonary hemorrhage with chronic inflammation (sero-sanguinous fluid with 42% neutrophils, 23% lymphocytes, and 35 % macrophages with phagocytosed red blood cells). Few free and phagocytosed bacilli were observed. Initial aerobic and anaerobic bacterial and fungal culture results were negative. Standing left lateral thoracic radiographs[2] revealed a well-marginated soft tissue mass (12 × 15cm) with a dorsal gas cap in the caudodorsal lung field. The fluid line observed in the structure was undulated, indicative of viscous content. A marked peribronchial infiltration with a mild alveolar pattern was observed over the ventral lung field. Thoracic ultrasonography[3] only revealed pleural surface irregularity of the left lung. Differential diagnoses for the imaging findings included a pulmonary abscess, neoplasia, or fungal granuloma.

Three percutaneous, ultrasound-guided biopsies were collected from the left caudodorsal lung at the site most affected by pleural irregularity. Direct ultrasound-guided biopsy of the pulmonary mass was not possible due to its depth and ultrasound reverberation artefact. Histopathological examination of the lung biopsies showed chronic fibrinous pleurisy of the superficial lung, but was not diagnostic. The owner declined further diagnostic procedures to sample the pulmonary mass and the gelding was discharged with treatment for suspected pulmonary bacterial abscess or fungal granuloma with a course of enrofloxacin[4] (7.5 mg/kg PO q24h for 8 weeks) and Potassium Iodide(KI[5])(10 g PO q24h for 6 months), with paddock rest.

Three months later, the horse was re-examined and was found to be in good body condition. The owner reported that there had been no further epistaxis or coughing. Clinical examination was normal and there was no respiratory abnormality detected on auscultation. CBC and fibrinogen results were within reference range. Thoracic radiographs showed moderate reduction in size of the pulmonary mass (9 cm diameter) which was of homogeneous soft tissue opacity, with no gas cap evident. A mild to moderate, focal broncho-interstitial pattern was present caudodorsal to the cardiac silhouette, but was markedly improved compared to previous examination. In view of the reduction in size of the mass, bacterial or fungal granuloma were still considered the most likely differential diagnoses, with neoplasia considered unlikely. The horse was discharged with a further 3-month course of KI. Resumption of ridden walking exercise was recommended with continued monitoring for coughing and epistaxis.

A BAL sample from the initial examination had been subjected to mycobacterial culture according to the laboratory standard operating procedure at the Tuberculosis Laboratory of ARC-Onderstepoort Veterinary Institute. Briefly, the sample was decontaminated for 10 min using 4 % NaOH, centrifuged at 3500 rpm for 10 min and the pellet neutralized with sterile distilled water and centrifuged as before. The resulting pellet was inoculated onto Löwenstein-Jensen media slopes, supplemented with glycerol and pyruvate known to promote growth of *Mycobacterium bovis (M. bovis)*, and incubated at 37 °C.

Mycobacterial identification of acid-fast colonies was done as previously described [11]. In brief, the mycobacterial isolates were confirmed as members of the *Mycobacterium tuberculosis* complex (MTBC) by using PCR amplification of the MTBC specific 372 bp product and as *M. bovis* by amplification of the 206 bp product within the RD9 region of difference in MTBC organisms. These results were available only 4 months after initial presentation and treatment of the horse, and by which time radiographic evaluation had indicated reduction in size of the pulmonary mass. The zoonotic implications of this condition were discussed with the owner as soon as mycobacterial involvement was confirmed but further testing and isolation could not be enforced.

Spoligotyping, spacer oligonucleotide typing, which detects variability in the direct repeat region in the DNA of MTBC species including *M. bovis*, and VNTR typing based on variation in the number of tandem repeat sequences in the chromosomes of MTBC species, were used for retrospective molecular characterization of the isolate as previously described [12, 13]. Spoligotyping also confirmed the isolates as *M. bovis*, based on the lack of spacers 3, 9, 16, 39–43. Additional spacers absent were 4, 5 and 13. This pattern was consistent with spoligotype SB0868 reported in the international *M. bovis* database (www.mbovis.org). VNTR typing based on a 13 loci VNTR panel was performed as described previously [13], and revealed a unique VNTR profile (6425346436553) which has not been detected in South Africa before.

Six years after initial examination the then 15-year-old gelding was admitted by a new owner for colic and standing, laparoscope-assisted surgery for left dorsal displacement of the large colon was performed. No link was made to the previous admission due to the new owner being unaware of the previous diagnosis. No respiratory tract abnormalities were reported or detected, however, and the horse made an uneventful recovery from surgery and was discharged. The gelding was again re-examined 2 years later as a routine follow-up in this study. He had been in full work with no report of epistaxis or coughing. Physical examination disclosed no abnormalities. Thoracic ultrasonography[6] revealed mild, bilateral pleural surface irregularity of the ventral lung fields, considered incidental. CBC and serum amyloid A were within reference range. The owner declined further diagnostics and respiratory tract sampling to support bacteriological status or cure.

The present report describes the unusual clinical presentation of epistaxis in a horse with a pulmonary mass and ante-mortem detection of a *M. bovis* strain not previously identified in South Africa. Epistaxis as a presenting clinical sign has not previously been reported with tuberculosis in horses. More common causes of epistaxis in horses, that were excluded in this case, include trauma, exercise induced pulmonary hemorrhage, ethmoid hematoma, guttural pouch mycosis and coagulopathy [14]. The case reported was treated with a 2-month course of fluoroquinolone antimicrobial, which was associated with resolution of clinical signs and concurrent reduction in size of the pulmonary mass. In human medicine, fluoroquinolones are classified as second line drugs for the treatment of tuberculosis [15]. The bactericidal activity of fluoroquinolones against *M. tuberculosis* is important to provide a rapid reduction in infective load and to sterilize the infection [16]. Furthermore, use of moxifloxacin fluoroquinolone in a combination treatment regimen with rifampin and pyrazinamide shortened the time to negative lung cultures, compared to a standard regimen in a murine model [17]. Whilst fluoroquinolones are currently regarded as protected antimicrobials in horses [18], the murine efficacy results may explain the positive clinical response to empirical therapy in the equine case reported. Definitive diagnosis of equine tuberculosis generally relies on post-mortem examination with histopathology, culture and PCR of tissue samples [9].

Infection with *M. bovis* in horses appears to occur mostly by ingestion and the most common site of infection is the gastro-intestinal tract [3]. This is considered unlikely in the reported case since the lesion was associated with the lungs, suggesting the respiratory route as the most probable mode of transmission. Pulmonary granulomatous infection has been reported previously in a -year-old Camargue stallion that had direct contact with infected cattle and shared potentially contaminated pasture [5]. The previous history of this horse and disease status of cograzing individuals was not known.

Genotyping results of the *M. bovis* isolated revealed a spoligopattern (SB0868) and VNTR profile not previously identified in South African wildlife or livestock. The affected horse had been born and was resident in another province, with one of the lowest incidences of bovine tuberculosis in the country, before being relocated after purchase. Based on the time frame between the dates of purchase and presentation for epistaxis, it is highly improbable that the horse had contracted the disease while in the possession of the new owner. Unfortunately, no further historical details were available which could assist in tracing back the origin of the *M. bovis* strain.

M. bovis can be transmitted from horses to humans, and a rare case of zoonotic transmission of *M. bovis* associated with the skin of a horse has been described [6]. This report emphasized the importance of public awareness and control of the disease with special attention to those domesticated animals with close contact to humans such as horses. Horses, like cats, dogs and sheep, are considered incidental spill-over hosts and infection is not sustained within the population concerned [19]. In the present case, *M. bovis* was isolated from a respiratory tract sample, signifying that the horse could have been shedding the organism in respiratory secretions. Before laboratory confirmation of the diagnosis, which was delayed due to the prolonged culture time for MTBC, the horse had multiple contacts with other horses and humans, raising the possibility of disease transmission. While antemortem diagnosis of *M. bovis* infection is difficult, it is recommended that horses presenting with similar lesions should be kept isolated until laboratory exclusion of mycobacterial infection, preferably using a more rapid diagnostic method such as PCR.

Conclusion

In conclusion, this report describes the unusual presentation of epistaxis in a horse secondary to pulmonary tuberculosis, and supports that horses may contract and harbor *M. bovis* despite their reported lower susceptibility compared to other domestic animals. The source of this infection is unknown as the *M. bovis* strain has not previously been detected in domestic animals or wildlife in South Africa. The organism was isolated from a BAL sample, indicating that the horse could have been shedding the organism and thereby presenting the risk of forward transmission at the time. Because of the contagious and zoonotic nature of the disease, it is of outmost importance to ensure that measures are taken to prevent transmission of *M. bovis* between potentially infected horses and in-contact persons.

Endnotes

[1]Olympus Medical System Corporation, Tokyo, Japan.
[2]Siemens Polydoros 100, Siemens, Forchheim, Germany.
[3]Aloka SSD 630, Aloka, Tokyo, Japan.
[4]Baytril 10 %, Bayer Animal Health, Isando, South Africa.
[5]KI powder, Kyron laboratories, Johannesburg, South Africa.
[6]Sonorite A6V, Sonoscape Co. Ltd, China.

Acknowledgements
We thank Ms Sussie Murray and Dr Claude Sabeta (ARC-Onderstepoort Veterinary Institute) for assisting with the isolation of *Mycobacterium bovis* and for critically reviewing the manuscript, respectively.

Funding
This work was funded by the ARC-Onderstepoort Veterinary Institute and Equine Clinic of the Onderstepoort Veterinary Academic Hospital.

Authors' contributions
TM conceived the study, identified the Mycobacteria, carried out molecular typing of the *M. bovis* isolate, analysed and interpreted results, and was involved in drafting the manuscript and critically reviewing it. DS was involved in the clinical examination and treatment and participated in drafting the manuscript and critically reviewing it. PP analysed and interpreted results, and was involved in drafting and critically reviewing the manuscript. AL was involved in the conception of the study, data analysis, and in the drafting and critical review of the manuscript. All authors read and approved the final manuscript.

Authors' information
TM is a Researcher at the ARC-Onderstepoort Veterinary Institute with an interest in Tuberculosis diagnostics and molecular epidemiology.

Competing interests
The authors declare that they have no competing interest.

Consent for publication
Not applicable.

Author details
[1]Zoonotic Diseases Section, ARC-Onderstepoort Veterinary Institute, Soutpan Rd., Onderstepoort 0110, South Africa. [2]Department of Companion Animal Clinical Studies, Faculty of Veterinary Science, University of Pretoria, Soutpan Rd., Onderstepoort 0110, South Africa. [3]The Weipers Centre Equine Hospital, School of Veterinary Medicine, University of Glasgow, Glasgow, UK. [4]Department of Veterinary Tropical Diseases, Faculty of Veterinary Science, University of Pretoria, Soutpan Rd., Onderstepoort 0110, South Africa.

References

1. Humblet M-F, Boschiroli ML, Saegerman C. Classification of worldwide bovine tuberculosis risk factors in cattle: a stratified approach. Vet Res. 2009;40:50.
2. O'Reilly LM, Daborn CJ. The epidemiology of *Mycobacterium bovis* infections in animals and man: a review. Tuberc Lung Dis. 1995;76(1):1–46.
3. Pavlik I, Jahn P, Dvorska L, Bartos M, Novotny L, Halouzka R. Mycobacterial infections in horses: a review of the literature. Vet Med. 2004;49:427–40.
4. Pavlik I, Jahn P, Moravkova M, Matlova L, Treml F, Cizek A, et al. Lung tuberculosis in a horse caused by *Mycobacterium avium subsp. avium* of serotype 2: a case report. Vet Med. 2008;53:111–6.
5. Keck N, Dutruel H, Smyej F, Nodet M, Boschiroli ML. Tuberculosis due to *Mycobacterium bovis* in a Camargue horse. Vet Rec. 2010;166:499–500.
6. Garba HS, Almed H, Galadima M. *Mycobacterium bovis* infection in a horse and man: a case of cross-infection. J Vet Sci. 2001;3:47–9.
7. Monreal L, Segura D, Segalés J, Garrido JM, Prades M. Diagnosis of *Mycobacterium bovis* infection in a mare. Vet Rec. 2001;149:712–4.
8. Sarradell JE, Alvarez J, Biscia M, Zumarraga M, Wunschmann A, Armien AG, Perez AM. *Mycobacterium bovis* infection in a horse with granulomatous enterocolitis. J Vet Diagn Invest. 2015;27:203–5.
9. Lyashchenko KP, Greewald R, Esfandiari J, Lecu, A, Waters WR, Posthaus, H, et al. Pulmonary disease due to *Mycobacterium tuberculosis* in a horse: Zoonotic concerns and limitations of ante mortem testing. Vet Med Int. 2012; Article ID 642145. Doi: 10.1155/2012642145.
10. Maas M, Michel AL, Rutten VP. Facts and dilemmas in diagnosis of tuberculosis in wildlife. Comp Immunol Microbiol Infect Dis. 2013;36:269–85.
11. Alexander KA, Pleydell E, Williams MC, Lane EP, Nyange JFC, Michel AL, et al. *Mycobacterium tuberculosis*: an emerging disease of free-ranging wildlife. Emerg Infect Dis. 2002;8:592–5.
12. Kamerbeek J, Schouls LM, Kolk A, Van Agterveld M, Van Soolingen D, Kuijper S, et al. Simultaneous detection and strain differentiation of *Mycobacterium tuberculosis* for diagnosis and epidemiology. J Clin Microbiol. 1997;35:907–14.
13. Hlokwe TM, van Helden P, Michel A. Evaluation of the discriminatory power of variable number of tandem repeat typing of *Mycobacterium bovis* isolates from southern Africa. Transbound Emerg Dis. 2013;60(1):111–20.
14. Barakzai SZ, Dixon PM. Epistaxis in the horse. Equine Vet Educ. 2004;16:207–17.
15. World Health Organization 2010. Multidrug and extensively drug-resistant TB (M/XDR-TB): 2010 global report on surveillance and response. WHO/HTM/TB/2010.3.
16. Gosling RD, Uiso LO, Sam NE, Bongard EG, Kanduma M, Nyindo RW, et al. The bactericidal activity of moxifloxacin in patients with pulmonary tuberculosis. Am J Respir Crit Care Med. 2003;168:1342–5.
17. Nuermberger EL, Yoshimatsu T, Tyagi S, Williams K, Rosenthal I, O'Brien R, et al. Moxifloxacin-containing regimen greatly reduces time to culture conversion in murine tuberculosis. Am J Respir Crit Care Med. 2004;169:421–6.

11

Visual evoked potentials in the horse

L. Ström* and B. Ekesten

Abstract

Background: Electrical potentials generated in the central nervous system in response to brief visual stimuli, flash visual evoked potentials (FVEPs), can be recorded non-invasively over the occipital cortex. FVEPs are used clinically in human medicine and also experimentally in a number of animal species, but the method has not yet been evaluated in the horse. The method would potentially allow the ophthalmologist and equine clinician to evaluate visual impairment caused by disorders affecting post-retinal visual pathways. The aim was to establish a method for recording of FVEPs in horses in a clinical setting and to evaluate the waveform morphology in the normal horse.

Methods: Ten horses were sedated with a continuous detomidine infusion. Responses were recorded from electrodes placed on the scalp. Several positions were evaluated to determine suitable electrode placement. Flash electroretinograms (FERGs) were recorded simultaneously. To evaluate potential contamination of the FVEP from retinal potentials, a retrobulbar nerve block was performed in two horses and transection of the optic nerve was performed in one horse as a terminal procedure.

Results: A series of positive (P) and negative (N) peaks in response to light stimuli was recorded in all horses. Reproducible wavelets with mean times-to-peaks of 26 (N1), 55 (P2), 141 (N2) and 216 ms (P4) were seen in all horses in all recordings. Reproducible results were obtained when the active electrode was placed in the midline rostral to the nuchal crest. Recording at lateral positions gave more variable results, possibly due to ear muscle artifacts. Averaging ≥100 responses reduced the impact of noise and artifacts. FVEPs were reproducible in the same horse during the same recording session and between sessions, but were more variable between horses. Retrobulbar nerve block caused a transient loss of the VEP whereas transection of the optic nerve caused an irreversible loss.

Conclusions: We describe the waveform of the equine FVEP and our results show that it is possible to record FVEPs in sedated horses in a clinical setting. The potentials recorded were shown to be of post-retinal origin. Further studies are needed to provide normative data and assess potential clinical use.

Keywords: Visual evoked potentials, Visual cortical evoked potentials, Flash visual evoked potentials, VEP, FVEP, Horse, Equine, Visual impairment

Background

Techniques currently available to evaluate visual impairment in the horse are limited to reflex testing, falling cotton-ball testing, ability to navigate an obstacle course and evaluation of findings detected during a routine ophthalmic examination. The results from these tests can be difficult to interpret and visual dysfunction may have to be severe before it can be diagnosed. Objective methods for evaluation of the function of visual pathways, such as visual evoked potentials (VEPs), would be a useful addition to the armamentarium of the veterinary ophthalmologist and equine clinician, to detect and evaluate disorders affecting post-retinal pathways in this species.

In 1954, Adrian & Matthews [1] reported that electrical potentials generated by neurons in the central nervous system in response to visual stimuli, VEPs, can be recorded from electrodes placed over the human occipital cortex. Dawson [2] developed a superimposition technique, called signal averaging, to extract the VEP waveform from the electroencephalogram (EEG) and subsequently, Cigánek [3] described the waveform morphology of the human VEP. In the years following further work was performed to explore the VEP in

* Correspondence: lena.strom@slu.se
Department of Clinical Sciences, Swedish University of Agricultural Sciences, PO Box 7054, SE-750 07 Uppsala, Sweden

human beings, improve the technique and implement recording of VEPs as a clinical, diagnostic aid.

Diseases or trauma affecting neurons in the retina or the post-retinal visual pathways can alter the waveform of the VEP. Therefore this technique can be used to investigate the functional integrity of post-retinal visual pathways, including the optic nerves, optic tract and optic radiation to the visual cortex. The method is used as a complement to the electroretinogram (ERG) and allows functional assessment of the visual pathways, while imaging techniques, such as magnetic resonance imaging (MRI) and computer tomography (CT), mainly are used to obtain information about structural integrity in patients. VEPs are used in human medicine to evaluate visual impairment due to several pathological conditions, such as cortical trauma or anoxia, meningitis, optic neuritis, optic neuropathies, demyelinating diseases and compression of post-retinal pathways due to tumors [4].

The International Society for Clinical Electrophysiology of Vision (ISCEV) regularly updates the human standard protocols for clinical electrophysiological examinations [5]. Guidelines are also issued by the American Clinical Neurophysiology Society [6]. In human patients, VEPs are usually recorded non-invasively using skin electrodes on the scalp overlying the visual cortex. In routine testing the VEP scalp electrodes are normally placed according to either the International 10/20 system [7] or the Queen Square System [8]. Midline electrodes over the visual cortex are used to assess prechiasmal function, while additional lateral electrode positions are used to assess chiasmal and postchiasmal dysfunction.

Usually one eye at a time is stimulated by flashes of white light (flash-VEP; FVEP) or a reversing, isoluminant pattern (pattern-VEP; PVEP). In human subjects, PVEPs are preferred in most clinical situations due to less variability than the FVEPs and PVEPs will also enable a better quantitative assessment of visual function. However, when using a pattern stimulus it is critical that the subject focuses on the pattern and in infants and patients with poor cooperation, poor fixation or poor acuity, the FVEP can be more useful [5].

While VEPs have been evaluated in a number of animal species such as the dog [9, 10], cat [11–13], cow [14], pig [15], sheep [16] and a large number of laboratory animal species [17], the use of VEP in the horse has only been very scantily described [18]. A simple protocol for recording the equine VEP in a clinical setting would be a useful tool to assess function of post-retinal pathways in this species and also of use in the investigation of neurological disorders.

Methods

The aim of this study was to establish a method for recording FVEP in horses in a clinical setting and to evaluate the waveform morphology in the normal horse. Electrode positions and the number of averaged responses needed to produce robust and reproducible VEP waveforms were also assessed. Additionally, recording of FVEPs after retrobulbar nerve block and transection of the optic nerve was performed to evaluate possible contamination of the FVEP by retinal potentials (ERGs).

Horses and procedures

Ten Swedish Standardbred Trotters, seven mares and three geldings, aged 3 to 19 years (median age: 11 years) were included in the study (Table 1). All horses were deemed to be healthy on the basis of a physical examination prior to the recordings. The regional Ethical Committee (Uppsala Djurförsöksetiska nämnd, Sweden, dnr C254/10 and dnr C39/12) approved the use of the horses in the study and the experiments were carried out following the guidelines of the ARVO guidelines for animal experimentation.

Table 1 FVEPs and FERGs were performed in ten healthy Swedish Standardbred Trotters

Horse	Age at examination (years)	Gender	Eye(s)	ERG	Number of averages	Electrode positions	Lateral positions	Transection	Retro bulbar nerve block	Reproducibility
A	19	M	OD	X	4–196	$P_{z\text{-}0}$ $P_{z\text{-}15}$ $P_{z\text{-}30}$ $P_{z\text{-}45}$ $P_{z\text{-}60}$	P_1 P_2 P_3 P_4	-	-	X
B	10, 11	G	OS	X	144	$P_{z\text{-}0}$ $P_{z\text{-}15}$ $P_{z\text{-}30}$ $P_{z\text{-}45}$ $P_{z\text{-}60}$	P_1 P_2 P_3 P_4	-	-	X
C	16, 17	M	OD	X	144	$P_{z\text{-}0}$ $P_{z\text{-}15}$ $P_{z\text{-}30}$ $P_{z\text{-}45}$ $P_{z\text{-}60}$	P_1 P_2 P_3 P_4	-	-	-
D	16, 17	M	OS (OD)	X	144	$P_{z\text{-}0}$ $P_{z\text{-}15}$ $P_{z\text{-}30}$ $P_{z\text{-}45}$ $P_{z\text{-}60}$	P_1 P_2 P_3 P_4	-	-	X
E	10, 11	M	OD	X	4–196	$P_{z\text{-}0}$ $P_{z\text{-}15}$ $P_{z\text{-}30}$ $P_{z\text{-}45}$ $P_{z\text{-}60}$	P_1 P_2	-	-	X
F	5	G	OS	X	4–196	$P_{z\text{-}45}$	P_1 P_2 P_3 P_4	-	-	X
G	17	M	OS	X	144	$P_{z\text{-}45}$	P_1 P_2	-	-	-
H	3	M	OS (OD)	X	144	$P_{z\text{-}45}$	P_1 P_2	-	-	-
I	4	M	OS (OD)	X	144	$P_{z\text{-}45}$	P_1 P_2	X	X	-
J	5	G	OD (OS)	X	144	$P_{z\text{-}45}$	P_1 P_2	-	X	-

Recordings from one, randomly selected eye were performed in six horses and from both eyes in four horses. "X" indicates that a certain procedure was performed. There were no statistical differences comparing eyes in this study

In five horses (horses A-E) five electrode positions in the midline, and two to four lateral positions were evaluated (Table 1). In the remaining five horses (horses F-J), one position in the midline and two to four lateral positions were evaluated. FVEPs were recorded at two separate sessions in five horses (horses A-B and D-F). The minimum number of responses averaged to obtain a waveform with clearly distinguishable wavelets was evaluated in three horses (horses A, E and F). For comparison between eyes in the same horse, both eyes were evaluated in horses D and H-J. Unilateral retrobulbar nerve blocks were performed in two horses (horses I and J) and transection of the optic nerve was performed in one horse (horse I). This was performed as a terminal procedure.

Ophthalmic examination

An ophthalmic examination including a cotton-ball test, reflex testing, slit-lamp biomicroscopy (Kowa SL-15; Kowa Co.Ltd., Tokyo, Japan), direct and indirect ophthalmoscopy (Heine Beta 200 and Heine Omega 500; Heine Optotechnik, Herrsching, Germany) and tonometry (TonoVet®, Icare Finland Oy, Helsinki, Finland) was performed in all horses. Furthermore, all horses were evaluated in a simple obstacle course, with five obstacles, under room-light conditions to assess vision prior to the recordings. No findings indicating visual impairment, ocular or neurological disease were observed in any of the horses.

Preparations

Pupils were dilated with 1–2 drops of tropicamide (Mydriacyl, 0.5 %, Alcon, Stockholm, Sweden). Recordings were started when pupils were fully dilated. The size of the pupils was monitored repeatedly during the recording sessions. The cornea was kept moist throughout the experiment by repeated instillation of artificial tears (ZilkEye, Evolan Pharma AB, Stockholm, Sweden).

The horses were sedated with a bolus injection of detomidine, 0.01 mg/kg (Domosedan vet, 10 mg/ml, Orion Pharma Animal Health, Sollentuna, Sweden) intravenously, followed by maintenance of sedation throughout the recording sessions using a continuous intravenous infusion of 2 % detomidine in physiologic saline solution (Natriumklorid, 7 mg/ml, Fresenius Kabi, Uppsala, Sweden) (2.0–2.6 mg detomidine hydrocloride/100 kg*h). The depth of sedation was monitored continuously and the infusion rate was adjusted to maintain a stable level of sedation where the horses kept their heads resting heavily on a padded headstand without becoming unsteady.

Akinesia and partial analgesia of the eyelids was induced with subcutaneous injections of 2.5 ml mepivacaine (Carbocain, 20 mg/ml, AstraZeneca, Södertälje, Sweden) over the auriculopalpebral and supraorbital nerves. A local infiltration of mepivacaine (Carbocain, 20 mg/ml, AstraZeneca, Södertälje, Sweden) was performed at each electrode position to reduce muscle contractions that potentially could give rise to artifacts in the FVEP. The cornea was anaesthetized with topical application of 2–3 drops of tetracaine (Tetrakain Chauvin, 1 %, Bausch & Lomb Nordic AB, Stockholm, Sweden).

The contralateral eye was covered by a black, opaque plastic eye shield during recordings (Fig. 1). Wads of cotton were stuffed in the ear canals to reduce noise-induced artifacts.

Retrobulbar nerve block and transection of the optic nerve

Horses I and J were prepared as for a transpalpebral enucleation in the standing, sedated horse [19, 20]. A single dose of flunixin meglumine (Flunixin N-vet, 50 mg/ml, N-vet, Uppsala, Sweden), 1.1 mg/kg, was administered intravenously pre-operatively. Akinesia of the eyelids, anesthesia at electrode positions and topical

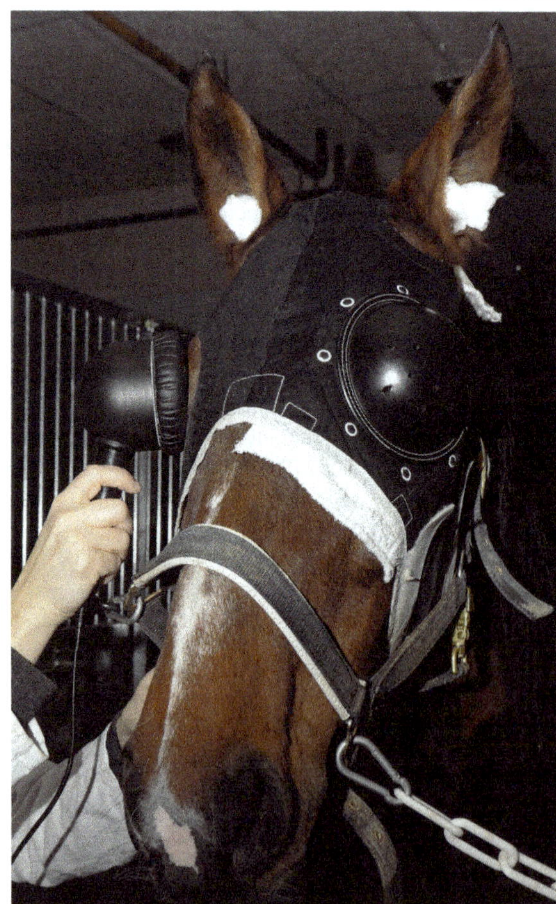

Fig. 1 FVEP in a horse using a handheld flash photostimulator. An opaque plastic eye shield covers the fellow eye and cotton wads in the ears are used to reduce auditory stimuli that could influence the level of consciousness

anesthesia were performed and sedation maintained as previously described. FERGs and FVEPs were recorded. A retrobulbar nerve block was performed as has been described by Gilger & Davidson [21] and the surgical site was infiltrated with mepivacain (Carbocain, 20 mg/ml, AstraZeneca, Södertälje, Sweden). Transection of the optic nerve was performed (horse I) 45 min after the retrobulbar nerve block. FERGs and FVEPs were recorded and rebound tonometry performed before and after the retrobulbar block in both horses, as well as before and after transection of the optic nerve in horse I. Both horses (I and J) were euthanized after the recordings in accordance with the ethical approval.

Electrophysiological testing

Light-adapted FERGs and FVEPs were recorded simultaneously. The recordings were performed in an examination room at the horse clinic of the University Animal Hospital, SLU, Uppsala. All electronic equipment not required for the study was disconnected to avoid mains current interference, but no other adjustments were made to the room.

A handheld dome-shaped photostimulator (Retiport mini-Ganzfeld, Acrivet GmbH, Hennigsdorf, Germany) with a background light intensity of 25 cd/m^2 and a flash intensity of 3 cd/m^2/s was used to light-adapt and stimulate the retina (Fig. 1). The stimuli were presented at a frequency of 1.09 Hz. The sweep duration was 500 ms post-stimulus. The room was kept dark during recordings to avoid interference by stray light.

Responses were amplified (amplifier set to x10^4), band-pass filtered (0.1–300 Hz for FERGs and 1–100 Hz for FVEPs), stored and analyzed using an Acrivet RETI*port* (Acrivet GmbH, Hennigsdorf, Germany, software version 5.9.7.0) and a laptop computer.

FERGs

Light-adapted FERGs were recorded using corneal electrodes (Gold-foil corneal electrodes, CH electronics, Bromley, UK). Metal corkscrew electrodes (Stainless Steel Disposable Corkscrew Electrode, Cephalon A/S, Nørresundby, Denmark) served as ground and reference electrodes and were placed at the forehead and approximately 3 cm caudal to the lateral canthus, respectively. Electrode impedance was kept below 3 kΩin all FERG recordings.

FVEPs

Electrode positions were essentially selected based on a combination of the International 10–20 system [7] and Queen Square System [8] for human beings. Figure 2 shows the position of evaluated electrode positions in the midline in relation to the equine brain and the primary visual cortex heralded by the stria of Gennari in our postmortem specimens. The electrodes were placed at distances relative to bony landmarks on the head to adjust for head size. The distance between the nuchal crest and a line connecting the supraorbital foramina was measured and the electrodes were positioned at preselected percentages along this distance (Fig. 3), where the nuchal crest was the starting point (0 %) and the level of the supraorbital foramina was at 100 %. The first active electrode was placed on the nuchal crest in the midline ($P_{z\text{-}0}$; z = in the sagittal midline, 0 = 0 % rostral

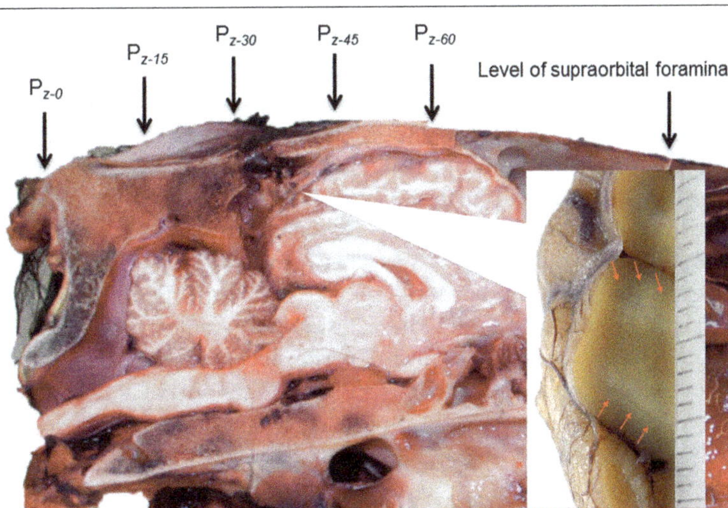

Fig. 2 The evaluated electrode positions along the midline shown relative to the equine brain. The subscript. "z" denotes a position in the sagittal midline and the numerical subscript reflects a percentage of the distance between the nuchal crest and the connecting line between the supraorbital foramina. The insert shows the approximate position of the striate cortex, or primary visual cortex. Red arrows indicate the stria of Gennari, which represents myelinated axons from the lateral geniculate body terminating in the gray matter in the primary visual cortex

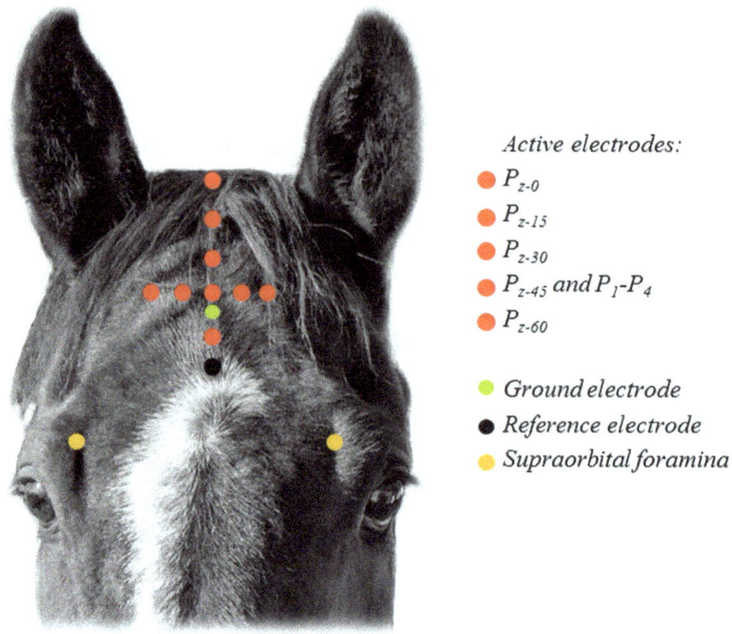

Fig. 3 The first active electrode was placed on the nuchal crest in the midline ($P_{z\text{-}0}$). The following positions along the midline were placed in front of the nuchal crest at regular intervals ($P_{z\text{-}0}$ to $P_{z\text{-}60}$). Lateral positions, P_1 to P_4, were evaluated with electrodes placed two and four centimeters lateral to the midline electrode at $P_{z\text{-}45}$. Photo: Dr Måns Michanek

to the nuchal crest). The following positions of active electrodes along the midline were placed in front of the nuchal crest at intervals of 15 % ($P_{z\text{-}0}$ to $P_{z\text{-}60}$). Lateral positions, P_1 to P_4, were evaluated with electrodes placed two and four centimeters lateral to the midline electrode at $P_{z\text{-}45}$. The ground and reference electrodes were positioned in the midline at 50 % and 70 %, respectively, of the distance from the nuchal crest and a line connecting the supraorbital foramina. Electrode impedance was kept below 2 kΩ in all FVEP recordings.

Averaged responses of 4, 16, 32, 64, 100, 144 and 196 sweeps were evaluated in horse A, E and F. The duration of a recording was therefore 3.7, 15, 29, 59, 92, 132 and 180 s respectively (frequency of 1.09 Hz). Averaged responses of 144 sweeps were evaluated in the remaining horses (horses B-D and G-J) and the duration of each averaged response was 2.2 min (132 s).

Monocular recordings were obtained from one randomly selected eye in all horses. In addition to this, recordings from the fellow eye were obtained in four horses (horses D and H-J to be able to enable comparison of recordings between eyes of the same horse.

Evaluation of ERGs and VEPs

FERG a- and b-wave amplitudes and times-to-peak (latencies) were measured according to convention [22]. The wavelets in the recorded FVEP waveform were named according to the nomenclature by Harding [23], a classification that was adopted in veterinary neurophysiology by Strain et al. in 1986 [14]. FVEP wavelet amplitudes and times-to-peak were measured as shown in Fig. 4. Results from recordings before and after retrobulbar nerve block (horse I-J) and transection of the optic nerve (horse I) were compared to evaluate if retinal potentials were recorded at the electrode positions on the scalp, thus contaminating the waveform, or if the recorded FVEP only represented post-retinal potentials.

Data analyses

Descriptive data; means, standard deviations (SDs) and ranges are reported for FVEP wavelet peak-to-peak amplitudes (μV) and times-to-peaks (ms). Data were analyzed using the non-parametric Kruskal-Wallis one-way analysis of variance by ranks and by regression analysis. Levene´s test was used to assess the equality of variances between groups. P-values ≤0.05 were considered statistically significant. Bonferroni correction was used to adjust the p-values when multiple comparisons were performed. Statistical analysis was performed with JMP® Pro 11 (Version 11.0.0, SAS Institute Inc., Cary, NC).

Results

Reproducible FVEPs and light-adapted FERGs were readily recorded from all ten, sedated horses. It was not possible to obtain reproducible recordings with acceptable quality from non-sedated horses due to movement and muscle artifacts. The waveform of the equine FVEP consisted of three major positive, P2-P4, and two major

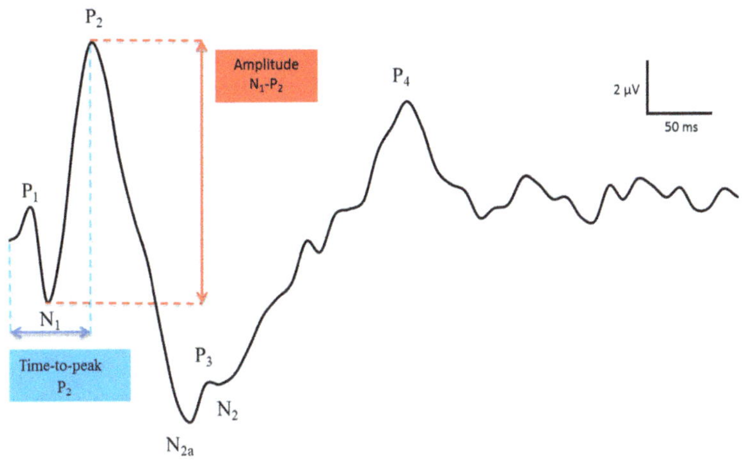

Fig. 4 Measurements of amplitudes and times-to-peak in the equine FVEP. Amplitudes were measured from the peak or trough of wavelet preceding the trough or peak of interest. Time-to-peak measurements were made from the onset of the stimulus to the maximum amplitude of the peak or trough

negative wavelets, N1-N2 (Fig. 5). The first negative wavelet, N1 and the most prominent positive wavelet, P2, was present in all recordings in all horses, as well as the large negative N2-complex and subsequent positive P4-wavelet. An early positive peak, P1, with a time-to-peak between 12–20 ms, was present in all horses, but only in approximately 50 % of the recordings in each horse. A small positive wavelet, P3, splitting the N2-complex into two parts, N2a and N2, was observed in all horses and in 82 % of recordings on average. A late positive wavelet, P5, with a time-to-peak between 275–375 ms was present in 74 % of recordings in nine out of the ten horses. Times-to-peak and peak-to-peak amplitudes are shown in Table 2.

The waveform was reproducibly recorded and no significant differences in amplitudes or times-to-peaks were found when comparing recordings from the same recording session and at the following session ($p > 0.05$; Fig. 6). There were no significant differences in times-to-peaks or amplitudes regardless of eye stimulated.

The overall waveform morphology did not differ between the electrode positions in the midline ($P_{z\text{-}0}$, $P_{z\text{-}15}$, $P_{z\text{-}30}$, $P_{z\text{-}45}$ and $P_{z\text{-}60}$) but the FVEP waveform was somewhat difficult to evaluate at the most caudal positions (Fig. 7). Average times-to-peak did not differ significantly between electrode positions but there were significant differences comparing amplitudes N1P2, P2N2 and N2P4 from recordings at $P_{z\text{-}0}$ and $P_{z\text{-}60}$ to recordings at $P_{z\text{-}30}$

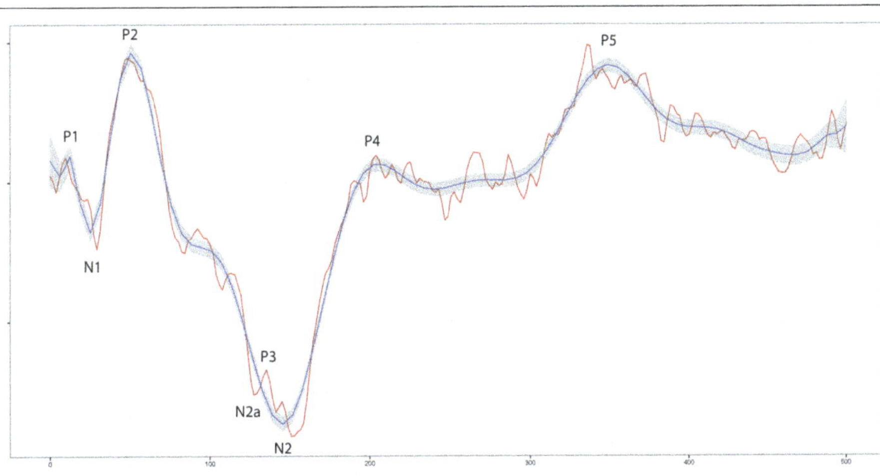

Fig. 5 Equine FVEP waveform. An equine FVEP waveform with typical peaks and troughs indicated (from horse B; position $P_{z\text{-}30}$). The red curve shows one recording (144 averaged responses). Data from 40 recordings (with 144 responses each) are averaged into the blue curve and shown with a 95 % confidence interval. Vertical division = 5 µV

Table 2 FVEP amplitudes and times-to-peaks in ten horses with the active electrode at P_{z-45}

		Time-to-peak (ms)								Peak-to-peak amplitude (μV)			
Horse	Eye	P1	N1	P2	N2a	P3	N2	P4	P5	N1-P2	P2-N2	N2a-P3	N2-P4
A	OD	13 ± 1.4	28 ± 1.2	59 ± 2.0	124 ± 3.5	137 ± 8.7	150 ± 4.6	273 ± 8.6	Missing	9.6 ± 1.0	11.9 ± 1.8	2.5 ± 1.2	8.4 ± 2.9
B	OS	12 ± 3.5	26 ± 1.1	54 ± 2.3	113 ± 4.2	123 ± 3.5	145 ± 8.8	218 ± 13.8	373 ± 31.4	7.4 ± 0.7	15.7 ± 3.6	0.4 ± 0.1	13.5 ± 4.9
C	OD	14 ± 0.1	28 ± 1.0	62 ± 2.5	104 ± 4.1	125 ± 5.6	153 ± 7.5	207 ± 13.8	354 ± 15.8	6.1 ± 1.2	5.9 ± 1.4	1.5 ± 1.0	3.7 ± 1.1
D	OS	18 ± 1.0	25 ± 2.0	47 ± 1.5	87 ± 12.0	107 ± 10.0	138 ± 8.8	200 ± 15.3	260 ± 7.2	2.2 ± 0.8	4.5 ± 1.0	1.5 ± 1.0	4.5 ± 1.1
E	OD	16 ± 3.5	29 ± 0.1	55 ± 4.0	99 ± 1.4	116 ± 2.8	153 ± 6.8	234 ± 24.6	375 ± 10.2	3.8 ± 1.5	4.6 ± 1.4	2.9 ± 1.1	4.5 ± 1.5
F	OS	12 ± 2.3	27 ± 1.4	54 ± 4.6	105 ± 4.6	122 ± 7.6	148 ± 6.4	213 ± 18.2	361 ± 26.2	7.3 ± 1.8	13.8 ± 3.9	0.4 ± 0.3	11.1 ± 3.7
G	OS	17 ± 1.2	30 ± 2.7	58 ± 3.0	104 ± 22.2	111 ± 18.9	137 ± 5.5	213 ± 13.3	355 ± 30.3	2.6 ± 0.6	6.2 ± 1.2	2.8 ± 4.7	8.3 ± 2.5
H	OD	20 ± 1.1	32 ± 5.9	57 ± 4.0	84 ± 28.9	95 ± 27.0	133 ± 7.9	202 ± 13.7	337 ± 32.7	2.5 ± 0.5	5.7 ± 1.5	0.9 ± 0.4	8.0 ± 2.6
I	OS	12 ± 3.1	17 ± 3.5	48 ± 2.2	103 ± 6.2	110 ± 8.2	130 ± 3.0	193 ± 7.1	305 ± 12.1	1.8 ± 0.2	3.5 ± 0.7	0.2 ± 0.1	4.5 ± 0.7
J	OD	6 ± 2.6	22 ± 5.9	52 ± 4.8	94 ± 12.5	107 ± 12.9	140 ± 6.8	206 ± 20.0	347 ± 19.8	2.2 ± 0.6	5.0 ± 1.5	4.8 ± 1.5	4.8 ± 1.7
95 % CI		12–14	26–28	55–57	99–105	113–120	137–142	213–224	324–345	4.3–5.5	6.1–7.8	1.3–2.3	5.9–7.4

A minimum of 5 recordings (144 averaged responses each) are included from each horse
Data are shown as means ± SDs

and P_{z-45} ($p < 0.001$). Amplitudes increased when moving the electrode position rostrally from the most caudal position at the nuchal crest, reaching maximum amplitudes at the positions P_{z-30} and P_{z-45} (Fig. 8). Moving further rostrally decreased the amplitudes.

At lateral positions (P_1 to P_4), both amplitudes and times-to-peak showed a greater variability compared to recordings in the midline but there were no significant differences between means of times-to-peaks and amplitudes in our material.

When averaging 4 and 16 responses, the waveform was very difficult to evaluate and most recordings were discarded. Times-to-peaks and amplitudes from recordings with 32 and 64 averaged responses did not differ statistically compared to recordings with 100, 144 and 196 averages, but the waveform was more challenging for the examiner to evaluate due to artifacts. By averaging no less than 100 responses, the background noise was reduced, which resulted in more easily discernible peaks and reduced number of peaks split by large artifacts.

The FVEP was affected by the retrobulbar nerve block (Figs. 9 and 10). FVEP amplitudes were gradually reduced in both horses (I and J) and after 25 min, only a minuscule remnant of P2 was discernible, despite that FERG a- and b-wave times-to-peaks were within normal limits and b-wave amplitudes were only marginally reduced. Intraocular pressures (IOPs) in the examined eye were 42 mmHg (horse J) and 56 mmHg (horse I) 25 min after the block (IOPs before retrobulbar block; 19 and 22 mmHg respectively). In horse J, the peaks and troughs of the equine FVEP were clearly visible again approximately 90 min after the nerve block, although FVEP amplitudes and times-to-peaks were not yet within normal limits. In horse I, the FVEP disappeared when the optic nerve was transected (Fig. 10). FERG a- and b-wave times-to-peaks were within normal limits after the transection, but amplitudes were somewhat

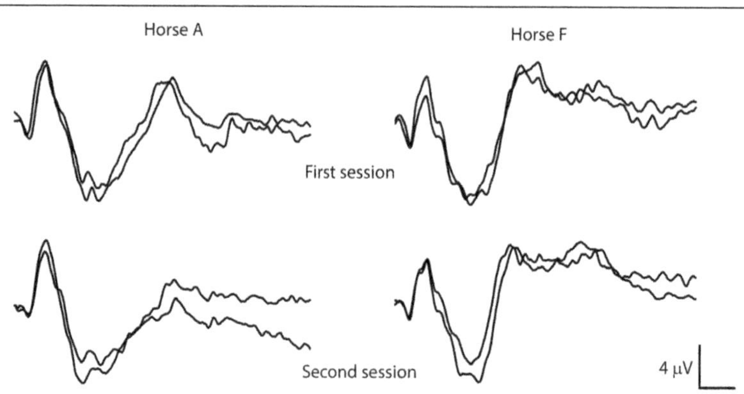

Fig. 6 Reproducibility of equine FVEPs. FVEPs recorded from two horses (horses A and F) with the active electrode at P_{z-45}. Two recordings from the first (top row) and second sessions several weeks later (bottom row) are shown

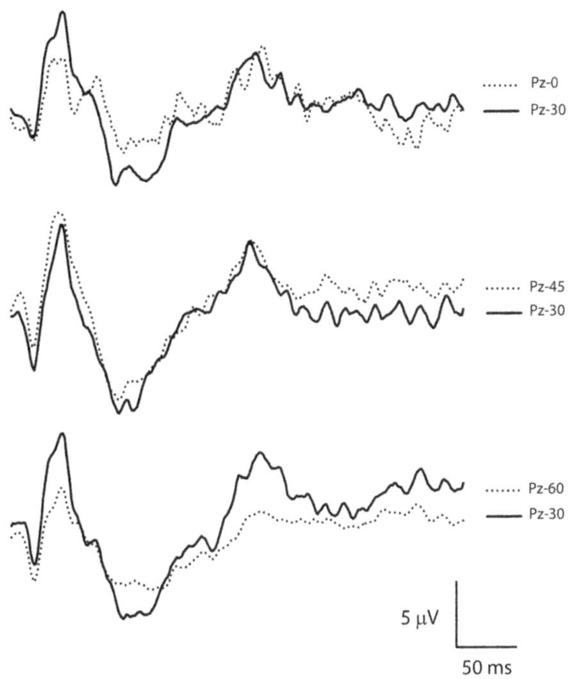

Fig. 7 FVEPs from different electrode positions. The overall waveform morphology did not differ between electrode positions in the midline but amplitudes were significantly reduced at the most caudal ($P_{z\text{-}0}$) and rostral ($P_{z\text{-}60}$) positions and it was often more difficult to obtain a reasonably smooth waveform due to artifacts. Recordings from horse A

reduced. The intraocular pressure was measured to 57 mmHg at this point. When the IOP rose above 70 mmHg due to retrobulbar hemorrhage and oedema (65 min after the nerve block), FERG a- and b-waves were also abolished.

Light-adapted FERGs were recorded from all eyes included in the study (Table 3). Times-to-peaks of the a- and b-waves were highly consistent both within and between horses while peak-to-peak amplitudes were more variable. Means for times-to-peaks of the a- and b-waves were 13 ± 1 ms and 30 ± 1 ms respectively. The mean a- and b-wave amplitudes were 10 ± 3 and 63 ± 15 μV respectively.

Discussion

VEPs were easily recorded in sedated horses under standard clinical settings and the overall waveform resembled those recorded in other mammalian species [5, 9–11, 13, 14, 16]. It has been shown in dogs that the signal recorded from VEP scalp electrodes can include a far-field conducted ERG [24, 25]. On the other hand, Sims et al. [9] have shown that transection of the optic nerve completely abolishes the light-adapted canine FVEP and that the recorded potentials are of post-retinal origin under light-adapted conditions. The horse has a large retina and the potentials generated are sizable. Thus it was important to evaluate if the equine FVEP recorded over the scalp consisted of post-retinal potentials only, or if a far-field conducted FERG was included. It is known in humans that a retrobulbar nerve block can cause temporary blindness due to a complete block of transmission in the optic nerve [26, 27] and we used retrobulbar anaesthesia and optic nerve transection to show that our recordings of the equine FVEP must be of post-retinal origin. Although the intraocular pressures were increased and FERG amplitudes were somewhat affected during the experiments, it has been shown in other species that increased intraocular pressures will result in reduced b-wave amplitudes [28–30], but simultaneous FVEP recordings will be more resistant to the pressure change [31]. Thus, it is highly unlikely that the increased intraocular pressure was causing the loss of the FVEPs in our recordings.

By using the FVEP we have also verified that the retrobulbar nerve block causes a transient loss of vision in the horse which should be considered when this method of anesthesia is employed for performing standing ocular surgery in this species.

Waveform morphology, times-to-peaks and peak-to-peak amplitudes were reproducible between recording sessions in the same horse and also similar between horses, although some differences in times-to-peaks and especially amplitudes were observed. It is well known from human beings [5] and other species [11] that the FVEP is highly variable between individuals. Four wavelets (N1, P2, N2 and P4) were observed in all FVEPs from all horses whereas additional wavelets were present in some recordings in all horses (P1, N2a and P3). A late, positive component (P5) was present in the majority of recordings in most horses. The differences in waveform morphology might represent the variability of the FVEP between individuals. However, in our study, these differences might also be due to varying depth of sedation, or that the individual horse might react differently to external disturbances in the clinical setting. The most reliable wavelets in the equine FVEP were the N1, P2, N2 and P4, which indicate that these peaks could be of use when the FVEP is employed as a diagnostic tool to diagnose and localize abnormal function in post-retinal visual pathways.

Choosing the suitable electrode position enhanced detection of the individual wavelets composing the equine FVEP. The wavelets became more obvious and distinct when the active electrodes were positioned well in front of the nuchal crest at electrode positions $P_{z\text{-}30}$ and $P_{z\text{-}45}$. These positions correspond well to the position of the occipital cortex and presumed anatomical location of the visual cortex in the horse [32], which we confirmed using the stria of Gennari as our landmark in postmortem specimens (Fig. 2). As expected, the electrode

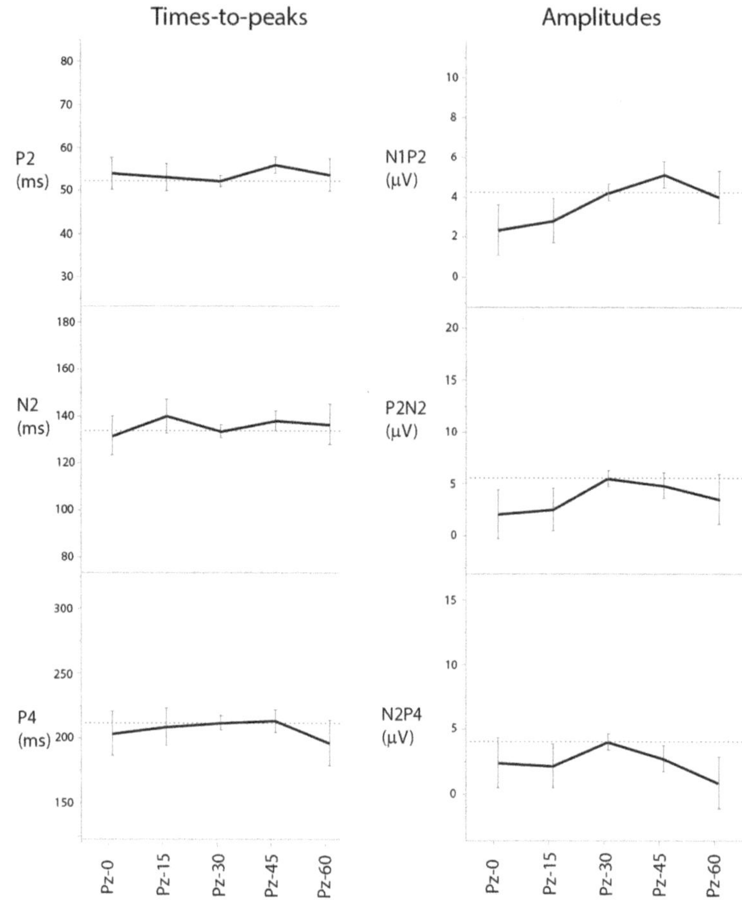

Fig. 8 Amplitudes and times-to-peaks at different electrode positions. Amplitudes increased when moving the electrode position rostrally from the most caudal position at the nuchal crest, reaching maximum amplitudes at the positions $P_{z\text{-}30}$ and $P_{z\text{-}45}$. Moving further rostrally decreased the amplitudes. Times-to-peaks did not differ significantly between any of the positions tested in this material

positions providing the largest amplitudes in the horse differ considerably from the positions recommended in the guidelines for clinical VEPs in human beings [5], reflecting the substantial anatomical differences between man and horse. An asymmetry was expected when recording the FVEP at ipsi- and contralateral positions due to the high degree of decussation of optic fibers in the horse of more than 80 % [33]. It was thus somewhat surprising that results from lateral positioning of the active electrodes were inconclusive, with regards to the separation of signals from the right and left hemispheres. The reason for this may be due to the close proximity to the ears of the horse. The lateral electrode positions were close to the base of the pinnae and the large muscles controlling ear movements in this species [34]. However, while muscle artifacts due to ear movements may have masked more subtle differences between lateral and midline positions, a method for obtaining FVEPs from the more lateral electrode positions without picking up artifacts from the ear muscles would be useful, because these positions may be important for differing between pre- and postchiasmal lesions in certain horses with visual impairment.

Sufficient and stable depth of sedation enhanced recording of FVEPs and FERGs in our study, which is in accordance with previous studies when FERGs were recorded in the standing, sedated horse [35–37]. Movement artifacts did occasionally overshadow a response, but the stable level of sedation obtained by continuous infusion of detomidine kept the horses sufficiently immobile to allow recording of reproducible FERGs and FVEPs. It was obvious that the depth of sedation influenced the amount of artifacts and the quality of recordings. When only light sedation was used, ear movements and head movements in response to sudden sounds caused muscle movement artifacts, which could wipe out the normal waveform. The use of earplugs reduced the episodes of increased alertness due to undesired auditory stimuli affecting the level of sedation. In summary, we conclude that a sufficiently stable level and depth of sedation can be accomplished by a bolus dose followed by a continuous infusion of detomidine.

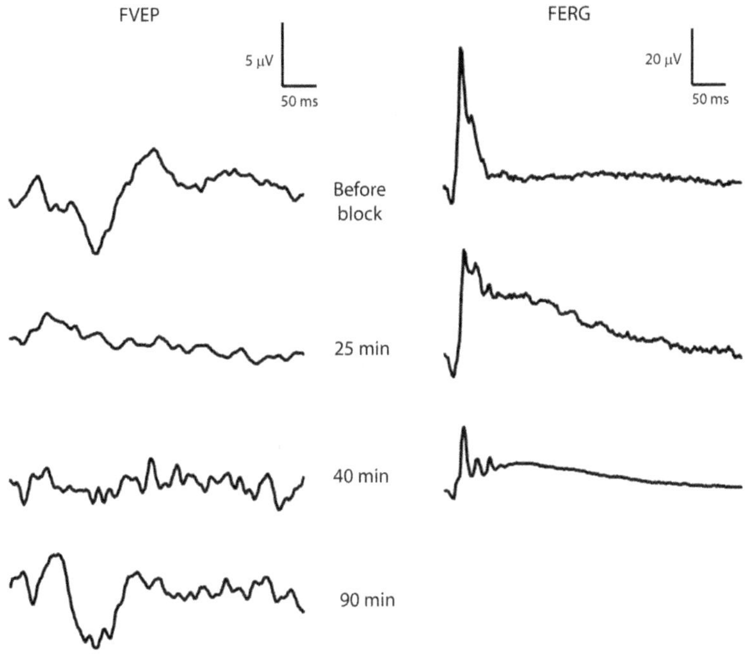

Fig. 9 FVEPs after retrobulbar nerve block. FVEPs recorded at P_{z-45} in horse J from the right eye (left column) before retrobulbar nerve block (uppermost tracing), 25, 40 and 90 min after retrobulbar nerve block (lower tracings). Simultaneous FERG recordings from the right eye are shown in the right column

However, it is important to note that in human beings and other species, some sedatives have been shown to affect the VEP [38], causing reduced amplitudes and somewhat prolonged times-to-peak. To our knowledge, the specific effects of detomidine on the VEP has not yet been evaluated. It is reasonable to believe that amplitudes and times-to-peaks may be affected by sedation with alfa-2-agonists, but we were unable to obtain recordings with acceptable quality from non-sedated horses. Therefore, we recommend performing recordings under sedation. To be able to compare results between horses, it is important to continuously monitor the level of sedation during the recordings.

According to our results, at least 100 sweeps are needed in sedated horses to suppress electrical noise and obtain curves with easily discernible, reproducible peaks and troughs. This might be especially important for the inexperienced examiner. Overall, the equine FVEP appears to require more averaged responses than suggested by the ISCEV guidelines, which is likely to reflect that both the amount of potentially disturbing auditory stimuli in a busy equine clinic is higher than in a human ophthalmology or neurology clinic, and that our equine patients may be less cooperative and docile than the average adult human patient. However, it is important to note that 32–64 averaged responses in the horse may also produce acceptable results. Although there might be more noise and artifacts affecting the quality of the recordings, our results indicate that times-to-peaks and amplitudes will not be significantly affected when measured by an experienced examiner. The advantage of averaging fewer responses is that the time to perform the examination will be reduced, which might be important when recording the VEP in a critically ill patient.

The corkscrew electrodes used were applied without difficulties and were well tolerated by the horses and maintained good contact between electrodes and horse (impedance <2 kΩ) throughout the recordings. Other technical considerations include keeping the connecting wires as short as possible to avoid mains interference from electric equipment in the examination room and ensuring equipment not necessary for the procedure are unplugged to reduce sources of electromagnetic noise.

Although this work confirmed that the potentials in the equine FVEP are of post-retinal origin, the exact sources of the potentials producing each of the wavelets in the equine VEP are still unknown. The FVEP has been a diagnostic aid in human medicine for decades, but the origins of some wavelets seen in the human FVEP are still not clearly identified. Further studies are needed in the horse to evaluate the components of the equine VEP with the aim of establishing the anatomical location of lesions causing certain aberrations in the VEP waveform.

The first study of the human VEP in different age groups was performed by Dustman and Beck in 1969

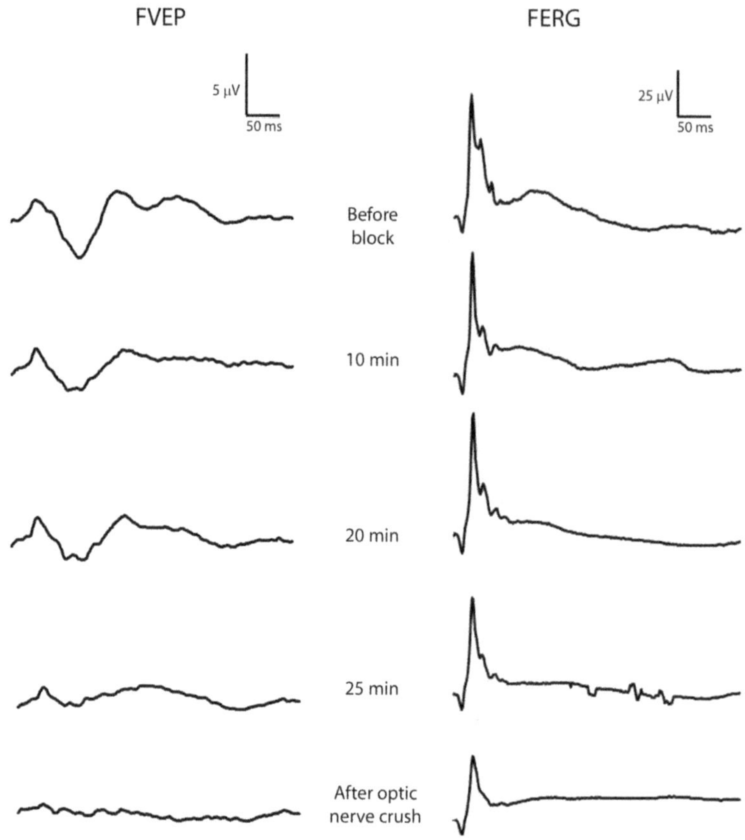

Fig. 10 FVEPs after retrobulbar nerve block and transection of the optic nerve. FVEPs recorded at $P_{z\text{-}45}$ in horse I from the right eye (left column) before retrobulbar nerve block (uppermost tracing), 10, 20 and 25 min after retrobulbar nerve block (middle rows) and after transection of the optic nerve (lowermost tracing). Simultaneous FERG recordings from the right eye are shown in the right column

[39] who showed that with increasing age, the human VEP alters in regards to times-to-peak and amplitudes, although the overall morphology stays the same throughout the adult life-span. Studies on the age-related development of VEPs have been performed in several animal species such as for example in cats [13], dogs [40], ruminants [16, 41, 42] and pigs [15]. As we have only few horses at each age in this study, further studies are needed to evaluate the normal variation of the equine VEP related to increasing age.

The FVEP in combination with concurrent FERGs provide an opportunity for objective, functional assessment of the post-retinal visual pathways in the standing, sedated equine patient. Equine FVEPs would be valuable for evaluating similar types of pathological conditions affecting the visual system as in human patients, such as cortical trauma, optic neuritis, tumors and demyelinating diseases. Additionally, FVEPs offer an opportunity to detect persistent visual impairment or blindness after retrobulbar nerve block, which has been reported as a rare complication in human patients [43]. As well the technique could be an important additional diagnostic tool to rule out visual impairment in cases of abnormal behavior.

Table 3 Flash electroretinograms

	a-wave	b-wave
Implicit time (ms)	13 ± 1	30 ± 1
Amplitude (μV)	10 ± 3	63 ± 15

Light-adapted FERG amplitudes and times-to-peak in ten healthy horses. Data are shown as means ± SDs

Conclusions

We have recorded FVEPs in healthy, sedated horses in a clinical setting. Active electrodes positioned at $P_{z\text{-}30}$ to $P_{z\text{-}45}$ provided a good signal-to-noise ratio and reproducible waveforms. Results from recordings after retrobulbar anaesthesia and transection of the optic nerve showed that the recorded responses were of post-retinal origin. Our technique for FVEP in the horse is relatively easily mastered and opens up for objective, functional assessment of the post-retinal visual pathways in this species.

Acknowledgements
We wish to thank Dr. John Pringle, Dr. Katarina Nostell, Dr. Marie Rhodin and Dr. Pia Haubro-Andersen for comments on the draft of the manuscript. We also wish to thank Dr. Ove Wattle for performing retrobulbar nerve blocks and transection of the optic nerve. We are grateful to the Mari Wallbring, Kenneth Larsson, Dennis Larsson and Carola Jansson in the Department for Clinical Sciences, SLU, for their excellent assistance during all the examinations of the horses.

Authors' contributions
LS participated in the design of the study, performed ophthalmic and electrophysiological examinations and drafted the manuscript. BE proposed the study, assisted in ophthalmic and electrophysiological examinations and in the drafting of the manuscript. Both authors read and approved the final manuscript.

Competing interests
The authors declare that they have no competing interests.

Consent for publication
Not applicable.

References

1. Adrian ED, Matthews BH. The interpretation of potential waves in the cortex. J Physiol. 1934;81(4):440–71.
2. Dawson GD. A summation technique for the detection of small evoked potentials. Electroencephalogr Clin Neurophysiol. 1954;6(1):65–84.
3. Ciganek L. The EEG response (evoked potential) to light stimulus in man. Electroencephalogr Clin Neurophysiol. 1961;13:165–72.
4. Young B, Eggenberger E, Kaufman D. Current electrophysiology in ophthalmology: a review. Curr Opin Ophthalmol. 2012;23(6):497–505.
5. Odom JV, Bach M, Brigell M, Holder GE, McCulloch DL, Tormene AP, Vaegan. ISCEV standard for clinical visual evoked potentials (2009 update). Doc Ophthalmol. 2010;120(1):111–9.
6. American Clinical Neurophysiology S. Guideline 9B: guidelines on visual evoked potentials. Am J Electroneurodiagnostic Technol. 2006;46(3):254–74.
7. Jasper HH. The ten-twenty electrode system of the International Federation. Electroencephalogr Clin Neurophysiol. 1958;10:371–5.
8. Blumhardt LD, Barrett G, Halliday AM. The asymmetrical visual evoked potential to pattern reversal in one half field and its significance for the analysis of visual field defects. Br J Ophthalmol. 1977;61(7):454–61.
9. Sims MH, Laratta LJ, Bubb WJ, Morgan RV. Waveform analysis and reproducibility of visual-evoked potentials in dogs. Am J Vet Res. 1989; 50(11):1823–8.
10. Strain GM, Jackson RM, Tedford BL. Visual evoked potentials in the clinically normal dog. J Vet Intern Med. 1990;4(4):222–5.
11. Creel DJ, Dustman RE, Beck EC. Visually evoked responses in the rat, guinea pig, cat, monkey, and man. Exp Neurol. 1973;40(2):351–66.
12. Padnick LB, Linsenmeier RA. Properties of the flash visual evoked potential recorded in the cat primary visual cortex. Vision Res. 1999;39(17):2833–40.
13. Rose GH, Gruenau SP, Spencer JW. Maturation of visual electrocortical responses in unanesthetized kittens: effects of barbiturate anesthesia. Electroencephalogr Clin Neurophysiol. 1972;33(2):141–58.
14. Strain GM, Olcott BM, Hokett LD. Electroretinogram and visual-evoked potential measurements in Holstein cows. Am J Vet Res. 1986;47(5):1079–81.
15. Strain GM, Tedford BL, Gill MS. Brainstem auditory evoked potentials and flash visual evoked potentials in Vietnamese miniature pot-bellied pigs. Res Vet Sci. 2006;80(1):91–5.
16. Strain GM, Claxton MS, Prescott-Mathews JS, LaPhand DJ. Electroretinogram and visual-evoked potential measurements in sheep. Can J Vet Res. 1991; 55(1):1–4.
17. Ridder W, J.R H, G.B A. Visual Evoked Potentials in Animals. In: Principles and Practice of Clinical Electrophysiology of Vision. 2nd ed. USA: MIT Press; 2006. p. 935–47.
18. Brooks DE. Equine Ophthalmology. In: Gelatt KN, editor. Veterinary Ophthalmology, vol. II. 3rd ed.: Philadelphia: Lippincott Williams & Wilkins; 1999. p. 1108.
19. Hewes CA, Keoughan GC, Gutierrez-Nibeyro S. Standing enucleation in the horse: a report of 5 cases. Can Vet J. 2007;48(5):512–4.
20. Pollock PJ, Russell T, Hughes TK, Archer MR, Perkins JD. Transpalpebral eye enucleation in 40 standing horses. Vet Surg. 2008;37(3):306–9.
21. Gilger BC, Davidson MG. How to prepare for ocular surgery in the standing horse. In: Annual Convention of the AAEP. Orlando: IVIS; 2002.
22. Ekesten B, Komaromy AM, Ofri R, Petersen-Jones SM, Narfstrom K. Guidelines for clinical electroretinography in the dog: 2012 update. Doc Ophthalmol. 2013;127(2):79–87.
23. Harding GFA. The visual evoked response. In: Roper-Hall MJea, editor. Advances in Ophthalmology. Basel: S Karger AG; 1974. p. 2–28.
24. Bichsel P, Oliver Jr JE, Coulter DB, Brown J. Recording of visual-evoked potentials in dogs with scalp electrodes. J Vet Intern Med. 1988;2(3):145–9.
25. Malnati GA, Marshall AE, Coulter DB. Electroretinographic components of the canine visual evoked response. Am J Vet Res. 1981;42(1):159–63.
26. Atkinson WS. Local anesthesia in ophthalmology. Am J Ophthalmol. 1948; 31(12):1607–18.
27. Cyriac IC, Pineda 2nd R. Postoperative complications of periocular anesthesia. Int Ophthalmol Clin. 2000;40(1):85–91.
28. Uenoyama K, McDonald JS, Drance SM. The effect of intraocular pressure on visual electrical responses. Arch Ophthalmol. 1969;81(5):722–9.
29. Uenoyama K, McDonald JS, Drance SM. The effect of artificially elevated intraocular pressure on the electroretinogram of the cat. Can J Ophthalmol. 1968;3(2):154–8.
30. Howard DR, Sawyer DC. Electroretinography of acute hypoxic and increased intraocular pressure status in the dog. Am J Vet Res. 1975;36(1):81–4.
31. Tsai TI, Bui BV, Vingrys AJ. Effect of acute intraocular pressure challenge on rat retinal and cortical function. Invest Ophthalmol Vis Sci. 2014;55(2):1067–77.
32. Takeuchi T, Sugita S. Cytoarchitectonic study of the cerebral cortex in the horse brain–classification of the cortex area. Kaibogaku Zasshi. 2001;76(2): 213–21.
33. Duke-Elder S. The eye in evolution. In: System of Ophthalmology, vol. I. London: Henry Kimpton; 1958. p. 446–504.
34. Budras KD. Anatomy of the Horse. 6th ed. Hannover: Schluetersche; 2012.
35. Ben-Shlomo G, Plummer C, Barrie K, Brooks D. Characterization of the normal dark adaptation curve of the horse. Vet Ophthalmol. 2012;15(1):42–5.
36. Church ML, Norman JC. Electroretinogram responses of the normal thoroughbred horse sedated with detomidine hydrochloride. Vet Ophthalmol. 2012;15 Suppl 2:77–83.
37. Komaromy AM, Andrew SE, Sapp Jr HL, Brooks DE, Dawson WW. Flash electroretinography in standing horses using the DTL microfiber electrode. Vet Ophthalmol. 2003;6(1):27–33.
38. Sannita WG. Neuropsychiatric drug effects on the visual nervous system. In: Heckenlively JR, Arden GB, editors. Principles and practice of clinical electrophysiology of vision. USA: Mosby Year Book; 1991. p. 167–73.
39. Dustman RE, Beck EC. The effects of maturation and aging on the wave form of visually evoked potentials. Electroencephalogr Clin Neurophysiol. 1969;26(1):2–11.
40. Strain GM, Jackson RM, Tedford BL. Postnatal development of the visual-evoked potential in dogs. Am J Vet Res. 1991;52(2):231–5.
41. Strain GM, Graham MC, Claxton MS, Olcott BM. Postnatal development of brainstem auditory-evoked potentials, electroretinograms, and visual-evoked potentials in the calf. J Vet Intern Med. 1989;3(4):231–7.
42. Takeuchi T, Suzuki M, Sitizyo K, Saito T. Postnatal development of visual evoked potentials in Japanese black calves. Jpn J Physiol. 1993;43(6):809–15.
43. Kumar CM, Dowd TC. Complications of ophthalmic regional blocks: their treatment and prevention. Ophthalmologica. 2006;220(2):73–82.

12

Seasonal fluctuations in body weight during growth of Thoroughbred racehorses during their athletic career

Yuji Takahashi* and Toshiyuki Takahashi

Abstract

Background: Domesticated horses adapt to environmental conditions through seasonal fluctuations in their metabolic rate. The seasonal change of metabolic rates of domesticated horses in pastures is documented. However, there are few investigations on seasonal body weight change of domesticated horses housed in stables, which are provided constant energy intake throughout the year. Both seasonal changes and gain in body weight of racehorses during their athletic career is known to a lesser extent because their body weight are not measured in most countries. Here, we used a seasonal-trend decomposition method to conduct a time series analysis of body weight of Thoroughbred racehorses participating in flat races held by the Japan Racing Association from 1 January 2002 to 31 December 2014.

Results: We acquired 640,431 body weight measurements for race starts and included 632,540 of these in the time series analysis. Based on seasonal component analysis, the body weight of male and gelding horses peaked in autumn and winter and reached its nadir in summer. In contrast, the body weight of female horses peaked in autumn and reached the nadir in spring. Based on trend component analysis, most of the increase in body weight was observed when all sexes approached 5 years of age. The slope of the body weight gain was smaller after that, and an approximately 30 kg gain was observed during their careers.

Conclusion: These results indicate that the body weight of a Thoroughbred racehorse fluctuates seasonally, and that there may be sex differences in energy balance mechanisms. Moreover, the present results suggest that the physiological development of Thoroughbred racehorses is completed just before they reach 5 years of age.

Keywords: Body weight, Growth, Racehorse, Seasonal change, Sex difference

Background

Seasonal changes in food availability and quality are inevitable. Because of changes in forage in the wild, the body weight of a wild herbivore varies seasonally [1, 2]. Przewalski horses, an ancestor of domesticated horses, which live in a semi-natural environment, exhibit annual fluctuations in body weight that peak in autumn and reach the nadir in spring [3]. These fluctuations are associated with energy quality and quantity derived from dry matter intake or with dietary composition [4]. Further, the energy expenditure of Przewalski horses is low in winter to adjust to food shortages and high in spring owing to pregnancy [5]. Energy balance varies with seasonal fluctuations depending on the relationship between energy intake and expenditure [6]. Therefore, body weight increases during an energetically abundant season and decreases during an energetically deficient season [3, 6].

In contrast to wild animals, the amount of forage available to domesticated animals is not affected by the season. However, recent studies reveal that domesticated mammals can change their energy expenditure depending on seasonal environmental changes such as temperature or photoperiod [7–9]. For example, the metabolic rate of a Shetland pony mare is high in summer and low in winter, according to climate change [8]. This seasonal metabolic change suggests that the body weight of a domesticated horse can change with seasonal fluctuations that are high

* Correspondence: yuji_takahashi@equinst.go.jp
Sports Science Division, Equine Research Institute, Japan Racing Association, 1400-4, Shiba, Shimotsuke, Tochigi 329-0412, Japan

in winter and low in summer, despite constant feeding. Although some studies investigated seasonal changes of the body weight of domesticated horses, including racehorses [7, 8, 10–12], most of the horses were kept on pastures with amounts of forage that varied between seasons. Therefore, little is known about seasonal changes of body weight that occur when energy intake is constant throughout the year.

In the equine industry, many investigations report growth curves from birth to the yearling stage [13–16] as well as the change in the body weight of mares [10, 17]. These studies show how horses grow from birth to approximately 700 days of age and how body weight changes during reproduction. This information would be helpful for providing appropriate nutrition during these times to prevent diseases such as laminitis or metabolic syndrome [3, 18, 19].

During a horse's athletic career, controlling body weight is considered important, because body weight can be associated with the risk of injury [20] or performance level [21]. From the perspective of skeletal development, we can expect an increase in body weight until the horse approaches 5 years of age, the time of the latest epiphysis closure [22]. However, few published investigations measured body weight changes over several years during a horse's athletic career [11] because body weight is not measured in most countries, except for some Asian countries, including Japan.

In Japan, there is no off-season for racing and about 65 flat races, from Maiden Races up to Group One (the highest class), are held every week throughout the year. The horses are all given an official birthday of January 1st to keep the age groups easily defined for race conditions; horses aged 2 years are allowed to debut in June, although most horses, which cannot win a Maiden Race until the end of September aged 3 years, are forced to retire due to the lack of their prize money. The Japan Racing Association (JRA) records body weight data for all horses participating in races. Therefore, the analysis of these data provides an opportunity to improve our understanding of the growth and seasonal body weight changes of racehorses.

Although Cho et al. investigated the average body weight of Thoroughbred horses of all sexes according to month and age separately [11], it is difficult to identify the component that determines body weight change during growth. This is because body weight during growth can be affected by seasonal effects, as described above, or by growth, genetic effects, nutrition, and so on. Therefore, dividing body weight data into seasonal and growth components is valuable and could have important implications for planning the nutritional management of athletic horses to prevent injury, increase performance, or both.

To investigate how the body weight of Thoroughbred racehorses changes during their careers, we conducted a time-series analysis by dividing the data into seasonal, trend and remainder components. We hypothesized that body weight changes between seasons and increases just before the age of 5 years.

Methods

We acquired body weights of racehorses at flat races held by the JRA from 1 January 2002 to 31 December 2014 from the JRA's official database. Permission to use this dataset for the present study was given by the Equine Research Institute of JRA. Each year, approximately 3400 flat races are held by the JRA, including 48,000 race starts. The JRA operates racecourses at Sapporo, Hakodate, Fukushima, Niigata, Tokyo, Nakayama, Chukyo, Kyoto, Hanshin and Kokura, which range in latitude from N 34° to N 43°.

In the present study, all horses were stabled at the Miho (N 36, E 140°) or the Ritto (N 35°, E 136) Training Centre in Japan for at least 10 days before races. Except during training, the horses were housed individually in stalls (2.8 × 4.0 m) under natural photo-thermoperiod conditions and at the ambient temperature. Training was typically performed for 90 to 120 min each day, 6 days a week, and workout training was performed once or twice each week; this is classified as very heavy work according to the National Research Council [23]. Stable staff controlled the care of the racehorses. However, we recommended to staff that the nutritional energy requirements of the horses should be calculated according to the following equation, and stable staff should feed the horses accordingly. The equation, which is for horses undergoing very heavy work, is as follows [23]:

$$\text{Digestible energy (Mcal/day)} = (0.0363 \times \text{body weight}) \times 1.9$$

The horses received their daily quantity of food as either two or three meals and water was available ad libitum in each stall. Generally, the dietary treatment consisted of mixed feed at 0.8%–1.2% body weight, oats at 0.5%–1.0% body weight, timothy or alfalfa hay at 1%–1.25% body weight as fresh matter, and small quantities of vitamin and mineral supplements; however, it is likely that the quantity of feed provided would differ somewhat between the stables. There was no pasture at either Training Centre. Because training and general animal care were performed by stable staff not associated with the research team, the feeding practice was not controlled precisely. All horses were transported to the racecourse in a horse trailer on the day before or the day of the race. All racehorses were Thoroughbreds, and their body weights were measured approximately 80 min before post time (i.e., the time the horses entered the starting gate). Body weight was measured at the racecourse using regularly calibrated electronic scales and recorded to the nearest 2 kg. Body weight, age and sex of each horse were recorded. The average body weight and standard error in each month were calculated for time series analysis. The JRA allows horses, which are 2 years of age, to debut in June. Therefore, data were collected after that time. We excluded data for horses ≥8 years of age because of the relatively small sample size of females and geldings. Further, the data for 2-year-old geldings between June and September were not used because of small sample size.

To investigate the seasonal change of body weight and growth as a function of age, we used a seasonal-trend decomposition procedure based on locally weighted regression (STL), which decomposes the time series into seasonal, trend and remainder components [24]. STL is a filtering procedure that iteratively applies locally weighted regression to the observations of the smoothing process in moving time windows, which allows analysis of large numbers of trends and seasonal smoothing [24]. For smoothing parameters, we used the algorithm implemented in the R language. We used STL to investigate seasonal cycles and trends for males, geldings and females, applying it first to all the data and then, in a subgroup analysis, to horses aged 2–4 years and those over 5 years for each sex. These analyses were performed using 2.13.0 R software [25].

Results

We acquired 640,431 body weight measurements for race starts between 2002 and 2014. This included horses that competed in several races (range 1–84 races; median, 6 races). The age of the horses ranged from 2 to 13 years. For STL decomposition, we used 632,540 body-weight measurements of race starts for horses ranging in age from 2 to 7 years, comprising 377,301 males, 19,100 geldings (except for horses 2 years of age from June to September) and 236,139 females. The distribution of age in each month is shown in Table 1. Figs. 1, 2 and 3 show the STL decomposition analyses of body weight for all ages according to sex. The data split by age subgroups is shown in Table 2. Table 3 shows the mean average monthly temperature during the study period at the Miho and Ritto Training Centres.

The mean body weight of the horses increased from the time of their debuts, with seasonal fluctuations, in all sexes. Over the course of their athletic careers, the mean body weights changed as follows: males, from 461 ± 0.7 kg to 493 ± 0.6 kg; geldings, from 458 ± 2.5 kg to 484 ± 1.7 kg; and females, from 442 ± 0.7 kg to 472 ± 2.4 kg (Figs. 1a, 2a and 3a, respectively). For the male horses, the seasonal component shown in Fig. 1b indicates that their body weight increased in winter, peaked in January and decreased in summer to its lowest value in August. The body weight changes in geldings were similar to those of the intact male horses, although they showed broader peaks in autumn and winter. The

Table 1 Distribution of horses by age and sex competing in Japan Racing Association races, by month

Age (y)	Sex	January	February	March	April	May	June	July	August	September	October	November	December
2	Male						1480	4378	6067	7037	9303	12,702	13,493
	Gelding						(14) [a]	(40) [a]	(51) [a]	(53) [a]	102	174	218
	Female						1121	3218	4632	5160	6436	8816	9283
3	Male	14,801	13,914	17,045	16,342	17,386	14,659	13,957	13,166	11,475	8600	6948	6797
	Gelding	281	291	435	435	551	505	553	605	493	333	225	273
	Female	10,311	9729	12,636	12,262	13,059	11,139	11,905	12,043	10,003	5860	4194	3764
4	Male	6699	5893	7353	6775	6925	6052	6233	5683	5104	5876	5957	5598
	Gelding	278	279	375	344	375	348	369	374	334	408	399	423
	Female	3471	3144	4025	3702	3957	3430	4117	4044	3308	3421	3303	3089
5	Male	5326	4725	5623	4872	5078	4033	3811	3250	3071	3808	3850	3744
	Gelding	362	347	392	394	456	339	324	350	320	397	381	373
	Female	2602	2358	2790	2470	2631	1967	2161	2190	1782	1888	1803	1690
6	Male	3299	2889	3219	2857	2914	2211	2218	1857	1539	1939	2036	1936
	Gelding	289	260	324	276	293	256	271	253	205	253	230	255
	Female	1309	1159	1193	796	752	573	632	618	536	554	510	451
7	Male	1635	1423	1548	1366	1391	1081	1019	853	654	854	883	791
	Gelding	187	151	212	162	157	136	133	118	97	122	129	116
	Female	339	261	271	194	191	136	171	150	101	118	113	97

[a]The data for 2-year-old geldings between June and September were not used for the seasonal-trend decomposition analysis because of the small sample size

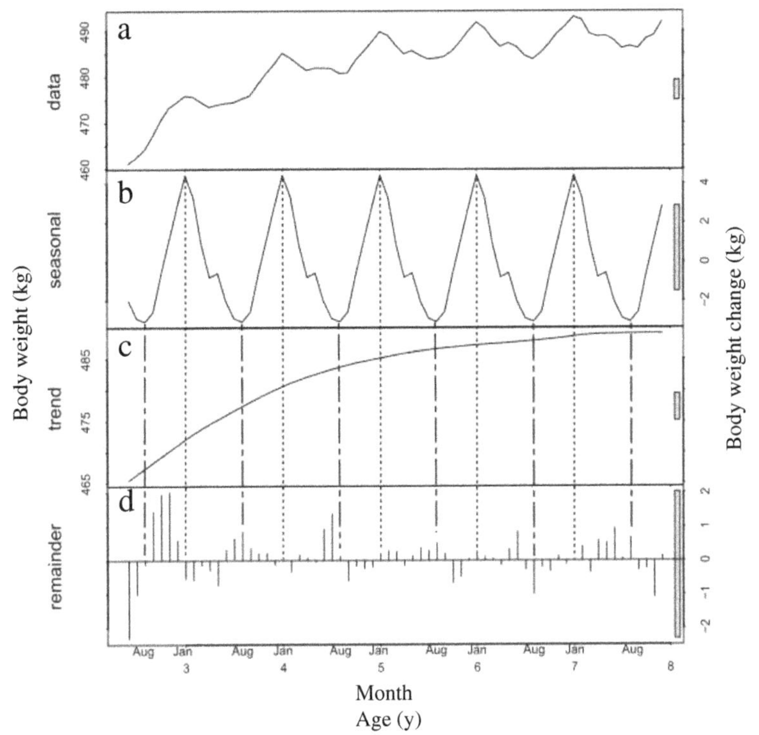

Fig. 1 Seasonal-trend decomposition analysis of the body weights of male racehorses. The data are for male horses aged 2–7 years that competed in races held by the Japan Racing Association in the years 2002–2014 (n = 377,301). **a** The mean body weight of the horses by age and month. **b** The seasonal component. **c** The trend component. **d** The remainder component after fitting the seasonal and trend components. The dotted vertical lines indicate the month each year when body weight peaked, and the dashed vertical lines indicate the month when the body weight was at its nadir. The grey bars to the right of each panel show the relative scales of the components. Each grey bar represents the same length, but because the plots are on different scales, the bars vary in size

body weight of the geldings reached its peak in November and decreased to its lowest value in July (Fig. 2b). The seasonal pattern for the female horses differed from those of the males and geldings. The seasonal component shows that the body weight of females increased in autumn and winter, particularly in October, and decreased in spring, particularly in March (Fig. 3b). The magnitudes of the seasonal fluctuations were 7 kg, 8 kg and 6 kg for the males, geldings and females, respectively.

The plots of the STL trend components show that body weight increased approximately linearly from the horse's debut until nearly 5 years of age in all sexes (Figs. 1c, 2c, 3c). The trend component in all sexes increased by around 20 kg up to the end of 4 years of age, and by a further 5 kg (i.e., an overall 25 kg increase) at the end of 7 years of age.

In males, there was the same seasonal pattern in both younger horses and older horses, which reached its peak in January and nadir in August (Table 2). In geldings, the peak month was October for younger horses and December for older horses and the nadir month was June in both groups (Table 2). In females, the peak months for younger and older horses were October and September, respectively, and the nadir months were April and February (Table 2).

Discussion

The present study demonstrates that the body weight of a Thoroughbred racehorse that consumes a relatively constant diet varied circannually. The present study shows that a horse's sex is associated with the seasonal cycle of body weight. Furthermore, although body weight increased up to approximately 7 years of age, most of the increase occurred before the age of approximately 5 years.

Body weight change depends on energy balance, which is defined as the relationship between energy intake and energy expenditure [26, 27]. This applies to horses [28]. The energy intake of Przewalski horses, which were originally wild herbivores of Central Asia, peaks in autumn and reaches its nadir in late winter [4], whereas energy expenditure is particularly low in winter compared with that in spring and summer [5]. The energy balance of Przewalski horses is positive in autumn, indicating that energy intake is higher than expenditure, and is negative in spring, indicating lower energy intake compared with expenditure. The consequence of these seasonal energy

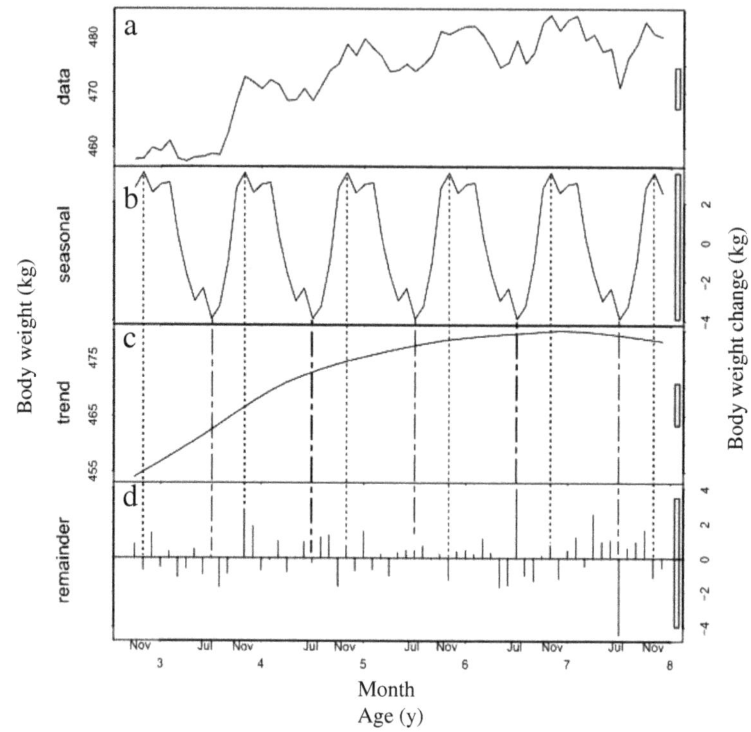

Fig. 2 Seasonal-trend decomposition analysis of the body weights of gelding racehorses (n = 19,100). **a** The mean body weight of the horses by age and month. **b** The seasonal component. **c** The trend component. **d** The remainder component after fitting the seasonal and trend components. For further details, see the legend for Fig. 1

balances would lead to a seasonal change of body weight, which is high in autumn and low in spring [3].

In the present study, the body weights of the Thoroughbred male and gelding racehorses that received sufficient annual nutrition showed seasonal variations that peaked in autumn and winter and reached their nadir in summer. Unlike the Przewalski horses, the racehorses should have received a constant amount of food throughout the year. However, a limitation of the present study is its observational design. Although it is recommended that racehorses should be fed diets according to the results of the equation described in the Methods section, the racehorses studied here were managed by individual stable staff and so we lacked detailed information of the actual energy intake of each horse during the study period. Although establishing the detailed energy intake information by precise feeding control would be ideal, investigating a large sample size of racehorses throughout their athletic career would be difficult. Indeed, because this study analyzed data for a very large number of horses over a period of 13 years, any local or short-term variations in feeding would be expected to be "averaged out" and unlikely to result in noticeable effects. To produce a systematic seasonable effect as we observed would require a consistent, widespread seasonable variation in feed provision that lasted throughout the study period. However, we are unaware of any stable staff changing the feeding protocol according to the season (personal communication). In addition, the annual fluctuation in the body weight of the horses in this study was within 8 kg, which is equivalent to less than 2% of their mean body weight. This compares with 22 kg fluctuations in the annual mean amplitude of the body weight of Przewalski horses in a semi-natural condition, equivalent to 7% of their mean body weight [3]. This suggests that the horses in the present study were fed more consistently than horses housed under semi-natural conditions.

Thus, the results of this study suggest that male and gelding racehorses were energetically abundant in autumn and winter, and deficient in summer. The assumption that there was little change in energy intake suggest that these results are due to the seasonal changes in energy expenditure (high in summer and low in winter); this is consistent with a previous report [8].

Seasonal environmental factors such as temperature or photoperiod may explain the seasonal changes in metabolic rate. The range in average monthly temperature over the year at both training centres was about 23 °C, with the highest temperatures in August and the lowest in January. The horses were stabled at the ambient temperature, so the high temperatures in summer may

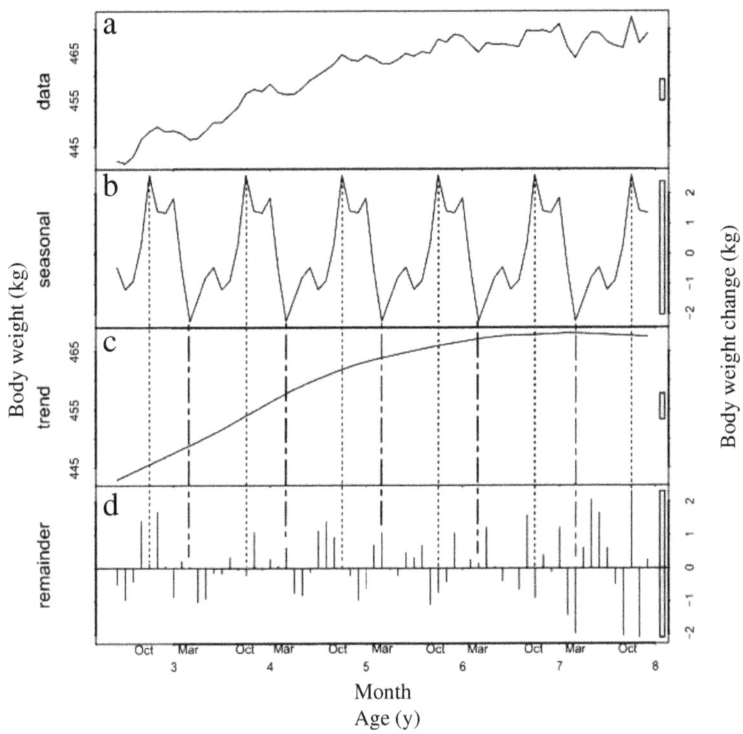

Fig. 3 Seasonal-trend decomposition analysis of the body weights of female racehorses (n = 236,139). **a** The mean body weight of the horses by age and month. **b** The seasonal component. **c** The trend component. **d** The remainder component after fitting the seasonal and trend components. For further details, see the legend for Fig. 1

have increased their metabolic rate and the low temperatures in winter may have reduced it, which would be consistent with the results of previous studies [8, 29, 30]. Although a long photoperiod induces a higher metabolic rate than a shorter photoperiod in rats and cats [9, 31], there are no published studies, to our knowledge, on the direct relationship between photoperiod and energy expenditure by horses. Further studies are required to confirm this potential relationship.

In contrast to male and gelding horses, the body weight of female horses peaked in autumn and reached the nadir in spring, consistent with a previous report [11]. These findings suggest that female horses employ a mechanism that maintains energy balance that differs from that of male and gelding horses. The sexual cycle of female horses may provide an explanation. For example, the locomotor activity of female Thoroughbred horses is higher during breeding season [32]. The metabolic rate can be higher in breeding season, similar to behavioural changes, because Thoroughbred racehorses stabled in the training centres maintain their oestrous cycle during training [33]. Further studies are required to identify sex-specific mechanisms that regulate body weight.

Table 2 The months corresponding to the peaks and nadirs of body weight, by age subgroup

		Peak	Nadir
Male	All ages	January	August
	2–4 y	January	August
	≥5 y	January	August
Gelding	All ages	November	July
	2–4 y	October	June
	≥5 y	December	June
Female	All ages	October	March
	2–4 y	October	April
	≥5 y	September	February

The seasonal fluctuations in body weight may have important implications for equine clinicians, racehorse trainers, or both. Our previous study shows that racehorses that are heavy at race time are at higher risk of superficial digital flexor tendon injury compared with horses that weigh less [20]. Further, increases in body weight might affect the results of the submaximal exercise test [21]. Therefore, equine clinicians and racehorse staff should adjust the amount of feed according to seasonal body weight changes such as the reduction of feeding amount in autumn and winter in males and geldings, and in autumn in females.

Table 3 The average monthly temperatures (°C) at the Miho and Ritto Training Centres (mean ± SEM values for 2002–2014)

	January	February	March	April	May	June	July	August	September	October	November	December
Miho	3.8 ± 0.3	4.8 ± 0.3	8.2 ± 0.3	13.0 ± 0.3	17.5 ± 0.2	21.1 ± 0.2	24.8 ± 0.5	26.4 ± 0.3	22.9 ± 0.3	17.4 ± 0.2	11.6 ± 0.3	6.1 ± 0.4
Ritto	3.8 ± 0.2	4.6 ± 0.3	7.5 ± 0.3	13.0 ± 0.3	18.0 ± 0.1	23.2 ± 0.8	26.3 ± 0.4	27.4 ± 0.3	23.7 ± 0.3	17.6 ± 0.3	11.6 ± 0.3	6.3 ± 0.3

We show here that the body weight of Thoroughbred racehorses increased 25 to 30 kg during their athletic career. According to the trend component, most of the increase was observed until horses approaches approximately 5 years of age. To our knowledge, this is the first report that determined the time interval associated with the increase in body weight of Thoroughbred racehorses during their athletic career. This finding is reasonable because the last epiphysis closure in a cervical vertebra occurs at the age of 4–5 years [22], indicating that horses mature by the end of their fourth year. Moreover, racing performance or average racing speed peaks at approximately 4.5–5 years of age [34, 35]. Together, the present and previous studies indicate that the physiological development of Thoroughbred racehorses is complete just before 5 years of age. It would be interesting to investigate the association between body weight increase and anatomical development, such as the development of bones and joints. However, this would be difficult to achieve for a large sample size. The mean body weights of the Thoroughbred racehorses at the completion of physiological development were approximately 490 kg, 480 kg and 465 kg for males, geldings and females, respectively. We propose the use of these values as standards for Thoroughbred racehorses in Japan.

The remainder component is an indication of the residual data after subtracting the seasonal and trend components [24] and shows variations due to random features. However, there appeared to be a small element of seasonality in the remainder component for the young male horses, especially those aged 2–3 years (Fig. 1d). Another age-related factor was that there were fewer older horses than younger ones, especially among the females (Table 1). It is possible that different number between older and younger horses may have had different seasonal patterns according to ages. For these reasons, we divided the data into two groups for each sex, younger horses (2–4 years) and older horses (those over 5 years). However, the results showed almost the same seasonal pattern as the undivided datasets, with the body weight of the males and geldings reaching a peak in autumn and winter, and their nadir in summer whereas the body weight of the females peaked in autumn and was at its lowest in spring, although the divided data showed a slightly wider range than the combined data for all ages. These additional results suggest that the datasets were appropriately divided into seasonal, trend and remainder components.

We should take care to correctly interpret the data acquired from the analysis of body weight change that occurs each month or season. For example, overall average body weight in JRA may be lower in June compared with May, because 2-year-old horses with lighter body weights compared with older horses are admitted to the JRA in June. To avoid such a misleading analysis, we applied STL techniques to body weight data classified according to age, which is a useful technique in diverse disciplines [36, 37]. The STL technique is an effective tool for visualizing and clarifying time series events by dividing them into seasonal, trend and remainder components [24]. We used this technique here to identify the seasonal change associated with growth.

Due to the JRA system described in the Introduction section, the distribution of age and month relatively changed according to the season. Especially after August, the number of 2-year-old horses increased while the number of 3-year-old horses decreased. If there were seasons specific for any age or gender, racing system can have possible role on body weight change. For example, if autumn and winter season were for only 2-year-old horses, reduction of workload for over 3-year-old horses might cause overall increase of body weight. However, races from Maiden to Group One are held every week regardless of age and gender in JRA. Therefore, we speculate that JRA system did not affect our interpretation.

Conclusions

The present study shows that Thoroughbred racehorses exhibited annual rhythms of body weight, suggesting that they maintain a seasonal energy balance. Further, there was a sex difference in the seasonal pattern of body weight changes, that is, the body weights of the male horses and geldings peaked in autumn and winter and reached their nadir in summer whereas the body weight of the female horses peaked in autumn and reached its nadir in spring. Additionally, most of the increase of body weight of Thoroughbred racehorses during their athletic careers is completed just before the age of 5 years. These results should be useful for optimizing the nutritional management of athletic horses.

Acknowledgments

The authors would like to thank Enago (www.enago.jp) for the English language review.

Funding

This study was supported by the Japan Racing Association.

Author's contributions
YT performed the analysis of data and drafted the manuscript. TT collected the data and revised the manuscript. We all read and approved the final manuscript.

Consent for publication
Not applicable

Competing interests
The authors declare that they have no competing interests.

References

1. Mitchell B, McCowan D, Nicholson IA. Annual cycles of body weight and condition in Scottish Red deer. J Zool. 1976;180(1):107–27.
2. Adamczewski JZ, Flood PF, Gunn A. Seasonal patterns in body composition and reproduction of female muskoxen (*Ovibos moschatus*). J Zool. 1997; 241(2):245–69.
3. Scheibe KM, Streich WL. Annual rhythm of body weight in Przewalski horses (*Equus ferus przewalskii*). Biol Rhythm Res. 2003;34(4):383–95.
4. Kuntz R, Kubalek C, Ruf T, Tataruch F, Arnold W. Seasonal adjustment of energy budget in a large wild mammal, the Przewalski horse (*Equus ferus przewalskii*) I. Energy intake. J Exp Biol. 2006;209(22):4557–65.
5. Arnold W, Ruf T, Kuntz R. Seasonal adjustment of energy budget in a large wild mammal, the Przewalski horse (*Equus ferus przewalskii*) II. Energy expenditure. J Exp Biol. 2006;209(22):4566–73.
6. Parker KL, Gillingham MP, Hanley TA, Robbins CT. Foraging efficiency: energy expenditure versus energy gain in free-ranging black-tailed deer. Can J Zoolog. 1996;74(3):442–50.
7. Brinkmann L, Gerken M, Riek A. Adaptation strategies to seasonal changes in environmental conditions of a domesticated horse breed, the Shetland pony (*Equus ferus caballus*). J Exp Biol. 2012;215(7):1061–8.
8. Brinkmann L, Gerken M, Hambly C, Speakman JR, Riek A. Saving energy during hard times: energetic adaptations of Shetland pony mares. J Exp Biol. 2014;217(24):4320–7.
9. Kappen KL, Garner LM, Kerr KR, Swanson KS. Effects of photoperiod on food intake, activity and metabolic rate in adult neutered male cats. J Anim Physiol Anim Nutr. 2014;98(5):958–67.
10. Fitzgerald BP, McManus CJ. Photoperiodic versus metabolic signals as determinants of seasonal anestrus in the mare. Biol Reprod. 2000;63(1):335–40.
11. Cho KH, Son SK, Cho BW, Lee HK, Kong HS, Jeon GJ, et al. Effects of change of body weight on racing time in Thoroughbred racehorses. J Anim Sci Technol. 2008;50(6):741–6.
12. Giles SL, Rands SA, Nicol CJ, Harris PA. Obesity prevalence and associated risk factors in outdoor living domestic horses and ponies. Peer J. 2014;2:e299.
13. Staniar WB, Kronfeld DS, Treiber KH, Splan RK, Harris PA. Growth rate consists of baseline and systematic deviation components in Thoroughbreds. J Anim Sci. 2004;82(4):1007–15.
14. Brown-Douglas CG, Parkinson TJ, Firth EC, Fennessy PF. Bodyweights and growth rates of spring-and autumn-born Thoroughbred horses raised on pasture. New Zeal Vet J. 2005;53(5):326–31.
15. Morel PCH, Bokor A, Rogers CW, Firth EC. Growth curves from birth to weaning for Thoroughbred foals raised on pasture. New Zeal Vet J. 2007; 55(6):319–25.
16. Onoda T, Yamamoto R, Sawamura K, Inoue Y, Matsui A, Miyake T, et al. Empirical growth curve estimation using sigmoid sub-functions that adjust seasonal compensatory growth for male body weight of Thoroughbred horses. J Equine Sci. 2011;22(2):37–42.
17. Lawrence LM, DiPietro J, Ewert K, Parrett D, Moser L, Powell D. Changes in body weight and condition of gestating mares. J Equine Vet Sci. 1992;12(6):355–8.
18. Geor RJ. Metabolic predispositions to laminitis in horses and ponies: obesity, insulin resistance and metabolic syndromes. J Equine Vet Sci. 2008;28(12):753–9.
19. Wylie CE, Collins SN, Verheyen KLP, Newton JR. Risk factors for equine laminitis: a case-control study conducted in veterinary-registered horses and ponies in Great Britain between 2009 and 2011. Vet J. 2013;198(1):57–69.
20. Takahashi T, Kasashima Y, Ueno Y. Association between race history and risk of superficial digital flexor tendon injury in Thoroughbred racehorses. J Am Vet Med Assoc. 2004;225(1):90 3.
21. Ellis JM, Hollands T, Allen DE. Effect of forage intake on bodyweight and performance. Equine Vet J Suppl. 2002;34:66–70.
22. Butler JA, Colles CM, Dyson SJ, Kold SE, Poulos PW. The spine. In: Clinical radiology of the Horse. Oxford: Blackwell Scientific; 1993. p. 355–98.
23. NRC. Nutrient requirement of horses 6th edition (online). Washington, DC: National Academy Press; 2007. https://www.nap.edu/read/11653/chapter/3. Accessed 3 Dec 2016.
24. Cleveland RB, Cleveland WS, McRae JE, Terpenning I. STL: a seasonal-trend decomposition procedure based on loess. J Off Stat. 1990;6(1):3–73.
25. R Development Core Team, 2011; R: a language and environment for statistical computing. Vienna; R Foundation for Statistical Computing. ISBN 3-900051-07-0. http://www.r-project.org. Accessed 7 June 2017.
26. Edholm OG, Adam JM, Best TW. Day-to-day weight changes in young men. Ann Hum Biol. 1974;1(1):3–12.
27. Ma Y, Olendzki BC, Li W, Hafner AR, Chiriboga D, Hebert JR, et al. Seasonal variation in food intake, physical activity, and body weight in a predominantly overweight population. Eur J Clin Nutr. 2006;60:519–28.
28. Amato C, Martin L, Dumon H, Jaillardon L, Nguyen P, Siliart B. Variations of plasma leptin in show horses during a work season. J Anim Physiol Anim Nutr. 2012;96(5):850–9.
29. Brinkmann L, Gerken M, Riek A. Seasonal changes of total body water and water intake in Shetland ponies measured by an isotope dilution technique. J Anim Sci. 2013;91(8):3750–8.
30. McBride GE, Christopherson RJ, Sauer W. Metabolic rate and plasma thyroid hormone concentrations of mature horses in response to changes in ambient temperature. Can J Anim Sci. 1985;65(2):375–82.
31. Boon P, Visser H, Daan S. Effect of photoperiod on body mass, and daily energy intake and energy expenditure in young rats. Physiol Behav. 1997; 62(4):913–9.
32. Bertolucci C, Giannetto C, Fazio F, Piccione G. Seasonal variations in daily rhythms of activity in athletic horses. Animal. 2008;2(7):1055–60.
33. Takahashi Y, Akai M, Murase H, Nambo Y. Seasonal changes in serum progesterone levels in Thoroughbred racehorses in training. J Equine Sci. 2015;26(4):135–9.
34. Gramm M, Marksteiner R. The effect of age on thoroughbred racing performance. J Equine Sci. 2010;21(4):73–8.
35. Takahashi T. The effect of age on the racing speed of Thoroughbred racehorses. J Equine Sci. 2015;26(2):43–8.
36. Ohshige K. Reduction in ambulance transports during a public awareness campaign for appropriate ambulance use. Acad Emerg Med. 2008;15(3): 289–93.
37. Lee HS, Levine M, Guptill-Yoran C, Johnson AJ, Kamecke P, Moore GE. Regional and temporal variations of Leptospira seropositivity in dogs in the United States, 2000–2010. J Vet Int Med. 2014;28(3):779–88.

13

Effect of intralesional platelet-rich plasma (PRP) treatment on clinical and ultrasonographic parameters in equine naturally occurring superficial digital flexor tendinopathies

Florian Geburek[1*], Moritz Gaus[1], Hans T. M. van Schie[2], Karl Rohn[3] and Peter M. Stadler[1]

Abstract

Background: Regenerative and anti-inflammatory effects on tendinopathies have been attributed to blood-derived biologicals. To date the evidence for the efficacy of autologous platelet-rich plasma (PRP) treatment of naturally occurring equine tendinopathies is limited. The purpose of this placebo-controlled clinical trial was to describe the effect of a single treatment of equine superficial digital flexor tendon (SDFT) disease with PRP on clinical and ultrasonographic parameters. Twenty horses with naturally occurring tendinopathies of forelimb SDFTs were randomly assigned to the PRP-treated group ($n = 10$) or control group ($n = 10$) after clinical and ultrasonographic examination. The SDFTs received an intralesional treatment with autologous PRP or were injected with saline, respectively (day 0). All horses participated in a standardized exercise programme and were re-examined clinically, with B-mode ultrasonography (5 times at regular intervals) and ultrasound tissue characterization (week 12 and 24 after treatment) until week 24. Long-term performance was estimated via telephone inquiry.

Results: Compared to day 0, lameness decreased significantly by week 8 after treatment with PRP and by week 12 in the control group. Ultrasonographically there was no difference in the summarized cross sectional area between the groups at any time point. Ultrasound tissue characterization showed that echo types representing disorganized matrix decreased significantly throughout the observation period in the PRP-treated group. Echo type II, representing discontinuous fascicles, not yet aligned into lines of stress was significantly higher 24 weeks after PRP treatment. Eighty percent of the PRP treated horses reached their previous or a higher level of performance after 12 months compared to 50 % in the CG. After 24 months these proportions were 60 % and 50 %, respectively.

Conclusions: A single intralesional treatment with PRP up to 8 weeks after onset of clinical signs of tendinopathy contributes to an earlier reduction of lameness compared to saline treatment and to an advanced organization of repair tissue as the fibrillar matrix is getting organized into fascicles while remodelling continues. Long term, PRP treatment has the potential to increase the number of horses reaching their previous level of performance. Earlier treatment of tendinopathy with PRP should be considered to enhance these effects.

(Continued on next page)

* Correspondence: florian.geburek@tiho-hannover.de
[1]Clinic for Horses, University of Veterinary Medicine Hannover, Foundation, Bünteweg 9, 30559 Hannover, Germany
Full list of author information is available at the end of the article

(Continued from previous page)
Keywords: Horse, Tendon, Lameness, Ultrasonography, B-mode, Ultrasound tissue characterization, UTC, Platelet-rich plasma, PRP

Abbreviations: ACD-A, Acid citrate dextrose-A; CG, Control group; DICOM, Digital imaging and communications in medicine; EDTA, Ethylendiamintetraacetate; G, Gauge; IV, Intravenously; MIZ, Maximal injury zone; PDGF-BB, Platelet derived growth factor-BB; PPP, Platelet poor plasma; PRP, Platelet-rich plasma; PRPG, Platelet-rich plasma-treated group; SDFT, Superficial digital flexor tendon; SEM, Standard error of the mean; T-CSA, Total cross-sectional area; TES, Total echo score; T-FAS, Total fibre alignment score; TGC, Time gain compensation; TGF-ß, Transforming growth factor-ß; US, Ultrasound; UTC, Ultrasound tissue characterization.

Background

Tendinopathy of the superficial digital flexor tendon (SDFT) is a common injury in Thoroughbred racehorses and other horse breeds [1, 2] and is regarded as a career-limiting disease [3]. Clinical injury is mostly strain induced and characterized by chronic degeneration after repetitive microtrauma in sport horses [3]. Tendinopathy may also be caused by a single external percutaneous trauma, such as a kick [4]. A plethora of substrates for intralesional injection with a potentially regenerative effect on tendinopathy are currently under investigation [5, 6]. Among these are platelet concentrates such as platelet-rich plasma (PRP) [7].

Concentrated platelets release numerous cytokines and growth factors, e.g. platelet derived growth factor-BB (PDGF-BB), transforming growth factor-ß (TGF-ß) and vascular endothelial growth factor. These factors are known to exercise specific actions during tendon healing (for review see Docheva et al. 2015) [6, 8]. PDGF-BB, e.g. stimulates tendon healing depending on its concentration [9]. PRP has been shown to enhance tenocyte proliferation [10], collagen and matrix synthesis [11, 12] and to influence vascular density [13].

PRP has shown significant enhancing effects on tendon healing such as improved biomechanical properties in a surgical model of equine SDFT lesions [13, 14] and is increasingly used for intralesional treatment of tendinopathy and desmopathy in humans [15] and horses [16–19] in clinical practice. However, the efficacy of PRP treatment on tendinopathy is seen controversially in human studies: In a randomized controlled clinical trial on chronic human Achilles tendinopathy intralesional PRP treatment showed no beneficial effects compared to saline injection [20]. These results are supported by a further randomized controlled study demonstrating no differences in elasticity modulus of PRP- versus non-treated Achilles tendons [21]. In other clinical studies without control groups PRP treatment of chronic Achilles and patellar tendinopathy significantly improved symptoms and function [22, 23]. To the best of our knowledge the effect of a single intralesional treatment with autologous PRP on equine naturally occurring SDF tendinopathy has not been documented in a prospective randomized placebo-controlled clinical study with long term follow-up in the literature to date (for review see Brossi et al. 2015) [18].

Autologous platelet concentrates are prepared by centrifugation or by gravitational cellular filtration [24]. Blood samples from different horses and the use of different non-standardised and commercial kits for the preparation of PRP lead to differences in the platelet, leucocyte and growth factor content [24]. Different breed, age and gender influences growth factor and cytokine release of platelets and leucocytes [25, 26]. The optimal platelet and leucocyte contents in PRP are a point of debate. Recent investigations have shown that a moderate increase in platelets seems to enhance equine tenocyte growth and collagen synthesis more effective than high platelet concentrations [27, 28]. High leucocyte counts in PRP were observed to enhance the inflammatory reaction in rabbit tendons [29].

The process of tendon healing is mainly divided into three phases which merge into each other: The acute inflammatory phase (<10–14 days) is characterized by phagocytosis of disrupted tendon tissue and demarcation of injured tendon tissue. A fibroproliferative callus is formed during the proliferative phase (4–45 days), while collagen fibrils are organised into tendon bundles during the phase remodelling (45–120 days; < 3 months) which may be divided into an consolidation (earlier) and maturation (later) phase [3, 30].

A critical parameter to determine the success of tendinopathy treatment is functionality, which can be characterized by lameness evaluation, long term recurrence rate [2, 31] and biomechanical testing [32]. To determine the quality of repair tissue tendon needle biopsies have been used successfully [33]. Ultrasound based modalities such as B-mode ultrasonography [34] and colour Doppler ultrasonography [13] have been established to monitor the process of tendon healing non-invasively. However, B-mode ultrasonography has several limitations, e.g. lack of axial information, operator-dependence, influence of ultrasound beam angle and limited resolution that impair its sensitivity [35, 36].

Ultrasound tissue characterization (UTC) is a new technique to quantify tendon integrity based on a computerized analysis of the stability of echo-patterns in contiguous US images [37, 38]. Based on the echo-pattern stability, 4 different echo types can be discriminated, with histo-morphology of tendon specimen as reference test [37, 39]. Ultrasound tissue characterization has been shown a viable diagnostic tool to monitor experimental tendinopathy in horses [39–42] and is increasingly used for the quantification of Achilles and patellar tendon integrity in humans [43, 44].

Aim of current study

The aim of the present study was to support the hypothesis that a single intralesional injection of autologous PRP into SDFT lesions up to 8 weeks after clinical onset (1) has a clinically detectable effect and (2) leads to improved ultrasonographic parameters (3) influences long term functionality.

Methods

Inclusion criteria for client-owned adult horses was an anamnesis of clinical signs of uni- or bilateral SDFT disease in front limbs for up to 8 weeks (56 days) prior to the presentation at the Equine Clinic of the University of Veterinary Medicine, Hannover, Foundation, or to collaborating veterinarians. Horses were only included if the clients agreed to the study design and tendons had not received intralesional injections before. Twenty horses with a mean age of 8.46 years (range: 4–21 years) and a mean bodyweight of 548 kg (range: 398–644 kg) met the inclusion criteria (Table 1). Horses were randomly assigned to the group treated with PRP (PRPG, $n = 10$) or the control group (CG, $n = 10$). The PRPG comprised 7 Warmbloods (70 %), 1 Haflinger (10 %), 1 New Forest Pony (10 %) and one Pinto (10 %). Eight Warmbloods (80 %), 1 Andalusian (10 %) and 1 German Riding Pony (10 %) were included in the CG (Table 1). The study was carried out between 2012 and 2014.

Clinical examination

All horses were examined clinically on the day of first presentation (day 0). This examination included assessment of lameness (5 grade score) [45] and palpable signs of inflammation scored semi-quantitatively by palpation (skin surface temperature in the palmar metacarpal region, sensitivity of the SDFT to palpation: 0 = no abnormality, 1 = mild abnormality, 2 = moderate abnormality, and 3 = severe abnormality) [46]. All clinical examinations throughout the study were performed by the same person (M.G.).

B-mode ultrasonography

Horses were sedated with romifidine (0.04–0.08 mg/kg intravenously [IV]) and butorphanol (0.01 mg/kg [IV]). Injured and contralateral SDFTs were examined by one examiner with B-mode ultrasound on day 0 in a transverse and longitudinal fashion with a linear 6–15 MHz linear scanner (Logiq E9, GE Healthcare, Wauwatosa, WI, USA) using a standoff (GE 12 L 2302652 Standoff, Veterinary Sales & Service Inc., Stuart, USA), according to the seven zone designations as previously described [47, 48]. Settings were 13 MHz, gain 52, depth 25 mm, focus position 15 mm. Images were stored digitally and analysed retrospectively with a DICOM workstation program (easyVET®, IFS Informationssysteme, Hannover, Germany) by one observer (M.G.) being unaware of the treatment modality. The following parameters were evaluated to determine the degree- and time-related changes of the lesions: maximal injury zone (MIZ), summarized cross sectional areas of tendon (total cross-sectional area, T-CSA). Echogenicity and fibre alignment were graded semiquantitatively at each zone and the scores for all levels were summarized (total echo score = TES, total fibre alignment score = T-FAS). Echogenicity was assigned to 0 (normoechoic), 1 (hypoechoic), 2 (mixed echogenicity), and 3 (anechoic), and fibre alignment was graded according to the estimated percentage of parallel fibres in the lesion: 0 (>75 %), 1 (50–74 %), 2 (25–49 %), and 3 (<25 %) [34, 48].

Ultrasound tissue characterization (UTC)

Injured SDFTs were scanned with the commercially available ultrasound tissue characterization (UTC) unit (UTC scan unit, configuration 2011, UTC Imaging B.V., 6171 GD Stein, Netherlands) on day 0. It consisted of 5–10 MHz linear transducer (LA T Transducer, Terason Ultrasound, Teratech Corporation, Burlington, USA) which was fixed in transverse position, perpendicular to the integrated stand-off, in a motorized tracking device (UTC scan unit, configuration 2011, Fa. UTC Imaging B.V., GD Stein, Netherlands) that moves the transducer automatically along the tendon. Within the UTC protocol the instrumental settings for the SDFT were selected which facilitated standard settings like persistence, depth, focal point, gain, TGC-curve, to be used for all scans. During scanning, transverse US images were captured at regular distances of 0.2 mm over a distance of 12 cm and stored real-time in a high-capacity laptop computer (MacBook Pro® 17", Apple, Cupertino, USA). Compilation of these images created a 3-D block of US information that was used for quantification of stability of contiguous echo-patterns. Based on the echo-pattern stability, 4 different echo-types were discriminated, with histo-morphology of tendon specimen as reference test: type I, generated by intact and fully aligned fascicles (secondary collagen bundles); type II, generated by discontinuous, waving, not (yet) aligned and/or swollen fascicles (secondary collagen bundles); type III, generated

Table 1 Signalement, clinical history, diagnostic data and treatment of 20 horses with SDFT lesions

Horse number	Breed	Age (y)	Gender	Purpose used for	Reported duration of SDFT tendinopathy until initial exam (w)	Reported initiating event	Limb affected	Maximal injury zone (MIZ)	Lesion type
PRP-group									
1	Hannoverian	4	G	Dressage	2	Unknown	LF	2a, lat	Marginal
2	Hannoverian	8	M	Dressage	1	Training	LF	3a, palm	Marginal
3	Haflinger	21	G	Trained horse	2	Pasture turnout	LF	2b	Diffuse
4	Trakehner	5	S	Dressage	4	Pasture turnout	RF	3b, med	Marginal
5	Oldenburger	16	G	Police horse	2	Ride	RF	2b	Diffuse
6	Rhenish Warmblood	13	M	Dressage	2	Unknown	RF	3a	Core
7	Hannoverian	6	M	Dressage	2	Running free	LF	2b, palm	Marginal
8	New Forest Pony	13	G	Pleasure	3	Pasture turnout	LF	2b	Diffuse
9	Hannoverian	11	G	Eventing	8	Training	RF	3a	Core
10	Pinto	20	G	Pleasure	7	Unknown	LF	2b, lat	Marginal
		Ø 11.7							
Control group									
1	Oldenburger	9	M	Jumping	4	Jumping	LF	3a, lat	Marginal
2	Hannoverian	5	G	Dressage	6	Unknown	LF	3a, med	Marginal
3	Andalusian	18	M	Pleasure	3	Pasture turnout	LF	2b	Diffuse
4	Hannoverian	15	M	Dressage, jumping	2	Training	LF	2b, med	Marginal
5	German Riding Pony	9	M	Jumping	1	Jumping	LF	3a, lat	Marginal
6	Hannoverian	12	G	Police horse	2	Running free	RF	1b, lat	Marginal
7	Hannoverian	20	M	Pleasure	2	Unknown	RF	2a	diffuse
8	Rhenish Warmblood	7	G	Eventing	2	Training	LF	3a	Core
9	Hannoverian	10	G	Eventing	6	Jumping	LF	2b, lat	Marginal
10	Hannoverian	6	G	Pleasure	4	Unknown	RF	3a	Diffuse
		Ø 11.1							

SDFT superficial digital fexor tendon, *w* week(s), *y* years, *S* stallion, *M* mare, *G* gelding, *LF* left front, *RF* right front, *PRP-group* SDFT treated with intralesional injection of platelet-rich plasma, *Control group* SDFT treated with intralesional saline injection, *lat* lateral, *med* medial, *palm* palmar, Ø mean

by a mainly fibrillar matrix (collagen fibrils not/no yet organized into fascicles) and type IV, generated by a mainly amorphous matrix and/or fluid [37, 39].

Scanning for UTC was performed in standing, fully sedated horses while all limbs were weightbearing. As the UTC device allows to scan a metacarpal segment of approximately 12 cm, the device was applied to the metacarpal area in a way during the initial exam that the zone of maximal injury (MIZ) was centered in the middle of the standoff. The distance from the most prominent point of the accessory carpal bone to the proximally located edge of the standoff was measured and recorded to ensure that the same segment would be scanned during following UTC scans. Additionally this point was marked in the horse's latero-palmar metacarpal haircoat with a shaving blade. A corresponding segment of the SDFT of the opposite front limb was scanned in the same manner.

With the help of the software, the stability of the echo pattern of corresponding pixels over 9 contiguous transverse images was analysed by UTC algorithms. Images were controlled for movement artifacts and repeated if necessary. Data sets were stored digitally on the computer until final analysis.

A single scan of each tendon was analyzed retrospectively with the analyzing-software (UTC2011® Analyser V1.0.1, Fa. UTC Imaging, 6171 GD Stein, The Netherlands) by one observer (M.G.) being blinded to the treatment modality: A 6 cm long tendon segment was defined from 3 cm distally and proximally to the MIZ, respectively, on the colour coded longitudinal image produced during the first examination (day 0). Within this segment, the entire cross sectional area of the SDFT was analyzed using every 15th consecutive transverse image, i.e. every 3 mm. Ratios of echo types were analyzed quantitatively as fractions of the entire cross sectional area and mean values for the proportion of each type were calculated. The distance from the center of MIZ to the proximal end of the scan was measured to retrieve the MIZ and thereby the segment to be analyzed in control scans during the remaining examination period.

Preparation of PRP, Intralesional treatment, controlled exercise and follow-up examinations

Fiftyfour millilitres of autologous blood were collected by a single venipuncture of one jugular vein into a 60 ml syringe preloaded with 6 ml of the anticoagulant acid citrate dextrose (ACD-A). Approximately 5 ml of whole blood was aspirated into a tube containing EDTA (Vacuette®, Greiner Bio-One International AG, Kremsmünster, Austria) for later cell counts. To ensure that the whole blood and anticoagulant homogenously mix, the syringe was inverted gently 4 times. The content was transferred aseptically into bag A of a commercially available PRP preparation system (Osteokine®, Orthogen, Düsseldorf, Germany). The bag system was inserted in a swingout bucket of a centrifuge (Universal 300®, Andreas Hettich GmbH & Co. KG, Tuttlingen, Germany) and a corresponding swingout bucket was filled with a counterweight. According to the manufacturer's instruction the first centrifugation step was performed at a relative centrifugation force of 900 g for 3 min. The plasma including the buffy coat was transferred via the connecting tube to bag B by gently rolling the bottom of bag A upwards with a clamp. After closing the ports between bag A and B the system was centrifugated for 10 min at a relative centrifugation force of 1470 g. The supernatant platelet poor plasma (PPP) was aspirated via the withdrawal port. The remaining pellet of platelets and residual erythrocytes was resuspended by reinjecting a volume of 3 ml of PPP into bag B. The resulting PRP was completely aspirated from bag B which led to a volume of 4 ml. An aliquot of 1 ml PRP was transferred to a tube containing EDTA (Vacuette®, Greiner Bio-One International AG, Kremsmünster, Austria), while the remaing 3 ml were used for intralesional injection. Platelet- and leucocyte content was determined from whole blood and PRP with an automated cell counter (KX-21 N®, Sysmex, Norderstedt, Germany).

Horses were sedated for the intralesional injections with detomidine hydrochlorid (0.01–0.03 mg/kg [IV]) and butorphanol (0.04–0.05 mg/kg [IV]), and the medial and lateral palmar nerves were anaesthetized 2 cm distal to the carpometacarpal joints with 2,5 ml of a 2 % mepivacain solution, respectively.

After aseptic preparation of the skin, superficial digital tendon lesions were injected under sonographic guidance from the lateral aspect of the tendon perpendicularly to its long axis directly into the most hypoechoic areas through a 22G (Ø 0.7 mm, 30 mm) canula (BD Microlance^{TM} 3, Becton Dickinson S.A., Fraga, Huesca, Spain) while the limb was weight-bearing. SDFTs allocated to the PRPG received an intralesional treatment of 3 ml into the tendon defect (day 0). Tendons in the CG were injected intralesionally with 3 ml 0,9 % sterile saline solution (Isotone Kochsalzlösung 0,9 %®, B. Braun Melsungen, Melsungen, Germany). The volume of PRP or saline was equally distributed to 3 sites. The first injection was performed at the maximal injury zone. Further injection sites were 1–2 cm distally and proximally to the first injection. A padded distal limb bandage was applied and left in place during a period of 3 days box rest in all horses. The contralateral SDFT was not injected. All front hooves of all horses were shod with a closed horse shoe with a straight bar [49]. All horses participated in a gradually increasing exercise programme adapted from Bosch et al. [14]. Depending on the anamnestically reported duration of clinical SDF tendinopathy of less than 4 weeks or 5–8 weeks, horses were either given box rest for another 4 weeks or commenced with handwalking for 10 min, respectively (Table 2). The horses were re-examined clinically and with B-mode ultrasonography at 4, 8, 12, 18 and 24 weeks after injection. Ultrasound tissue characterization was repeated 12 and 24 weeks after treatment.

All owners were asked about the performance of their horses via telephone inquiry 12 and 24 months after treatment according to the following categories: reached previous or higher level of performance; was ridden at a lower level of performance; was retired; died.

Statistical analysis

Analysis of data was performed using SAS® Version 9.3 (SAS Institute, Cary, NC, USA). The level of significance

Table 2 Gradually increasing exercise programme adapted from Bosch et al. [14] and modified

Exercise/day	Period
Box rest	4 weeks
10 min walk	Weeks 5–8
20 min walk + 2 × 3 min trot	Weeks 9–12
30 min walk + 15 min trot	Weeks 13–15
30 min walk + 15 min trot + 3 × 1 min gallop	Weeks 16–18
35 min walk + 15 min trot + 3 × 5 min gallop	Weeks 19–24

min minutes

was set at $p < 0.05$. All values in the graphs are expressed as arithmetic mean values with standard error ($\overline{X} \pm$ SEM). The assumption of normality was tested using the Kolmogorov-Smirnov test and visual assessment of qq-plots of model residuals. In the case of rejection of normal distribution, distribution-free nonparametric methods were applied. Fisher's exact test was applied by evaluation of contingency tables to test the differences between groups (PRP-treated group and control group) on each examination day with regard to the parameters degree of lameness, sensitivity to palpation and skin surface temperature. To work out the differences of these parameters within a group between examination days, non-adjusted p-values were used provided that the global test was significant ($p < 0{,}05$) or showed a tendency to significance ($p = 0{,}05$ - 1). The influence of the groups and time points on the ultrasonongraphic parameters (T-CSA, T-FAS and TES) was tested using a two-way analysis of variance for independent samples (groups) and repeated measurements (time points), followed by the Tukey *post hoc* test for multiple pairwise comparisons. P-values were used in terms of comparison to assess differences of parameters between individual days of examination within a group and *vice versa*, and to determine the differences between the two groups on the respective examination day.

Results

Clinical examination

Lameness

On day 0, 60 % ($n = 6$) of the horses included in the PRPG were lame. Fifty percent ($n = 5$) of the control horses showed a lameness. In all horses it was the lame limb where tendinopathy was diagnosed. After 24 weeks 2 horses in the PRPG were still lame and 1 horse in the CG was lame. The mean degree of lameness did not differ between groups on any day of examination. Compared to day 0 lameness decreased significantly by week 8 after treatment within the PRPG ($p = 0.011$) and it decreased significantly by week 12 in the CG ($p = 0.014$) (Fig. 1a).

Clinical signs of inflammation

No statistically significant differences between the two groups with regard to scores for sensitivity to palpation and skin surface temperature were observed on day 0 and during the entire observation period (Fig. 1b, c). Within the PRPG scores for sensitivity to palpation of the SDFTs decreased significantly for the first time between week 4 and week 8 ($p = 0.003$) and in the CG between day 0 and week 4 ($p = 0.02$). From week 12 until the end of the observation period no painful reaction could be elicited in all horses (Fig. 1b). Scores for skin surface temperature (Fig. 1c) decreased significantly between day 0 and week 4 ($p = 0.001$) in the PRPG. Within the CG it took until week 8 that skin surface temperature decreased significantly ($p = 0.001$). From week 8 onwards scores for this parameter remained at a low level up to 24 weeks in both groups.

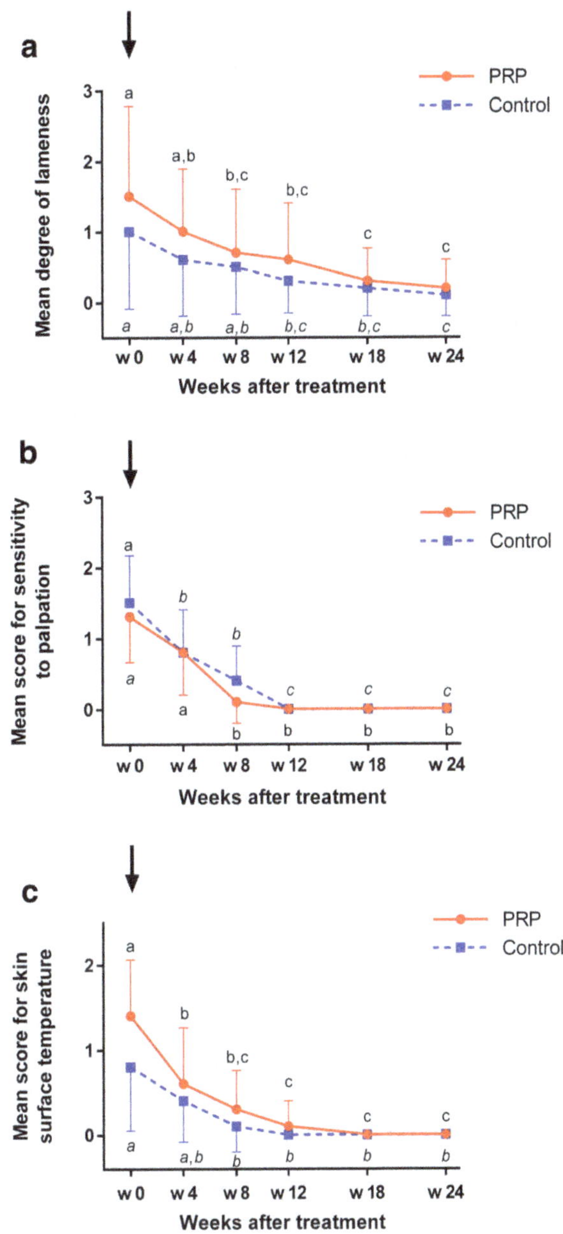

Fig. 1 Clinical findings after PRP and saline treatment of SDFT lesions over time. **a** Degree of lameness. **b** Scores for sensitivity to palpation. **c** Scores for skin surface temperature in the palmar metacarpal region. Mean ± SE; global test for PRPG and CG $p < 0.001$; Different letters (PRP normal and control italic) indicate significant differences ($p < 0.05$) within groups; PRPG = PRP-group: $n = 10$ limbs, SDFTs treated intralesionally with PRP; CG = control group: $n = 10$ limbs, SDFTs treated intralesionally with saline; black arrow = day 0: diagnosis, intralesional injection of PRP/saline; PRP = platelet-rich plasma; w = weeks; SDFT = superficial digital flexor tendon

B-mode ultrasonography

The horses included were presented with core lesions (3 horses), marginal lesions (11 limbs) or diffuse lesions (6 limbs) of the SDFT (Table 1). Control horses no. 3 and 7 had ultrasonographic signs of scarring of the SDFT in the contralateral non-lame limb on day 0. The MIZ of most lesions was located in zones 2b and 3a (80 % of horses in PRPG and CG, respectively), followed by zone 2a (10 % of horses in PRPG and CG, respectively), and zones 1b (10 % of horses in PRPG) and 3b (10 % of horses CG), respectively). There was no difference in T-CSA between the groups at any time point (Fig. 2a). Compared to the contralateral SDFT, T-CSA was significantly higher in PRP treated and in control limbs than in the respective contralateral limbs during the whole observation period ($p < 0.05$). Within the PRP group T-CSA was significantly higher ($p = 0.024$) only in week 4 as compared to week 18 (Fig. 2a). TES was significantly higher in the PRPG than in the CG at weeks 4, 8, 12 and 24 ($p = 0.0397$, $p = 0.0069$, $p = 0.00297$, $p = 0.0424$) (Fig. 2b); and T-FAS was significantly higher in the PRPG than in the CG at weeks 4, 8 and 12 ($p = 0.0387$, $p = 0.0140$, $p = 0.0283$) (Fig. 2c). Regarding the progression of TES and T-FAS they decreased significantly between day 0 and week 12 in the PRPG (TES: $p = 0.002$; T-FAS: $p = 0.001$) and between day 0 and week 8 the CG (TES: $p < 0.001$, T-FAS: $p = 0.023$) (Fig. 2b, c).

Ultrasound tissue characterization

The percentages of echo types I, III, IV (Fig. 3a, c, d), combined types I + II and combined types III + IV (Fig. 4) did not differ between groups at any time point. The percentage of echo type II was significantly higher ($p = 0.0492$) in the PRPG than in the CG at the end of the observation period (Fig. 3b).

In the PRPG percentages of combined type I + II pixels representing fascicular structures increased significantly between week 12 and 24 ($p = 0.009$) (Fig. 4a). Combined types III + IV percentages representing disorganized matrix decreased significantly between day 0 and week 12 ($p < 0.001$) and again between weeks 12 and 24 ($p = 0.024$) in the PRPG (Fig. 4b). In the CG both, combined type I + II and combined type III + IV did not change throughout the observation period ($p > 0.05$) (Fig. 4).

In the CG echo type I, i.e. intact and fully aligned fascicles increased significantly between day 0 and week 12 ($p = 0.001$) and after PRP treatment between week 12 and 24 ($p = 0.012$) (Fig. 3a). Echo type III representing mainly fibrillary matrix decreased significantly in both groups between day 0 and week 12 ($p < 0.001$). It further decreased significantly between week 12 and 24 in the PRPG ($p = 0.006$) while it remained on the same level in the CG (Fig. 3c). The percentage of echo type IV, i.e. amorphous matrix/fluid decreased siginificantly between day 0 and week 12 in the PRPG ($p < 0.001$). In the CG this type remained on the same level throughout the whole observation period (Fig. 3d).

Concentration of platelets and leucocytes

The mean number of platelets was $157.3 \pm 35.9 \times 10^3/\mu l$ in whole blood and $892.37 \pm 364.7 \times 10^3/\mu l$ in PRP. Leucocyte content was $7.8 \pm 1.5 \times 10^3/\mu l$ in whole blood and $14.1 \pm 7.0 \times 10^3/\mu l$ in PRP. Compared to whole blood platelets and leucocytes were concentrated significantly by factor 5.67 ($p = 0.0001$) and 1.81 ($p = 0.0139$), respectively in PRP.

Long-term follow-up

One horse allocated to the PRPG and one control horse developed recurrence of tendon injury in the treated limb within 2 years post diagnosis. One PRP treated horse developed tendinopathy in the SDFT of the contralateral front limb. Twelve months after treatment 80 % (8/10) of the horses allocated to the PRPG performed at the previous or at a higher level while this was the case in 50 % (5/10) of the control horses. Twenty-four months after treatment 60 % (6/10) were still ridden at the previous or higher level of performance in the PRPG while this was the case in 50 % (5/10) of the control horses. Horses that were ridden at a lower level of performance made up 10 % (1/10) of the PRP treated horses after 12 months and 20 % (2/10) after 24 months. In the CG 40 % (4/10) of the horses performed at a lower level after 12 months and 20 % (2/10) after 24 months. One horse included in the PRPG was retired within 12 months while one control horse was retired between 12 and 24 months after treatment. One PRP treated horse died of reasons unrelated to tendinopathy between 12 and 24 months and one control horse died within 12 months after treatment. Long term outcome did not differ significantly between groups.

Discussion

Results of this controlled clinical trial demonstrate that, compared to controls, single intralesional PRP treatment leads to an earlier reduction of the degree of lameness until week 8 and to an earlier decrease in palpable skin temperature of the SDFT region until week 4 after treatment. At 24 weeks after PRP treatment ultrasound tissue characterization showed a significantly higher percentage of type II echoes which, in combination with decrease of type III and IV, is indicative for advanced repair as the fibrillar matrix is getting organized into fascicles, although not yet aligned into lines of stress. Eighty percent of the PRP treated horses reached their previous or a higher level of performance after 12 months and 60 % continued to perform at this level after 24 months compared to 50 % in the CG at both time points.

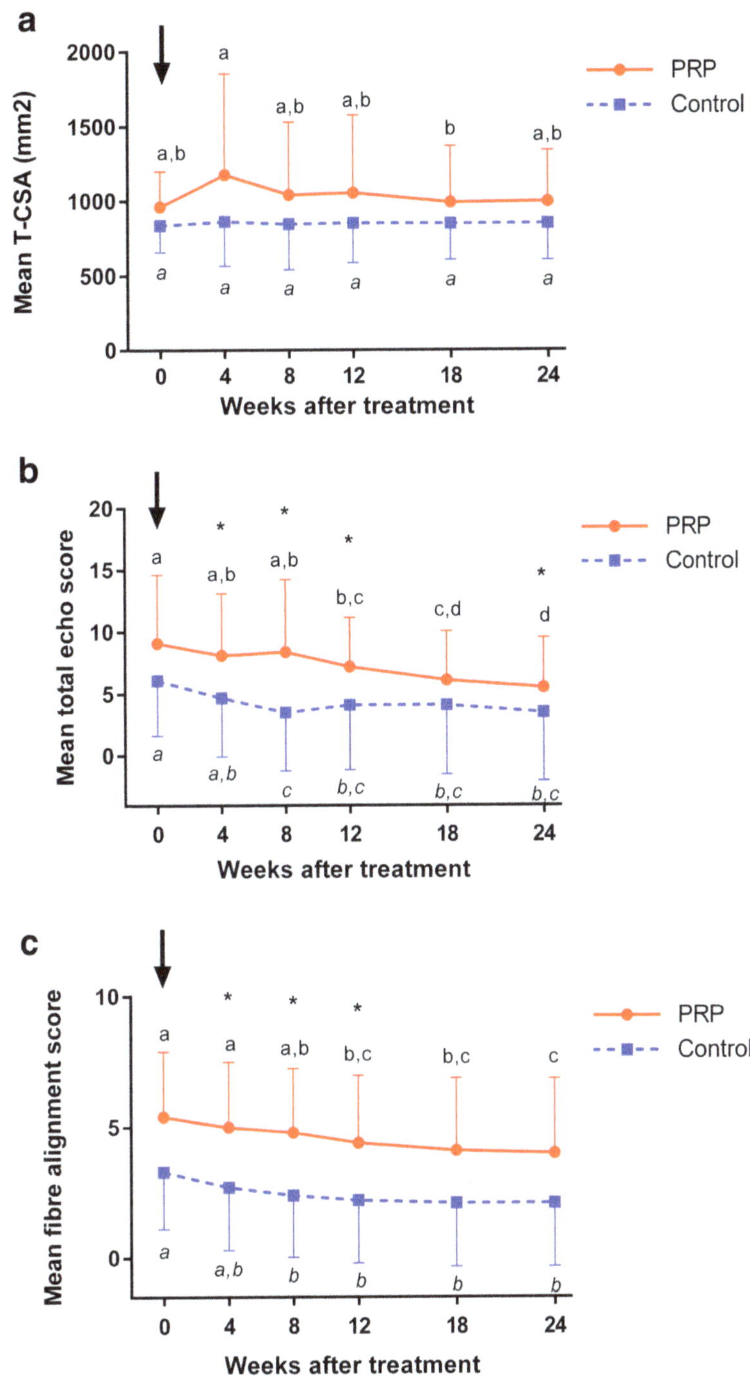

Fig. 2 B-mode ultrasonographic measurements. **a** Total cross sectional area of PRP- and saline treated SDFTs over time (global test: PRPG $p = 0.079$, CG $p = 0.999$). **b** Total echo scores of PRP- and saline treated SDFT lesions over time (global test: PRPG and CG $p < 0.001$). **c** Fiber alignment scores of PRP- and saline treated SDFT lesions over time (global test: PRPG and CG $p < 0.001$). Mean ± SE; Values labelled with asterisk (*) differ significantly ($p < 0.05$) between groups. Different letters (PRP normal and control italic) indicate significant differences ($p < 0.05$) within groups; PRPG = PRP-group: $n = 10$ limbs, SDFTs treated intralesionally with PRP; CG = control group: $n = 10$ limbs, SDFTs treated intralesionally with saline; black arrow = day 0: diagnosis, intralesional injection of PRP/saline; PRP = platelet-rich plasma; FAS = fiber alignment score; SDFT = superficial digital flexor tendon; TCSA = total cross sectional area; TES = total echo score; w = weeks

Because of the generally limited availability of adequate patients for a controlled experimental study in a clinical setting, horses of different ages, breeds and types of use were included in the current study. It is established that the potential for tendon healing is greater in younger horses [50] and that among others

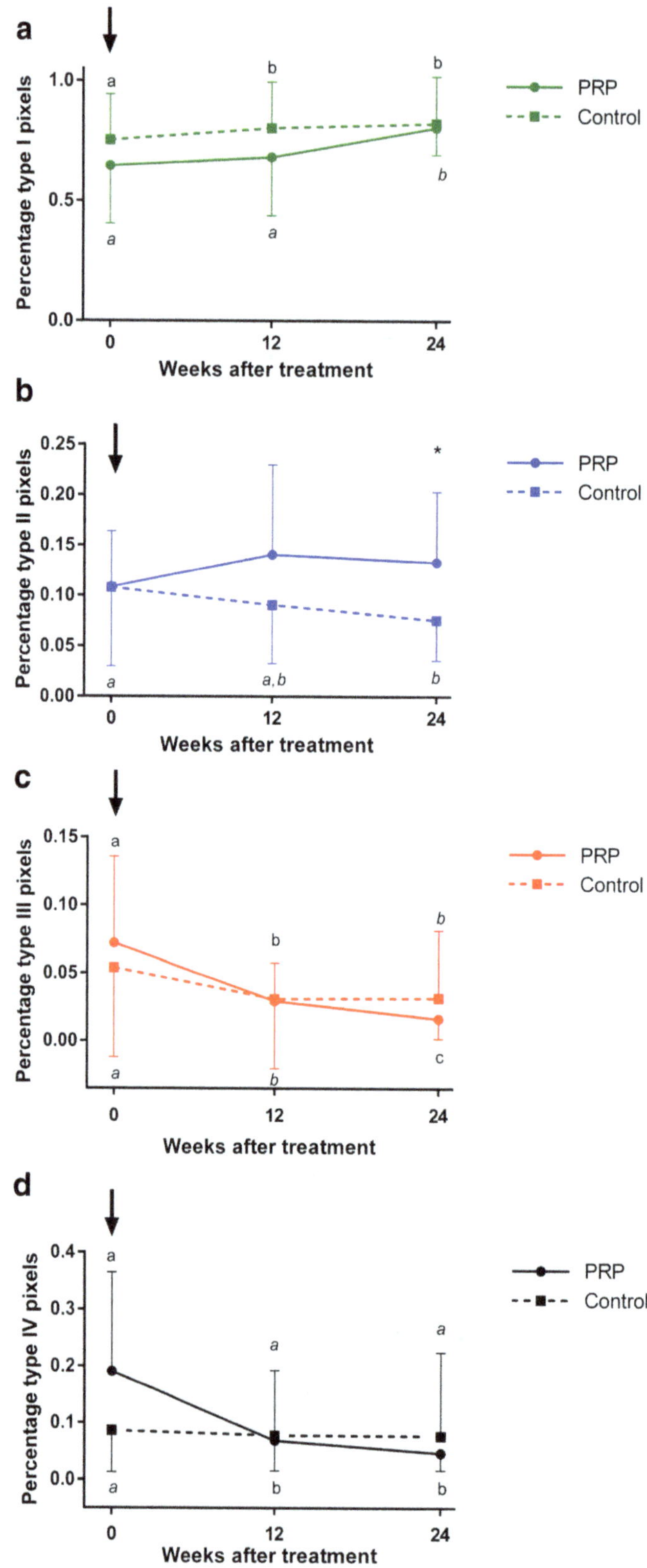

Fig. 3 (See legend on next page.)

(See figure on previous page.)

Fig. 3 Ultrasound tissue characterization: Proportion of echo-types I-IV. Proportion of echo types **a** I, **b** II, **c** III and **d** IV for PRP and saline treated SDFTs; PRP-group: solid lines; Control group: dotted lines; Mean ± SE; Values labelled with asterisk (*) differ significantly ($p < 0.05$) between groups. Global tests: echo type I: PRPG $p = 0.099$, CG $p = 0.004$; echo type II: PRPG $p = 0.204$, CG $p = 0.057$; echo type III: PRPG $p < 0.001$, CG $p = 0.002$; echo type IV: PRPG $p < 0.001$, CG $p = 0.940$; Different letters (PRP normal and control italic) indicate significant differences ($p < 0.05$) within groups; PRPG = PRP-group: $n = 10$ limbs, SDFTs treated intralesionally with PRP; CG = control group: $n = 10$ limbs, SDFTs treated intralesionally with saline; PRP = platelet-rich plasma; SDFT = superficial digital flexor tendon; w = weeks

male gender and high body weight are risk factors for tendinopathy [51]. The CG contains more horses used for show jumping and eventing which generally implies a higher tendon load and a potentially higher risk for self-inflicted blunt trauma than the use as e.g. dressage horse [52]. This has a potential impact on the severity of tendon lesions and during the long term rehabilitation after 24 weeks.

Fiftyfive percent of the horses included in the current study had ultrasonographic signs of marginal/peripheral SDFT lesions which was considered as a high proportion compared to centrally located tendon lesions frequently diagnosed in race- and performance horses [4]. The etiology of peripheral tendon lesions has not been investigated separately. However, it has been assumed that these lesions typically occur in show jumpers, dressage horses [52] and cutting horses [53]. They may be attributed to degeneration or blunt trauma, e.g. self-kicking with the ipsilateral hind hoof, or to excessive strain on the lateral aspect of the affected limbs [53]. By contrast centrally located ("core") lesions are the result of repetitive micro-injuries at high speed exercise and consecutive repair with insufficient tissue [3]. This lesion pattern was detected in only 3 horses in the current study

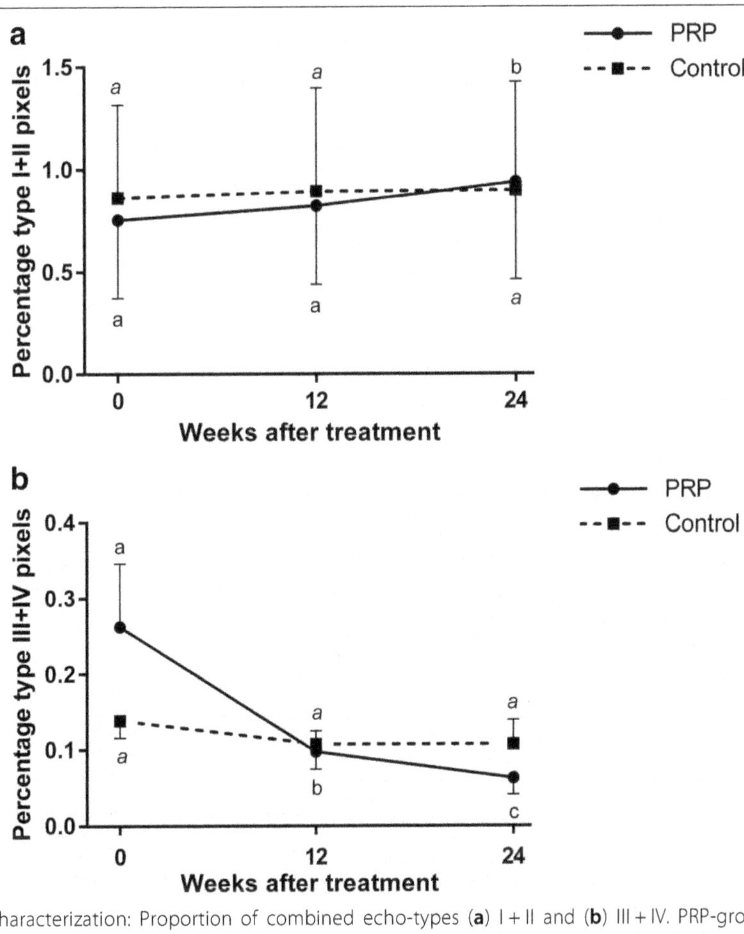

Fig. 4 Ultrasound tissue characterization: Proportion of combined echo-types (**a**) I + II and (**b**) III + IV. PRP-group: solid lines; Control group: dotted lines; Mean ± SE; Global tests: combined echo type I + II: PRPG $p = 0.0826$, CG $p = 0.318$; combined echo type I + II: PRPG $p < 0.001$; CG $p = 0.362$; Different letters (PRP normal and control italic) indicate significant differences ($p < 0.05$) within groups; PRPG = PRP-group: $n = 10$ limbs, SDFTs treated intralesionally with PRP; CG = control group: $n = 10$ limbs, SDFTs treated intralesionally with saline; PRP = platelet-rich plasma; SDFT = superficial digital flexor tendon; w = weeks

population which predominantly consisted of warmblood horses used for jumping and dressage purposes.

This might explain why the effect of a single PRP injection on several parameters of tendon healing study was less profound in the current than in the surgical model used by Bosch et al. (2010) [14] that mimics central core-lesions after single macro-trauma in young mature horses, thus no effects of underlying ageing and/or degeneration. A recent systematic literature review revealed that generally more experimental, especially *in vitro* PRP studies yield positive results than clinical trials do, which proves that experimental settings only imperfectly replicate conditions of natural tendon repair [18]. Although the number of peripheral tendon lesions was similar in both groups of the current study, different lesion patterns potentially respond differently to intralesional injections. Fluid might more easily reflux to the subcutis after injection into marginally compared to centrally located lesions as the former are only surrounded by the peritendineum at their peripheral aspect. At the same time larger tendon lesions generally have a worse prognosis for functional repair [54] and CSA of peripheral lesions is small in most cases. It has been shown that peripheral tendon lesions in cutting horses required a mean convalescent period of 4 months before horses returned to full exercise [53] which is shorter than the usual rehabilitation period for other SDFT injuries [2].

In the current study all tendon lesions were injected with the same volume of PRP or saline to avoid an impact of a variable volume on the outcome. This was practiced inconsistently in previous studies including injections of naturally occurring, i.e. non-standardized tendon or ligament lesions with variable dimensions [16, 55]. A volume of 3 ml was chosen based on encouraging results of an equine study using the same volume in an experimental model of SDFT tendinopathy [14]. Volumes used in previous case series mostly focusing on suspensory ligament desmopathy varied between 0.5 and 12 ml [16, 17, 19, 55]. The volume chosen in the current study seemed to be appropriate as no resistance of the syringe plunger occurred during injection of the SDFTs being slightly under tension in a weightbearing position.

The volumes of PRP and saline were evenly distributed to three injection sites in the current study. A comparable approach was chosen in a human study comparing the effect of PRP and saline on chronic Achilles tendinopathy [20]. Saline led to similar improvements of the tendon structure as PRP which might indicate that also multiple injections with tiny volumes of sterile saline at one single time-point may trigger a healing response.

The number of horses with owner consent for a controlled clinical trial is generally limited and the current study was conducted in an equine referral clinic where horses are usually presented within several weeks after onset of clinical signs of tendinopathy. This led to the decision to include horses with a history of clinical signs of tendinopathy for up to 8 weeks. It had to be accepted that some tendons were most probably already in the late proliferative or even in the remodelling phase of tendon healing while most were in the late inflammatory and early proliferative phase. By contrast mechanically induced core lesions were treated as early as 1 week after creation of lesions, i.e. at the end of a well-defined acute inflammatory phase in the experiment by Bosch et al. (2011) [13]. There is evidence that timing of intralesional tendon treatment has a significant influence on outcome supported by a comparative experimental equine investigation showing that PRP treatment 7 days after SDFT lesion creation led to an earlier improvement of ultrasonographic parameters than treatment on day 14 [56]. It is known that growth factors from the α-granula of platelets such as PDGF and TGF-ß have a positive influence during the inflammatory phase of tendon healing: [57–59]. In an experimental model of rat collateral ligament injury the effectiveness of PDGF dropped markedly if it was administered more than 24 h after injury [60]. This is in accordance with results after treatment of chronic human Achilles tendinopathy which showed no beneficial effects of PRP versus placebo treatment with sterile saline [20]. At the same time PRP injections have been reported to be beneficial in chronic human tendon disorders refractory to other treatment modalities in several uncontrolled clinical studies [23, 61]. During the proliferation and remodelling phase of tendon healing Vascular Endothelial Growth Factor, which is a major component of PRP, might play a role as promotor of angiogenesis [58].

Horses in the current study received a single PRP treatment. This decision was based on the finding that growth factor and cytokine release from platelets continues from their mRNA reserves for at least 7 days after activation [62] and on a significant and long-lasting effect of a single injection approach in an experimental equine tendinopathy study [14]. Another reason was the intention to investigate a low dose of PRP as a basis for further research in equine naturally occurring tendinopathies [33], because to date no dose dependent studies are available with regard to treatment of equine tendinopathies. The limited long term effect in the current study may have been influenced by the fact that most growth factors contained in PRP are *per se* short lived which probably contributed to a low concentration over time in the clinical setting chosen. In a study using a rodent experimental model it was also shown that a single injection of heterologous PRP immediately after Achilles tendon transection only had time-limited effects on tendon healing during the observation period of up to 6 weeks [63]. Results of another experimental study in a rodent model of tendinosis suggested that a single intratendinous injection of PRP does not lead to a local and systemic increase in several cytokines and growth factors over the observation period of 25 days [64].

The adequate number of injections over time is also a point of debate in naturally occurring human tendinopathy: In a long term clinical trial in humans it was shown that a second early PRP injection does not rapidly improve clinical signs of tendinopathy in case of incomplete resolution after the first treatment [65]. However, it has been shown in a controlled human clinical trial that patients with chronic patellar tendinopathy receiving two injections of a leucocyte poor platelet concentrate (autologous conditioned plasma®) showed better improvement in outcomes when compared to a monoinjection [66]. Accordingly application of 3 consecutive PRP injections significantly improved clinical symptoms and function of human athletes with chronic patellar tendinopathy [22]. Summarily it cannot be excluded that more than one intralesional treatment might have enhanced the clinical effects observed in the current study.

Based on whole blood platelets and leucocytes were concentrated by a mean factor of 5.67 and 1.81, respectively in PRP in the current study. Compared to other PRP systems the bag system used in this study leads to an intermediate platelet and low leucocyte concentration [24]. By contrast platelets and leucocytes were enriched with factors 3.78 and 6, respectively, utilizing a different double centrifugation system in an equine surgical model of tendinopathy [14]. Among various other factors the different concentrations of platelets and leucocytes might have contributed to the differences in outcome between the latter and the current study.

Low platelet counts have been demonstrated to be inefficient in bone regeneration [67] and increasing platelet concentrations in a leucocyte reduced PRP preparation leads to delivery of more anabolic and less pro-inflammatory cytokines *in vitro* [28]. However, with increasing platelet concentrations the synthesis of collagen type I and III decreases suggesting a diminishing effect on tendon metabolism [28]. This observation corresponds to a dose dependent *in vitro* investigation showing that intermediate platelet concentrations, such as used in the current study, have stronger effects on tenocyte proliferation, migration and collagen production than highest concentrations [68].

While some beneficial effects such as anti-infectious properties [69], growth factor content [70] and promotion of chemotaxis, proliferation and differentiation of cells [71] have been attributed to leucocytes they also contribute to a greater acute inflammatory response [29, 72] and to the expression of catabolic factors, e.g. MMPs and IL-1, that may influence tendon healing negatively [27, 73, 74], so that a low leucocyte content seems to be preferable to enhance anabolic effects during tendon healing.

In summary PRP characteristics vary significantly depending on the technique and preparation kit used for its production [24, 75] which has a significant impact on clinical outcome and makes comparison between clinical trials difficult [61]. The optimal platelet to leucocyte ratio for treatment of tendinopathy is unknown to date and most probably dependent on the stage of tendon healing [76].

Clinical parameters did not differ between the PRPG and controls at any time point which corresponds to the results of an equine PRP study using an experimental model of tendinopathy [14]. However, clinical signs of inflammation such as the degree of lameness and scores for skin surface temperature decreased earlier in the PRPG than in the CG which may be attributed to anti-inflammatory and analgesic effects of PRP [40, 77, 78]. This correlates well to reduced pain scores in humans after PRP treatment of tendinopathy [79, 80] and to uncontrolled observations in two horses that returned to competition level performance as soon as 4,5 months after PRP treatment of SDFT lesions [17]. However, mean scores for sensitivity to palpation decreased earlier in controls than in PRP treated tendons despite a similar curve progression in both groups. This is potentially attributed to a high interindividual variation of score values due to the inclusion of different lesion patterns. Established semi-quantitative clinical score systems were used to monitor clinical parameters in the current study. Accuracy could have been increased by the use of computerized gait analysis and thermography [81].

With regard to B-mode ultrasonography total cross sectional area (T-CSA) decreased significantly between week 4 and 18 after PRP treatment while it did not change throughout the observation period in the CG. Sensitivity of CSA is potentially low to detect minor changes as shown by routine ultrasound assessment of racehorses [82]. However, a delayed decrease of T-CSA after the inflammatory phase of tendon healing can be interpreted as a therapeutic effect of the PRP injection.

In contrast to controls, scores for echogenicity were significantly higher which implies a low echogenicity of the tendon lesions at 4, 8 and 12 weeks after PRP treatment and at week 24, i.e. at the end of the observation period. Similarly scores for fiber alignment were significantly higher in the PRPG than in the CG at 4, 8 and 12 weeks after treatment suggesting a lower degree of continuity of fibrous structures. A potential explanation for the differences between groups is that TES and FAS as determined by B-mode were higher in the PRP group from the beginning of the experiment onwards, as comparison of the different time points reveals a tendency to a significant difference ($p = 0.05$–0.1) for most of the remaining time points. Consequently the intermittent significant difference between groups should be interpreted with caution. However, it cannot be excluded that PRP injection effectively induced a transient inflammatory response [29, 83] which might have contributed to a temporary decrease in echogenicity and in alignment of fibrous structures. This contrasts with results of an experimental equine study showing no differences at all for several B-mode parameters between SDFTs treated with a leucocyte poor single centrifugation plasma product and saline [84]. Although echogenicity and fiber alignment scoring using B-mode ultrasonograms are established tools in clinical settings, they have a limited sensitivity to adequately reflect tendon intergrity [35]. Additionally lesion types included in the current study were heterogenous and the number of cases per group was relatively low. These factors made B-mode ultrasonography not the ideal modality to comparatively monitor especially subtle changes during the process of tendon repair in the current study. It could be proved that echogenicity and fibre alignment scores based on B-mode ultrasonograms do not correspond to the degree of echo continuity as determined by UTC implying a higher sensitivity of the latter technique [35, 37].

During ultrasound tissue characterization of PRPG tendons there was a significant drop in the proportion of non-structure related echo-type type IV representing a mainly amorphous matrix and/or free fluid between day 0 and week 12 while proportions for this echo type remained on the same level in the CG throughout 24 weeks. This phenomenon was previously observed in an experimental equine study after a single PRP injection and may be attributed to acute anti-inflammatory effects exerted by PRP [40, 77, 78].

The decreasing proportions of non-structure related echo types III and IV between day 0 and week 12 after PRP treatment in the current study rather resembles the course between week 4 and 12 after surgical induction of SDFT lesions without treatment [39] and the progression between week 5 and 18 after PRP treatment in another experimental equine study [40] and might therefore be an indicator for the chronicity of some tendon lesions included in the current study population. Hence, the delayed treatment up to 8 weeks after the onset of clinical signs might have contributed to a right-shift of the healing pattern as determined by UTC compared to experimental tendon lesions. However, more frequent UTC examinations between day 0 and week 12 would have been necessary to further prove this. This could not be realized due financial constraints and organisatory reasons as all horses were client owned and horses have to be sedated for 30–60 min during UTC scanning.

Between week 12 and week 24 combined echo-types I and II (fascicular structures) increased significantly within the PRPG. This resulted in a significantly higher percentage of echo type II being representative for the organization of a fibrillary matrix into fascicles that are still discontinous and not yet aligned, thus still remodelling after 24 weeks in PRP treated compared to control tendons. An echo-type II ratio described for normal tendon tissue, i.e. approximately 0.18 [39], was almost reached. In combination with a significant decreases of summarized echo-types III and IV between week 12 and week 24 this indicates an advanced organization of fibrillar and amorphous matrix into fascicles that are less continuous, more swollen and not aligned yet. The latter interpretation is supported by a lack of significant differences between groups with regard to echo-type I proportions representing intact and fully aligned fascicles (secondary tendon bundles).

In contrast to the current study PRP treated SDFTs had a significantly lower percentage of echo type II than controls in a surgical tendon model at the end of the observation period of 24 weeks [40]. This indicates that in the Bosch et al. study, using a single macro-trauma, the PRP-treated tendons passed already the remodelling stage while during the experiment described in this manuscript the fascicles were still not aligned yet and still requiring remodelling. In general the higher proportion of echo-type II in the PRPG is an indicator of an active process of remodelling 24 weeks after treatment [40].

The proportion of echo type III being representative for mainly fibrillar matrix continued to decrease significantly between week 12 and 24 only in the PRPG. Comparison of the proportion of this echo type to others in the PRPG suggests that the decrease in echo type III is rather in favour of echo type I than in favour of echo type II between week 12 and 24 as could be expected from a previous study [39]. Main reason for this observation is that in our study there are only limited time-points for UTC scanning, missing some detailed information on stages of repair. Anyhow, this finding suggests a transformation from fibrillar components into intact and aligned tendon bundles during the remodelling phase after PRP treatment of naturally occurring tendinopathies.

All horses included in the current study underwent the same controlled exercise regimen as it is known that controlled exercise has a therapeutic effect on tendon healing [85]. The duration of the controlled exercise prescribed for the included horses started on the basis of the estimated duration of tendinopathy (<4 weeks or 5–8 weeks) to adequately address the potentially therapeutic effect of gradually increasing controlled exercise on the process of tendon healing in each individual. To avoid inadequate loading of the tendons immediately after treatment all horses were given 3 days box rest and the first actual exercise level was restricted to 10 min walk.

Similarly all horses were shod with a closed horse shoe with a straight bar because this type of shoeing has been described as adequate during rehabilitation in cases of SDFT tendinopathy [49]. Despite potential alternative approaches to decrease strain in the SDFT via orthopaedic shoeing [86] authors intended to assure that rehabilitation conditions including shoeing were as similar as possible for all horses which seemed to be achievable most consistently with the type of shoeing chosen.

Recurrence rate is one of the most critical parameters of long-term functionality after tendon injury [31]. Only 1 out of 10 horses in either group developed recurrence of tendinopathy in the treated limb within 24 months after treatment. This is a lower recurrence rate than that previously reported after conventional intralesional treatment of SDF tendinopathy in different types of performance horses [2]. However, it has to be considered that several previous equine tendon studies mainly included racehorses typically developing centrally located core lesions [3, 31] which probably have a different etiology than most of the tendon lesions in the current study [53]. Due to the relatively low number of horses included and different types of use, recurrence rate in the current study should be interpreted cautiously. Biomechanical testing using tendon explants is the gold standard to determine elasticity and strength of tendon tissue. Due to the inclusion of client owned horses it could not be performed in the current study.

The performance level which is another important indicator of functionality did not differ statistically between groups at 12 and 24 months after treatment. However, the current study revealed that 8 versus 5 horses reached their previous level of performance 12 months after PRP and saline treatment respectively. After another 12 months only 6 of the PRP treated and 5 control horses performed at their previous level. This finding reflects the results of a clinical study including racehorses with midbody suspensory ligament demopathies [16]. Horses treated with PRP had fewer starts than control horses delayed only during the third year after return to racing.

Conclusions

This controlled clinical trial shows that a single intralesional injection of PRP up to 8 weeks after onset of clinical signs of tendinopathy contributes to an earlier reduction of lameness compared to a single intralesional treatment with saline. Compared to controls fibrillar matrix in PRP treated tendons is getting organized into fascicles that are not aligned yet after six months which is a sign of advanced tendon repair while remodelling continues. PRP treatment has the potential to increase the number of horses reaching their previous or a higher level of performance after 12 months which is not sustained after 24 months. Earlier treatment of tendinopathy with PRP should be considered to enhance these effects. Future controlled clinical studies should include higher numbers of horses.

Acknowledgements

We are grateful to all horse owners for their co-operation and to the veterinary staff of the Tierklinik Großmoor, Adelheidsdorf for their support. We thank Orthogen, Düsseldorf for providing ten Osteokine® sets free of charge.

Funding

No funding was obtained for this study.

Authors' contributions

FG had the idea of performing the study, designed the study and co-ordinated it. He participated in the collection of clinical and ultrasonographic data and their analyses and wrote the manuscript. MG collected the clinical and ultrasonographic data and participated in their analyses and revised the manuscript critically. KR performed the statistical analysis and revised the manuscript critically. HTMvS participated in the design of the study, assisted in the interpretation of the data and revised the manuscript critically. PS participated in the design of the study, contributed to the analyses of the data and revised the manuscript critically. All authors read and approved the manuscript for publication.

Authors' information

Results of the current study are part of the Dr. med. vet. thesis submitted by Moritz Gaus to the University of Veterinary Medicine Hannover, Foundation, Germany.

Competing interests

HTMvS is the inventor of the UTC device. He has not given any financial support for this study and has no financial interests in relation to this study. No non-financial conflicts of interests exist for any of the authors.

Consent for publication

Not applicable.

Author details

[1]Clinic for Horses, University of Veterinary Medicine Hannover, Foundation, Bünteweg 9, 30559 Hannover, Germany. [2]Department of Equine Sciences, Faculty of Veterinary Medicine, Utrecht University, Yalelaan 112, 3584 CM Utrecht, Netherlands. [3]Institute for Biometry, Epidemiology and Information Processing, University of Veterinary Medicine Hannover, Foundation, Bünteweg 2, 30559 Hannover, Germany.

References

1. Gibson KT, Snyder JR, Spier SJ. Ultrasonographic diagnosis of soft tissue injuries in horses competing at the Sydney 2000 Olympic Games. Equine Vet Educ. 2002;14(3):149–56.
2. Dyson SJ. Medical management of superficial digital flexor tendonitis: a comparative study in 219 horses (1992–2000). Equine Vet J. 2004;36(5):415–9.
3. Patterson-Kane JC, Firth EC. The pathobiology of exercise-induced superficial digital flexor tendon injury in Thoroughbred racehorses. Vet J. 2009;181(2):79–89.

4. Avella CS, Smith RKW. Diagnosis and management of tendon and ligament disorders. In: Auer JA, Stick JA, editors. Equine Surgery. 4th ed. St. Louis: Elsevier Saunders; 2011. p. 1157–79.
5. Geburek F, Stadler P. Regenerative Therapie von Sehnen- und Banderkrankungen bei Pferden. Terminologie, Herstellung, biologisches Potential und *in vitro* Effekte. (Regenerative therapy for tendon and ligament disorders in horses. Terminology, production, biologic potential and *in vitro* effects). Tierarztl Prax Ausg G Grosstiere Nutztiere. 2011;39(6):373–83.
6. Docheva D, Muller SA, Majewski M, Evans CH. Biologics for tendon repair. Adv Drug Deliv Rev. 2015;84:222–39. doi:10.1016/j.addr.2014.11.015.
7. Textor J. Autologous biologic treatment for equine musculoskeletal injuries: platelet-rich plasma and IL-1 receptor antagonist protein. Vet Clin North Am Equine Pract. 2011;27(2):275–98.
8. Kaux JF, Drion P, Croisier JL, Crielaard JM. Tendinopathies and platelet-rich plasma (PRP): from pre-clinical experiments to therapeutic use. J Stem Cells Regen Med. 2015;11(1):7–17.
9. Solchaga LA, Bendele A, Shah V, Snel LB, Kestler HK, Dines JS, et al. Comparison of the effect of intra-tendon applications of recombinant human platelet-derived growth factor-BB, platelet-rich plasma, steroids in a rat achilles tendon collagenase model. J Orthop Res. 2014;32(1):145–50.
10. Mazzocca AD, McCarthy MB, Chowaniec DM, Dugdale EM, Hansen D, Cote MP, et al. The positive effects of different platelet-rich plasma methods on human muscle, bone, and tendon cells. Am J Sports Med. 2012;40(8):1742–9.
11. Smith JJ, Ross MW, Smith RK. Anabolic effects of acellular bone marrow, platelet rich plasma, and serum on equine suspensory ligament fibroblasts *in vitro*. Vet Comp Orthop Traumatol. 2006;19(1):43–7.
12. Schnabel LV, Mohammed HO, Miller BJ, McDermott WG, Jacobson MS, Santangelo KS, et al. Platelet rich plasma (PRP) enhances anabolic gene expression patterns in flexor digitorum superficialis tendons. J Orthop Res. 2007;25(2):230–40.
13. Bosch G, Moleman M, Barneveld A, van Weeren PR, van Schie HT. The effect of platelet-rich plasma on the neovascularization of surgically created equine superficial digital flexor tendon lesions. Scand J Med Sci Sports. 2011;21(4):554–61.
14. Bosch G, van Schie HT, de Groot MW, Cadby JA, van de Lest CH, Barneveld A, et al. Effects of platelet-rich plasma on the quality of repair of mechanically induced core lesions in equine superficial digital flexor tendons: a placebo-controlled experimental study. J Orthop Res. 2010;28(2):211–7.
15. Alsousou J, Thompson M, Hulley P, Noble A, Willett K. The biology of platelet-rich plasma and its application in trauma and orthopaedic surgery: a review of the literature. J Bone Joint Surg (Br). 2009;91(8):987–96.
16. Waselau M, Sutter WW, Genovese RL, Bertone AL. Intralesional injection of platelet-rich plasma followed by controlled exercise for treatment of midbody suspensory ligament desmitis in Standardbred racehorses. J Am Vet Med Assoc. 2008;232(10):1515–20.
17. Arguelles D, Carmona JU, Climent F, Munoz E, Prades M. Autologous platelet concentrates as a treatment for musculoskeletal lesions in five horses. Vet Rec. 2008;162(7):208–11.
18. Brossi PM, Moreira JJ, Machado TSL, Baccarin RYA. Platelet-rich plasma in orthopedic therapy: a comparative systematic review of clinical and experimental data in equine and human musculoskeletal lesions. BMC Vet Res. 2015;11.
19. Bazzano M, Piccione G, Giannetto C, Tosto F, Di Pietro S, Giudice E. Platelet Rich Plasma Intralesional Injection as Bedside Therapy for Tendinitis in Athletic Horse. Acta Sci Vet. 2013;41.
20. de Vos RJ, Weir A, van Schie HT, Bierma-Zeinstra SM, Verhaar JA, Weinans H, et al. Platelet-rich plasma injection for chronic Achilles tendinopathy: a randomized controlled trial. Jama. 2010;303(2):144–9.
21. Schepull T, Kvist J, Norrman H, Trinks M, Berlin G, Aspenberg P. Autologous platelets have no effect on the healing of human achilles tendon ruptures: a randomized single-blind study. Am J Sports Med. 2011;39(1):38–47.
22. Charousset C, Zaoui A, Bellaiche L, Bouyer B. Are multiple platelet-rich plasma injections useful for treatment of chronic patellar tendinopathy in athletes? a prospective study. Am J Sports Med. 2014;42(4):906–11.
23. Monto RR. Platelet rich plasma treatment for chronic Achilles tendinosis. Foot Ankle Int. 2012;33(5):379–85.
24. Hessel LN, Bosch G, van Weeren PR, Ionita JC. Equine autologous platelet concentrates: A comparative study between different available systems. Equine Vet J. 2015;47(3):319–25.
25. Schnabel CL, Steinig P, Schuberth HJ, Koy M, Wagner B, Wittig B, et al. Influences of age and sex on leukocytes of healthy horses and their *ex vivo* cytokine release. Vet Immunol Immunopathol. 2015;165(1–2):64–74.
26. Giraldo CE, Lopez C, Alvarez ME, Samudio IJ, Prades M, Carmona JU. Effects of the breed, sex and age on cellular content and growth factor release from equine pure-platelet rich plasma and pure-platelet rich gel. BMC Vet Res. 2013;9:29.
27. McCarrel TM, Minas T, Fortier LA. Optimization of leukocyte concentration in platelet-rich plasma for the treatment of tendinopathy. J Bone Joint Surg Am. 2012;94(19):e143(1–8).
28. Boswell SG, Schnabel LV, Mohammed HO, Sundman EA, Minas T, Fortier LA. Increasing platelet concentrations in leukocyte-reduced platelet-rich plasma decrease collagen gene synthesis in tendons. Am J Sports Med. 2014;42(1):42–9.
29. Dragoo JL, Braun HJ, Durham JL, Ridley BA, Odegaard JI, Luong R, et al. Comparison of the acute inflammatory response of two commercial platelet-rich plasma systems in healthy rabbit tendons. Am J Sports Med. 2012;40(6):1274–81.
30. Jann H, Stashak TS. Equine wound management. In: Stashak TS, Theoret CL, editors. Equine Wound Management. Ames: Wiley-Blackwell; 2008. p. 489–508.
31. O'Meara B, Bladon B, Parkin TD, Fraser B, Lischer CJ. An investigation of the relationship between race performance and superficial digital flexor tendonitis in the Thoroughbred racehorse. Equine Vet J. 2010;42(4):322–6.
32. Crevier-Denoix N, Collobert C, Pourcelot P, Denoix JM, Sanaa M, Geiger D, et al. Mechanical properties of pathological equine superficial digital flexor tendons. Equine Vet J Suppl. 1997;23:23–6.
33. Geburek F, Lietzau M, Beineke A, Rohn K, Stadler PM. Effect of a single injection of autologous conditioned serum (ACS) on tendon healing in equine naturally occurring tendinopathies. Stem Cell Res Ther. 2015;6:126.
34. Reef VB, Genovese RL, Davis WM. Initial long-term results of horses with superficial flexor tendinitis treated with intralesional beta-aminoproprionitrile fumarate. 43rd Annual Convention of the AAEP. Phoenix, Arizona; 1997
35. van Schie JT, Bakker EM, van Weeren PR. Ultrasonographic evaluation of equine tendons: a quantitative *in vitro* study of the effects of amplifier gain level, transducer-tilt, and transducer-displacement. Vet Radiol Ultrasound. 1999;40(2):151–60.
36. van Schie HT, Bakker EM, Jonker AM, van Weeren PR. Ultrasonographic tissue characterization of equine superficial digital flexor tendons by means of gray level statistics. Am J Vet Res. 2000;61(2):210–9.
37. van Schie HT, Bakker EM, Jonker AM, van Weeren PR. Computerized ultrasonographic tissue characterization of equine superficial digital flexor tendons by means of stability quantification of echo patterns in contiguous transverse ultrasonographic images. Am J Vet Res. 2003;64(3):366–75.
38. van Schie HT, Bakker EM, Jonker AM, van Weeren PR. Efficacy of computerized discrimination between structure-related and non-structure-related echoes in ultrasonographic images for the quantitative evaluation of the structural integrity of superficial digital flexor tendons in horses. Am J Vet Res. 2001;62(7):1159–66.
39. van Schie HT, Bakker EM, Cherdchutham W, Jonker AM, van de Lest CH, van Weeren PR. Monitoring of the repair process of surgically created lesions in equine superficial digital flexor tendons by use of computerized ultrasonography. Am J Vet Res. 2009;70(1):37–48.
40. Bosch G, Rene van Weeren P, Barneveld A, van Schie HT. Computerised analysis of standardised ultrasonographic images to monitor the repair of surgically created core lesions in equine superficial digital flexor tendons following treatment with intratendinous platelet rich plasma or placebo. Vet J. 2011;187(1):92–8.
41. Docking SI, Daffy J, van Schie HT, Cook JL. Tendon structure changes after maximal exercise in the Thoroughbred horse: use of ultrasound tissue characterisation to detect *in vivo* tendon response. Vet J. 2012;194(3):338–42.
42. Cadby JA, David F, van de Lest C, Bosch G, van Weeren PR, Snedeker JG, et al. Further characterisation of an experimental model of tendinopathy in the horse. Equine Vet J. 2013;45(5):642–8.
43. van Schie HT, de Vos RJ, de Jonge S, Bakker EM, Heijboer MP, Verhaar JA, et al. Ultrasonographic tissue characterisation of human Achilles tendons: quantification of tendon structure through a novel non-invasive approach. Br J Sports Med. 2010;44(16):1153–9.

44. de Vos RJ, Weir A, Tol JL, Verhaar JA, Weinans H, van Schie HT. No effects of PRP on ultrasonographic tendon structure and neovascularisation in chronic midportion Achilles tendinopathy. Br J Sports Med. 2011;45(5):387–92.
45. Edinger J. Orthopädische Untersuchung der Gliedmaßen und der Wirbelsäule. In: Wissdorf H, Gerhards H, Huskamp B, Deegen E, editors. Praxisorientierte Anatomie und Propädeutik des Pferdes. Hannover: M. u. H. Schaper; 2010. p. 890–926.
46. Schmidt H. Die Behandlung akuter und chronischer Sehnenerkrankungen beim Pferd mit hochmolekularer Hyaluronsäure (Dr. med. vet. thesis). Hannover: Tierärztliche Hochschule Hannover; 1989.
47. Genovese RL, Rantanen NW, Hauser ML, Simpson BS. Diagnostic ultrasonography of equine limbs. Vet Clin North Am Equine Pract. 1986;2(1):145–226.
48. Rantanen NW, Jorgensen JS, Genovese RL. Ultrasonographic evaluation of the equine limb: technique. In: Ross MW, Dyson SJ, editors. Diagnosis and Management of Lameness in the Horse. 1st ed. St. Louis: Elsevier; 2003. p. 166–88.
49. Höppner S. Orthopädische Beschläge bei Sehnenerkrankungen. Der praktische Tierarzt. 2010;91(4):326–9.
50. Jorgensen JS, Genovese RL, Ross MW. Superficial digital flexor tendonitis in racehorses. In: Ross MW, Dyson SJ, editors. Diagnosis and Management of Lameness in the Horses. 2nd ed. St. Louis: Elsevier, Saunders; 2011. p. 706–15.
51. Takahashi T, Kasashima Y, Ueno Y. Association between race history and risk of superficial digital flexor tendon injury in Thoroughbred racehorses. J Am Vet Med Assoc. 2004;225(1):90–3.
52. Dyson SJ. Superficial digital flexor tendonitis in event horses, show Jumpers, dressage horses and pleasure horses. In: Ross MW, Dyson SJ, editors. Diagnosis and Management of Lameness in the Horses. 2nd ed. St. Louis: Elsevier, Saunders; 2011. p. 721–6.
53. Tipton TE, Ray CS, Hand DR. Superficial digital flexor tendonitis in cutting horses: 19 cases (2007–2011). J Am Vet Med Assoc. 2013;243(8):1162–5.
54. Marr CM, Love S, Boyd JS, McKellar Q. Factors affecting the clinical outcome of injuries to the superficial digital flexor tendon in National Hunt and point-to-point racehorses. Vet Rec. 1993;132(19):476–9.
55. Castelijns G, Crawford A, Schaffer J, Ortolano GA, Beauregard T, Smith RK. Evaluation of a filter-prepared platelet concentrate for the treatment of suspensory branch injuries in horses. Vet Comp Orthop Traumatol. 2011;24(5):363–9.
56. Fonseca FA, Oliveira FTA, Rajao MD, Dumont CBS, Santos-Leonardo A, Lima EMM et al. Does time matter for platelet-rich plasma treatment of equine tendinitis? 23rd Scientific Meeting of the European College of Veterinary Surgeons. Copenhagen, Denmark; 2014
57. Kashiwagi K, Mochizuki Y, Yasunaga Y, Ishida O, Deie M, Ochi M. Effects of transforming growth factor-beta 1 on the early stages of healing of the Achilles tendon in a rat model. Scand J Plast Reconstr Surg Hand Surg. 2004;38(4):193–7.
58. Molloy T, Wang Y, Murrell G. The roles of growth factors in tendon and ligament healing. Sports Med. 2003;33(5):381–94.
59. Thomopoulos S, Zaegel M, Das R, Harwood FL, Silva MJ, Amiel D, et al. PDGF-BB released in tendon repair using a novel delivery system promotes cell proliferation and collagen remodeling. J Orthop Res. 2007;25(10):1358–68.
60. Batten ML, Hansen JC, Dahners LE. Influence of dosage and timing of application of platelet-derived growth factor on early healing of the rat medial collateral ligament. J Orthop Res. 1996;14(5):736–41.
61. Filardo G, Kon E, Di Matteo B, Di Martino A, Tesei G, Pelotti P, et al. Platelet-rich plasma injections for the treatment of refractory Achilles tendinopathy: results at 4 years. Blood Transfus. 2014;12(4):533–40.
62. Senzel L, Gnatenko DV, Bahou WF. The platelet proteome. Curr Opin Hematol. 2009;16(5):329–33.
63. Parafioriti A, Armiraglio E, Del Bianco S, Tibalt E, Oliva F, Berardi AC. Single injection of platelet-rich plasma in a rat Achilles tendon tear model. Muscles, Ligaments and Tendons J. 2011;1(2):41–7.
64. Dallaudiere B, Louedec L, Lenet MP, Pesquer L, Blaise E, Perozziello A, et al. The molecular systemic and local effects of intra-tendinous injection of Platelet Rich Plasma in tendinosis: preliminary results on a rat model with ELISA method. Muscles, Ligaments Tendons J. 2015;5(2):99–105.
65. Dallaudiere B, Meyer P, Hummel V, Perozziello A, Peuchant A, Moreau-Durieux MH, et al. Efficacy of second intra-tendinous platelet-rich-plasma injection in case of incomplete response of the first injection: three-year follow up experience. Diagn interv Imaging. 2013;94(9):871–7.
66. Zayni R, Thaunat M, Fayard JM, Hager JP, Carrillon Y, Clechet J, et al. Platelet-rich plasma as a treatment for chronic patellar tendinopathy: comparison of a single versus two consecutive injections. Muscles, Ligaments Tendons J. 2015;5(2):92–8.
67. Weibrich G, Hansen T, Kleis W, Buch R, Hitzler WE. Effect of platelet concentration in platelet-rich plasma on peri-implant bone regeneration. Bone. 2004;34(4):665–71.
68. Giusti I, D'Ascenzo S, Manco A, Di Stefano G, Di Francesco M, Rughetti A, et al. Platelet concentration in platelet-rich plasma affects tenocyte behavior *in vitro*. Biomed Res Int. 2014;2014:630870.
69. Lopez C, Carmona JU, Giraldo CE, Alvarez ME. Bacteriostatic effect of equine pure platelet-rich plasma and other blood products against methicillin-sensitive Staphylococcus aureus. An *in vitro* study. Vet Comp Orthop Traumatol. 2014;27(5):372–8.
70. Grainger DJ, Mosedale DE, Metcalfe JC. TGF-beta in blood: a complex problem. Cytokine Growth Factor Rev. 2000;11(1–2):133–45.
71. Wrotniak M, Bielecki T, Gazdzik TS. Current opinion about using the platelet-rich gel in orthopaedics and trauma surgery. Ortop Traumatol Rehabil. 2007;9(3):227–38.
72. Wasterlain AS, Braun HJ, Harris AH, Kim HJ, Dragoo JL. The systemic effects of platelet-rich plasma injection. Am J Sports Med. 2013;41(1):186–93.
73. Pifer MA, Maerz T, Baker KC, Anderson K. Matrix metalloproteinase content and activity in low-platelet, low-leukocyte and high-platelet, high-leukocyte platelet rich plasma (PRP) and the biologic response to PRP by human ligament fibroblasts. Am J Sports Med. 2014;42(5):1211–8.
74. Zhou Y, Zhang J, Wu H, Hogan MV, Wang JH. The differential effects of leukocyte-containing and pure platelet-rich plasma (PRP) on tendon stem/progenitor cells - implications of PRP application for the clinical treatment of tendon injuries. Stem Cell Res Ther. 2015;6(1):173.
75. Oh JH, Kim W, Park KU, Roh YH. Comparison of the Cellular Composition and Cytokine-Release Kinetics of Various Platelet-Rich Plasma Preparations. Am J Sports Med. 2015;43(12):3062–70.
76. Mautner K, Malanga GA, Smith J, Shiple B, Ibrahim V, Sampson S, et al. A call for a standard classification system for future biologic research: the rationale for new PRP nomenclature. PM R. 2015;7(4 Suppl):S53–9.
77. El-Sharkawy H, Kantarci A, Deady J, Hasturk H, Liu H, Alshahat M, et al. Platelet-rich plasma: growth factors and pro- and anti-inflammatory properties. J Periodontol. 2007;78(4):661–9.
78. Mazzocca AD, McCarthy MB, Intravia J, Beitzel K, Apostolakos J, Cote MP, et al. An *in vitro* evaluation of the anti-inflammatory effects of platelet-rich plasma, ketorolac, and methylprednisolone. Arthroscopy. 2013;29(4):675–83.
79. Mishra A, Pavelko T. Treatment of chronic elbow tendinosis with buffered platelet-rich plasma. Am J Sports Med. 2006;34(11):1774–8.
80. Kon E, Filardo G, Delcogliano M, Presti ML, Russo A, Bondi A, et al. Platelet-rich plasma: new clinical application: a pilot study for treatment of jumper's knee. Injury. 2009;40(6):598–603.
81. Turner TA. Thermography as an aid to the clinical lameness evaluation. Vet Clin North Am Equine Pract. 1991;7(2):311–38.
82. Avella CS, Ely ER, Verheyen KL, Price JS, Wood JL, Smith RK. Ultrasonographic assessment of the superficial digital flexor tendons of National Hunt racehorses in training over two racing seasons. Equine Vet J. 2009;41(5):449–54.
83. Textor JA, Tablin F. Intra-articular use of a platelet-rich product in normal horses: clinical signs and cytologic responses. Vet Surg. 2013;42(5):499–510.
84. Estrada RJ, van Weeren R, van de Lest CHA, Boere J, Reyes M, Ionita JC, et al. Effects of Autologous Conditioned Plasma® (ACP) on the healing of surgically induced core lesions in equine superficial digital flexor tendon. Pferdeheilkunde. 2014;30(6):633–42.
85. Gillis CL. Rehabilitation of Tendon and Ligament Injuries. 43rd Annual Convention of the AAEP. Phoenix, Arizona; 1997
86. Lawson SE, Chateau H, Pourcelot P, Denoix JM, Crevier-Denoix N. Effect of toe and heel elevation on calculated tendon strains in the horse and the influence of the proximal interphalangeal joint. J Anat. 2007;210(5):583–91. doi:10.1111/j.1469-7580.2007.00714.x.

14

Effects of two alfalfa preparations with different particle sizes on the gastric mucosa in weanlings: alfalfa chaff versus alfalfa pellets

Sarah Vondran[1], Monica Venner[2] and Ingrid Vervuert[1*]

Abstract

Background: Feeding alfalfa hay is often recommended for its buffering components, like protein and calcium, to prevent lesions of the gastric mucosa in horses. Until now, there has been no information regarding the influence of alfalfa particle size on the gastric mucosa. The aim of this study was to investigate the effects of feeding two alfalfa preparations with different particle sizes (alfalfa chaff vs alfalfa pellets) in comparison with grass hay on the gastric mucosa in weanling horses. We hypothesized that feeding a high proportion of fine alfalfa particles would negatively impact gastric mucosa and that feeding long alfalfa chaff would improve gastric mucosal health in weanlings.

Results: Before weaning, the prevalence of gastric mucosa lesions (one or more lesions considering all locations in the stomach) was 84.3 %; at 14 days after weaning, it was almost 100 %. Before and after weaning, most of the lesions were found at the greater curvature of the squamous mucosa and at the lesser curvature. After weaning, gastric mucosal lesions at the pylorus were significantly more severe in the group fed alfalfa chaff ($p = 0.002$). In the other regions, no differences related to the feeding regimes were observed.

Conclusions: Feeding alfalfa failed to improve gastric mucosal lesion scores in weanlings. Furthermore, foals fed alfalfa chaff had higher lesion scores at the pylorus. Alfalfa leaves contain a superior protein source and high amounts of calcium and magnesium, providing extra nutritional advantages in growing horses. At this time, either traditional grass hay rations or grass hay with alfalfa pellets can be recommended.

Keywords: Squamous, Glandular, Stomach, Gastric lesions, Horse

Background

Gastric ulceration is commonly identified in horses and foals. The prevalence of gastric ulcers in Thoroughbred racehorses is estimated to be >80 % in the squamous mucosa [1]. In weanlings it ranges between 32 and 94 % [2, 3]. Risk factors for gastric mucosa lesions, specifically for equine squamous gastric ulcer disease, are stall confinement, strenuous exercise, transport stress in adult horses (as reviewed by Andrews and others [4]), and the weaning process in foals [2, 3]. Nonsteroidal anti-inflammatory drugs have been demonstrated to be a risk factor for the equine glandular region in adult horses and foals [5, 6].

The relationship between feeding and gastric mucosal health has been demonstrated. Dietary factors that may effect squamous gastric mucosa in horses include buffering substances [7], the level of starch intake [8], or the type and daily amount of food [8, 9]. Furthermore, the particle size of the diet appears to be a factor in glandular gastric mucosa [2]. In foals, feeding alfalfa chaff resulted in glandular mucosal lesions, which may have been related to mechanical irritation [2]. Furthermore, no favorable effect was found on the squamous mucosa in weanlings. However, other authors observed beneficial

* Correspondence: ingrid.vervuert@vetmed.uni-leipzig.de
[1]Institute of Animal Nutrition, Nutrition Diseases and Dietetics, Faculty of Veterinary Medicine, University of Leipzig, D-04103 Leipzig, Germany
Full list of author information is available at the end of the article

effects of feeding alfalfa hay on the squamous mucosa in foals [10] and adult horses [7]. In pigs fed a diet of finely ground pellets, the squamous gastric ulcer score was significantly higher than for those fed a diet of larger particles [11]. Furthermore, feeding a coarse ground feed reduced mucosa lesions of the pars oesophagea in growing pigs [12].

The aim of this study was to investigate the effects of feeding two alfalfa preparations with different particle sizes (alfalfa chaff vs alfalfa pellets) in comparison with grass hay on the gastric mucosa in weanling horses. We hypothesized that feeding a high proportion of fine particles (alfalfa pellets) would negatively impact gastric mucosa in foals and that foals receiving alfalfa chaff would have better gastric mucosal lesion scores.

Results

None of the foals in the study demonstrated any clinical signs commonly associated with the presence of gastric ulcers such as colic, inappetence, or depression, as reviewed by Andrews and others [4].

The daily average consumption of grass hay per foal was 4.3 kg in the alfalfa chaff group, 5.0 kg in the alfalfa pellets group, and 8.3 kg in the grass hay group (Table 1). In addition to the grass hay intake, the mean daily feed intake (± SD) was 5.95 ± 0.13 kg in the alfalfa chaff group, 5.47 ± 0.18 kg in the alfalfa pellets group, and 3.66 kg in the hay group.

In the alfalfa chaff group, 91 % of alfalfa chaff particles were longer than 2 mm; in the alfalfa pellets group, 60 % of alfalfa pellets particles were smaller than 0.25 mm (Table 2).

Mean (± SD) body weight increased in all groups (alfalfa chaff group: 4.8 ± 1.9 %; alfalfa pellets group: 5.5 ± 2.5 %; hay group: 4.3 ± 2.3 %). There was no significant difference ($p = 0.49$) in weight gain between groups.

Before weaning ($T = 0$), the prevalence of gastric mucosa lesions (one or more lesions considering all locations in the stomach) was 84.3 %; at 14 days after weaning ($T = 16$), it was almost 100 %. Before and after weaning, most of the lesions were found at the greater curvature of the squamous mucosa and at the lesser curvature (Table 3, Figs. 1, 2, 3, 4 and 5).

Effect of weaning on gastric mucosa

Only very few foals had gastric mucosa lesions in the dorsal squamous fundus before and after weaning in the three diet groups. In the squamous region of the greater curvature, the median lesion score was 1 (0/1) before and 0 (0/2) after weaning in the hay group ($p = 0.78$), 0 (0/1) before and 0 (0/1) after weaning in the alfalfa chaff group ($p = 0.21$), and 1 (0/2) before and 2 (1/2) after weaning in the alfalfa pellets group ($p = 0.17$) (Fig. 1). In the squamous region of the lesser curvature, the median lesion score increased from 1 (0/2) before to 2 (1.75/2) after weaning in the hay group ($p = 0.03$), increased from 1 (0/2) before to 2 (1/3) after weaning in the alfalfa chaff group ($p = 0.02$), and was 2 (1/2) before and 2 (0/3) after weaning in the alfalfa pellets group ($p = 0.14$) (Fig. 2).

In the glandular region of the greater curvature, the median lesion score was 0 (0/1) before and 0 (0/1) after weaning in the hay group ($p = 1$), 0 (0/0) before and 0 (0/0) after weaning in the alfalfa chaff group ($p = 0.48$), and 0 (0/1) before and 0 (0/0) after weaning in the alfalfa pellets group ($p = 0.35$) (Fig. 3). In the antrum, the median lesion score was 0 (0/0) before and 0 (0/0) after weaning in the hay group ($p = 0.18$), 0 (0/0) before and 0 (0/1) after weaning in the alfalfa chaff group ($p = 0.01$), and 0 (0/0) before and 0 (0/1) after weaning in the alfalfa pellets group ($p = 0.03$) (Fig. 4). At the pylorus, the median lesion score was 0 (0/0) before and 0 (0/0) after weaning in the hay group ($p = 1$), 0 (0/0) before and 1 (0/2) after weaning in the alfalfa chaff group ($p < 0.001$), and 0 (0/0) before and 0 (0/0) after weaning in the alfalfa pellets group ($p = 0.56$) (Fig. 5).

Effect of diet on gastric mucosa

Before weaning ($T = 0$), the gastroscopic findings of each region did not differ significantly between the three diet groups (Table 3). After weaning ($T = 16$), gastric mucosal lesions at the pylorus were significantly more severe in the group fed alfalfa chaff ($p = 0.002$) (Fig. 5). In the other regions, no differences related to the feeding regimes were observed.

Discussion

Various methods have been used to induce gastric ulcers. In this study we used the weaning process as a

Table 1 Mean (± SD) daily dry matter and nutrient intake for each foal according to diet

Diet	DM	Ash	CP	CF	NDF	Starch	Ca	P	Mg
AC	9383 ± 120	461 ± 9	1190 ± 19.5	2978 ± 54	5265 ± 75	1410 ± 7	82 ± 1.6	27 ± 0.4	16 ± 0.2
AP	9798 ± 167	608 ± 21	1232 ± 31	2937 ± 54	5585 ± 79	1410 ± 9.5	86 ± 4	26 ± 0.4	16 ± 0.3
HA	10,800	457	1270	3286	6729	1404	89	29	20

Intake is expressed as grams

AC: diet including 3 kg alfalfa chaff, 4.3 kg grass hay, 2.7 kg oats, 240 g soybean meal, 70 g calcium oxide and 40 g of a commercial trace element mixture; AP: diet including 3 kg alfalfa pellets, 5.0 kg grass hay, 2.7 kg oats, and 40 g of a commercial trace element mixture; HA: diet including 8.3 kg grass hay, 3 kg oats, 0.5 kg soybean meal, 120 g $CaCO_3$ and 40 g of a commercial trace element mixture

Ca calcium, *DM* dry matter, *CF* crude fiber, *CP* crude protein, *HA* diet including hay, *Mg* magnesium, *NDF* neutral detergent fiber, *P* phosphorus

Table 2 Percentages of different particle sizes of alfalfa pellets and alfalfa chaff

Feedstuff	>2 mm	>1 mm	>0.5 mm	>0.25 mm	<0.25 mm
Alfalfa chaff	90.8 %	6.62 %	1.94 %	0.28 %	0.31 %
Alfalfa pellets	4.63 %	6.95 %	12.4 %	16.1 %	59.9 %

model to induce gastric ulcers in foals to determine the effects of feeding. Previous studies have shown that the weaning process is a stressful event in a foal's life and may increase gastric lesions. Dahlkamp and others [3] reported that ulcer scores of the squamous region, as examined by gastroscopy, increased from 48 % before weaning to 78 % 2 weeks after weaning. This study revealed an initial prevalence of gastric lesions in glandular and squamous regions of 84.3 % prior to weaning. The changes in feeding and housing management 1 week before weaning may have resulted in high gastric lesion scores. The introduction to new stables and housing groups was performed to ensure standardized experimental conditions.

The aim of the study was to evaluate the impact of feeding different particle sizes to weanlings. Gastric findings of each region of the stomach were scored separately because we assumed that diet regime might have various influences on the gastric mucosa of different regions.

One food source recommended to prevent gastric lesions in horses is alfalfa hay. Nadeau and others [7] found a lower incidence of gastric lesions in horses fed alfalfa hay. The reason for the beneficial effects of feeding alfalfa is related to its buffering components, like protein and calcium. High calcium intake reduced the basal HCl secretion in rats. This effect was suspected to be a result of higher extracellular and intracellular calcium concentrations in parietal and G cells. Higher extracellular and intracellular calcium concentrations may lower the cAMP concentration, thus reducing the production of HCl [13]. Exposure of the equine gastric mucosa to HCl and short-chain fatty acids significantly decreased sodium transport of the cells. The addition of calcium carbonate decreased the sodium transport to baseline [14]. From these results, the authors proposed that calcium has a protective effect in the development of gastric lesions. Nadeau and others [7] found significantly lower scores of the squamous mucosa in horses fed an alfalfa hay/grain diet compared to horses fed a brome hay diet. The authors concluded that high amounts of protein and the quality of the protein may have buffering effects in the stomach, as previously seen in cattle [15].

Table 3 Grading of the different stomach regions before weaning for the different feeding protocols

Diet	Squamous region			Glandular region		
	Dorsal fundus	Lesser curvature	Greater curvature	Greater curvature	Antrum	Pylorus
AC	0 (0/0)	1 (0/2)	0 (0/1)	0 (0/0)	0 (0/0)	0 (0/0)
AP	0 (0/0)	2 (1/2)	1 (0/2)	0 (0/1)	0 (0/0)	0 (0/0)
HA	0 (0/0)	1 (0/2)	1 (0/1)	0 (0/1)	0 (0/0)	0 (0/0)
p value	0.39	0.20	0.18	0.31	0.25	0.94

Data expressed as median (25th/75th percentiles)

Alfalfa is believed to have beneficial effects on gastric mucosa by buffering gastric pH because it contains large amounts of calcium, magnesium, and protein. In the present study, calcium and protein intake were approximately equal among the different feeding groups (Table 1), but particle size between the two alfalfa preparations was different. Former studies have demonstrated the impact of the particle size on the stomach mucosa in different species. Saliva production is related to the particle structure of a diet, and saliva has a buffering effect due to its potassium, chloride, and bicarbonate [16]. For example, feeding 1 kg of hay results in 3 to 6 L of saliva production and feeding 1 kg of grain results in 1 to 1.7 L of saliva production in adult horses [17]. The concentration of bicarbonate in saliva may impact stomach pH [18]. These effects may explain the lower gastric lesion scores in weanlings fed hay in our study. However, lesion scores of weanlings in the alfalfa pellets group were not significantly different from those in the hay group. It is possible that although the foals fed alfalfa pellets may have produced less saliva, the high-quality protein in the alfalfa may have resulted in ulcer scores similar to those in the hay group.

Foals fed alfalfa chaff had higher ulcer scores at the pylorus than those fed alfalfa pellets or hay. These results were surprising because alfalfa chaff has been suggested to be associated with higher saliva production due to the more intensive chewing involved; increased saliva flow is known to have a buffering effect on the stomach. The findings in the alfalfa chaff group were similar to those of Fedtke and others [2]. These authors noted that feeding alfalfa chaff resulted in significantly greater ulcer scores at the pylorus following weaning. They speculated that the pyloric ulcers might be related to the small particles of the alfalfa chaff, similar to results obtained in swine [2]. Mößeler and others [11] fed pigs four different diets with different grinding intensities and different physical forms (pellets vs meal) for 3 days. Animals were examined post-mortem. Samples of the frozen gastric contents were taken from 15 standardized locations of the stomach. Mößeler and others [11] demonstrated that a finely ground pellet diet resulted in more liquid gastric contents and that pH values were similar in all regions of the stomach (mean ± SD pH difference between the regions: 0.175 ± 0.140). In contrast, a coarsely ground diet resulted in stratification of the gastric chyme content, with a pH difference of 2.22 ± 1.04 (mean ± SD). In the squamous region, the gastric ulcers score was significantly higher in pigs fed a

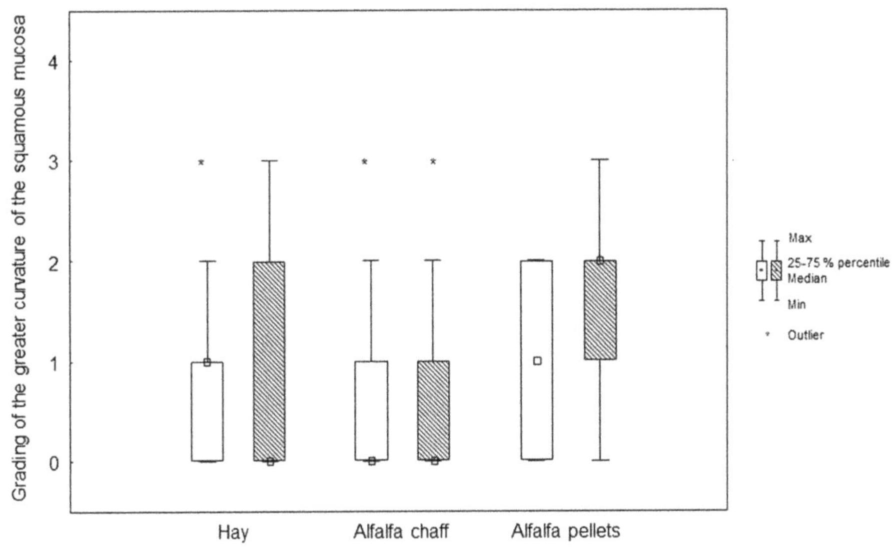

Fig. 1 Box (median) and whisker (25th/75th percentiles) plots of lesions grades for the greater curvature of the squamous mucosa before and after weaning for the different feeding protocols (white plots before weaning; striped plots after weaning)

finely ground pellet diet in comparison with pigs fed a coarsely ground diet without pellets [19]. All studies performed on pigs focused on the squamous region, which is the most common region for development of gastric ulceration in pigs [20]. Pigs fed a diet of finely ground pellets also showed greater histological evidence of inflammation compared to pigs fed other diets [21].

However, our results differed from those noted in pigs. Higher ulcer scores were observed after feeding alfalfa chaff compared to hay or alfalfa pellets. In our study alfalfa pellets with a particle size smaller than 1 mm did not induce pyloric lesions. This might be due to the fact that all foals in our study had free access to hay and straw bedding as sources of food. This factor may have masked the negative effects of fine particles in the diet. However, due to the large sample size number, we could not provide individual feeding, but due to the very close monitoring of the foals, we can ensure a similar feed intake within the groups and between the different diets.

It is possible that the harsh acanthous structure of alfalfa chaff may cause mechanical injury at the pylorus. The pyloric region is an area of the stomach with high motility. We assume that the movement of the alfalfa stems may excoriate the mucosa during passage. This

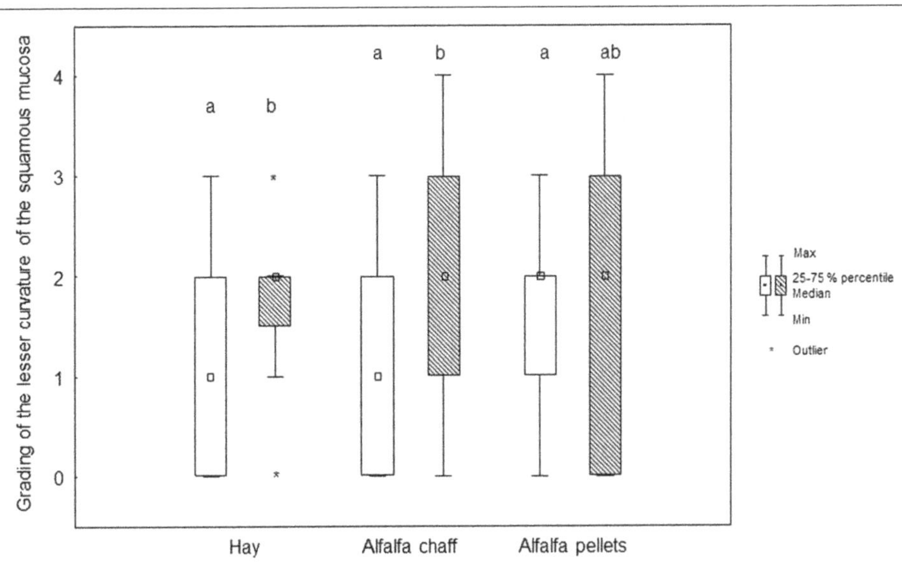

Fig. 2 Box (median) and whisker (25th/75th percentiles) plots of lesions grades for the lesser curvature of the squamous mucosa before and after weaning for the different feeding protocols (white plots before weaning; striped plots after weaning). Unlike letters are different with $p < 0.05$

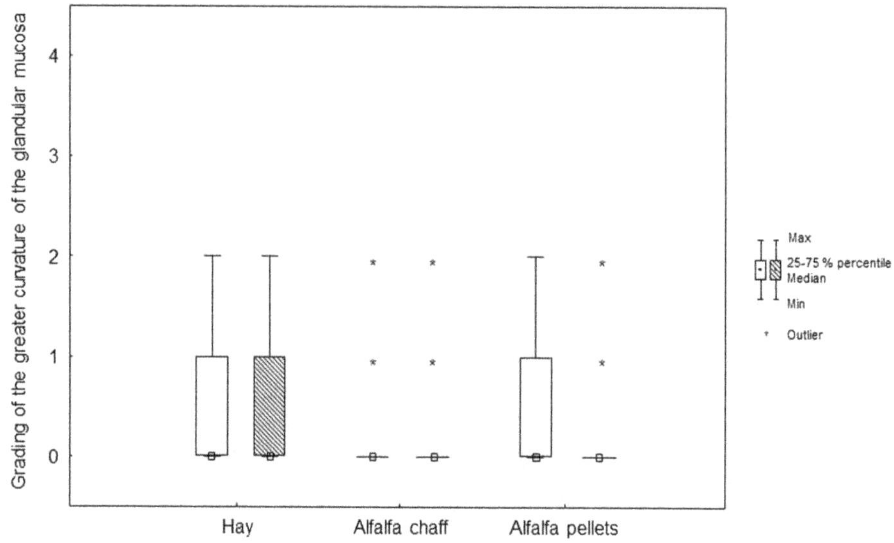

Fig. 3 Box (median) and whisker (25th/75th percentiles) plots of lesions grades for the greater curvature of the glandular mucosa before and after weaning for the different feeding protocols (white plots before weaning; striped plots after weaning)

initial injury of the glandular mucosa might leave the pylorus more vulnerable to the insults of short-chain fatty acids, hydrochloric acid, and/or bile salts. Pyloric lesions are of particular clinical concern because damage to the pylorus may result in pyloric stenosis with delayed gastric emptying [22]. However, further studies are required to determine whether feeding the whole alfalfa plant may result in similar findings.

Conclusions

Foals fed alfalfa chaff had higher lesion scores at the pylorus. These findings stress the importance of scoring all gastric regions separately. Furthermore, in the past, particle size has been neglected in equine nutrition; however, our data seem to show this might be an issue in the occurrence of pyloric lesions. It remains unclear whether the mucosa injuries can be observed only in weanlings during the stressful weaning process as a result of impaired mucosal defence or whether the damage can also be induced in adult horses. Nevertheless, alfalfa leaves contain a superior protein source and high amounts of calcium and magnesium [23], providing extra nutritional advantages in growing horses. At this time, either traditional grass hay rations or grass hay with alfalfa pellets can be recommended.

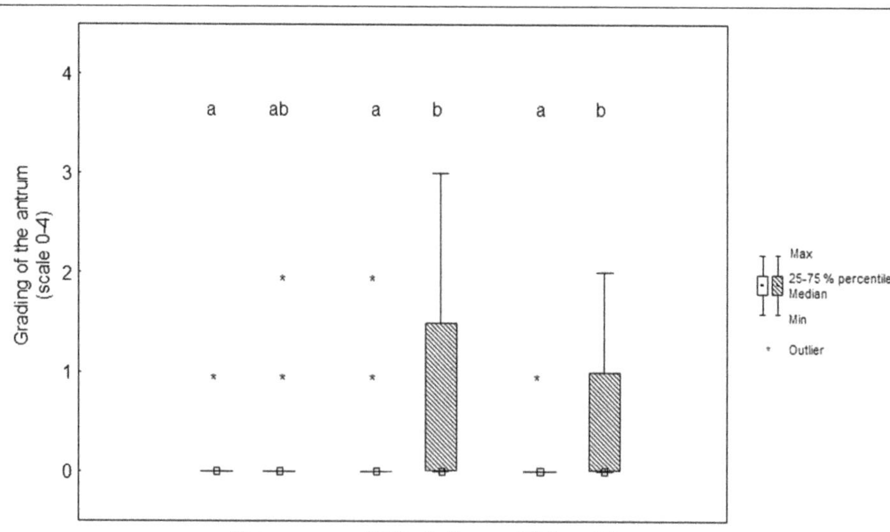

Fig. 4 Box (median) and whisker (25th/75th percentiles) plots of lesions grades for the antrum before and after weaning for the different feeding protocols (white plots before weaning; striped plots after weaning). Unlike letters are different with $p < 0.05$

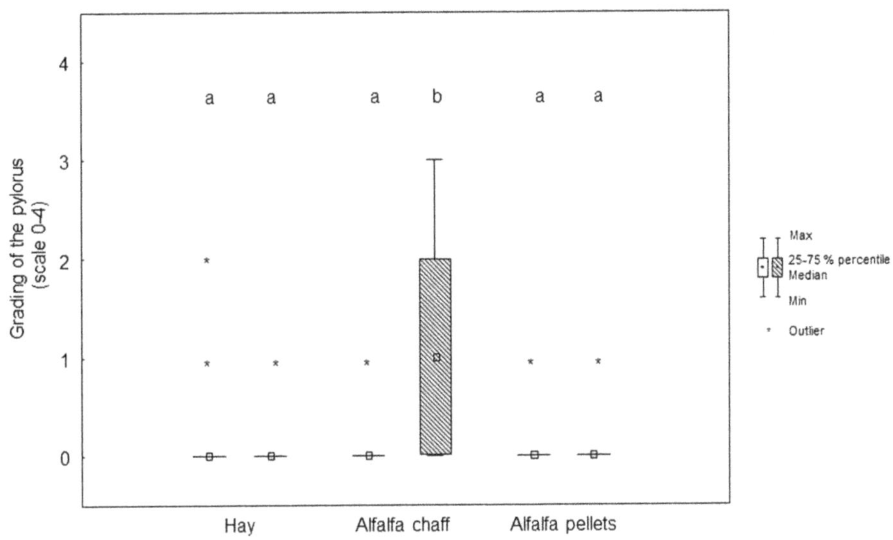

Fig. 5 Box (median) and whisker (25th/75th percentiles) plots of lesions grades for the pylorus before and after weaning for the different feeding protocols (white plots before weaning; striped plots after weaning). Unlike letters are different with $p < 0.05$

Methods

Animals

Seventy warmblood foals (39 males, 31 females), 164 to 234 days of age, with a mean body weight (± SD) of 256 ± 24 kg were included in the study. All foals were born and raised at a stud farm in Germany. Inclusion criteria for the foals were minimum age of 150 days, no findings at clinical examination and physiological white blood cell count, and no medication 10 days prior to initiation of the study. At T = -7, the foals and mares were moved into covered barns with straw bedding and free access to concrete runs. Mares and foals were fed a total mixed ration (TMR) once per day (approximately 13 kg per mare and foal per day) to meet or exceed the energy and nutrient requirements of the mares. The TMR comprised 3 kg corn silage, 6 kg grass silage, 2 kg oats, 0.5 kg straw, 0.3 kg soybean meal, 0.05 kg of a commercial mineral vitamin supplement (Vilomix Biolex; Deutsche Vilomix Tierernährung GmbH, Neuenkirchen-Vörden, Germany), and 0.04 kg $CaCO_3$. Horses had access to grass hay and water ad libitum.

Foals were weaned at $T = 0$ and grouped with respect to their dietary treatment. All groups were housed as described. Sample size calculation was performed with PASS 2002 (NCSS, Statistical Software). The required sample size was 15 foals. To ensure a proper sample size at the end of study, and taking into account that some foals might have to be excluded during the study period due to reasons not related to the study design, we increased the groups to up to 25 foals. During the study we had to exclude five foals because of orthopedic injuries. Foals were allocated to each group according to the homogenous distribution of gastric findings at the first gastroscopy.

During the study period the foals were monitored three times daily by a veterinarian for signs of discomfort, depression, inappetence, bruxism, or colic.

Feeding

Before weaning, foals were introduced to their respective diets from $T = -3$ to $T = 0$ (day of weaning) without being separated from their dam.

After weaning, the foals were separated from their dam and allocated to the three diets. In the alfalfa chaff group ($n = 25$), foals were fed daily with 3 kg alfalfa chaff per foal and had free access to grass hay. Additionally, foals were offered 2.7 kg oats, 240 g soybean meal, 70 g calcium oxide and 40 g of a commercial trace element mixture (see above) mixed with the alfalfa chaff. To ensure uniform consumption, alfalfa chaff was mixed with 400 ml of water for each foal to bind alfalfa chaff to the other feed components.

In the alfalfa pellets group ($n = 21$), each foal was fed daily with 3 kg alfalfa pellets composed of finely ground alfalfa leaves. Additionally, each foal was fed daily with 2.7 kg oats and 40 g of a commercial trace element mixture (see above) and had free access to grass hay. The alfalfa pellets were mixed with oats and the commercial trace element mixture.

The hay group ($n = 24$) had free access to grass hay and received 3 kg oats, 0.5 kg soybean meal, 120 g $CaCO_3$ and 40 g of a commercial trace element mixture (see above).

Each diet was standardized to supply a similar nutrient intake per day in each feeding group. The feed was offered in two equal portions twice daily (7:00 AM and 3:30 PM) in a continuous trough providing enough room for each foal. Feed intake was monitored several times daily and remaining feed was weighed after 24 h. In total, the different diets were fed for 16 days after the weaning process. The nutrient intake is summarized in Table 1.

Gastroscopy

A gastroscopy with a flexible gastroscope (Karl Storz, Tuttlingen, Germany) with a working length of 3 m was performed immediately prior to weaning ($T = 0$) and again after the feeding period of 16 days ($T = 16$). Prior to gastroscopy, foals were fasted by using muzzles for 9 to 12 h, but they had water ad libitum. The foals were sedated with 0.02 mg/kg body weight intravenous detomidinhydrochloride (Cepesedan®; CP Pharma, Burgdorf, Germany). The stomach was insufflated with air until the mucosal folds vanished. The following regions of the stomach were evaluated separately: dorsal squamous fundus; lesser curvature; greater curvature of the squamous region; greater curvature of the glandular region; antrum; and pylorus. Each region and mucosal type was given a score from 0 to 4. Squamous mucosa was scored according to a proposal of the European College of Equine Internal Medicine [24] (Table 4). Glandular gastric mucosa including the antrum and pylorus was evaluated according to a modified scoring system (Table 5). Gastric mucosa was evaluated during gastroscopy by the same blinded and experienced investigator (MV).

Scaling

Body weight was measured by an electronic weight scale (Müller, Jagstzell, Germany) immediately before each gastroscopy. Feedstuffs were weighed using an automatic scale (Beurer, Ulm, Germany and Waagen-Schmitt GmbH, Hamburg, Germany).

Nutrient analysis

Dry matter (DM) was determined after oven-drying (103 °C) to a constant mass (Table 6). Crude ash was measured by ashing the feeds in a muffle furnace (6 h, 600 °C) [25]. Starch content was estimated polarimetrically (Polartronic E; Schmidt and Haensch, Berlin, Germany).

Table 4 Scoring system of the squamous regions of the equine stomach. Adapted from the proposal of the European College of Equine Internal Medicine [24]

Grade	Characteristics
0	Epithelium intact and no appearance of hyperkeratosis
1	Mucosa intact, but areas of hyperkeratosis
2	Small, single or multifocal lesions
3	Large single or extensive superficial lesions
4	Extensive lesions with areas of apparent deep ulceration

Table 5 Scoring system of the glandular regions including the antrum and pylorus of the equine stomach

Grade	Characteristics
0	Epithelium intact and no appearance of hyperemia (reddening) or fibrinosupperative areas
1	Intact flat mucosa, but with small single or multifocal areas of reddening
2	Raised mucosa with large single or multifocal areas of reddening or fibrinosupperative areas, no signs of bleeding
3	Raised mucosa with hemorrhagic and fibrinosupperative areas
4	Ridged or depressed mucosa with severe signs of bleeding or with large and distinct fibrinosupperative areas

Sugar contents (glucose and sucrose) were determined by the Luff Schoorl method. Crude nutrients were assayed by the Weende system [25]. Neutral detergent fiber was analyzed by the Fibertec® (Tectator, Rellingen, Germany) [26].

Sieving

To determine particle sizes, 50 g of alfalfa pellets were soaked with 1 L water for 24 h prior to sieving. Samples were sieved for 5 min with an extrusion of 1.5 mm and running water. Samples were dried (60 °C) before weighing. Fifty grams of dry alfalfa chaff were sieved for 5 min with an extrusion of 1 mm. Sizes of the sieves were 2 mm, 1 mm, 0.5 mm, and 0.25 mm.

Statistical analysis

Statistical analysis was performed using a statistical software program (STATISTIKA, StatSoft). Body weight was analyzed for normal distribution by the Shapiro-Wilk W test. Stomach scores were calculated using medians, 25th and 75th percentiles, and ranges. The Wilcoxon signed rank test was used to compare gastroscopic scores within a group before and after weaning. Kruskal-Wallis ANOVA was performed to compare the gastroscopic scores between the treatment groups. A value of $p < 0.05$ was considered significant.

Table 6 Chemical composition of feed

		Alfalfa chaff	Alfalfa pellets	Hay	Oats
Ash	g/kg DM	71	117	45	26
CP	g/kg DM	150	172	95	123
CF	g/kg DM	412	302	372	132
NDF	g/kg DM	578	441	732	355
Ca	g/kg DM	12.3	20.9	5.2	1.2
P	g/kg DM	2.74	2.3	1.8	4.6
Mg	g/kg DM	1.65	1.8	1.7	1.7

Ca calcium, CF crude fiber, *CP* crude protein, *DM* dry matter, *NFE* nitrogen-free extractives, *Mg* magnesium, *P* phosphorus

Abbreviations

DM, dry matter; Fig, figure; HCl, hydrochloric cid; L, liter; SD, standard deviation; T, time point; TMR, total mixed ration

Acknowledgments

The authors acknowledge support from German Research Foundation (DFG) and University of Leipzig within the program of Open Access Publishing.

Funding

Not applicable.

Authors' contributions

SV carried out the feeding of the foals and participated in the gastroscopies, and helped to draft the manuscript. MV carried out the gastroscopies, and participated in its design and drafted the manuscript. IV designed the study and performed the statistical analysis and drafted the manuscript. All authors read and approved the final manuscript.

Competing interests

The authors declare that they have no competing interests.

Consent for publication

Not applicable.

Author details

[1]Institute of Animal Nutrition, Nutrition Diseases and Dietetics, Faculty of Veterinary Medicine, University of Leipzig, D-04103 Leipzig, Germany. [2]Equine Veterinary Clinic, D-38162 Destedt, Germany.

References

1. Vatistas NJ, Snyder JR, Carlson G, Johnson B, Arthu RM, Thurmond M, Zhou H, Lloyd KLK. Cross-sectional study of gastric ulcers of the squamous mucosa in thoroughbred racehorses. Equine Vet J. 1999;31:34–9.
2. Fedtke A, Pfaff M, Volquardsen J, Venner M, Vervuert I. Effects of alfalfa chaff on gastric mucosa in weanling foals. Pferdeheilkunde. 2015;6:596–602.
3. Dahlkamp M, Feige K, Venner M. Incidence of gastric ulcers in weanling foals and the treatment with omeprazole. Pferdeheilkunde. 2012;28:561–9.
4. Andrews F, Bernard W, Byars D, Cohen N, Divers T, MacAllister C, McGladdery A, Merritt A, Murray M, Orisini J, Snyder J, Vatistas N. Recommendations for the diagnosis and treatment of equine gastric ulcer syndrome (EGUS). Equine Vet Educ. 1999;11:262–72.
5. Monreal L, Sabaté D, Segura D, Mayós I, Homedes J. Lower gastric ulcerogenic effect of suxibuzone compared to phenylbutazone when administered orally to horses. Res Vet Sci. 2004;26:145–9.
6. Meschter CL, Gilbert M, Krook L, Maylin G, Corradino R. The effects of phenylbutazone on the morphology and prostaglandin concentrations of the pyloric mucosa of the equine stomach. Vet Pathol. 1990;27:244–53.
7. Nadeau JA, Andrews FM, Mathew AG, Argenzio RA, Blackford JT, Sohtell M, Saxton AM. Evaluation of diet as a cause of gastric ulcers in horses. Am J Vet Res. 2000;61:784–90.
8. Luthersson N, Nielsen KH, Harris P, Parkin TD. Risk factors associated with equine gastric ulceration syndrome (EGUS) in 201 horses in Denmark. Equine Vet J. 2009;41:625–30.
9. Coenen M, Kienzle E, Vervuert I, Zeyner A. Recent German developments in the formulation of energy and nutrient requirements in horses and the resulting feeding recommendations. J Equine Vet Sci. 2011;31:219–29.
10. Lybbert TC. Gastric ulcer syndrome in exercising horses fed different types of hay [master thesis]. Texas: A&M University; 2007.
11. Mößeler A, Köttendorf S, Große Liesner V, Kamphues J. Impact of diets' physical form (particle size; meal/pelleted) on the milieu within the stomach content (dry matter content, pH, chloride concentration) of pigs. Livest Sci. 2010;134:146–8.
12. Millet S, Kumar S, De Boever J, Meyns T, Aluwé M, De Brabander D, Ducatelle R. Effect of particle size distribution and dietary crude fibre content on growth performance and gastric mucosa integrity of growing-finishing pigs. Vet J. 2012;192:316–21.
13. Fisher H, Kaufman RH, Hsu HC, Kasziba E, Farmanfarmaian A, Flancbaum LJ. Inhibition of gastric acid secretion in the rat by high calcium. Nutr Res. 1990;10:1441–53.
14. Andrews FM, Buchanan BR, Smith SH, Elliott SB, Saxton AM. In vitro effects of hydrochloric acid and various concentrations of acetic, propionic, butyric, or valeric acids on bioelectric properties of equine gastric squamous mucosa. Am J Vet Res. 2006;67:1873–82.
15. Haaland G, Tyrrell H, Moe P, Wheeler W. Effect of crude protein level and limestone buffer in diets fed at two levels of intake on rumen pH, ammonia-nitrogen, buffering capacity and volatile fatty acid concentration in cattle. J Anim Sci. 1982;55:943–50.
16. Breves G. Nahrungsaufnahme und Speichelsekretion. In: von Engelhardt W, Breves G, Hrsg, editors. Physiologie der Haustiere. 3.Aufl. Stuttgart: Verlag Enke; 2005. p. 332-8
17. Meyer H, Coenen M, Probst D. Futtereinspeichelung und -passage im Kopfdarm des Pferdes. Beiträge zur Verdauungsphysiologie des Pferdes. Japan. 1986;56:171–83.
18. Eckersall PD, Aitchison T, Colquhoun KM. Equine whole saliva: variability of some major constituents. Equine Vet J. 1985;17:391–3.
19. Mößeler A, Wintermann M, Sander SJ, Kamphues J. Effect of grinding and pelleting fed either dry or liquid feed on dry matter and pH in the stomach of pigs and the development of gastric ulcers. J Anim Sci. 2012;90:343–5.
20. Große Liesner V. Investigations on the effects of diet's physical form (particle size, meal vs. pellets) and addition of lignocellulose on the integrity of gastric mucosa in reared piglets [PhD Dissertation med. vet.]. Hannover: Tierärztliche Hochschule Hannover; 2008. http://elib.tihohannover.de/dissertations/grosseliesnerv_ss08.pdf. Accessed 27 May 2008.
21. Ganter M. Magenulzera beim Schwein aus klinischer Sicht. Deutsche Tierärztl Wochenschr. 1999;106:75.
22. Andrews FM, Nadeau JA. Clinical syndroms of gastric ulceration in foals and mature horses. Equine Vet J Suppl. 1999;29:30–3.
23. Cuddeford D. Artificially dehydrated lucerne for horses. Vet Rec. 1994;29:426–9.
24. Sykes BW, Hewetson M, Hepburn RJ, Luthersson N, Tamzali Y. European college of equine internal medicine-consensus statement: equine gastric ulcer syndrome (EGUS) in adult horses. J Vet Intern Med. 2015;29:1288–99.
25. Naumann C, Bassler R. Methoden der landwirtschaftlichen forschungs- und untersuchungsanstalt biochemische untersuchung von futtermitteln. Methodenbuch III (mit ergänzungslieferungen bis 2004). Darmstadt: Verlag VDLUFA; 1976.
26. Van Soest PJ, Roberston JB, Lewis BA. Methods for dietary fiber, neutral detergent fiber, and nonstarch polysaccharides in relation to animal nutrition. J Dairy Sci. 1991;74:3583–97.

15

Procalcitonin as a biomarker in equine chronic pneumopathies

Ann Kristin Barton[1*], Anna Pelli[1], Martin Rieger[2] and Heidrun Gehlen[1]

Abstract

Background: Procalcitonin (PCT), a precursor protein of the hormone calcitonin, is a sensitive inflammatory marker in human medicine, which is primarily used for diagnosis of bacterial sepsis, but is also useful in diagnosis of exacerbation of asthma and COPD. In this study, PCT was evaluated as a potential biomarker for different chronic pneumopathies in the horse using an equine specific ELISA in comparison to established clinical markers and different interleukins.

Sixty-four horses were classified as free of respiratory disease, recurrent airway obstruction (RAO), inflammatory airway disease (IAD) or chronic interstitial pneumopathy (CIP) using a scoring system. PCT concentrations were measured in plasma ($n = 17$) and in the cell-free supernatant of bronchoalveolar lavage ($n = 64$). PCT concentrations were correlated to interleukins IL-1ß and IL-6 in BALF, clinical findings and BALF cytology.

Results: The median PCT concentrations in plasma were increased in respiratory disease (174.46 ng/ml, $n = 7$) compared to controls (13.94 ng/ml, $n = 10$, $P = 0.05$) and correlated to PCT in BALF supernatant (rs = 0.48). Compared to controls (5.49 ng/ml, $n = 15$), median PCT concentrations in BALF supernatant correlated to the overall clinical score (rs = 0.32, $P = 0.007$) and were significantly increased in RAO (13.40 ng/ml, $n = 21$) and IAD (16.89 ng/ml, $n = 16$), while no differences were found for CIP (12.02 ng/ml, $n = 12$). No significant increases were found for IL-1 and IL-6 between controls and respiratory disease in general as well as different disease groups.

Conclusions: Although some correlations were found between PCT in plasma, BALF supernatant and clinical scores, PCT in BALF does not seem to be a superior marker compared to established clinical markers. PCT in plasma seems to be more promising and a greater number of samples should be evaluated in further studies.

Keywords: Horse, Recurrent airway obstruction, Inflammatory airway disease, Chronic interstitial pneumopathy, Procalcitonin, Biomarker

Background

Since the 1970s, hypocalcemia and its correlation to sepsis have been in the focus of research [1]. Procalcitonin (PCT) is a precursor protein of the hormone calcitonin, which regulates the calcium homeostasis by inhibition of osteoclastic activity. In health, preprocalcitonin (prePCT) is exclusively produced in the thyroid c-cells. Low concentrations of <0.1 ng/ml are found in human serum [2].

During sepsis, PCT is found in high concentrations in blood and almost all tissues [3], but PCT is not only a precursor of calcitonin leading to hypocalcemia. It seems to have another pathophysiologic role as an inflammatory mediator and is found in almost all inflammatory processes independent from hypocalcemia. Its synthesis can be triggered by TNF-α and several interleukins [4, 5]. Despite lower PCT concentrations in plasma compared to endotoxemia and sepsis, differentiation between different forms of pneumonia is possible [6–8] and chronic respiratory diseases like asthma or COPD (chronic obstructive pulmonary disease) are also characterized by increases in PCT concentrations. As acute exacerbation of asthma is often caused by bacterial infections of the lower airways, PCT can be used for the decision pro or contra the initiation and duration of antibiotic therapy [9] and can help in the interpretation of indifferent thoracic radiographs [10]. Similar results have been found for COPD, where PCT measurement can support the decision for individual

* Correspondence: Ann-Kristin.Barton@fu-berlin.de
[1]Equine Clinic, Freie Universitaet Berlin, Oertzenweg 19b, 10163 Berlin, Germany
Full list of author information is available at the end of the article

therapy involving antibiotics or glucocorticoids and is considered to be helpful in long-term management [11, 12].

Equine RAO (recurrent airway obstruction) is known for parallels to human asthma (respiratory hypersensitivity, good response to bronchodilators and glucocorticoids) as well as COPD (airway neutrophilia, epithelial metaplasia and hypersecretion into the lower airways), resembling what is called "wheezy bronchitis" in men [13]. During disease exacerbation, increased inflammatory markers may be found in plasma as described for haptoglobin and serumamyloid A [14], but local neutrophila in bronchoalveolar lavage fluid (BALF) is considered the most reliable feature [15]. Inflammatory airway disease (IAD), a possible precursor of RAO [16], shows a lower grade of inflammation including airway neutrophilia and/or increases in mast cell and eosinophil counts [17], while interstitial pneumopathies are characterized by increases in macrophage percentages in BALF cytology [18, 19]. As systemic markers were only increased in RAO exacerbation, measurement of biomarkers may be more rewarding out of BALF in chronic respiratory disease. High disease prevalence and economic impact have been described for equine chronic respiratory disease, therefore new biomarkers may help to differentiate these pneumopathies and to identify cases of subclinical disease. A species specific ELISA for equine PCT (ePCT) was established [20], which allows quantitative measurements instead of gene expression with a high specificity and sensitivity. High ePCT concentrations were found in plasma of endotoxemic horses suffering from colic [21, 22].

In this study, we aimed to compare ePCT concentrations in BALF with clinicals findings, BALF cytology and other biomarkers, namely interleukins 1ß and 6, which have been shown to stimulate hyperprocalcitonemia in other species [4, 23]. Additionally, ePCT concentrations were measured in plasma. We hypothesized that ePCT correlates with clinical scores, BALF cytology and interleukins in RAO, IAD and CIP and may be a superior marker in cases of low-grade inflammation.

Methods

Preparticipation examination

A total of 71 horses were examined, of which 15 had no clinical signs or history of respiratory disease and 56 were presented to the clinic with a history of chronic lower airway disease.

The pre-participation examination included anamnesis documentation, clinical examination, exercise test, blood gas analysis, bronchoscopy, BALF cytology and thoracic radiography. Using a modified clinical score system [24, 25], endoscopy score results, parameters of gas exchange, BALF cytology and thoracic radiography results, horses were classified as free of respiratory disease (controls, group I), Recurrent airway obstruction in exacerbation (RAO, group II), Inflammatory airway disease (IAD, group III), chronic interstitial pneumopathy (CIP, group IV) or were excluded from the study, if they could not be assigned to these groups ($n = 7$). In detail, groups were defined as follows:

- Group I: No history of respiratory disease, clinical score < 2, no tracheal secretions, low cellular density and neutrophils ≤ 8% in BALF, $AaDO_2 \leq 8$ mmHg, exclusion of acute signs of infection (leukocytosis, fever, depression).
- Group II: History of recurrent cough or dyspnea, clinical score > 6, high amount or viscosity of tracheal secretions, high cellular density and neutrophils ≥ 25% in BALF, $AaDO_2 > 8$ mmHg, exclusion of acute signs of infection (leukocytosis, fever, depression) according to *Robinson* [15].
- Group III: History of cough or exercise insufficiency, clinical score 2–6, low to moderate amount or viscosity of tracheal secretions, increased cellular density and neutrophils ≥ 8% or mast cells ≥ 2% or eosinophils ≥ 0.1% in BALF, exclusion of acute signs of infection (leukocytosis, fever, depression) according to *Couëtil* et al. [17].
- Group IV: History of exercise insufficiency, clinical score 2–6, low to moderate amount or viscosity of tracheal secretions, increased cellular density and ratio of macrophages:neutrophils ≥ 2.5:1 in BALF, increased interstitial opacity of thoracic radiographs, exclusion of acute signs of infection (leukocytosis, fever, depression) according to *Dieckmann* et al. [18].

BALF collection and processing

During endoscopy, 20 ml of 2% lidocaine (Bela-Pharm GmbH, Vechta, Germany) were infused around the tracheal bifurcation. The catheter (Silicone Bronchoalveolar Lavage Catheter 300 cm, Smiths Medical ASD, Inc, USA) was wedged into the bronchus by mean of an air balloon. Five hundred milliliters of pre-warmed phosphate buffered saline (Phosphate buffered saline, Lonza, Verviers, Belgium) were infused as recommended by the International Workshop on Equine Chronic Airway disease [15] and immediately aspirated.

BALF was divided into 2 portions for cytological and biochemical examination. After centrifugation at 1500 rpm for 10 min at 4 °C the cell-free supernatant was stored at −80 °C until assayed. Cytology was performed using Wright-Giemsa staining and counting 500 cells at 500× magnification.

ELISA for quantification of ePCT in plasma and BALF

As the ELISA for equine PCT was only validated for plasma, it was adapted to BALF according to the guidelines of the American Food and Drug Administration for Validation of bioanalytic methods (2013) by partial validation which was done here by reanalyzing intra-assay (IaA) and inter-assay (IeA) coefficients of variation (CV) and recovery in BALF matrix (Table 1).

Measurements of PCT in plasma

In 17 horses (10 controls, 7 horses with respiratory disease), PCT was measured in plasma using a specific ELISA for equine PCT [20]. As this was not part of the original study, we did not have plasma samples available from all horses.

Measurements of PCT in BALF

In 64 horses, PCT was measured in undiluted BALF supernatant samples using a specific ELISA for equine PCT [20] after adaption to this substrate.

Measurements of interleukins

In 64 horses, interleukins was measured in undiluted BALF samples using commercially available specific ELISAs for equine IL-1ß and 6 (ELISA Kit for Interleukin 1 Beta (IL1b) and ELISA Kit for Interleukin 6 (IL6), Uscn Life Science Inc, USA) according to the manufacturer's manual.

Statistical analysis

Data were statistically analyzed using SPSS (SPSS Statistics, Version 17.0 released 2008, SPSS Inc., USA) and expressed as median (min-max). The data were tested for normal distribution using the Kolmogoronov-Smirnov and Shapiro Wilks Test. The level of significance was set at P 0.05.

Kruskal Wallis H test was used to compare between controls and different disease groups followed by Post-Hoc testing using Mann-Whitney U Test for 2-group comparison to determine intergroup differences.

Spearman rank correlation coefficients were calculated between clinical parameters, cytologic data, PCT and interleukin concentrations. Correlations were classified as irrelevant (rs = 0–0.25), weak (rs = 0.25–0.5), moderate (rs = 0.5–0.75) and strong (rs > 0.75).

Results

Clinical scoring

According to the results of clinical scoring and BALF cytology, the 71 horses (42 geldings, 29 mares, age 12.5 ± 5.31 years, BDW 470.8 ± 91.3 kg) presented for participation in this study were classified as follows: 15 horses were classified as free of respiratory disease (group I, controls), 21 as RAO (group II), 16 as IAD (group III), 12 as chronic interstitial pneumopathy (group IV), 4 horses suffered from acute respiratory infections and 3 could not be clearly assigned to groups I-IV. Therefore, the later 7 were excluded, leaving 64 horses for statistical analysis.

Hematology and ionized calcium

In all 64 horses, controls and horses affected by respiratory disease, hematology was unremarkable. Leucocytes ($8.1 \pm 2.2 * 10^3/\mu l$), hematocrit (35 ± 5.1%), total protein (6.7 ± 0.5 g/dl) and ionized calcium (1.64 ± 0.10 mmol/l) were within normal limits. There was no difference between in ionized calcium between controls (1.58 ± 0.11 mmol/l) and horses affected by respiratory disease in groups II-IV (1.65 ± 0.09 mmol/l).

Measurements of PCT in plasma

In 17 horses (10 controls, 7 affected by respiratory disease), PCT was measured in plasma using a specific ELISA for equine PCT [20]. Overall PCT concentrations in respiratory disease (174.46 ng/ml, $n = 7$) were higher than in group I (controls, 13.94 ng/ml, $n = 10$). The median concentrations in group II (RAO) was even 482.23 ng/ml ($n = 4$).

Adaption of PCT ELISA to BALF

According to the guidelines of the *American Food and Drug Administration for Validation of Bioanalytic Methods*

Table 1 Concentrations spiked ($Conc_{spik}$) and found ($Conc_{found}$), intra-assay (IaA) and inter-assay (IeA) coefficients of variation (CV) and recovery-values for equine PCT ELISA in BALF

Sample	$Conc_{spik}$[ng/ml]	$Conc_{found}$[ng/ml]	IaA-CV (%)	IeA-CV (%)	Recovery (%)
1	10	15.6 ± 4.7	30.4	10.9	156
2	**25**	24.9 ± 0.7	**2.7**	**8.4**	**99.2**
3	**50**	43.2 ± 2	**4.7**	**3.1**	**86.2**
4	**100**	102.6 ± 13.9	**13.6**	**11.4**	**102.5**
5	**250**	377 ± 22.3	**5.9**	**7**	**150.8**
6	500	658.5 ± 248	37.7	16.1	131.6
7	1.000	*	*	*	*
8	5.000	*	*	*	*
9	10.000	*	*	*	*

The working range is marked in bold

Table 2 Median values of PCT and interleukin concentrations in BALF supernatant over different disease groups, significance ($P < 0.05$) is indicated by*

Diagnosis	PCT [ng/ml]	IL-1β [pg/ml]	IL-6[pg/ml]
Controls ($n = 15$)	5.49 (1.49–23.32)	5.7 (5.7–104)	2.5 (2.5–25)
RAO ($n = 21$)	13.40* (1.32–681.66)	25 (5.7–122)	11 (2.5–53)
IAD ($n = 16$)	16.89* (1.49–493.72)	22 (5.7–84)	3.5 (2.5–41)
CIP ($n = 12$)	12.02 (3.82–1761.86)	33.5 (5.7–121)	10.5 (2.5–63)

(2013) the variation coefficients in medical ELISAs need to be below 15%, therefore the working range for equine BALF was defined as 25–250 ng/ml, as shown in Table 1.

Measurements of PCT in BALF

In 64 horses, PCT was measured in undiluted BALF supernatant using a specific ELISA for equine PCT [20] after adaption to this substrate. The median concentration in group I (controls, 5.49 ng/ml) as well as in groups II-IV was below the defined working range of the ELISA (25–250 ng/ml). PCT was significantly increased in groups II (RAO, median13.40 ng/ml) and III (IAD, median 16.89 ng/ml), while no differences were found for group IV (CIP, median 12.02 ng/ml), Table 2 and Fig. 1. Significant inter-group differences were found between groups I (controls) and II (RAO, $P = 0.033$) as well as groups I and III (IAD, $P = 0.006$).

Correlation of PCT to clinical parameters

A weak correlation was found between PCT concentrations in plasma and BALF supernatant (rs = 0.48, $P =$ 0.060). The highest correlation was found between PCT in plasma and the respiratory rate (rs = 0.53, $P = 0.025$). Negative correlations were found between PCT in plasma and the arterial PaO_2 (rs = −0.60, $P = 0.009$). A weak correlation was found between PCT concentration in BALF and airway obstruction (rs = 0.42, $P = 0.010$) as well as overall clinical score (rs = 0.32, $P = 0.007$). Neither PCT in plasma nor in BALF supernatant correlated to the percentage of neutrophils in BALF cytology, but PCT in plasma with the eosinophils (rs = −0.49, $P = 0.039$).

Measurements of interleukins in BALF

In 64 horses, interleukin concentrations were measured in undiluted BALF samples using a specific ELISA for equine IL-1ß and IL-6. No significant increases were found for IL-1ß or IL-6 between group I (controls) and groups II-IV in general ($P = 0.122$) or between controls and single disease groups ($P = 0.365$). Results are shown in detail in Table 2.

Discussion

In the late 1990s, it has been shown that procalcitonin is a sensitive marker for systemic inflammatory processes caused by bacterial infection, but not of other pathogenesis [26–28]. While exacerbations of asthma and COPD in men are often triggered by viral and bacterial infection of the lower airways [29, 30],

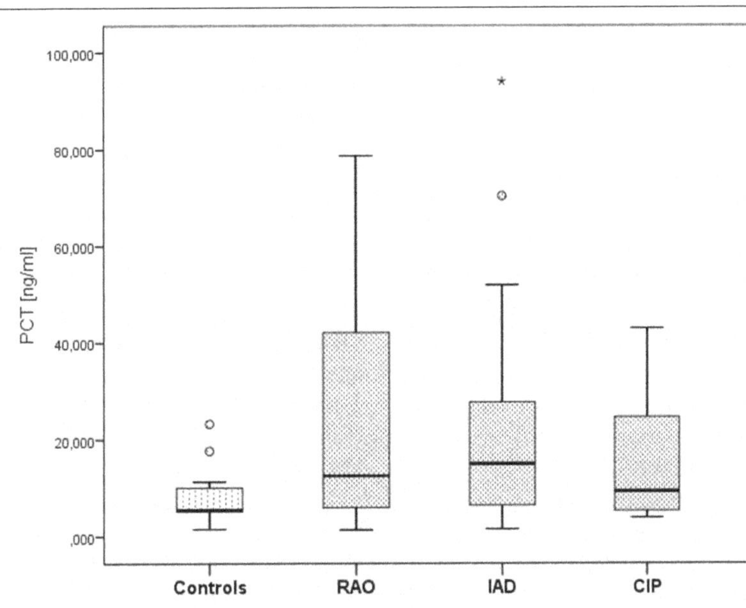

Fig. 1 PCT concentrations (0–250 ng/ml) in BALF over different disease groups ($n = 59$). Five samples had PCT values > 250 ng/ml and were excluded from this graph, but not from statistical analysis. ° shows outliers 1.5–3 times out of the interquartile range, * shows extreme outliers > 3 times out of the interquartile range

this is not a common feature in RAO [31]. In IAD, however, microbiologic examinations of tracheal aspirates are often positive despite no evidence of systemic infection [32]. Interstitial pneumonia may also be the consequence of bacterial infection, but in the phase of chronic interstitial disease it is usually impossible to find evidence of bacterial disease [19].

Equine PCT was characterized in the early 2000s [33]. Hypocalcemia in case of acute systemic disease was also found in horse [34]. Low plasma levels of ionized calcium were found in severe colic, gastrointestinal inflammation and induced endotoxemia [35, 36]. Studies in horses suffering from acute or chronic respiratory disease have not been published so far. In our study, concentrations of ionized calcium were within normal limits, both in healthy controls and in horses affected by chronic pneumopathies. Of course, chronic respiratory disease is not commonly associated with endotoxemia, but ePCT may have a pro-inflammatory function independent from its role in calcium metabolism, possibly playing a role in chronic respiratory disease. It was shown in other species that anti-PCT antibodies increase the chance of survival after induced endotoxemia [37–39].

For the quantification of ePCT in plasma and BALF a validated sandwich ELISA using human anti-PCT Antibodies and equine recombinant PCT (erPCT) as standard was used [20]. Rieger et al. [20] showed that the assay has a working range of 25–1000 ng/mL. The authors stated parallelism up to a concentration of 10.000 ng/mL. Higher concentrations of ePCT led to irregularities in quantification regarding different dilutions. However, the authors showed acceptable values for IaCv and Recovery resulting in a working range of 25–1000 ng/mL. Changing the matrix for validated immunoassays can be done by partial validation which was done here by reanalyzing IaCV/IeCV and recovery in BALF matrix. Although the working range was defined to be 25–250 ng/mL, lower concentrations can be reported with this assay, but results must be regarded with caution, as variability at 10 ng/mL (which was approximately the BALF PCT concentration within this study) is higher (30%). For future studies in BALF, the method has to be improved e.g., by immunoaffinity enrichment of ePCT before analyzing the samples in the assay or the development of a more sensitive method, for example electrochemiluminescence (ECl).

In human medicine, PCT concentrations are routinely measured systemically from blood samples. A good correlation has been found between PCT in serum and BALF [40, 41]. Studies focusing on PCT in BALF samples only, however, have led to disappointing results. In some cases, very low concentrations were found in the alveolar space making it impossible to use PCT in the differentiation of pulmonary disease [40–44]. Low sensitivity of methods of detection and the dilution effect of BALF may have been the reasons for this [40, 43]. In equine medicine, bronchoalveolar lavage is an easy to perform and safe procedure to characterize airway inflammation and is recommended for the diagnosis of common respiratory disease like RAO or IAD [15, 17]. Much higher ePCT concentrations were found in serum of horses compared to men [20]. Therefore, it seemed logical that alveolar concentrations might also be higher in this species. Several biomarkers have been evaluated in equine BALF, as it has been shown that chronic respiratory disease does not always have a systemic component and inflammatory processes may be localized to the lung in case of minor disease like RAO in remission [14]. As PCT in plasma is only increased in case of systemic inflammation [45], we suspected that increases in ePCT would be most obvious in the alveolar space, but the results of our study show that it might be better to measure ePCT concentrations in plasma. This might be an advantage, as blood samples are much easier to obtain than BALF, but should be confirmed in a higher number of samples, as correlations based on different numbers of samples have to be interpreted with caution. ePCT in BALF allowed differentiating between controls and chronic respiratory disease, while no differentiation was possible between different disease groups. The highest concentrations were found in RAO in exacerbation and IAD, but inter-group-differences were insignificant. Again, a higher number of samples may allow to establish reasonable cut-off values for different types of disease.

A week positive correlation was found between PCT and clinical score. In human asthma, a correlation between PCT and the severity of disease has also been described [9]. Pro-inflammatory cytokines including IL-1ß and IL-6 are involved in stimulation of PCT synthesis [4, 46]. As these mediators also play a role in acute and chronic pulmonary disease, we evaluated their concentration and correlation to PCT in equine BALF. Nevertheless, no correlation was found between PCT and these interleukins in our study. Therefore, our results do not support their role in triggering PCT synthesis in the alveolar space.

For IL-1ß, no significant differences were found between healthy controls and horses affected by chronic respiratory disease in general and single disease groups, while in former studies increased transcription and protein concentrations have been found in severe RAO [47–50]. Similar results have been found for IAD [51, 52] and human asthma and COPD [53, 54]. In our study, the highest concentrations were found in CIP, where IL-1ß is known to stimulate the fibronectin and collagen synthesis. Therefore, it is a direct mediator of pulmonary fibrosis formation [54]. IL-1ß is produced by activated macrophages, which are the dominant cell type in BALF cytology in CIP.

For IL-6, no significant differences were found between healthy controls and horses affected by chronic respiratory disease either. The highest median concentration was found in group II (RAO in exacerbation). Former studies have led to contrasting results. While some authors found no significant increases in IL-6 were found in RAO exacerbation [50, 55, 56], others describe increases about three days after natural challenge [48, 52].

A weak point of this study was group definition, as samples were obtained from clinic patients. Therefore disease status was not as uniform as in experimental studies, where samples were obtained after defined disease induction. On the other hand, biomarkers are used in a clinical setting, therefore it seems logical to evaluate their usefulness in the same situation. Although IAD and RAO in remission were planned as two distinct groups, it was not possible to differentiate clearly between these two. Anamnestic information of recurrent respiratory distress was often unreliable and the majority of owners did not agree to a natural challenge test. Descriptions of equine CIP are rare in the literature and an international consensus statement is missing, so definition of this group was based on a quite old clinical case series including only 12 horses [18]. Thoracic radiography showing interstitial patterns is not very specific for CIP and may also be found in RAO and IAD [57, 58]. Again, the majority of owners did not agree to lung biopsies. We tried to face these problems by calculating correlations between PCT and interleukins with clinical and cytologic parameters over all 64 horses independent of diagnosis.

Conclusions

In conclusion, correlations between PCT concentrations in plasma and BALF supernatant were found and also with clinical data, but PCT in BALF does not seem to be a superior marker compared to established clinical markers, in particular in cases of low-grade inflammation. Following the definition by Couëtil [17], a lower grade of inflammation can be assumed in IAD compared to RAO, but PCT was also not able to differentiate between these two. There were significant differences between controls and respiratory disease in general, but differentiation between different forms of chronic pneumopathies was not possible. PCT in plasma seems to be a more promising marker, but its usefulness should be evaluated in a higher number of cases.

Abbreviations

$AaDo_2$: Arterio-alveolar pressure difference; BALF: Bronchoalveolar lavage fluid; BDW: Body weight; CIP: Chronic interstitial pneumopathy; COPD: Chronic obstructive pulmonary disease; ELISA: Enzyme-linked immunosorbent assay; IAD: Inflammatory airway disease; IL: Interleukin; LaGeSo: State Office of Health and Social Affairs Berlin; PCT: Procalcitonin; RAO: Recurrent airway obstruction; Rpm: Rounds per minute; SD: Standard deviation; TNF-α: Tumer-necrosis-factor α

Acknowledgements

The authors acknowledge R. Merle for statistical support, Tarek Shety, Caroline Wirth and Henrike Heinemann, who helped to carry out the clinical examinations. We thank the owners of the horses for participation in this study.

Funding

This study was financed by a research grant of Freie Universitaet Berlin.

Authors' contributions

AKB carried out the clinical examinations, participated in the conceivement, design and coordination of the study and drafted the manuscript. AP carried out the laboratory assays and performed the statistical analysis. MR participated in the coordination of the study and participated in the laboratory assays, HG conceived of the study, participated in its design and coordination. All authors read and approved the final manuscript.

Competing interests

The authors declare that they have no competing interests.

Consent for publication

Not applicable.

Author details

[1]Equine Clinic, Freie Universitaet Berlin, Oertzenweg 19b, 10163 Berlin, Germany. [2]Research unit microbe-plant interactions, Helmholtz Zentrum Muenchen, Ingolstädter Landstraße 1, 85764 Neuherberg, Germany.

References

1. Holowaychuk MK, Martin LG. Review of hypocalcemia in septic patients. J Vet Emergency Crit Care. 2007;17:348–58.
2. Russwurm S, Oberhoffer M, Zipfel PF, et al. Procalcitonin—a novel biochemical marker for the mediator-directed therapy of sepsis. Mol Med Today. 1999;5:286–7.
3. Müller B, White JC, Nylen ES, et al. Ubiquitous expression of the calcitonin-I gene in multiple tissues in response to sepsis. J Clin Endocrinol Metabol. 2001;86:396–404.
4. Oberhoffer M, Stonans I, Russwurm S, et al. Procalcitonin expression in human peripheral blood mononuclear cells and its modulation by lipopolysaccharides and sepsis-related cytokines in vitro. J Lab Clin Med. 1999;134:49–55.
5. Whang KT, Vath SD, Becker KL, et al. Procalcitonin and proinflammatory cytokine interactions in sepsis. Shock. 2000;14:73–8.
6. Berg P, Lindhardt BØ. The role of procalcitonin in adult patients with community-acquired pneumonia - a systematic review. Dan Med J. 2012;59:A4357.
7. Pereira JM, Teixeira-Pinto A, Basílio C, et al. Can we predict pneumococcal bacteremia in patients with severe community-acquired pneumonia? J Crit Care. 2013;28:970–4.
8. Julián-Jiménez A, Timón Zapata J, Laserna Mendieta EJ, et al. Diagnostic and prognostic power of biomarkers to improve the management of community acquired pneumonia in the emergency department. Enferm Infecc Microbiol Clin. 2014;32:225–35.
9. Tang J, Long W, Yan L, et al. Procalcitonin guided antibiotic therapy of acute exacerbations of asthma: a randomized controlled trial. BMC Infect Dis. 2013;13:596.
10. Walsh EE, Swinburne AJ, Becker KL, et al. Can serum procalcitonin levels help interpret indeterminate chest radiographs in patients hospitalized with acute respiratory illness? J Hosp Med. 2013;8:61–47.
11. Brightling CE. Biomarkers that predict and guide therapy for exacerbations of chronic obstructive pulmonary disease. Ann Am Thorac Soc. 2013;10(Suppl):214–9.
12. Zhao YF, Jiang YP, Zhou LF, et al. Prognostic value of chronic obstructive pulmonary disease assessment test, serum copeptin, procalcitonin and C-

reactive protein: six months of outcome in patients with acute exacerbation of chronic obstructive pulmonary disease. Am J Med Sci. 2014;347:393–9.
13. Barnes PJ. Mechanisms in COPD – Differences fromasthma. Chest. 2000;117(Suppl):10–4.
14. Lavoie-Lamoureux A, Leclere M, Lemos K, et al. Markers of systemic inflammation in horses with heaves. J Vet Intern Med. 2012;26:1419–26.
15. Robinson NE. International workshop on equine chronic airway disease, Michigan State University 16–18 June 2000. Equine Vet J. 2001;33:5–19.
16. Leclere M, Lavoie JP. "(Dis) Similarities between IAD and RAO." Proceedings of the 2nd Havemeyer Workshop on IAD, Cabourg (France) 2014: 87–89.
17. Couëtil LL, Hoffman AM, Hodgson J, et al. Inflammatory airway disease of horses. J Vet Intern Med. 2007;21:356–61.
18. Dieckmann MP, Klein HJ, Deegen E. Chronic interstitial lung disease in the horse – Findings in arterial bloodgas analysis, tracheobronchial mucus cytology and radiological examination of the thorax. Pferdeheilkunde. 1990;6:155–60.
19. Wilkins PA, Lascola KM. Update on interstitial pneumonia. Vet Clin North Am Equine Pract. 2015;31:137–57.
20. Rieger M, Kochleus C, Teschner D, et al. A new ELISA for the quantification of equine procalcitonin in plasma as potential inflammation biomarker in horses. Anal Bioanal Chem. 2014;406:5507–12.
21. Bonelli F, Meucci V, Divers TJ, et al. Procalcitonin in healthy and endotoxemic horses. Proceedings of the ECEIM-Congress, Prague 2014: 54.
22. Teschner D, Rieger M, Coopmann C, et al. Procalcitonin in horses with an acute colic. Pferdeheilkunde. 2015;31:317–77.
23. Redl H, Schlag G, Togel E, et al. Procalcitonin release patterns in a baboon model of trauma and sepsis: relationship to cytokines and neopterin. Crit Care Med. 2000;28:3659–63.
24. Gehlen H, Oey L, Rohn K, et al. Pulmonary dysfunction and skeletal muscle changes in horses with RAO. J Vet Intern Med. 2008;22:1014–21.
25. Ohnesorge B, Trötschel C, Deegen E. Diagnostic value of capnography in horses with RAO. Proceedings 5th World Equine Vet Assoc Congress 1998: 65–69.
26. Karzai W, Oberhoffer M, Meier-Hellmann A, et al. Procalcitonin—a new indicator of the systemic response to severe infections. Infection. 1997;25:329–34.
27. Russwurm S, Wiederhold M, Oberhoffer M, et al. Molecular aspects and natural source of procalcitonin. Clin Chem Lab Med. 1999;37:789–97.
28. Müller B, Becker KL, Schachinger H, et al. Calcitonin precursors are reliable markers of sepsis in a medical intensive care unit. Crit Care Med. 2000;28:977–83.
29. Chang CH, Tsao KC, Hu HC, et al. Procalcitonin and C-reactive protein cannot differentiate bacterial or viral infection in COPD exacerbation requiring emergency department visits. Int J Chron Obstruct Pulmon Dis. 2015;13:767–74.
30. Iikura M, Hojo M, Koketsu R, et al. The importance of bacterial and viral infections associated with adult asthma exacerbations in clinical practice. PLoS One. 2015;10:e0123584.
31. Pirie RS. Recurrent airway obstruction: a review. Equine Vet J. 2014;46:276–88.
32. Wood JL, Newton JR, Chanter N, et al. Association between respiratory disease and bacterial and viral infections in British racehorses. J Clin Microbiol. 2005;43:120–6.
33. Toribio RE, Kohn CW, Leone GW, et al. Molecular cloning and expression of equine calcitonin, calcitonin gene-related peptide-I, and calcitonin gene-related peptide-II. Mol Cell Endocrinol. 2003;199:119–28.
34. Toribio RE. Endocrine dysregulation in critically ill foals and horses. Vet Clin North Am Eq Pract. 2011;27:35–47.
35. Garcia-Lopez JM, Provost PJ, Rush JE, et al. Prevalence and prognostic importance of hypomagnesemia and hypocalcemia in horses that have colic surgery. Am J Vet Res. 2001;62:7–12.
36. Toribio RE, Kohn CW, Hardy J, et al. Alterations in serum parathyroid hormone and electrolyte concentrations and urinary excretion of electrolytes in horses with induced endotoxemia. J Vet Intern Med. 2005;19:223–31.
37. Nylen E, Whang K, Snider RJ, et al. Mortality is increased by procalcitonin and decreased by an antiserum reactive to procalcitonin in experimental sepsis. Crit Care Med. 1998;26:1001–6.
38. Martinez JM, Wagner KE, Snider RH, et al. Late immunoneutralization of procalcitonin arrests the progression of lethal porcine sepsis. Surg Infect. 2001;2:193–203.
39. Wagner KE, Martinez JM, Vath SD, et al. Early immunoneutralization of calcitonin precursors attenuates the adverse physiologic response to sepsis in pigs. Crit Care Med. 2002;30:2313–21.
40. Linssen CFM, Bekers O, Drent M, et al. C-reactive protein and procalcitonin concentrations in bronchoalveolar lavage fluid as a predictor of ventilator-associated pneumonia. Annals Cli Biochem. 2008;45:293–8.
41. Stiletto RJ, Baacke M, Gotzen L, et al. Procalcitonin versus interleukin-6 levels in bronchoalveolar lavage fluids of trauma victims with severe lung contusion. Crit Care Med. 2001;29:1690–3.
42. Duflo F, Debon R, Monneret G, et al. Alveolar and serum Procalcitonin: diagnostic and prognostic value in ventilator-associated pneumonia. Anesthesiol. 2002;96:74–9.
43. Jung B, Embriaco N, Roux F, et al. Microbiogical data, but not procalcitonin improve the accuracy of the clinical pulmonary infection score. Intensive Care Med. 2010;36:790–8.
44. Lederer W, Stichlberger M, Hausdorfer J, et al. Alveolar neopterin, procalcitonin, and IL-6 in relation to serum levels and severity of lung injury in ARDS. Clini Chem Lab Med. 2013;51:e213–5.
45. Meisner M. Update on procalcitonin measurements. Annals Lab Med. 2014;34:263–73.
46. Nijsten MW, Olinga P, The TH, et al. Procalcitonin behaves as a fast responding acute phase protein in vivo and in vitro. Crit Care Med. 2000;28:458–61.
47. Giguère S, Viel L, Lee E, et al. Cytokine induction in pulmonary airways of horses with heaves and effect of therapy with inhaled fluticasone propionate. Vet Immunol Immunopathol. 2002;85:147–58.
48. Pietra M, Peli A, Bonato A, et al. Equine bronchoalveolar lavage cytokines in the development of recurrent airway obstruction. Vet Res Comm. 2007;3:313–6.
49. Sarli G, Peli A, Marocco R, et al. A comparison of IL-1β and IL-8 mRNA and their respective proteins in equinebronchoalveolar lavage fluid during recurrent airway obstruction. Online J Vet Res. 2011;15:215–28.
50. Padoan E, Ferraresso S, Pegolo S, et al. Real time RT-PCR analysis of inflammatory mediator expression in recurrent airway obstruction-affected horses. Vet Immunol Immunopathol. 2013;156:190–6.
51. Hughes KJ, Nicolson L, Da Costa N, et al. Evaluation of cytokine mRNA expression in bronchoalveolar lavage cells from horses with inflammatory airway disease. Vet Immunol Immunopathol. 2011;140:82–9.
52. Beekman L, Tohver T, Léguillette R. Comparison of cytokine mRNA expression in the bronchoalveolar lavage fluid of horses with inflammatory airway disease and bronchoalveolar lavage mastocytosis or neutrophilia using REST software analysis. J Vet Intern Med. 2012;26:153–61.
53. Arend WP. The balance between IL-1 and IL-1Ra in disease. Cytokine Growth Factor Rev. 2002;13:323–40.
54. Chung KF. Cytokines in chronic obstructive pulmonary disease. Eur Respir J. 2001;18:50–9.
55. Riihimäki M, Raine A, Art T, et al. Partial divergence of cytokine mRNA expression in bronchial tissues compared to bronchoalveolar lavage cells in horses with recurrent airway obstruction. Vet Immunol Immunopathol. 2008;122:256–64.
56. Riihimäki M, Raine A, Pourazar J, et al. Epithelial expression of mRNA and protein for IL-6, IL-10 and TNF-α in endobronchial biopsies in horses with recurrent airway obstruction. BMC Vet Res. 2008;4:8.
57. Tilley P, Sales Luis JP, Branco FM. Correlation and discriminant analysis between clinical, endoscopic, thoracic X-ray and bronchoalveolar lavage fluid cytology scores, for staging horses with recurrent airway obstruction (RAO). Res Vet Sci. 2012;93:1006–14.
58. Mazan MR, Vin R, Hoffman AM. Radiographic scoring lacks predictive value in inflammatory airway disease. Equine Vet J. 2005;37:541–5.

16

Analytical validation and establishment of reference intervals for a 'high-sensitivity' cardiac troponin-T assay in horses

E. Shields[1], I. Seiden-Long[2], S. Massie[1], S. Passante[1] and R. Leguillette[1*]

Abstract

Background: Cardiac troponin-I assays have been validated in horses.'High-sensitivity' cardiac troponin assays are now the standard in human cardiology. *Objective:* Appropriately validate the'high-sensitivity' cardiac Troponin-T (hscTnT) assay for clinical use in horses, establish reference intervals, determine the biological variation, and demonstrate assay utility in selected clinical cases. *Methods:* Analytical validation of the Roche hscTnT assay included within- and between-run precision, linear dose response, limit of quantitation (LoQ), stability, and comparison with cTn-I (iSTAT). Reference intervals and biological variation were determined using adult, healthy, Non-Competition Horses (N = 125) and Racing-Thoroughbreds (N = 178). HscTnT levels were measured in two horses with cardiac pathology.

Results: The hscTnT demonstrates acceptable within-run (L1 = 6.5 ng/L, CV 14.9 %, L2 = 10.1 ng/L, CV 8.7 %, L3 = 15.3 ng/L, CV 5.4 %) and between-run precision (L1 = 12.2 ng/L, CV 8.4 %, L2 = 57.0 ng/L, CV 8.4 %, L3 = 256.0 ng/L, CV 9.0 %). The assay was linear from 3 to 391 ng/L. The LoQ was validated at 3 ng/L. Samples demonstrated insignificant decay over freeze-thaw cycle. Comparison with cTnI assay showed excellent correlation (range: 8.0–3535.0 ng/L, $R^2 = 0.9996$). Reference intervals: The upper 95th and 99th percentile of the hscTnT population distribution were 6.8 and 16.2 ng/L in Non-Competition Horses, and 14.0 and 23.2 ng/L in Racing-Thoroughbreds. Between-breed, diurnal effect, and between-day variation was below LoQ. Two clinical cases with presumed cardiac pathology had hscTnT levels of 220.9 ng/L and 5723.0 ng/L.

Conclusions: This benchmark study is the first to comply with CLSI guidelines, thus further establishing the performance characteristics of the hscTnT assay, and reference intervals in healthy horses. Two clinical cases demonstrated further the clinical utility of the assay.

Keywords: Horse, Blood chemistry, Myocardium, Muscle

Background

As acknowledged in a recent joint consensus statement, subtle or occult cardiac abnormalities are often difficult to diagnose in horses [1]. Similarly, determining the impact of any cardiovascular abnormality on present or future performance, on rider or driver safety, and the long-term effects on health and longevity can be problematic [1]. Early detection of cardiac pathologies would provide the opportunity to recognize occult disease and allow intervention prior to potentially more serious outcomes such as cumulative cardiac damage or sudden death.

One cardiac diagnostic tool that has been adopted for use in veterinary medicine is the troponin assay. Of the three troponin subunits, only cardiac Troponin-T (cTnT) and cardiac Troponin-I (cTnI) have unique amino acid sequences expressed as cardiac muscle-specific isoforms, and are encoded by different genes than the troponins expressed in skeletal muscle [2]. Since 2000, after an extensive search for a biomarker of myocardial damage with sufficient analytical sensitivity and specificity, troponin assays have been deemed the test of choice for detection of acute myocardial injury (AMI) in humans [3]. The assays have evolved through

* Correspondence: rleguill@ucalgary.ca
[1]University of Calgary Faculty of Veterinary Medicine (UCVM), 3330 Hospital Dr. NW, Calgary T2N 4 N1, AB, Canada
Full list of author information is available at the end of the article

numerous generations, each of which has undergone improvements in analytical performance. Troponin-I and T assays with total imprecision ≤ 10 % at the 99th percentile, and measurable normal values below the 99th percentile in at least 50 % of healthy individuals are now classified as'high-sensitivity' assays in humans [4]. Older generation ('non-hs') troponin assay use in veterinary medicine has been fairly widespread (reviewed by Rossi et. al.) [5], and recently two reports use the hscTnT assay [6, 7]. There are problems however, associated with the clinical utility and application of the troponin assays reported in the equine literature to date [6, 8–12]. These include: 1)- The general lack of appropriate analytical validation which can lead to erroneous interpretation of results and subsequent designation of reference ranges and threshold cut-off points. 2)- The large number of commercially available troponin assays that differ from one another in terms of antibody-epitope specificity and preclude direct comparison of results from various studies. 3)- The use of older generation troponin assays that lack the sensitivity to detect occult or potentially cumulative myocardial injury with the degree of certainty needed in veterinary sports medicine to explore the effects of subclinical myocardial damage. With'high-sensitivity' (5th generation) cardiac troponin assays now available, our aim was to validate a human automated'high-sensitivity' cardiac Troponin-T (hscTnT) Roche Diagnostics assay for use in horse plasma, and to establish hscTnT reference intervals in adult, healthy, Non-Competition Horses and Racing-Thoroughbreds as presented in 2014 [13]. This validation study of the Roche hscTnT assay for use in horses provides additional valuable information by complying with the recommendations of the Clinical and Laboratory Standards Institute (CLSI), the National Academy of Clinical Biochemistry (NACB), and American Society of Veterinary Clinical Pathology (ASVCP) [14–17] for the first time.

Methods

1) Genetic homology

   Utilizing NCBI protein BLAST, *Homo sapiens* cardiac Troponin-T amino acid residues of epitopes recognized by capture MAb (M7) (125–131:DRIERR) and detection MAb (M11.7) (136–147:EQQRIRNEREKE) for the hscTnT assay were compared to *Equus caballus* cardiac and skeletal Troponin-T (Fig. 1).

2) Analytical validation of 'high-sensitivity' cardiac Troponin-T assay

   Roche Diagnostics cardiac Troponin-T 'high-sensitivity' assay, Cobas-e601 Analyzer

   HscTnT assay, a 5th generation electrochemiluminescence immunoassay, was used on the Cobas-e601 Analyzer for analysis of equine plasma samples, complying with manufacturer's instructions and CLS internal quality controls systems. The manufacturer determined the analytical characteristics for this assay in accordance with the CLSI-EP17-A2 requirements. The analyzer was calibrated using human cTnT standards supplied for use of the hscTnT assay kit with human plasma.

   Equine Troponin-T samples

   Purified equine cardiac troponin used in linearity and precision studies was obtained from harvested equine myocardium as previously described [18]. Plasma samples were collected from all live horses, by jugular venipuncture in 5 mL lithium-heparinized tubes. Specimens were centrifuged at 2000 x *g* for 10 min, separated, frozen within 90 min, and stored at–80 °C until batch analyzed. Degree of hemolysis in all samples was assessed using the serum indices instrument application on the Roche Cobas-e601 platform[2] and no specimen

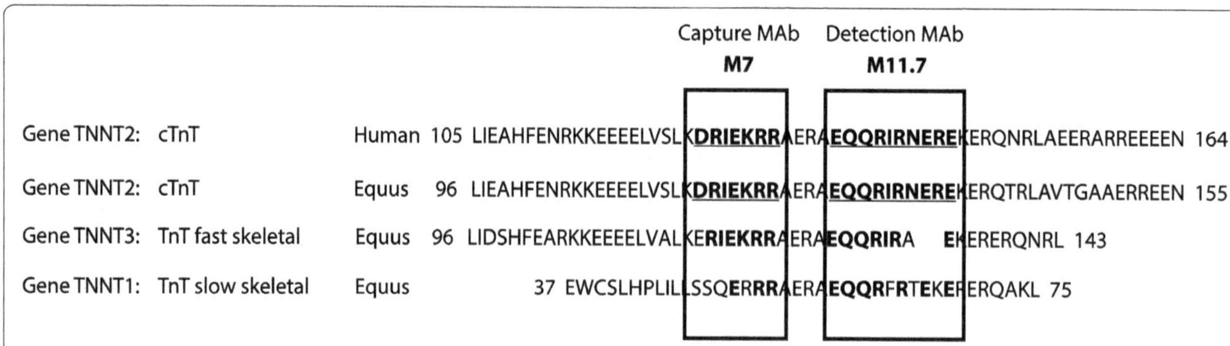

Fig. 1 Amino acid sequence alignment of human cardiac Troponin-T (Type 2) adult isoform (cTnT) with horse (*Equus caballus*) cardiac Troponin-T (Type 2) and homology with equine fast and slow skeletal muscle TnT using NCBI protein BLAST. Amino acid sequences include the epitope regions against which the Roche, Cobas-e601 capture (M7) and detection (M11.7) antibodies are directed

included in this study reached the hemolysis threshold to be excluded.

Tissue specificity

Homogenates of cardiac and skeletal muscle harvested from a healthy horse were prepared as previously described [19] and subsequently diluted.[3] Dilutions used were within the linear range of the hscTnT assay (cardiac: 100,000 fold, skeletal muscle: 10,000 fold). The tissue reactivities, expressed in ng/L wet weight, were corrected for the dilution factor and are presented as means ± SEM. Tissue Reactivity (ng/g of wet tissue) = x hscTnT(ng/L) x dilution factor ÷ weight of muscle sample(g) x dilution of original homogenate muscle stock.

Linear dose response

N = 10 dilutions were prepared from purified equine cardiac troponin stock by serial 1:2 dilution (from 1:100 to 1:0.2) using normal equine plasma (hscTnT 3.28 ng/L) as diluent. Triplicates of the resultant 11 samples (mean hscTnT levels ranging from 8.0 to 3526.7 ng/L) were analyzed to detect linearity over the expected measurable range.

Assay precision

Within-run precision was evaluated by assaying plasma samples from 3 horses containing 3 different previously determined (Roche Diagnostics hscTnT assay) concentrations of hscTnT (L1 = 6.5 ng/L, L2 = 10.1 ng/L, L3 = 15.3 ng/L) 10 times in the same run. Between-run precision was evaluated by assaying prepared quality control samples consisting of purified equine cardiac troponin diluted with equine plasma at 3 levels (L1 = 12.2 ng/L, L2 = 56.9 ng/L, L3 = 254.0 ng/L) over 3 months and 10 different runs.

Functional sensitivity

The limit of quantitation (LoQ), defined as the lowest analyte concentration that can be reproducibly measured with a between-run CV ≤ 10 %, was determined using 5 serial dilutions of a stock, diluted, purified equine cardiac troponin sample (hscTnT range 4-37 ng/L), and analysing each dilution 5 times in 1 day.

Stability study

Stability of samples was tested at–80 °C for a period of 24 months. Samples were measured at the start and end of the testing period and the average difference between the measured values before and after storage was calculated. Criteria for significant change: average difference of less than 2X the between-run standard deviation of the control level closest to the mean of samples measured.

Comparison study

Eleven diluted, purified equine cardiac troponin samples of various increasing, known hscTnT levels (previously determined using Roche Diagnostics assay), were run in duplicate on the iSTAT for equine cTnI analyte levels allowing for comparison of hscTnT to older generation cTnI results.

3) Reference intervals and biological variation of hscTnT levels in healthy horses

Two subset populations were included in the study and sampled by convenience (summer 2013): one group of Non-Competition Horses with varying levels of routine physical activity and a second group of Racing-Thoroughbred geldings (Table 1). These populations provide reference intervals of troponin levels for application of the assay in sports medicine and exercise physiology in addition to general application in clinical cardiomyopathy cases. The study was approved by the UCVM-Veterinary Sciences Animal Care Committee and consent was obtained from the animals' owners.

Non-Competition Horses: Plasma samples were taken from 125 non-performance, healthy horses (ages 2–24; median 5 years, 69 geldings, 56 mares) represented by Quarter horses, Quarter horse-crosses, Thoroughbreds, Warmbloods, Draft horses, and Arabians.

Racing-Thoroughbreds: Plasma samples were taken from 178 healthy, fit, actively competing Thoroughbred Chuckwagon racing geldings (ages 4–18; median 9 years) when the horses were at rest in the morning prior to races.

For both populations, a physical examination with heart auscultation was performed, and Telemetric ECG was run stall-side and observed for two minutes on all horses. Horses were excluded for abnormal physical exam findings, murmurs Grades III or greater, or any arrhythmia other than second-degree atrioventricular block. Horses had no known history of congenital or acquired cardiac abnormalities.

Breed, diurnal and intra-individual variation

Evaluation of differences in hscTnT levels between breed was determined by sample collection from 25 horses representing Warmbloods, Thoroughbreds, Quarter Horses, Arabians and Draft Horses (5 horses of each breed). In addition, diurnal and intra-individual variation was assessed by sample collection from each horse every morning and evening for 5 consecutive days.

4) Two selected case studies demonstrating clinical use of hscTnT assay

Table 1 Comparison of ages, sexes, breeds and resting heparin plasma hscTnT concentrations in horses

Number	125	178	1	1
	Non-Competition Horses	Racing- Thoroughbreds	Clinical Case I	Clinical Case II
Median Age (Range)	5 (2–24)	9 (4–18)	11	14
Sexes	56 Mares, 69 Geldings	178 Geldings	Gelding	Mare
Breed(s)	TB, QH, Drafts, Arabians, WB	TB	TB	QH
Resting hscTnT Mean (±SD), ng/L	3.6 (±2.1)	5.4 (±3.8)	221.0[a]	5723.0[b]
hscTnT Median, ng/L	3.0	4.0[c]	N/A	N/A
hscTnT Range, ng/L	3.0–17.0	3.0–24.0	N/A	N/A
hscTnT 95 % URL (90 % CI), ng/L	6.79 (6.0–12.0)	14.0 (10.0–18.0)	N/A	N/A
hscTnT 99 % URL (90 % CI), ng/L	16.2 (N/A)	23.2 (N/A)	N/A	N/A

Comparison of ages, sexes, breeds and resting heparin plasma hscTnT concentrations from 303 apparently healthy horses (Non-Competition Horses and Racing-Thoroughbreds) as well as two clinical cases
[a]Heparin plasma hscTnT sample taken 5 h after race-induced upper respiratory crisis event
[b]Heparin plasma hscTnT sample taken 41 h after initially presented to clinic
[c]Indicates a significant difference from Non-Competition Horses

Case one

An 11 year old Thoroughbred Chuckwagon gelding passed a mandatory racetrack veterinary physical and lameness examination on the morning of a race. He had no history of previously administered medications. The gelding later presented with near-collapse event at the end of his race secondary to an acute upper airway obstruction. The horse was diagnosed stall-side, via auscultation, with ventricular tachycardia immediately following racing. Telemetric ECG was subsequently run stall-side intermittently over 48 h. Plasma hscTnT analyte levels were measured at 5 and 72 h following the event.

Case two

Fourteen year old Quarter Horse mare, 3 months pregnant, diagnosed with *Neorickettsia ristícii* by PCR and showing acute clinical signs of cardiacimpairment, hypovolemic shock, and systemic inflammatory response syndrome (SIRS). Diagnostic testing was completed to document the status of the patient in light of the primary colitis pathology (venous hematologic, blood chemistry, venous/arterial blood gas, urinalysis, fractional excretion electrolyte ratios, and fecal PCR). Cardiac evaluation included physical examination, heart auscultation, 24-h Telemetric ECG, and plasma hscTnT analyte levels, but lacked cardiac ultrasonography (due to logistical restrictions associated with isolation hospitalization of a severe diarrhea case). Following euthanasia, post-mortem examination with selected histology was performed.

Statistical analysis

Linearity and LoQ were determined using Analyse-it software[5]. Linearity of the assay was assessed by linear and polynomial regression of the data and difference plot with Total Error criteria. A Weighted Deming fit was used to compare the fit between the hscTnT assay versus the cTnI assay. The hscTnT population distributions were not normal using the Kolmogorov-Smirnov test. CLSI-28A3C guidelines recommend Dixon's and Tukey's techniques for outlier detection, however both are based on the assumption that there is a normal distribution to the population data [14]. Due to the severity of the right-skewed population in this case, normalization of the data is unreliable with transformation techniques such as Box-Cox transformation. Consequently, visual inspection was selected as a screening method and no outliers were detected in the populations tested. The Mann-Whitney *U* test was utilized to test the difference between the hscTnT levels in the two horse sub-populations. Nonparametric methods, complying with CLSI guidelines, were used for determination of the 95th and 99th percentiles and 90 % confidence intervals for horses from each population.

Results

1) Analytical validation of 'high-sensitivity' cardiac Troponin-T assay

Genetic homology

The epitopes detected by this commercial hscTnT assay were conserved between humans and horses with 100 % homology detected when comparing human adult cardiac isoform cTnT and equine cTnT [XP_005614937.1], while only 80 % [XP_005898432.1] and 56 %

[XP_005896826.1] conservation was shown between human adult cTnT and equine fast and slow skeletal muscle respectively (Fig. 1).

Tissue specificity

Although there was some minimal detectable reactivity from equine skeletal muscle in the hscTnT immunoassay, hscTnT reactivity of cardiac muscle was 256.2 times greater than that in skeletal muscle (2.49 $x10^7$ and 9.75 $x10^4$ ng/g wet weight respectively).

Linear dose response

While linear dose response was tested in the range of 8–3527 ng/L, the assay was linear over the hscTnT range of 3–391 ng/L (±2 ng/L or 5 %). Above 391 ng/L there is bias in the regression with over-recovery of the analyte demonstrated and even when the linearity criteria are widened (to ±5 ng/L or 20 %) the response is significantly non-linear (Fig. 2).

Assay precision

Within-run precision was: L1 = 6.5 ng/L, CV 14.9 %, L2 = 10.1 ng/L, CV 8.7 %, L3 = 15.3 ng/L, CV 5.4 % and between-run precision was: L1 = 12.2 ng/L, CV 8.4 %, L2 = 57.0 ng/L, CV 8.4 %, L3 = 256.0 ng/L, CV 9.0 % (Table 2). In humans studies, the required precision is 10 % within-run CV at the upper limit of normal for the population. The horse specimens have < 10 % CV at the levels closest to the upper reference limit (99th percentile) in both horse populations tested (Table 2).

Functional sensitivity (Limit of Quantitation)

The LoQ was validated at 3 ng/L (using a 10 % CV).

Stability study

The stability of the samples was excellent and demonstrated slight, but not statistically significant decrease in hscTnT analyte over the average 24 month period between free-thaw cycles (mean = 15.8 ng/L, average difference = 1.75 ng/L).

Comparison study

Comparison with cTn-I assay showed excellent correlation (range: 8–3535 ng/L, $R^2 = 0.9996$). Bias was evident in the Deming regression

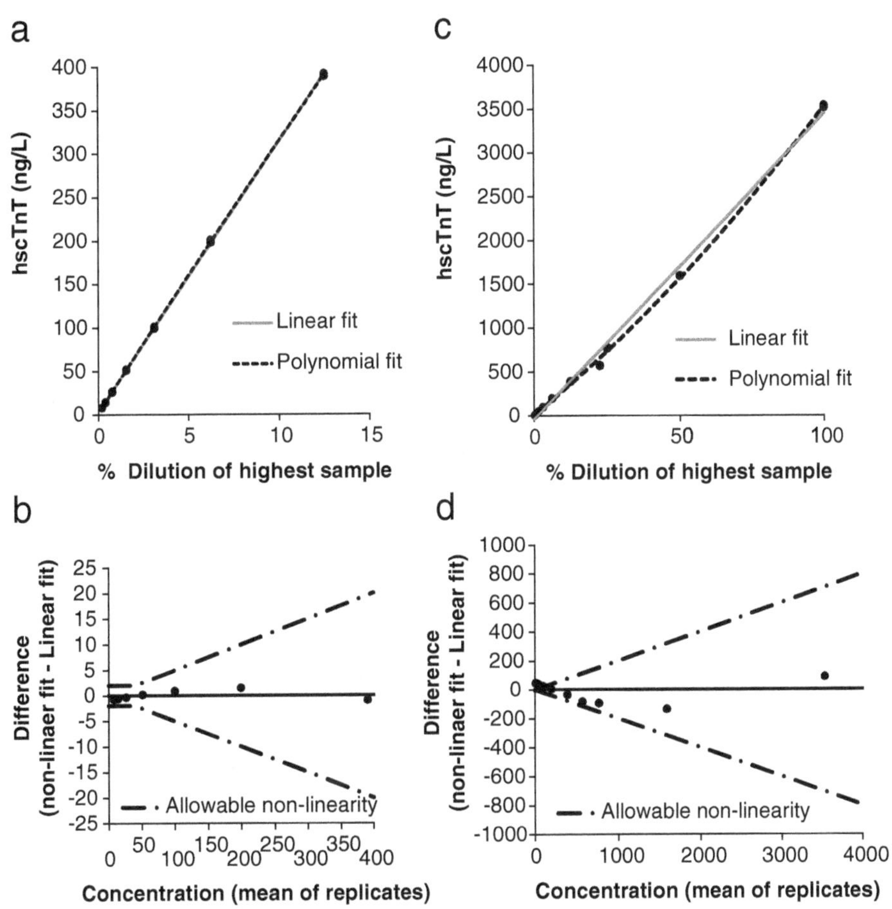

Fig. 2 Plot of the linearity (triplicates of increasing concentrations of equine hscTnT) of the Roche, Cobas-e601 hscTnT assay. **a**, **b** Linear to a level of 391 ng/L (±2 ng/L or 5 %). **c**, **d** Linearity run up to 3500 ng/L shows over-recovery

Table 2 Precision of the hscTnT assay (Roche Diagnostics, Cobas-e601) for measuring equine plasma

	Level 1 (L1)	Level 2 (L2)	Level 3 (L3)
Within-Run hscTnT Mean (CV), ng/L	6.5 (14.9 %)	10.1 (8.7 %)	15.3 (5.4 %)
Between-Run hscTnT Mean (CV), ng/L	12.2 (8.4 %)	57.0 (8.4 %)	256.0 (9.0 %)

Abbreviations: *CV* Coefficient of variation (in %)
Precision of the hscTnT assay (Roche Diagnostics, Cobas-e601) for measuring equine plasma hscTnT of three increasing levels (Level 1, 2, 3) on 10 separate occasions

results [hscTnT = (0.6 ± 0.0028)*(cTnI*1000)–(11.5 ± 5.5)] (Fig. 3).

2) Biological variation of hscTnT levels in healthy horses

Reference interval determination of two subset populations

HscTnT levels were different between the Non-Competition Horses and Racing-Thoroughbreds ($p < 0.0001$) (Table 1). As such, the populations have been considered separately with respect to upper reference limits. The upper 95th (90 % CI) and 99th percentile of the population distribution in Non-Competitive Horses (N = 125) is 6.8 (90 % CI:6.0–12.0) and 16.2 ng/L and for Racing-Thoroughbreds (N = 178) is 14.0 (90 % CI:10.0–18.0) and 23.2 ng/L, respectively (Table 1 and Fig. 4). Lower reference limits are not clinically relevant and are defined by the LoQ of the assay (3 ng/L). 90 % CI could not be calculated for the 99th percentile due N value restrictions [14]. Measureable hscTn analyte levels were obtained in 56.8 and 88.8 % for Non-Competition Horses and Racing-Thoroughbreds groups respectively.

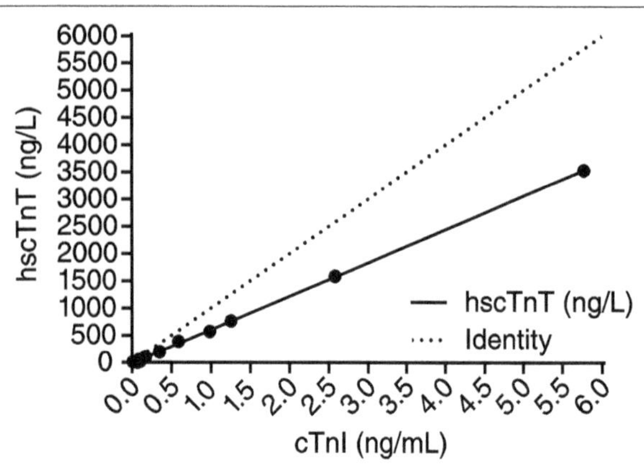

Fig. 3 Correlation between cTn concentration in duplicates of equine plasma samples of increasing levels as measured by the Roche, Cobas-e601 hscTnT assay and the iSTAT cTnI assay. Correlation between the 2 methods was high (range: 8–3535 ng/L, r = 0.9998). Bias was evident in the Deming regression results [hscTnT = (0.6 ± 0.0028)*(cTnI*1000)–(11.5 ± 5.5)]

Breed, diurnal and intra-individual variation in Non-Competition Horse population

The assay did not have sufficient sensitivity to assess between breed, diurnal effect and between-day variation in Non-Competition Horses partly due to low levels of hscTnT (43.2 % of this reference population had average values ≤ 3 ng/L) (Fig. 4).

3) Two selected case studies demonstrating clinical use of hscTnT assay

Case one

The 11 year old TB Chuckwagon horse had previously passed a veterinary physical and lameness examination on the morning of the race. The gelding finished the 0.5 mile race in distress and presented immediately for assessment. Examination showed cyanotic mucous membranes and persistent tachycardia (heart rate: 180 bpm). No cardiac murmurs were noted on auscultation. Ventricular tachycardia was confirmed on ECG that converted to atrial fibrillation within 30 min and spontaneously returned to sinus rhythm with supportive therapy, but no conversion treatment, within 12 h. The plasma sample taken 5 h after the race for hscTnT had a value of 221 ng/L; by 72 h the hscTnT value was 21 ng/L. Five weeks later, a standing and over-

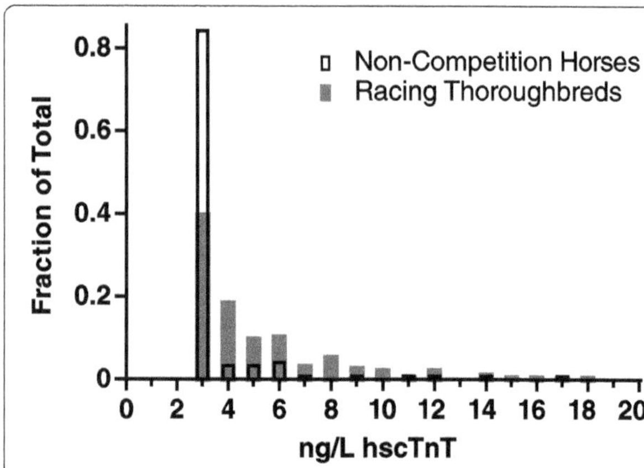

Fig. 4 Frequency distribution for hscTnT levels in Non-Competition Horses and Racing-Thoroughbreds

the-ground dynamic endoscopy during exercise revealed a subepiglottic cyst with a severe retroversion of the epiglottis during maximal effort.

Case two

The 14 year old QH mare was diagnosed with Potomac Horse Fever, and SIRS (based on tachycardia, fever, abnormal WBC count, as well as severe elevations in lactate and toxic, tacky mucous membranes) [20]. On admission the mare had severe electrolyte imbalances, endotoxemia (toxic neutrophils noted), acute renal failure, and liver impairments (Table 3). Despite emergency symptomatic treatment she remained unstable and showed deterioration in cardiovascular status (development of severe bradyarrhythmia with intermittent long sinusal pauses for up to 40 s, pale mucous membranes, and weak pulses), as well as ongoing severe diarrhea. A plasma sample taken for hscTnT 41 h following initial presentation measured 5723 ng/L. The mare was euthanized 44 h after initial presentation and post mortem findings included a moderately enlarged heart, failure of left ventricle to contract completely after rigor mortis, multifocal myocardial necrosis, and congestion of the liver all suggestive of myocardial function impairment.

Discussion

Adhering to the ASVCP guidelines based largely on the strict CLSI guidelines, our results indicate that the Roche Diagnostics cTnT assay (on the Cobas-e601 analyzer) can not only appropriately and adequately measure plasma concentrations of equine cTnT, but it can be classified as a'high-sensitivity' immunoassay fit for diagnostic use in horses. Meeting the CLSI guidelines, our study defined the reference intervals and determined the upper 95th (90 % CI) and 99th percentile of the population distribution in Non-Competitive Horses (N = 125) is 6.8 (90 % CI: 6.0–12.0) and 16.2 ng/L and for Racing-Thoroughbreds (N = 178) is 14.0 (90 % CI: 10.0–18.0) and 23.2 ng/L, respectively (Table 1, Fig. 4). This study provides additional information key to interpreting hscTnT results in clinical context as compared with recent reports [6, 7].

The epitopes detected by this hscTnT assay were conserved between humans and horses with 100 % homology detected when comparing human adult cTnTand equine cTnT (Fig. 1). Utilizing a series of validation experiments according to industry guidelines, the assay was challenged with detecting and measuring equine cTnT [15, 16]. Homogenates of equine cardiac and skeletal muscle allowed for the determination of specificity of the assay for hscTnT in cardiac versus skeletal muscle. Cross-reactivity with the skeletal muscle isoform of Troponin-T was minimal, indicating excellent assay specificity for the cardiac isoform. Purified equine cardiac troponin obtained from harvested equine myocardium allowed for the determination of linearity explored to levels exceeding the expected upper limit of the assay according to ASVCP guidelines (up to 3526.7 ng/L) [16]. This method differed from that used in the Van Der Vekens study [6] (in which diluted pooled samples from clinical cases were used to assess linearity up to 1098. 8 ng/L) and allowed assessment of assay linearity at higher analyte levels. Linearity of the assay in our study was assessed by linear and polynomial regression of the data and difference plot with Total Error criteria, whereas the Van Der Vekens group used simple linear regression analysis. Our work demonstrated good assay linearity over the low range of cTnT concentrations, but slightly over-recovers at high levels. However, 391 ng/L is > 10 times our defined URLs, so linearity to this level should confer good diagnostic sensitivity for distinguishing sick from healthy populations. For an accurate quantitative determination for clinical purposes it is therefore recommended to dilute specimens > 391 ng/L into the linear range for future studies. No such dilutions were performed on any clinical samples utilized throughout this study.

The within-run and between-run precision values were similar to those reported for measurement of human cTnT and were within CLSI standards [21]. In humans this assay has complied with the standards set forth by the International Federation of Clinical Chemistry and Laboratory Medicine to be defined as a'high-sensitivity' assay [4]. Based on the same stringent criteria, our study shows that this assay can be classified as a 'high-sensitivity' assay appropriate for diagnostic use in horses. Specifically we showed that the total imprecision was ≤ 10 % at the 99th percentiles for our two reference populations (16.22 and 23.21 ng/L), and measureable cTn analyte levels were obtained in 56.8 and 88.8 % for Non-Competition Horses and Racing-Thoroughbreds groups respectively.

It is critical for clinicians to understand certain basic characteristics of assays, development of reference intervals, and establishment of decision thresholds in order to critically interpret troponin assay use reported in the equine literature, and to successfully apply the assays available for use in practice. The limit of quantitation (LoQ) is the concentration above which quantitative results may be obtained with a specific degree of confidence (ie.CV ≤ 10 %), and according to the CLSI guidelines is recommended over the limit of detection (LoD) for setting the lower reporting limits of a test for clinical use. Importantly, only concentrations exceeding an assay's LoQ should be reported as a numerical value.

Table 3 Case two selected laboratory results

		Time of admission	36 h Post-adm.
COMPLETE BLOOD COUNT			
	RBC (x 10^{12}/L) [6.4–10.4]	10.9	5.7
	Hct (%) [30.0–47.0]	44	22.7
	WBC (x 10^{12}/L) [4.9–11.1]	13.6	7.1
	NEU (x 10^{12}/L) [2.5–6.9]	10.2	5.6
	LYM (x 10^{12}/L) [1.5–5.1]	2.4	1.1
	MONO (x 10^{12}/L) [0.2–0.6]	1.0	0.4
	EOS (x 10^{12}/L) [0.0–0.8]	0	0
	BASO (x 10^{12}/L) [0.0–0.1]	0.02	0.01
	PLT (K/μL) [100–250]	238	196
	Fibrinogen Manual (g/L)	7	5
CHEMISTRY			
	UREA (mmol/L) [3.6–8.9]	> 46.4	40.6
	CREA (μmol/L) [71–194]	Too high to report	Too high to report
	CA (mmol/L) [2.6–3.2]	2.1	2.7
	Total Protein (g/L) [56–79]	77	49
	ALB (g/L) [19–32]	29	18
	GLOB (g/L) [24–47]	48	31
	AST (U/L) [100–600]	410	442
	ALKP (U/L) [10–326]	195	134
	GGT (U/L) [0–87]	17	20
	TBIL (μmol/L) [0–60]	25	20
	CK (U/L) [10–350]	505	361
	LDH (U/L) [250–2070]	1694	2058
	Na (mmol/L) [133–150]	104	147
	K (mmol/L) [3.0–5.3]	2.3	2.4
	Cl (mmol/L) [97–109]	79	116
	HscTnT (ng/L)		5723
BLOOD GAS		Venous	Arterial
	pH (7.35–7.45)	7.3	7.3
	pCO_2 (mmHg) [3.6–8.9]	40.4	38.4
	PO_2 (mmHg)	48	61
	HCO_3 (mmol/L) [25.0–30.0]	18	18.9
	$T\ CO_2$ (mmol/L) [24–32]	19	20
	Base Excess [−5 to +5]	−9	−8
	sO_2 (%)	77	89
	Lactate (mmol/L) [0.3–1.5]	3.0	0.9
URINE			
	USG	1.009	
	Fraction of Excretion–Na (%)		40
	Fraction of Excretion–Cl (%)		68
	Fraction of Excretion–K (%)		157

Selected laboratory results for Case two, a 14 year old QH mare diagnosed with Potomac Horse Fever, and subsequent myocardial damage

The LoQ can, for example, be significantly greater than the LoD, as is reported in human plasma (LoD =3 ng/L, but LoQ = 13.5 ng/L) [21]. All equine studies to date using cardiac troponins mainly report values above manufacturers' defined LoDs, without verifying [6, 7, 9, 10], or adhering to a determined functional sensitivity (LoQ) [8]. The LoQ that we determined for equine plasma using Roche's hscTnT assay was validated at 3 ng/L (10 % CV). It is possible that the true LoQ may be at a level lower than 3 ng/L, but because the manufacturer limits all reported values to 3 ng/L, lower levels could not be validated. Additionally, the 10 % CV at 3 ng/L which is lower than what was observed in within-run precision Level 1 (14.9 % at 6.5 ng/L) may indicate that at 3 ng/L the assay is approaching non-linear dose response. Nevertheless, our results imply that any Roche hscTnT assay value reported by the e601-Cobas instrument is reliable for use in horse plasma.

The hscTnT assay reported values < 3 ng/L in 43.2 and 11.2 % of the Non-Competition Horses and Racing-Thoroughbreds, respectively, which is similar to the validation study in heathy humans (20.1 % at < 3 ng/L) [21]. This limited the determination of biological variation, measured as intra-individual, inter-individual variation (between-breed), reference change values (RCVs), and the index of individuality values. The ability of this assay to function at these low concentrations (LoQ level) is unique when compared to the only cTnI assay similarly validated appropriately by ASVCP and CLSI standards for use in horses [8], and thus continues to show promise for its' ability to detect myocardial dysfunction as well as the response of equine myocardium to various exercise regimes. Comparison of hscTnT analyte levels (measured on the Roche Diagnostics hscTnT assay) and cTnI analyte levels (measured on the the iSTAT[4]) in purified equine cardiac troponin samples, using a Deming regression, showed excellent correlation. Of note, a Blant-Altman graph represents a bias plot and was not used to compare the two assays as the numerical value of any bias between hsTnT and cTnI is not clinically interpretable when comparing the relative recoveries of these two entirely different molecules. As human laboratories trend toward only using'high-sensitivity' troponin assays, the manufacturing of older generation assays may discontinue.

While troponin assays' use continues to grow in veterinary fields clinicians must be aware that "all troponin assays are NOT created equal" [22]. In the thorough review by Rossi et al. the use of troponin I assays in horses, as well as their associated limitations and challenges, are highlighted [5]. The analysis and standardization for cTnT is beneficially more straightforward than for cTnI. All assays for cTnT are marketed by one manufacturer[1], and instruments are calibrated to the same reference material. It has been demonstrated that Roche's cTnT immunoassay detects binary (cTnT-I and cTnT-C), ternary complexes (cTnT-I-C) of troponin, and the free-cTnT form, as well as capably measures cTnT degradation by-products and phosphorylated-cTnT in circulation [23]. Therefore, cTnT degradation does not affect harmonization between different assays as previously reported for the cTnI assays [24]. The effect of EDTA in the cTnT assay seems to be minimal, whereas differences between serum and plasma values have been reported for a number of cTnI methods [4]. In human patient samples, cTnT appears to be very stable at room temperature, 4 °C, and when repeatedly frozen and thawed [21]. Similarly our study demonstrated excellent stability of equine samples frozen, stored, and then thawed over various time periods.

A goal for any assay is to establish decision thresholds to distinguish among different groups. In human medicine, an algorithm has been agreed upon to differentiate healthy individuals from those suffering an AMI that includes the use of cTn assays but importantly includes other criteria such as presence of clinical signs, and other diagnostic imaging findings. Furthermore it recommends obtaining individuals' cTn levels at a second time point to increase the specificity of the assay and promotes the use a delta cut-off instead of single diagnostic cut-off value [25]. Other factors, such as exercise exposure, must be considered when interpreting the results of individual hscTnT analyte levels. This will be particularly relevant when this assay is to be used on performance horses, and thereby warrants further study into the kinetics of hscTnT in the exercising horse.

Utilizing the ROC curve method, a calculated hscTnT 6.6 ng/L cut-off point for distinguishing healthy horses from those with primary myocardial disease has been recently published using the same Roche hscTnT assay [7]. Applying this cut-off point to our two defined reference populations would imply 5 % of the Non-Competition, and 22 % of the Racing-Thoroughbreds would be classified as having primary myocardial disease. This interpretation is unlikely, and indicates caution must be used when applying this cut-off point to various horse populations. The discrepancy may be partly explained by the inclusion of only 20 healthy horses in the reference population described by Van Der Vekens et al. [7], as compared to our N = 125 Non-Competition and N = 178 Racing-Thoroughbred reference populations. Including a minimum of 120 horses in each of our groups provided populations for which reference intervals could be defined by statistical methods in compliance with ASCVP guidelines and provide better whole population normal hscTnT level estimations. The use of only 20 horses in the reference population used by Van Der Vekens et. al. [7] led to a "tight" reference range, and significant overlap between their normal group and those classified with primary myocardial disease. Their low cut-off point was necessary to maintain acceptable sensitivity of the assay, enabling it to distinguish between their two groups, but is at the expense of possibly misclassifying an unacceptably high number of healthy horses as diseased. Their healthy horse group is most likely more similar to our Non-Competition group of horses (than our Racing-Thoroughbred group), but the authors did not describe the use or fitness status of the members of this group in which 10/35 were Trotters that may have been in training or racing. Regardless, a hscTnT 6.6 ng/L cut-off point differentiating healthy from those with primary myocardial is likely more appropriately applied to relatively sedentary horses rather than racing populations. Future studies may be warranted to determine cardiac troponin cut-off points specific to racing horses.

The inclusion of only two case studies in our study is few, but nevertheless demonstrate applications of the hscTnT assay unique to those recently presented [7]. In case one we report an adult Thoroughbred racing gelding that presented for near collapse event, distress, clinical signs of hypoxia (cyanosis), cardiac abnormalities identified on auscultation and ECG, and subsequently abnormally high levels of hscTnT. The later over-the-ground dynamic endoscopic confirmation of severe epiglottic retroversion with a subepiglottic cyst and dorsal displacement of the soft palate suggests a possible association between the clinical presentation of impaired gas exchange and cardiac function as documented by elevations in the myocardial biomarker hscTnT. We do however acknowledge that a cardiac ultrasonographic assessment is missing, which limited the full characterization of his cardiac status and the ability to determine the complete etiology of his presentation. The elevated value detected 72 h later demonstrates persistence of the biomarker cTnT further emphasizing its clinical utility, as the practitioner can take samples at time points slightly past onset of acute condition without missing the opportunity to detect myocardial insult. Case two demonstrates a severe, multi-organ system dysfunction likely related to SIRS and endotoxemia associated with Potomac horse fever. Increases in cardiac troponin have been previously reported in experimentally-induced endotoxemia [9]. The diagnosis of myocardial function impairment in this case was based on clinical presentation, ECG monitoring, hscTnT levels, and post-mortem evaluation but may have been strengthened by completion of cardiac ultrasonography. Case two exemplifies the level to which hscTnT may be seen clinically (5723 ng/L in this case as compared to the highest level of 1341 ng/L recorded by the Van de Vekens group in a horse with primary myocardial disease) [7]. Despite the fact that our linearity experiment showed the assay has slight over-recovery of the hscTnT analyte > 391 ng/L value, tracking the trend over time in severely elevated values in cases such as this would be of interest to the clinician with respect to case management and prognosis [11].

Additional limitations of our study include the abbreviated resting-ECG (2 min) on all horses included in the two reference populations, as well as the absence of cardiac ultrasonography. These methods reflect field-study condition constraints. More thorough screening may have further identified individuals that were inappropriate for study inclusion as "healthy horses". Our total samples numbers included, and the absence of significant outliers suggest however that the reference populations appropriately reflect more generalized healthy populations.

Conclusions

In conclusion, this report has validated, according to the rigorous recommendations of the CLSI, the only'high-sensitivity' troponin assay (Roche hscTnT, Cobas-e601) for use in horses. The current literature is lacking many of the validation experiments conducted in our study, and thus the data published here significantly adds to the conclusions of Van der Vekens et al. [6, 20]. In our study reference intervals for the hscTn-T assay in healthy adult Non-Competition and Racing Thoroughbred horses were established, as were assay performance characteristics, and sample collection protocols in equine plasma samples. While the assay remains insufficiently sensitive to provide biological variation information in mainly sedentary healthy horses at this time, it will prove extremely useful for assessment of subtle myocardial injury as well as the effects of exercise on equine myocardium.

Endnotes

[2]Cobas-e601, Roche Diagnostics, Indianapolis, IN.

[3]Elecsys diluent multi-assay, Roche Diagnostics, Indianapolis, IN.

[5]Televet-100, Engel Engineering, Offenbach, Germany.

[4]iSTAT-2, Heska Corp, Loveland, CO.

[1]Troponin-T hs, Roche Diagnostics, Indianapolis, IN.

Abbreviations

AMI, acute myocardial injury; ASVCP, American Society of Veterinary Clinical Pathology; Bpm, beats per minute; CI, confidence interval; CLSI, Clinical and Laboratory Standards Institute; cTn-I, cardiac Troponin-I; cTnT, cardiac Troponin-T; CV, coefficient of variation; ECG, electrocardiogram; EDTA, Ethylenediaminetetraacetic acid; hscTnT, high-sensitivity cardiac Troponin-T; L1, level 1; L2, level 2; L3, level 3; LoD, limit of detection; LoQ, limit of quantitation; NACB, National Academy of Clinical Biochemistry; PCR, polymerase chain reaction; RCVs, reference change values; ROC, receiver operating characteristic; SIRS, systemic inflammatory response syndrome; URL, upper reference limit; WBC, white blood cell

Acknowledgements

The authors thank contributing owners and Glennis Doiron and the CLS collaborators for technical assistance.

Funding
Funded by the University of Calgary, Faculty of Veterinary Medicine, Clinical Research Fund.

Authors' contributions
ES carried out the study design, data collection, data analysis, and drafting of the manuscript. SM contributed to data collection and data analysis. SP participated in data collection. IL and RL carried out the design of the study, data analysis and drafting of the manuscript. All authors read and approved the final manuscript.

Authors' information
ES: HBSc., DC, DVM, ACVMR (Sports Medicine and Rehabilitation)—Equine Resident UCVM/Moore Equine Veterinary Centre,
IL: PhD, DCC, FCACB, DABCC—Clinical Assistant Professor, Clinical Biochemist, CLS. Program Director, Clinical Biochemistry Fellowship Program. Department of Pathology & Laboratory Medicine.
RL: MSc., PhD, DMV, Dipl. ACVIM, Dipl. ACVSMR (Sports Medicine and Rehabilitation)—Associate Professor UCVM.

Competing interests
The authors declare that they have no competing interest.

Consent to publish
Not applicable.

Author details
[1]University of Calgary Faculty of Veterinary Medicine (UCVM), 3330 Hospital Dr. NW, Calgary T2N 4 N1, AB, Canada. [2]Foothills Medical Centre, University of Calgary Faculty of Medicine and Calgary Lab Services (CLS), Room C618B, 1403-29th St. NW, Calgary T2N 2 T9, AB, Canada.

References

1. Reef VB, Bonagura J, Buhl R, Mcgurrin MK, Schwarzwald CC, van Loon G, et al. Recommendations for management of equine athletes with cardiovascular abnormalities. J Vet Intern Med. 2014;28(3):749–61.
2. Katrukha IA. Human cardiac troponin complex. Structure and functions. Biochem Biokhimiia. 2013;78(13):1447–65.
3. Thygesen K, Alpert JS, Jaffe AS, Simoons ML, Chaitman BR, White HD, et al. Writing group on the joint ESC/ACCF/AHA/WHF: third universal definition of myocardial infarction. Eur Heart J. 2012;33(20):2551–67.
4. Apple FS, Collinson PO. Biomarkers ITFoCAoC: analytical characteristics of high-sensitivity cardiac troponin assays. Clin Chem. 2012;58(1):54–61.
5. Rossi TM, Pyle WG, Maxie MG, Pearl DL, Physick-Sheard PW. Troponin assays in the assessment of the equine myocardium. Equine Vet J. 2014;46(3):270–5.
6. Van Der Vekens N, van Dievoet MA, De Puydt H, Decloedt A, Ven S, De Clercq D, et al. Analytical validation of a high-sensitivity cardiac troponin T assay in horses. J Vet Diagn Inves. 2015;27(4):504–9.
7. Van Der Vekens N, Decloedt A, Ven S, De Clercq D, van Loon G. Cardiac troponin I as compared to troponin T for the detection of myocardial damage in horses. J Vet Intern Med. 2015;29(1):348–54.
8. Slack J, Boston R, Soma L, Reef V. Cardiac troponin I in Racing Standardbreds. J Vet Intern Med. 2012;26(5):1202-8.
9. Nostell K, Brojer J, Hoglund K, Edner A, Haggstrom J. Cardiac troponin I and the occurrence of cardiac arrhythmias in horses with experimentally induced endotoxaemia. Vet J. 2012;192(2):171–5.
10. Kraus MS, Jesty SA, Gelzer AR, Ducharme NG, Mohammed HO, Mitchell LM, et al. Measurement of plasma cardiac troponin I concentration by use of a point-of-care analyzer in clinically normal horses and horses with experimentally induced cardiac disease. Am J Vet Res. 2010;71(1):55–9.
11. Nath LC, Anderson GA, Hinchcliff KW, Savage CJ. Serum cardiac troponin I concentrations in horses with cardiac disease. Aust Vet J. 2012;90(9):351–7.
12. Trachsel DS, Schwarzwald CC, Bitschnau C, Grenacher B, Weishaupt MA. Atrial natriuretic peptide and cardiac troponin I concentrations in healthy warmblood horses and in warmblood horses with mitral regurgitation at rest and after exercise. J V Cardiol. 2013;15(2):105–21.
13. Shields E, Passante S, Massie S, Seiden-Long I, Leguillette R. Validation of a novel high-sensitivity cardiac troponin-T assay in horses. Equine Vet J. 2014;46(S46):25–5.
14. Defining, Establishing, and Verifying Reference Intervals in the Clinical Laboratory; Approved Guideline-3rd Ed.. Clinical and Laboratory Standards Institute. 2012. http://clsi.org/standards/documents-for-public-review/. Accessed 03 Dec 2015.
15. Evaluation of Detection Capability for Clinical Laboratory Measurement Procedures; Approved Guideline-2nd Ed.. Clinical and Laboratory Standards Institute. 2012. http://clsi.org/standards/documents-for-public-review/. Accessed 03 Dec 2015.
16. Principles of quality assurance and standards for veterinary clinical pathology. American Society for Veterinary Clinical Pathology; 2009. http://www.asvcp.org/pubs/pdf/ASVCPQualityControlGuidelines.pdf. Accessed 03 Dec 2015.
17. Guidelines for determination of reference intervals in veterinary species and related topics. American Society of Veterinary Clinical Pathology Quality Assurance and Laboratory Standards Committee; 2011. https://www.asvcp.org/pubs/pdf/RI%20Guidelines%20For%20ASVCP%20website.pdf. Accessed 03 Dec 2015.
18. Potter JD. Preparation of troponin and its subunits. Methods Enzymol. 1982; 85:241–63.
19. O'Brien PJ, Dameron GW, Beck ML, Brandt M. Differential reactivity of cardiac and skeletal muscle from various species in two generations of cardiac troponin-T immunoassays. Res Vet Sci. 1998;65(2):135–7.
20. Roy MF. Sepsis in adults and foals. Vet Clin North Am Equine Pract. 2004; 20(1):41–61.
21. Giannitsis E, Kurz K, Hallermayer K, Jarausch J, Jaffe AS, Katus HA. Analytical validation of a high-sensitivity cardiac troponin T assay. Clin Chem. 2010;56(2):254–61.
22. Christenson RH, Phillips D. Sensitive and high sensitivity next generation cardiac troponin assays: more than just a name. Pathology. 2011;43(3):213–9.
23. Cardinaels EP, Mingels AM, van Rooij T, Collinson PO, Prinzen FW, van Dieijen-Visser MP. Time-dependent degradation pattern of cardiac troponin T following myocardial infarction. Clin Chem. 2013;59(7):1083–90.
24. Vafaie M, Biener M, Mueller M, Schnabel PA, Andre F, Steen H, et al. Analytically false or true positive elevations of high sensitivity cardiac troponin: a systematic approach. Heart. 2014;100(6):508–14.
25. de Lemos JA. Increasingly sensitive assays for cardiac troponins: a review. JAMA. 2013;309(21):2262–9.

17

Serological evidence of equine arteritis virus infection and phylogenetic analysis of viral isolates in semen of stallions from Serbia

Sava Lazić[1], Diana Lupulović[1], Delphine Gaudaire[2], Tamas Petrovic[1], Gospava Lazić[1] and Aymeric Hans[2*]

Abstract

Background: Equine arteritis virus (EAV) is responsible for infections in equids. It can spread easily within the horse population and has a major impact on the horse breeding industry. No EAV outbreak has ever been reported in Serbia. To determine whether EAV is nonetheless circulating there, especially in the Vojvodina region, 340 horse serum samples were subjected to serology testing to detect EAV antibodies. In parallel, semen samples from three seropositive stallions were collected to evaluate their EAV status, using RT-qPCR and virus isolation on cell culture.

Results: Horse sera with EAV antibodies represented 15.88% (54/340) of the tested samples, 83.23% (283/340) being negative, and just three samples (0.89%) being uninterpretable due to cytotoxicity. Only 7.2% (10/138) of horses kept by private owners on their own property were seropositive for EAV, whereas 21.8% (44/202) of horses kept on stud farms had EAV antibodies. Phylogenetic analysis showed that the Serbian EAV isolate was most closely related to isolates from the neighbouring Hungary.

Conclusions: EAV is circulating in the Serbian horse population, especially among the breeding population certainly due to the use of EAV shedder stallions since there is no surveillance programme in Serbia and only limited checks on racehorses. Moreover, phylogenetic analysis indicates that the EAV isolated from a Lipizzaner stallion in Serbia is closely related to isolates from Hungary, and together form a new cluster.

Keywords: Horse, Equine arteritis virus, Epidemiology, Phylogeny, Serbia

Background

Equine arteritis virus (EAV), a member of the *Arteriviridae* family in the *Nidovirales* order [1], is the cause of an infectious disease affecting equids, including horses [2–4]. Phylogenetic analysis based on an ORF5 nucleotide sequence has grouped EAV strains into two clades: the North American group and the European group, itself divided into two subgroups named European subgroup-1 (EU-1) and European subgroup-2 (EU-2) [2]. EAV can be transmitted by respiratory or venereal routes. Although the majority of infections are subclinical, some infected animals can develop typical signs of the disease, i.e. fever up to 41 °C, depression, anorexia, oedema, nasal discharge and conjunctivitis. Young foals may lose weight and condition due to fulminating pneumonia with a lethal outcome [4]. The infection of a pregnant mare may lead to abortion, stillbirth or the delivery of a weak foal. Following primary infection, up to 70% of stallions may become persistently infected [4, 5]. Stallions shedding the virus in their semen are the reservoir of EAV and thus a key component of EAV epidemiology and transmission, since they can disseminate the virus among the horse population during breeding seasons [6].

Investigations conducted worldwide have revealed that EAV infection is present in North and South America, Europe, Australia, Africa and Asia [7–12]. Interestingly, a study performed in New Zealand concluded that there was no EVA in the New Zealand horse population [13]. The history of EVA in the Balkan region of Europe is

* Correspondence: aymeric.hans@anses.fr
[2]ANSES, Laboratory for Equine Diseases, Virology Unit, Dozulé, France
Full list of author information is available at the end of the article

unknown. Indeed, only one study has reported the characterisation of an EAV isolate from the semen of a Lipizzaner stallion imported in 1981 from former Yugoslavia [14].

The horse population in Serbia is estimated at around 16,000. Ten thousand horses are registered and live in Central Serbia and 6000 in Vojvodina Province, in the northern part of the country (*"Statistical Yearbook of the Republic of Serbia 2014"*, issued by the Statistical Office of the Republic of Serbia, abbreviation *STAT.YEARB.-SERB. 2014*). The horses are intended for racing, working, recreational riding and carriage rides, but there is also a trade in horsemeat. Currently, neither stallions nor their sperm are monitored, and there is no active plan to prevent EVA spreading among stallions and indeed the whole Serbian horse population. There is neither an EAV vaccination policy nor any registered vaccines in Serbia. The objective of our study was thus to investigate the circulation of EAV infection and complete the molecular characterisation of EAV isolated from the horse population registered in Serbia. To our knowledge, this is the first report of the genetic characterisation of an EAV isolate from a shedder stallion bred in Serbia.

Methods

Blood samples

Blood samples from 340 unvaccinated horses, including 168 mares and 172 stallions, were collected for serological examination from October 2013 to October 2014. Of these, 202 horses (94 mares and 108 stallions) were from nine stud farms and four riding schools, while 138 horses (74 mares and 64 stallions) were kept on the private property of their owners. The number of horses on any one stud farm or in any one riding school ranged from 20 to 100 and from 10 to 25 respectively. Private owners kept up to seven horses on their property. After collection, the samples were kept at −20 °C until testing.

The study encompassed different types and breeds: sport horses (English thoroughbreds or part-bred horses), Arabians, Lipizzaners, Standardbred horses, French Trotters, East Bulgarian sport horses, Hungarian sport horses, Holsteiners, Hanoverians, Koninklijk Warmbloed Paard Nederland (KWPNs), Haflingers, working horses (the Nonius, Gidran, Belgian or Bosnian Mountain horse), ponies for recreational riding and grade horses used for work or raised for the meat trade. The horses ranged in age from 1 to 26 years. None of the horses from which blood was collected showed any clinical signs of the disease at the time of sampling.

Serological examination by virus neutralisation test (VNT)

All sera samples were tested for the presence of anti-EAV antibodies by the virus neutralisation test (VNT) in accordance with chapter 2.5.10 of the OIE *Manual of Diagnostic Tests and Vaccines for Terrestrial Animals* (OIE, 2015). Briefly, serial two-fold dilutions of heat-inactivated sera from 1:2 to 1:256 were made in 96-well flat-bottom plates using Minimum Essential Media (MEM). Subsequently, an equal volume of the working dilution of stock virus with 30 to 300 tissue culture infective doses ($TCID_{50}$) of EAV Bucyrus strain (ATCC VR - 796) was added to the plates and incubated for 1 h at 37 °C. After incubation, 100 μl of cell suspension containing about 200,000 cells/ml of RK-13 (ATCC CCL - 37) in MEM with 10% foetal calf serum was added to each well. Duplicate positive and negative serum controls were included in the assay, as were controls for serum cytotoxicity, cell viability and viral infectivity. After 72 h of incubation at 37 °C in a humid atmosphere with 5% CO_2, the cytopathic effect (CPE) was checked under a microscope. Sera with a titre of 1:4 or higher were considered positive. Cytotoxic sera were retested using a one-day-old monolayer of RK-13 cells.

Semen samples

During this study, 17 semen samples from three Lipizzaner stallions bred in Vojvodina Province were collected using an artificial vagina as described by Lazic et al. [15]. Four of the 11 PCR-positive semen samples were subjected to sequencing.

Viral RNA extraction and polymerase chain reaction

RNA was extracted from the semen as described previously [16]. The eluted RNA was analysed by RT-qPCR targeting a portion of the EAV nucleoprotein (N) gene as described by Balasuriya et al. [17]. RNA from positive samples was reverse transcribed into cDNA using a SuperScript III kit (Invitrogen Corporation, Carlsbad, California, USA). The ORF5 (nucleotides 11,085–11,944 from GenBank accession number DQ846750) PCR amplification from 2.5 μl of cDNA products was performed using the PCR extender system—a kit including a high fidelity enzyme with proofreading activity (5Prime GmbH, Hamburg, Germany)—with primers 5′-TACCGCTTGGTTTTGTGGCTAT-3′ and 5′-TCACCTAAAATCCCGTCACC-3′. During the first cycle, samples were incubated at 94 °C for 2 min followed by 35 - cycles under the following conditions: 94 °C for 20 s, 55 °C for 20 s, 72 °C for 2 min. The program ended with one cycle at 72 °C for 10 min.

Sequencing and phylogenetic analyses

A total of four ORF5 PCR amplified products were sequenced (Beckman Coulter Genomics) using Applied Biosystems BigDye version 3.1. The sequences were assembled using software Ridom TraceEditPro 1.2.2., then compared to other EAV sequences using a BLAST web-based program (http://www.ncbi.nlm.nih.gov/BLAST). Nucleotide sequences were aligned in keeping with the Clustal W method. The phylogenetic trees were constructed using the Maximum Likelihood method and the tree's statistical robustness was assessed by bootstrap resampling (1000 datasets) of the multiple alignments. Phylogenetic reconstruction was carried out using MEGA software version 5.1. [18]. The sequence described in the article was submitted to GenBank and registered under accession number KX 645659.

Virus isolation

EAV was isolated from semen samples using an RK-13 cell line in accordance with chapter 2.5.10 of the OIE *Manual of Diagnostic Tests and Vaccines for Terrestrial Animals* (OIE, 2015). Briefly, serial ten-fold dilutions (10^{-1}–10^{-3}) from 1 ml of the seminal plasma were prepared in MEM, and 1 ml of each dilution was inoculated into each of two 25 cm^2 flasks containing confluent monolayers of 3-day-old RK-13 cells. Flasks were incubated at 37 °C for 1 h then 9 ml of medium containing 0.75% carboxymethyl cellulose (CMC) was added. Flasks were checked for the appearance of any CPE on day 4 post inoculation using a 1% crystal violet solution to stain the cell monolayer. When no CPEs were detectable, a second passage was performed using new RK-13 monolayers with 1 ml of supernatant from the first passage as the inoculum and incubated for an additional 4 days.

Statistical analysis

Statistical analyses were performed with Statistica 12 (StatSoft Inc., Dell). Differences in seropositivity between males and females; sport horses and privately-kept horses; and between breeds were calculated using the Chi-square test. A *p*-value less than 0.05 ($p < 0.05$) was considered statistically significant.

Results

Serological results

Horse serum samples were collected mainly from horses in the Vojvodina Province (northern part of Serbia), though a few were from horses in the cities of Belgrade and Požarevac in Central Serbia. The survey covered 37 locations in 21 municipalities (Fig. 1).

This study revealed that the overall percentage of EAV-seropositive horses tested was 15.88% (54/340), 83.23% (283/340) being negative. Only three samples (0.89%) were found to be cytotoxic. The antibody titres of the 54 positive sera detected ranged from 1:4 to over 1:512. The majority of animals, i.e. 70.37% (38/54) had an antibody titre value between 1:4 and 1:64, while 27.78% (15/54) reacted positively with a titre value over 1:96. Just one horse had an antibody titre higher than 1:512 (1.85%, 1/54). The population tested was composed of 168 mares and 172 stallions. The EAV seropositivity rate reached 18.45% (31/168) in mares with antibody titres from 1:4 to ≥1:512. A smaller percentage of stallions—13.37% (23/172)—were positive for

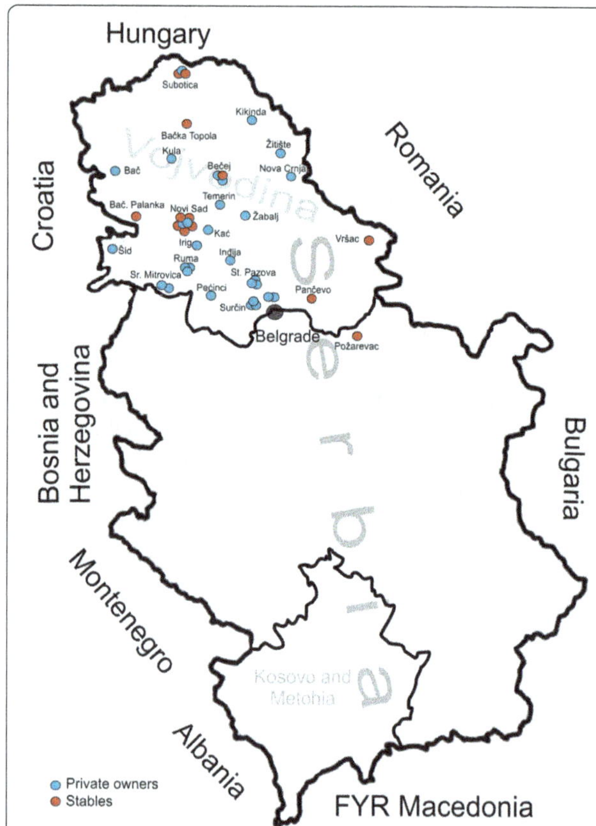

Fig. 1 Localities of the Vojvodina region from which horse serum samples were collected

EAV with antibody titres as high as 1:384. The seropositivity rate according to age category was evaluated by first dividing the equids up into three age groups. Seropositivity was seen to steadily increase with age, rising from 3.03% for younger horses (≤ 5 years old) to 34.21% for horses above 11 years old. Horses between 6 and 11 years of age had a seropositivity rate of 15.15%. These differences between the three age groups were statistically significant ($p < 0.05$).

Serological tests performed on the 202 horses bred and kept on nine stud farms or in four riding schools showed that 21.8% (44/202) were seropositive for EAV (Table 1). However, of the 13 professional structures analysed, only nos. 7, 11 and 12 had no EAV-seropositive horses. Two of these structures were riding schools and one was a stud farm breeding sport horses. Conversely, 20 out of 32 (62.5%) horses were positive for EAV on stud farm no. 6, specialising in the Lipizzaner breed (Table 1). Of seven stallions tested in stud farm no. 6, four were seropositive.

The percentage of EAV-seropositive equids according to the different breeds or types studied were as follows: 66.8% of ponies, 39.7% of Lipizzaners, 12.8% of sport horses and 9.1% of Nonius horses. Differences between breeds or types were statistically different ($p < 0.05$) The same analysis performed on samples from 138 horses kept by private owners

Table 1 Serological results of the virus neutralisation test (VNT) for equids kept in professional structures (stud farms or riding schools)

Stud farms and riding schools	Type/Breed	No. of horses tested	Positive (%)	Negative (%)	Uninterpretable (%)
1	Sport	22	2 (9.1%)	20 (90.9%)	0 (0.0%)
2	Lipizzaner	10	1 (10.0%)	9 (90.0%)	0 (0.0%)
3	Sport	24	1 (4.2%)	22 (91.6%)	1 (4.2%)
4	Sport	10	1 (10.0%)	9 (90.0%)	0 (0.0%)
5	Sport, Nonius, Lipizzaner	24	4 (16.7%)	20 (83.3%)	0 (0.0%)
6	Lipizzaner	32	20 (62.5%)	12 (37.5%)	0 (0.0%)
7	Sport	20	0 (0.0%)	20 (100.0%)	0 (0.0%)
8	Sport, Pony	17	7 (41.2%)	9 (52.9%)	1 (5.9%)
9	Lipizzaner	11	2 (18.2%)	9 (81.8%)	0 (0.0%)
10	Sport	12	3 (25.0%)	9 (75.0%)	0 (0.0%)
11	Sport, Nonius	7	0 (0.0%)	7 (100.0%)	0 (0.0%)
12	Sport	7	0 (0.0%)	7 (100.0%)	0 (0.0%)
13	Sport	6	3 (50.0%)	3 (50.0%)	0 (0.0%)
Total	/	202	44 (21.8%)	158 (77.2%)	2 (1.0%)

on their own property showed that only 7.2% of horses were positive for EAV according to the VNT results (Table 2). Again, this difference was statistically significant ($p < 0.05$). Of all the tested equids kept on their owner's private property, sport horses had the highest percentage of seropositive samples (28.57%). There were no positive results among Nonius horses, ponies, Belgian or Posavian working horses kept on their owner's property (Table 2).

The highest number of seropositive horses was reported in Subotica, a municipality near the Hungarian border, followed by Novi Sad in the central part of the Vojvodina region and Vršac municipality near the Romanian border. The lowest number of seropositive horses was detected in the municipalities of Požarevac, Irig, Bačka Palanka, Ruma, Bečej and Nova Crnja (Fig. 2).

Virus detection and genotyping

Seventeen semen samples in all from three seropositive stallions were collected between 2013 and 2014. Eleven of these samples were positive for EAV by RT-qPCR. Two out of the three stallions were shedding EAV in their semen. Unfortunately, viruses could not be isolated and amplified on RK-13 cells, probably due to the delay between the collection date and the freezing date. An attempt was therefore made at sequencing viral RNA directly extracted from the semen of shedder stallions. The virus was genotyped by sequencing a 518-nucleotide portion of ORF5 encoding the virus's GP 5. Phylogenetic analysis on this ORF5 sequence and the 145 EAV sequences retrieved from GenBank showed that the Serbian isolate, KX 645659 EAV-SER1, clusters with EAV strains isolated in Hungary [19] (Fig. 3).

Discussion

The goals of this study were to evaluate the presence of EAV in the Serbian horse population, especially in the northern part (Vojvodina Province) as well as in Belgrade and Požarevac cities (Central Serbia), and to genotype virus from unvaccinated stallions. Indeed, no EAV vaccines are either registered or used by practitioners

Table 2 Serological results of the virus neutralisation test (VNT) for equids kept by private owners on their own property

Private property	No. of private owners	Type/Breed	No. of horses tested	Positive (%)	Negative (%)	Cytotoxic (%)
A	12	Mixed breed	59	2 (3.39%)	57 (96.61%)	0 (0.0%)
B	33	Lipizzaner	54	4 (7.41%)	49 (90.74%)	1 (1.85%)
C	14	Sport	14	4 (28.57%)	10 (71.43%)	0 (0.0%)
D	3	Nonius	4	0 (0.00%)	4 (100.0%)	0 (0.0%)
E	3	Pony	3	0 (0.0%)	3 (100.0%)	0 (0.0%)
F	1	Posavian horse	3	0 (0.0%)	3 (100.0%)	0 (0.0%)
G	1	Belgian horse	1	0 (0.0%)	1 (100.0%)	0 (0.0%)
Total	67	/	138	10 (7.2%)	127 (92.0%)	1 (0.8%)

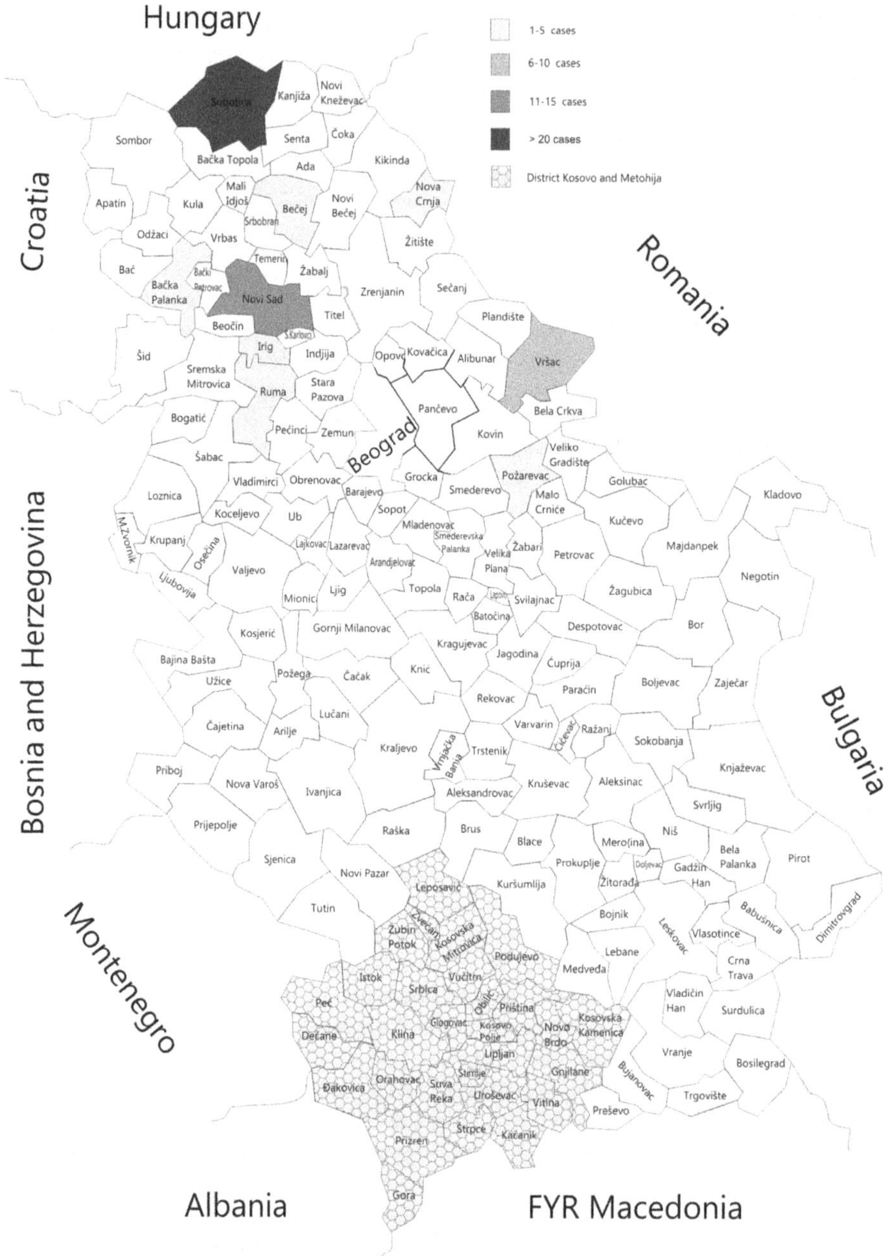

Fig. 2 Serological results of the virus neutralisation test for EAV in horses living in Serbian municipalities

in Serbia. Although some evidence of EAV circulation in the Serbian horse population has been published in the past few years [15], no viral description has ever been published to date.

Our study revealed that 15.88% (54/340) of the unvaccinated Serbian horses tested had EAV antibodies. This percentage of seropositive animals is in accordance with reports from other European countries where the percentage of positive horses ranged from 11.3% to 20% [20–25]. Moreover, our data indicate that mares were more likely to be positive for EAV than were stallions (18.45% vs 13.37%), although the difference was not statistically significant.

In our survey, the seropositivity rate increased with the age of tested equids, reaching 34.21% in the older population (>11 years old). These results confirm that EAV has been circulating in the Serbian horse population for several years and are in accordance with the investigations conducted in France, Poland, Spain, Algeria, Slovenia and Bulgaria that have also described a higher seropositivity rate in older horses [11, 20, 25–27]. This may be related to the re-infection of horses during their

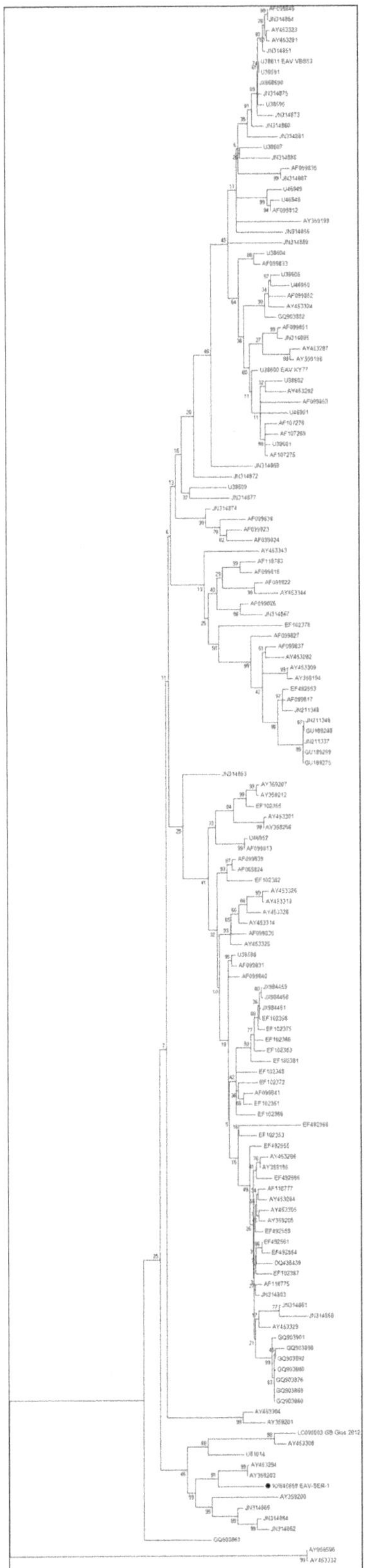

Fig. 3 Phylogenetic analysis of the ORF5 sequences (518 nucleotides) encoded by EAV. The Serbian isolate, KX 645659 EAV-SER1, clusters with EAV strains isolated in Hungary. A Maximum Likelihood tree was created using MEGA 5 [18]. The analysis involved 147 nucleotide sequences retrieved from GenBank. The percentage of trees in which the associated taxa clustered together is shown next to the branches

lifetime [2]. Young horses not used for breeding may be infected by the respiratory route after contact with diseased horses within the same stable [11, 14].

The percentage of seropositive horses found in professional structures such as stud farms or riding schools, varies from 0% to 62.5%. This result can be explained by various management factors and uncontrolled mating. Indeed, other studies have reported that management efficacy and control over reproduction have a crucial impact on viral transmission [25, 27]. Interestingly, a mean of 21.9% of horses kept on stud farms were seropositive for EAV compared to 7.2% of horses kept by private owners on their own property. These results indicate that EAV appears to be less prevalent in that part of the Serbian horse population not used for breeding purposes. EAV infections in the latter population thus appear most likely to occur via the respiratory route following direct contact with infected horses. In Serbia, horses kept on stud farms are used for in-hand breeding only, since artificial insemination has not yet been implemented in the country. Moreover, the semen of stallions used for reproduction in Serbia is not tested for any sexually transmitted disease such as EAV. Stallions shedding EAV in their semen may therefore transmit the virus to mares during mating and those covered mares are likely to transmit the virus to other horses in the stable by the respiratory route following direct contact. Our data indicate that the risk to the breeding population of contracting EAV is higher than the risk to horses kept by their owners on private property, reinforcing the importance of good practice as well as a strict application of health measures when managing horse breeding on stud farms.

Interestingly, the EAV isolate obtained from a Lipizzaner stallion appeared to differ from those available in GenBank. However, this Serbian isolate—KX 645659 EAV-SER1is closely related to a virus isolated in the neighbouring Hungary [19]. Moreover, our phylogenetic analysis showed that the latest strain described by Steinbach et al. [28] is also closely related to both a Hungarian strain [29] and a strain isolated in Kentucky, USA [30]. Taken together, the EAV strains described recently clustered together to form a new distinct group of viruses originating in the central European region.

Conclusions

This study is the first equine serological survey conducted in Serbia that encompasses data on type/breed, age, titre level and EAV geographical distribution. EAV is shown to be currently circulating in the Serbian horse population since 15.88% (54/340 tested animals) of the animals tested had EAV antibodies despite the fact that there are no registered vaccines and no vaccination policy in Serbia. Moreover, the sequence analyses and phylogenetic characterisation of EAV from a persistently infected stallion is also reported for the first time in Serbia. The isolate characterised here is closely related to the strain isolated in Hungary and, to a lesser extent, to the isolate described in 2015 by Steinbach et al. in the United Kingdom [28]. Moreover, these strains group together to form a new cluster.

Serbian authorities have not yet initiated a programme to control the spread of EAV within the horse population. Serological testing is basically carried out once a year in the case of racehorses; before an agricultural fair in the case of working horses; or on the owner's personal request, usually prior to mating. Clinical cases are neither registered nor declared to the competent authorities. There is furthermore a need to improve the cooperation of horse owners and veterinarians with official veterinary authorities in order to improve the reporting of actual or suspected cases of EAV and to clarify the epidemiology of the infection.

Our data show that horses used for breeding in Serbia are more likely to test positive for EAV than the rest of the horse population, probably due to the use of EAV shedder stallions. To prevent the further spread of EAV in the Serbian breeding horse population, it is essential to implement effective strategies and a surveillance programme to check the EAV carrier status of stallions.

Abbreviations

EAV: Equine arteritis virus; EU-1: European subgroup 1; EU-2: European subgroup 2; EVA: Equine Viral Arteritis; RT-qPCR: Reverse transcriptase quantitative polymerase chain reaction; VNT: Virus neutralisation test

Acknowledgements

The authors would like to thank official veterinary services in the field for conducting the epidemiological investigations and collecting samples from infected horses. We are also grateful to Delphine Libby-Claybrough, professional translator and native English speaker, for editorial assistance.

Funding

This study was supported by the Hubert Curien Partnerships (PHC-Pavle Savic), the European Reference Laboratory for Equine Diseases other than African Horse Sickness, ANSES's own institutional resources and the Ministry of Science and Technological Development of the Republic of Serbia (Grant no. TR31084). The funders had no role in study design, data collection and interpretation, or the decision to submit the work for publication.

Authors' contributions

SL participated in study design and coordination. DL performed experiments, assisted in study design and coordination and helped prepare the manuscript and figures. DG performed experiments and helped prepare the manuscript and figures. TP and GL performed experiments. AH conceived the study, participated in its design and coordination and edited the manuscript. All the authors read and approved the final manuscript.

Consent for publication

Not applicable.

Competing interests

The authors declare that they have no competing interests.

Author details

[1]Scientific Veterinary Institute "Novi Sad", Novi Sad, Serbia. [2]ANSES, Laboratory for Equine Diseases, Virology Unit, Dozulé, France.

References

1. Cavanagh D. Nidovirales: a new order comprising Coronaviridae and Arteriviridae. Arch Virol. 1997;142(3):629–33.
2. Balasuriya UB, Go YY, MacLachlan NJ. Equine arteritis virus. Vet Microbiol. 2013;167(1–2):93–122.
3. Stadejek T, Mittelholzer C, Oleksiewicz MB, Paweska J, Belak S. Highly diverse type of equine arteritis virus (EAV) from the semen of a south African donkey: short communication. Acta Vet Hung. 2006;54(2):263–70.
4. Timoney PJ, McCollum WH. Equine viral arteritis. Vet Clin North Am Equine Pract. 1993;9(2):295–309.
5. Timoney PJ, McCollum WH, Roberts AW, Murphy TW. Demonstration of the carrier state in naturally acquired equine arteritis virus infection in the stallion. Res Vet Sci. 1986;41(2):279–80.
6. Timoney PJ, McCollum WH. Equine viral arteritis: further characterization of the carrier state in stallions. J Reprod Fertil Suppl. 2000;56:3–11.
7. Hullinger PJ, Gardner IA, Hietala SK, Ferraro GL, MacLachlan NJ. Seroprevalence of antibodies against equine arteritis virus in horses residing in the United States and imported horses. J Am Vet Med Assoc. 2001;219(7):946–9.
8. Huntington PJ, Forman AJ, Ellis PM. The occurrence of equine arteritis virus in Australia. Aust Vet J. 1990;67(12):432–5.
9. Szeredi L, Hornyak A, Palfi V, Molnar T, Glavits R, Denes B. Study on the epidemiology of equine arteritis virus infection with different diagnostic techniques by investigating 96 cases of equine abortion in Hungary. Vet Microbiol. 2005;108(3–4):235–42.
10. Echeverria MG, Pecoraro MR, Galosi CM, Etcheverrigaray ME, Nosetto EO. The first isolation of equine arteritis virus in Argentina. Rev Sci Tech. 2003;22(3):1029–33.
11. Laabassi F, Amelot G, Laugier C, Zientara S, Nasri AM, Hans A. Prevalence of equine viral arteritis in Algeria. Rev Sci Tech. 2014;33(3):967–74.
12. Pagamjav O, Kobayashi K, Murakami H, Tabata Y, Miura Y, Boldbaatar B, Sentsui H. Serological survey of equine viral diseases in Mongolia. Microbiol Immunol. 2011;55(4):289–92.
13. McFadden AM, Pearce PV, Orr D, Nicoll K, Rawdon TG, Pharo H, Stone M. Evidence for absence of equine arteritis virus in the horse population of New Zealand. N Z Vet J. 2013;61(5):300–4.
14. Guthrie AJ, Howell PG, Hedges JF, Bosman AM, Balasuriya UB, McCollum WH, Timoney PJ, MacLachlan NJ. Lateral transmission of equine arteritis virus among Lipizzaner stallions in South Africa. Equine Vet J. 2003;35(6):596–600.
15. Lazic S, Lupulovic D, Vladimir P, Miroslav V, Lazic G, Enisa P, Petrovic T. Detection of equine arteritis virus in the semen of stallions in the republic of serbia. Acta Vet (Beogr). 2015;65(4):557–67.
16. Hans A, Gaudaire D, Manuguerra JC, Leon A, Gessain A, Laugier C, Berthet N, Zientara S. Combination of an unbiased amplification method and a resequencing microarray for detecting and genotyping equine arteritis virus. J Clin Microbiol. 2015;53(1):287–91.
17. Balasuriya UB, Leutenegger CM, Topol JB, McCollum WH, Timoney PJ, MacLachlan NJ. Detection of equine arteritis virus by real-time TaqMan reverse transcription-PCR assay. J Virol Methods. 2002;101(1–2):21–8.
18. Tamura K, Peterson D, Peterson N, Stecher G, Nei M, Kumar S. MEGA5: molecular evolutionary genetics analysis using maximum likelihood, evolutionary distance, and maximum parsimony methods. Mol Biol Evol. 2011;28(10):2731–9.
19. Hornyak A, Bakonyi T, Tekes G, Szeredi L, Rusvai M. A novel subgroup among genotypes of equine arteritis virus: genetic comparison of 40 strains. J Vet Med B Infect Dis Vet Public Health. 2005;52(3):112–8.
20. Moraillon A, Moraillon R. Results of an epidemiological investigation on viral arteritis in France and some other European and African countries. Ann Rech Vet. 1978;9(1):43–54.
21. de Boer GF, Osterhaus AD, van Oirschot JT, Wemmenhove R: Prevalence of antibodies to equine viruses in the Netherlands. Vet Q 1979, 1(2):65-74.

22. Glaser AL, de Vries AA, Rottier PJ, Horzinek MC, Colenbrander B. Equine arteritis virus: a review of clinical features and management aspects. Vet Q. 1996;18(3):95–9.
23. Kolbl S, Schuller W, Pabst J. Serological studies of the recent infections of Austrian horses with the equine arteritis virus. Dtsch Tierarztl Wochenschr. 1991;98(2):43–5.
24. Eichhorn W, Heilmann M, Kaaden OR. Equine viral arteritis with abortions: serological and virological evidence in Germany. Zentralbl Veterinarmed B. 1995;42(9):573–6.
25. Cruz F, Fores P, Mughini-Gras L, Ireland J, Moreno MA, Newton R. Seroprevalence and factors associated with seropositivity to equine arteritis virus in Spanish purebred horses in Spain. Equine Vet J. 2016;48(5):573–7.
26. Rola J, Larska M, Rola JG, Belak S, Autorino GL. Epizotiology and phylogeny of equine arteritis virus in hucul horses. Vet Microbiol. 2011;148(2–4):402–7.
27. Hostnik P, Mankoč S, Toplak I, Klobučar I, Malovrh T, Grom J. Control of equine arteritis virus (EAV) on stud farm. Veterinarski Arhiv. 2011;81(2):175–86.
28. Steinbach F, Westcott DG, McGowan SL, Grierson SS, Frossard JP, Choudhury B. Re-emergence of a genetic outlier strain of equine arteritis virus: impact on phylogeny. Virus Res. 2015;202:144–50.
29. Mittelholzer C, Stadejek T, Johansson I, Baule C, Ciabatti I, Hannant D, Paton D, Autorino GL, Nowotny N, Belak S. Extended phylogeny of equine arteritis virus: division into new subgroups. J Vet Med B Infect Dis Vet Public Health. 2006;53(2):55–8.
30. Balasuriya UB, Timoney PJ, McCollum WH, MacLachlan NJ. Phylogenetic analysis of open reading frame 5 of field isolates of equine arteritis virus and identification of conserved and nonconserved regions in the GL envelope glycoprotein. Virology. 1995;214(2):690–7.

The influence of hay steaming on clinical signs and airway immune response in severe asthmatic horses

Marie Orard[1,2], Erika Hue[1,2], Anne Courouce[3], Céline Bizon-Mercier[3], Marie-Pierre Toquet[1,2], Meriel Moore-Colyer[4], Laurent Couëtil[5], Stéphane Pronost[1,2], Romain Paillot[1,2], Magali Demoor[2] and Eric A. Richard[1,2*]

Abstract

Background: Avoidance of antigenic stimuli was found to significantly reverse airway obstruction of horses with severe equine asthma (sEA). To date, no published study investigated the influence of steaming hay on lower airway condition of sEA-affected horses. The objectives were to determine the clinical, cytological and cytokine respiratory responses of both sEA and control (CTL) horses experimentally exposed to steamed or dry hay.

Results: A cohort of 6 sEA horses and 6 CTL horses was involved in this field study. On day 0, both groups were fed with steamed hay for 5 consecutive days, followed by a wash-out period of 26 days prior to be fed with dry hay for 5 consecutive days. Investigations performed 2 days prior to and 5 days after each challenge included clinical score, tracheal mucus accumulation, and bronchoalveolar lavage fluid (BALF) cytology and cytokine mRNA expression. Feeding steamed hay significantly decreased its mould content ($P < 0.001$). Mucus score significantly increased when feeding dry hay ($P = 0.01$). No significant influence of challenge type was found on clinical score. Percentages of neutrophils ($P < 0.001$) as well as mRNA expression of IL-1β ($P = 0.024$), IL-6R ($P = 0.021$), IL-18 ($P = 0.009$) and IL-23 ($P = 0.036$) in BALF of sEA affected horses were significantly increased after both (steamed and dry hay) challenges. Relative mRNA expression of IL-1β, IL-6R and IL-23 in BALF were also significantly correlated to neutrophil percentages and both clinical and tracheal mucus score.

Conclusions: Steaming significantly decreased mould content but inconsistently influenced the respiratory response of sEA affected horses when fed hay. Based on BALF cytology and cytokine profiles, its relevance might be controversial as a non-medicinal therapy for sEA-affected horses.

Keywords: Equine asthma, Hay steaming, Inflammation, Cytology, Cytokines

Background

Severe equine asthma (sEA; previously known as recurrent airway obstruction) is a chronic disease of adult horses characterised by frequent coughing and increased respiratory effort at rest, as well as marked lower airway inflammation and reversible airway obstruction [1]. While neutrophils involvement in the pathophysiology of this disease is well defined, controversies still persist in terms of T-helper (Th)-1 and/or Th-2 polarisation, as determined by cytokines mRNA expression in BALF-derived cells [2, 3]. Involvement of Th-17 pathway [4, 5] and regulatory T cells (Treg; [6]) have also been suggested. Exposure to airborne environmental antigens is central in both initiation and maintenance of the disease, especially through stabling and exposure to hay and straw [7]. Feeding mouldy hay indeed represents a long-established model for sEA exacerbation in susceptible horses [2], and also allows differentiation from mild/moderate equine asthma (mEA; previously known as inflammatory airway disease) [3]. Inhalation challenges with aqueous mould extracts were previously found to induce neutrophilic inflammation in sEA affected horses but not in controls [8]. Results from experimental exposure of sEA affected

* Correspondence: eric.richard@laboratoire-labeo.fr
[1]LABÉO Frank Duncombe, Caen, France
[2]Normandie Université, UniCaen, BIOTARGEN, Caen, France
Full list of author information is available at the end of the article

horses to hay dust suspensions highlighted the synergistic effect of endotoxins and other dust components [9].

Environmental change, especially pasture turnout, with or without anti-inflammatory medication was found to significantly reverse airway obstruction of sEA affected horses [10]. On the other hand, corticosteroid therapy while maintaining the horse in a dusty environment leads to improved clinical signs and lung function but persistent airway inflammation [11, 12]. Feeding haylage and bedding wood shavings have been associated with significantly lower levels of both respirable dust (< 5 μm diameter) and endotoxins, within the horse's breathing zone, when compared to hay/straw environment [13, 14]. Alternatively, soaking and high-temperature steaming of hay for 16 h and 50 min respectively, significantly reduced respirable particles exposure; however endotoxin levels were not investigated [15, 16]. Steaming was also found to be effective at reducing mould content in hay, unlike soaking hay for 9 h [17]. Steaming hay indeed aims to reach and uniformly diffuse a temperature of 100 °C within the hay bale. To date, there is no published study that has investigated the potential influence of steaming hay on lower airway inflammation of sEA-affected horses.

The aim of the study was to determine clinical, cytological and cytokine respiratory responses of both sEA and control (CTL) horses experimentally exposed to steamed or dry hay. Our hypothesis was that feeding sEA affected horses with dry hay will result in higher respirable dust exposure, airway inflammation and clinical signs, as compared to feeding high-temperature steamed hay. Steaming hay indeed significantly decreased mould content but inconsistently influenced the respiratory response of sEA-affected horses. Both cytological and cytokine profiles actually revealed a significant airway inflammation when feeding hay (steamed or not).

Results

One sEA horse exhibited fever during the wash-out period and was subsequently excluded from the study. In the end, 5 sEA horses and 6 CTL horses completed both challenges (Additional file 1).

Hay and air sampling

Both bacterial and mould content were significantly lower ($P < 0.001$) in steamed hay (195 280 ± 465 270 and 1 507 ± 1 864 CFU/g, respectively), when compared to dry hay (4 042 000 ± 6 748 619 and 118 150 ± 187 624 CFU/g, respectively; Additional file 2). *Aspergillus* family (principally *A. glaucus* and *A. nidulens*) was identified in 9/10 samples of dry hay and 10/10 samples of steamed hay; *Aspergillus fumigatus* has been identified in one sample of dry hay only. Similarly, *Penicillium* spp. was identified in 3/10 samples of dry hay and 1/10 samples of steamed hay. Concentrations of respirable dust collected within the breathing zones (CTL and sEA horse) were 0.0015 and 0.0034 mg/m^3, respectively, during challenge #1 (steamed hay) vs. 0.0024 and 0.0057 mg/m^3 during challenge #2 (dry hay). Similarly, the inhalable fractions collected were 0.0045 and 0.0082 mg/m^3, respectively, during challenge #1 vs. 0.31 and 0.26 mg/m^3 during challenge #2. Endotoxin activities from respirable fraction were 0.08 and 0.98 EU/mL, respectively, during challenge #1, vs. 2.19 and 3.88 EU/mL during challenge #2. Levels of β-D-glucan were 340 and 1067 pg/mL, respectively, during challenge #1, vs. 895 and 2367 pg/mL during challenge #2.

Clinical score and tracheal mucus

Overall, the mean clinical scores were not significantly different between sEA and CTL horses ('disease status'; $P = 0.071$) and no significant influence on clinical scores was found for either 'challenge' or 'time' (Fig. 1), controlling for age. A significant interaction ($P = 0.049$) was found for clinical score between 'challenge' (steamed vs. dry hay) and 'time' (d + 5 vs. d-2); the post-hoc tests were however not significant for any further comparison. Mean mucus score was significantly higher ($P = 0.005$) for sEA horses when compared to CTL horses and overall significantly higher ($P = 0.024$) at d + 5 when compared to d-2 (Fig. 1). A significant interaction ($P = 0.022$) was also found for tracheal mucus between 'challenge' and 'time'; the score being significantly higher for dry hay at d + 5 when compared to d-2 ($P = 0.01$), but not significantly different between d + 5 and d-2 for steamed hay ($P = 0.98$).

BALF cytology

After controlling for age, no significant influence on the proportions of BALF volume recovered was found for either 'challenge', 'time' or 'disease status', nor any interaction between categories. Total cell counts were overall significantly higher ($P = 0.037$) for sEA compared to CTL horses (Additional file 3). The mean percentage of BALF neutrophils was significantly higher ($P = 0.011$) for sEA horses when compared to CTL horses and was overall significantly higher ($P < 0.001$) at d + 5 when compared to d-2 (Fig. 2), while no significant interaction was found between 'challenge' and 'time' ($P = 0.197$). The mean percentage of BALF lymphocytes was significantly lower ($P = 0.001$) at d + 5 when compared to d-2. A significant interaction ($P = 0.009$) was found between 'disease status' and 'time' for the percentage of BALF macrophages; the post-hoc tests being however not significant. The mean percentage of BALF metachromatic cells were significantly lower ($P = 0.001$) for sEA horses when compared to CTL horses (Additional file 3). No overall influence of the 'challenge' type (steamed vs. dry hay), or any interaction between 'challenge' and either

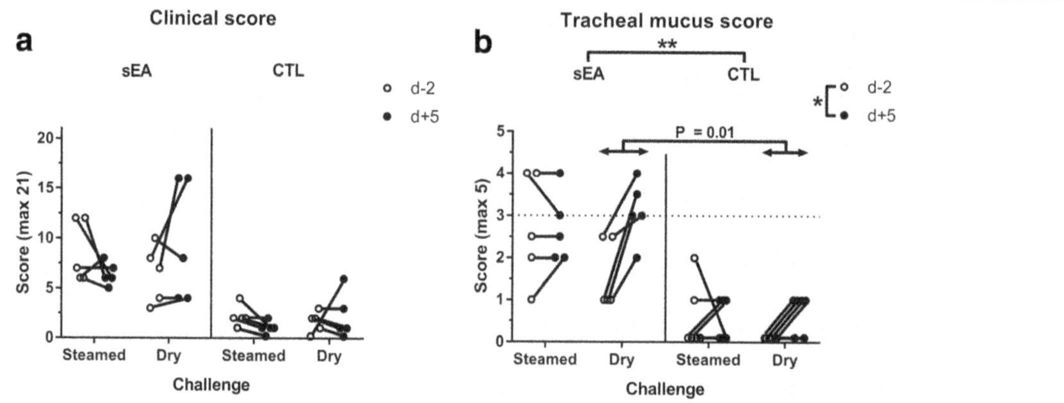

Fig. 1 **a** Clinical score and **b** tracheal mucus score, before and after the initiation of each challenge. sEA, severe equine asthma; CTL, control; d-2, 2 days before challenge; d + 5, 5 days after challenge. *, ** significant difference between groups ($P < 0.05$ and < 0.01), based on ANOVA investigation. Significant overall interactions ($P < 0.05$) were also found between 'challenge' (steamed, dry) and 'time' (d-2, d + 5); the p-value correspond to the subsequent Tukey-Kramer's post-hoc test

'time' or 'disease status' was found for any of the investigated cytological parameters.

BALF cytokines

After controlling for age, mean mRNA expression was significantly lower for IL-4 ($P = 0.022$) and significantly higher for IL-17 ($P < 0.001$) and TNF-α ($P = 0.006$) in BALF of sEA affected horses, when compared to CTL horses (Fig. 3). Overall mRNA expression of IL-10 was significantly higher ($P < 0.001$) at d + 5 when compared to d-2, irrespective of the horse disease status (Fig. 3). Significant interactions were found between 'disease status' and 'time' (higher at d + 5 than d-2 for sEA horses only) for relative mRNA expression of IL-1β ($P = 0.024$), IL-6R ($P = 0.021$), IL-18 ($P = 0.009$) and IL-23 ($P = 0.036$) in BALF (Fig. 4). No significant variation was found throughout challenges for relative mRNA expression of IL-2, IL-5, IL-6, IL-8, IL-13, IFN-γ and TGF-β (Additional file 4). No overall influence of the 'challenge' type (steamed vs. dry hay), or any interaction between 'challenge' and either 'time' or 'disease status' was found for any cytokine relative expression in BALF.

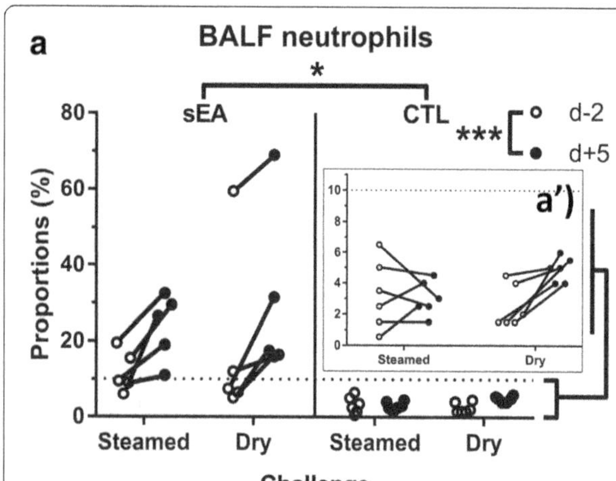

Fig. 2 **a**) Mean neutrophil percentages in bronchoalveolar lavage fluid (BALF), before and after the initiation of each challenge; a') focus (same data) on the control horses. sEA, severe equine asthma; CTL, control; d-2, 2 days before challenge; d + 5, 5 days after challenge. *, *** significant difference between groups or timepoints ($P < 0.05$ and 0.001, respectively), based on ANOVA investigation

Correlations

Relative mRNA expression of IL-1β, IL-6R, IL-8, IL-10 and IL-23 were significantly associated with BALF neutrophil percentages of sEA affected horses (Fig. 5), and mRNA expression of IL-1β, IL-6R, IL-8, IL-13, IL-23 and TGF-β in BALF were also significantly correlated with tracheal mucus score (Additional file 5). Relative mRNA expression of IL-6R was negatively correlated with the percentage of macrophages in BALF of sEA affected horses, and IL-4 was significantly correlated with metachromatic cell percentages (Additional file 5).

Discussion

This is, to our knowledge, the first study in which the inflammatory and immune airway responses of both sEA and CTL horses have been investigated through a controlled exposition challenge with steamed and dry hay. Horses with sEA had been on pasture for at least 6 weeks prior to the challenge initiation. Unsurprisingly and due to the persistent nature of this syndrome, some level of clinical and/or cytological abnormalities at the time of enrolment was observed for 2 out of the 5 sEA-affected horses. Interestingly, the initial clinical scores were indeed 12/21 for both horses, and decreased to 6/21 at the end of the first exposure period (to steamed hay). Despite a significant interaction between 'challenge' (steamed vs. dry hay) and 'time' (d + 5 vs.

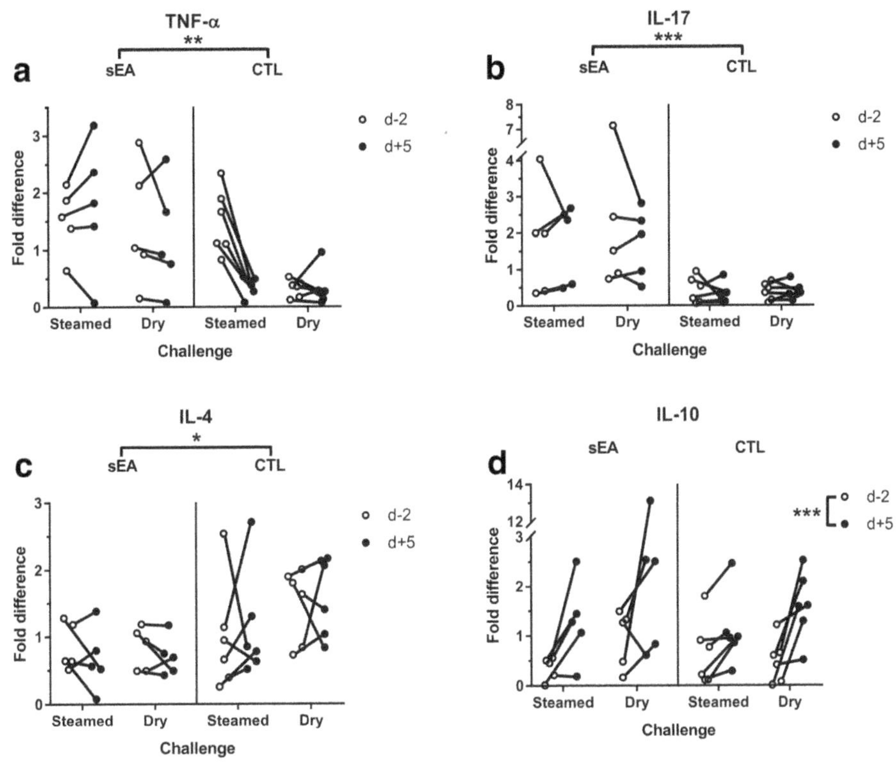

Fig. 3 Relative mRNA expression of cytokines in bronchoalveolar lavage fluid (BALF), before and after the initiation of each challenge: **a** tumour necrosis factor (TNF)-α; **b** interleukin (IL)-17; **c** IL-4; **d** IL-10. sEA, severe equine asthma; CTL, control; d-2, 2 days before challenge; d + 5, 5 days after challenge. *, **, *** significant difference between groups or timepoints ($P < 0.05$, 0.01 and 0.001, respectively), based on ANOVA investigation

d-2), the individual variability of clinical scores may have confounded the results. However, 4 out of the 5 sEA horses showed significantly ($P = 0.01$) elevated tracheal mucus score (≥ 3) after being fed dry hay, while the score remained < 3 for a majority of them (3 out of 5) after being fed steamed hay.

Percentages of neutrophils in BALF were overall higher at d + 5 when compared to d-2, irrespective of 'challenge' (steamed and dry hay) and 'disease status' (sEA and CTL). Induction of a significant neutrophilic airway inflammation has been previously reported in CTL horses through environmental challenges [18, 19]. In the present study, all BALF neutrophil percentages measured from CTL horses systematically remained < 10%, while the same "good quality" (non-mouldy) hay was used in both challenges. Steaming hay significantly decreased mould content by a hundred fold, as previously described [17]. The mould content in hay was investigated in the present study by mycological culture only; the presence of spores, antigenic fragments or mycotoxins has not been evaluated. Targeted and non-targeted methodologies, such as qPCR and Maldi-Tof mass spectrometry, respectively, would considerably increase both the sensitivity and broadness of aeroallergen detection.

Based on the inflammatory responses measured after both challenges, it might be hypothesised that other non-evaluated stimuli might still be present within the hay even after steaming (e.g. mould and bacterial wall fragments). Horses were kept in paddocks during exposure periods, in order to avoid the influence of environmental confinement [20] and associated management of stables ventilation. Alternatively, steaming hay may not have been sufficient to prevent the synergistic inflammatory activity of various hay dust components, especially including endotoxins, which has previously been demonstrated experimentally [9]. When considering air sampling within the breathing zone during the present study, the inhalable fraction was 100 times lower when feeding steamed hay compared to dry hay. The influence of steaming hay on the respirable particles was however more limited in the current study, while this fraction was found to be significantly associated with lower airway inflammation of horses [21]. Respirable dust, endotoxin and β-D-glucan levels may also have been affected by individual horse's behaviour when eating hay, as previously demonstrated for particulate concentrations [22]. The mean values measured for endotoxin activities within the breathing zones were 5.7 times lower with steamed hay, when compared to dry hay,

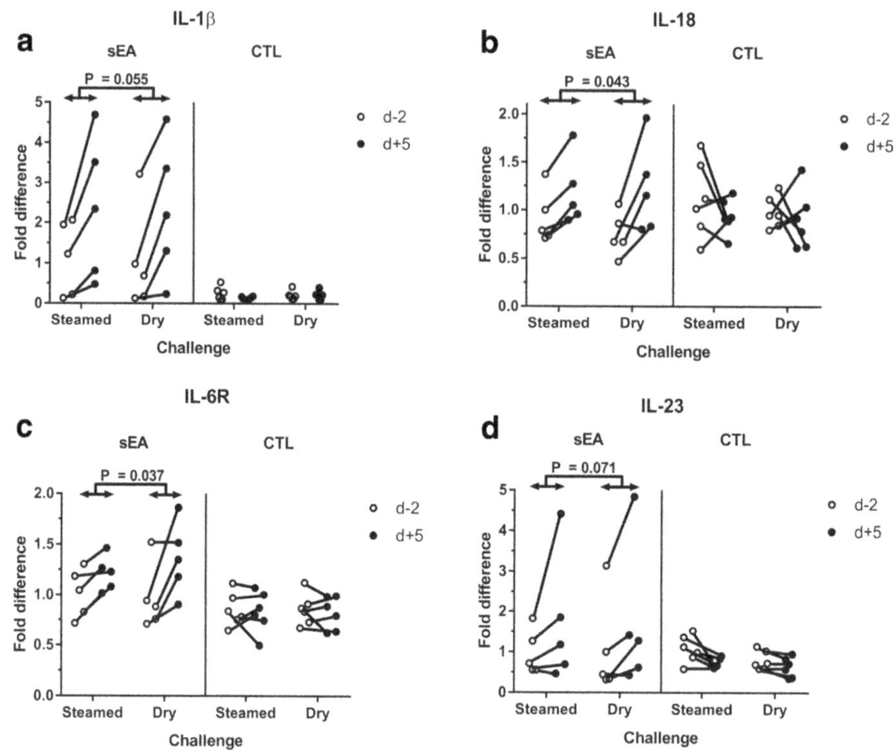

Fig. 4 Relative mRNA expression of cytokines in bronchoalveolar lavage fluid (BALF), before and after the initiation of each challenge: **a** interleukin (IL)-1β; **b** IL-18; **c** IL-6R; **d** IL-23. sEA, severe equine asthma; CTL, control; d-2, 2 days before challenge; d + 5, 5 days after challenge. Significant overall interactions ($P < 0.05$) were found between between 'disease status' (sEA, CTL) and 'time' (d-2, d + 5); the p-values correspond to the subsequent Tukey-Kramer's post-hoc tests

while a large variability was observed among horses. Interestingly, values for endotoxin activities within the breathing zone when feeding steamed hay were also comparable with previously published data for haylage/wood shavings combination [14].

No significant influence of the 'challenge' type (steamed vs. dry hay) was found for any cytokine mRNA expression in BALF. Significant interactions were found between 'disease status' (sEA vs. CTL) and 'time' (d + 5 vs. d-2) for mRNA expression of IL-1β and IL-18; relative mRNA expression of TNF-α was also significantly higher in BALF from sEA affected horses, when compared with CTL horses. Such observations are coherent with the measurable inflammatory response of sEA affected horses to both (steamed and dry) hay challenges. Interestingly, mRNA expression of IL-6R in BALF was also increased post-challenges for sEA affected horses only. To date, the relative expression of this receptor has not been investigated in BALF of horses. Interestingly, a genome-wide association study identified a significant association between a single nucleotide polymorphism in the IL-6R gene and the risk of asthma in humans [23]. Further investigations are warranted to characterize the IL- 6 signaling pathway involvement in equine asthma, especially in terms of subsequent T-helper (Th) polarisation as recently demonstrated in humans [24].

The previously suggested involvement of Th17 pathway in the airways of horses with severe asthma [4, 5], is supported by the present study. Overall IL-17 mRNA expression was indeed significantly higher in BALF of sEA affected when compared with CTL horses. The IL-23 mRNA expression in BALF was also increased post-challenges for sEA affected horses only, and was furthermore significantly correlated with both tracheal mucus score and BALF neutrophil percentages. Surprisingly, IL-8 mRNA expression was neither significantly different among groups ($P = 0.11$; controlling for age of the horses) nor significantly influenced by the challenge types. However, a significant correlation ($R = 0.688$) was found with neutrophil percentages in BALF. While overexpression has been associated with sEA chronicity [4, 5], it is likely that IL-8 contributes to neutrophil chemotaxis in the earlier stages of equine asthma [2]. The short duration of each challenge period in the current study might partly explain the limited amplitude of IL-8 mRNA expression in BALF.

The lower mRNA expression of IL-4 in BALF of sEA versus CTL horses was unexpected, mainly based on the

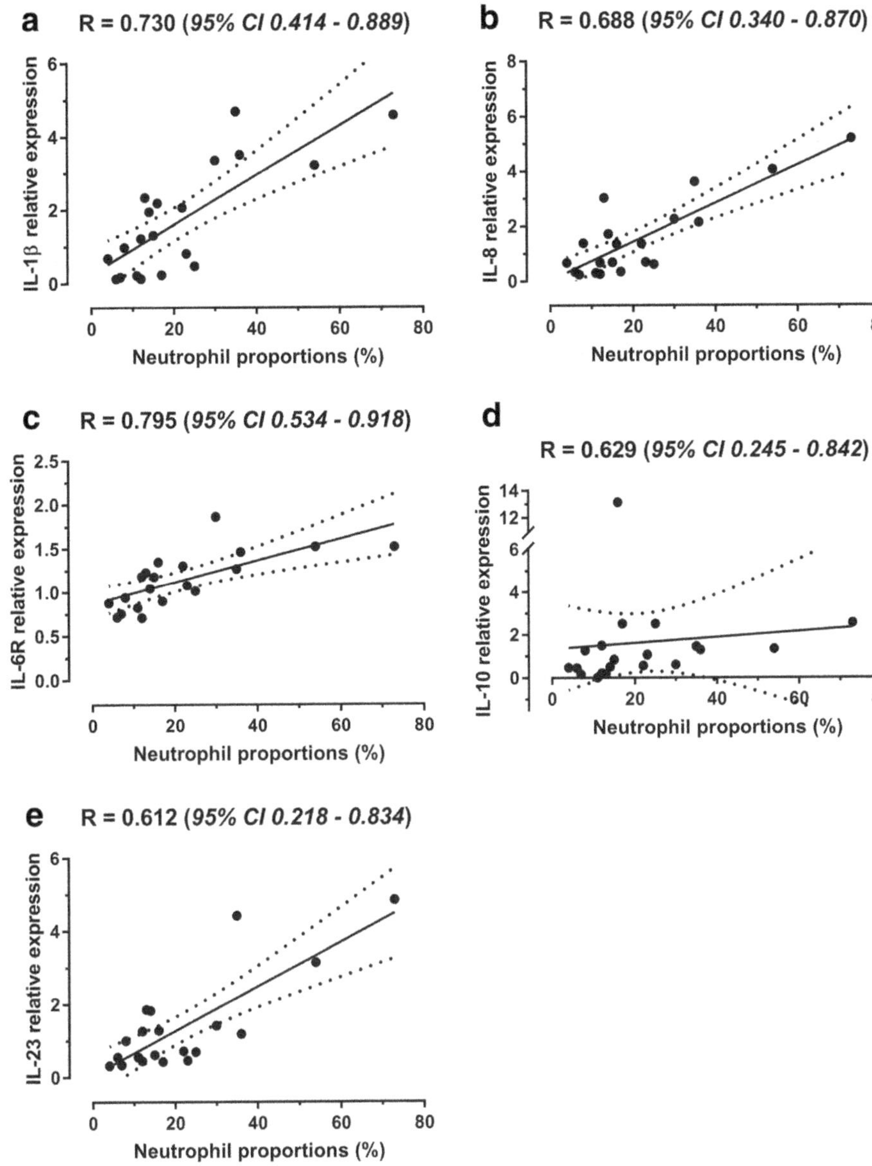

Fig. 5 Correlations (95% confidence interval) between relative mRNA expression of cytokines and neutrophil proportions in bronchoalveolar lavage fluid (BALF) of sEA affected horses, before and after the initiation of each challenge: **a** interleukin (IL)-1β; **b** IL-8; **c** IL-6R; **d** IL-10; **e** IL-23. Straight line, linear regression; dotted lines, 95% confidence

previously demonstrated Th2 polarisation for this syndrome [25]. Interestingly, mRNA expression of IL-4 in BALF of both sEA and CTL horses was also not significantly influenced by either challenge. The sEA group exhibited significantly lower percentages of metachromatic cells in BALF, when compared to CTL horses; and IL-4 mRNA expression was significantly correlated with both eosinophil and metachromatic cell percentages. When considering a possible Treg involvement in sEA, mRNA expression of TGF-β was interestingly not significantly modified throughout the study. On the other hand, IL-10 was the only cytokine which mRNA expression in BALF was significantly higher post-challenges and correlated to BALF neutrophil proportions, with however no significant difference between sEA and CTL horses. Surprisingly, mRNA expression of IL-10 in BALF from sEA affected horses was previously found not to be significantly influenced by various environmental challenges [26]. Alternatively, percentages of different Treg subpopulations, as characterised by flow cytometry, were found to be significantly higher in BALF of sEA horses during crisis exacerbation when compared to remission [6].

Study limitations

All 12 horses involved in this field trial were client-owned, with differences in terms of geographic origins prior to enrolment in the study. The limited number of horses enrolled in this study was consistent with similar works previously published [4, 8]. Based on the current results, the retrospective statistical power analyses highlights the variability of sample size required in relation to the multiple outcomes investigated. Values of power indeed ranged from 30% for clinical score to 82 and 98% for respectively mucus score and BALF neutrophil percentages. Unlike mucus and cytology (for which estimated sample size = 4–6), a minimum of 20 horses would have been required for clinical signs to reach a 80% power with a α-level of 0.05. The average age was significantly different between groups; the CTL horses being significantly younger than the sEA affected horses. This confounding factor was then taken into account in all further statistical analyses. In terms of design, both challenges (steamed and dry hay) were not performed as a cross-over study, since horses were initially fed with steamed hay (challenge #1) and subsequently fed dry hay (challenge #2). For ethical reasons, the design (i.e. steamed then dry hay) aimed at limiting the risk of horse exclusion (due to crisis exacerbation and subsequent treatment) at the end of the first exposure period, which would have precluded the horse to be involved in the second period. No significant difference was found for each group at d-2 (i.e. initiation of each exposure period) for all investigated parameters; suggesting that horses returned to "baseline level" prior to challenge #2. Also, clinical and tracheal mucus scoring were performed by clinicians not blinded to either challenge type (steamed vs. dry) or horse disease status (sEA vs. CTL), unlike all subsequent laboratory analyses, and lung function tests were not available for this study. Finally, the immune responses in BALF were investigated for the various cytokines through relative mRNA expressions only. Measuring BALF cytokine concentrations using commercially available ELISA kits however lacks sensitivity, since many BALF samples previously showed undetectable cytokine concentrations [27, 28].

Conclusions

Steaming hay significantly decreased mould content and induced less tracheal mucus in horses. However, both types of hay (steamed or not) induced BALF neutrophilia, and none induced respiratory clinical signs. The relevance of steaming hay however warrants further investigations both in the context of prevention/therapy for mEA horses at training and for long-term preclusion of lately developing sEA.

Methods

Horses

A cohort of 12 privately owned leisure horses were used in the study, and was subdivided into 2 separate groups. The control (CTL) group included 6 young horses (4 mares and 2 geldings, aged 2–5 years). These horses had no history of coughing or nasal discharge, exhibited no tracheal mucus upon endoscopy, and had less than 10% neutrophils in bronchoalveolar lavage fluid (BALF) from each lung when investigated 10 days prior to the trial. The other group included 6 adult horses (5 mares and 1 gelding, aged 9–17 years) that had all previously been diagnosed by the same clinician as suffering from sEA, based on clinical investigations, BALF cytology and reversible airway obstruction after medical/environmental change. Only horses kept in pasture and without any medical treatment or access to hay for at least 1 month prior to the trial were enrolled in the study. Recruitment for the study was made on a volunteer basis from private training centres (CTL horses) and from the caseload previously referred to the hospital (sEA horses; Oniris, Nantes). All owners signed an informed consent, and all procedures were performed by veterinarians and complied with relevant guidelines (Directive 2010/63/EU). The study was also approved by the Institutional Ethic Committee for Clinical Research (CERVO-2017-8-V).

Study design

This study was conducted during spring 2017. At the initiation of the trial, all horses were gathered and kept in a 4 ha pasture without access to hay for a duration of 2 weeks (Fig. 6). Since stabling was previously found to be associated with increased airway inflammation [29], horses were kept in 1 000 m^2 paddocks by subgroups of three individuals during both exposure periods. On day 0 of the trial, both groups (sEA and CTL) were fed on the ground with about 5 kg per horse of steamed hay (challenge #1), twice daily for 5 consecutive days (i.e. exposure period #1); followed by a wash-out period of 26 days in the 4 ha pasture without access to hay, prior to a second challenge with similar distribution of dry hay (challenge #2) for 5 consecutive days, (exposure period #2). Horses had access to water ad libitum and were also fed flaked cereals and dry pellets (Twenty Horse[1]) twice daily. Good quality (non-mouldy) grass hay was harvested as square bales (12–15 kg). For the challenge #1, the hay was steamed using a commercial device (HG-600[2]), according to manufacturer's recommendations, and immediately distributed to horses. Briefly, the hay bale was placed onto the steamer and pushed down firmly until the manifold spikes pierce the hay to their full length; the steam generator (containing water) was then activated and steam diffused in hay through the spikes. At the end of exposure period #2, asthmatic horses received dexamethasone (0.1 mg/kg IV for 2 days, then progressively decreasing doses over 1 week) and all horses (sEA and CTL) were returned to their owners. Two days before (d-2) and 5 days

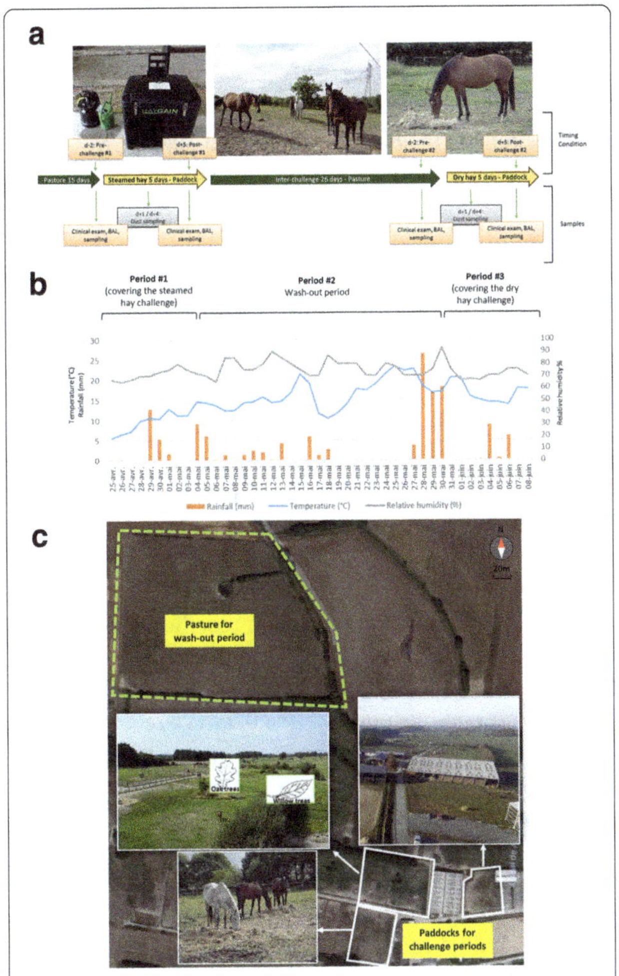

Fig. 6 Overview of the study: **a** experimental design, **b** climatic conditions, and **c** geographical repartition

after (d + 5) the initiation of each challenge, all horses underwent a full clinical evaluation, as well as a tracheal endoscopy and BALF sampling. The 2010 CONSORT guidelines for reporting clinical trial were used for this report (Additional files 1 and 6) [30, 31].

Hay characterisation

Hay samples (random sampling by hand for a total of 1 kg) were collected from 10 different square bales before and after the steaming procedure, and stored in dedicated bags[1]. All square bales originated from the same batch of hay (one single pasture), and all analyses were performed immediately after sampling. For bacteriology, 20 g of crushed hay were mixed with 180 ml of 0.1% peptone water and diluted 1/10 up to 10^{-6}. One ml of each dilution was plated onto a Plate Count Agar (PCA) and incubated at 37 °C. One ml of each dilution was also cultured in oxytetracycline-glucose-yeast Extract Agar (OGA) and incubated at 25 °C for fungal growth. Bacterial and fungal growths were expressed as colony forming units (CFUs) after 5 days of incubation. The fungal colonies were then isolated on Sabouraud agar in order to be identified.

Air quality

Air sampling within the breathing zone was performed continuously for 2-3 h during hay feeding, on d + 1 (one CTL horse) and d + 4 (one sEA horse) of each exposure period. Respirable and inhalable particulates were collected according to previously published procedures [21].

Particulates

Horses were equipped with two samplers. The respirable fraction was collected with a flow rate of 2.5 L/min (AirCheck XR5000[3]) onto 37 mm type AE glass fibre filters using aluminium cyclone. The inhalable fraction was collected with a flow rate of 2.0 L/min (AirCheck 3000[3]) onto 25 mm PVC filters using Institute of Occupational Medicine (IOM) personal sampler. Sampling pumps were calibrated (Defender Bios calibrator[3]) before and after sampling. Measurements of respirable and inhalable dust were assessed by gravimetric method, in triplicate measurements. The weight of particulates was divided by volume of air sampled to obtain airborne concentrations. Filters were placed in a desiccator for 24 h prior to any weight measurement. Negative controls were similarly prepared and only transported to and from the site of trial.

Endotoxins

Endotoxins were measured from the 37 mm type AE glass fibre filters, which were kept frozen (– 20 °C) after particulates measurements. Filters were eluted in 10 mL of 0.05% Tween 20[4] within pyrogen-free water. Samples were then shaken during 1 h (MS-NRK-30[5]). After elution, the suspension was centrifuged (1000 *g*; 15 min). The supernatant was then kept frozen (– 20 °C) until being analysed. The eluates provided from sample filters were diluted at 1/10 in pyrogen-free water. Endotoxin activities were assayed using Endosafe – PTS2005F,[6] according to manufacturer's recommendations.

β-D-glucan

Following endotoxin elution, heat extraction was performed in order to measure (1–3)-β-D-glucan content. Samples were then respectively diluted 10-fold for blank filters and 100-fold for sample filters in pyrogen-free water. Measures were carried out in duplicates, using a Glucatell test,[7] according to manufacturer's recommendations. The range of quantification was 5–40 pg/mL.

Clinical score, tracheal mucus and bronchoalveolar lavage fluid cytology

On d-2 and d + 5 for each exposure period, a clinical score, based on a 0–21 scale (Additional file 7) [32], was assigned to each horse. Detomidine hydrochloride (0.01 mg/kg IV) and butorphanol tartrate (0.01 mg/kg IV) was given prior to endoscopy. Airway endoscopy and BAL collection were performed using a flexible 3.2 m long, 12.8 mm tip diameter videoendoscope.[8] The amount of tracheal mucus was scored (grade 0–5) according to the previously published scale [33]. Left and right lungs were then sampled according to previously published procedures [34], with minor modifications. Briefly, a total of 500 mL of warmed isotonic saline solution (2 boluses of 250 mL each) was instilled and aspirated for each lung. Samples were conditioned (+ 4 °C in EDTA tubes) and processed (cytocentrifugation, May-Grünwald-Giemsa staining) as described previously [35]. Differential cell counts were performed on 300 leukocytes. Unlike clinical and mucus scores, cytological investigations of BALF from both lungs were conducted by investigators blinded to challenge type and horse status.

RNA isolation and reverse transcription

Each BALF sample obtained from the right lung was conditioned in order to determine cytokine relative expressions. Expression of 15 cytokines (representative of the different pathways previously associated with sEA) and one receptor (described in human allergic asthma) have been targeted in this study: interferon (IFN)-γ, interleukin (IL)-1β, IL-2, IL-4, IL-5, IL-6, IL-6R, IL-8, IL-10, IL-12, IL-13, IL-17, IL-18, IL-23, transforming growth factor (TGF)-β and tumour necrosis factor (TNF)-α.

Twenty milliliters of BALF was centrifuged and the cell pellets resuspended in RNA protect Cell Reagent.[9] Total RNA was extracted from cell pellets using the RNeasy Plus Mini Kit[9]. Concentration and purity of total extracted RNA was assessed using a NanoDrop 2000c Spectrophotometer[10]; and RNA integrity was evaluated using a 2100 Bioanalyzer[11] and the RNA 6000 Nano kit[11]. Mean value (± standard deviation) of RNA integrity number (RIN) for all samples was 9.7 ± 0.2. After extraction, 200 ng was retrotranscribed and cDNA generated using a Superscript Vilo cDNA synthesis kit,[12] according to the manufacturer's recommendations. All cDNA samples were stored at − 20 °C until further use. Apart from the cytokines of interest, three reference genes, namely β-actin (ACTB), glyceraldehyde-3-phosphate dehydrogenase (GAPDH) and β-glucuronidase (β-GUS), were also assessed. For each reaction, cDNA was amplified in a 25 μl standard reaction (Taqman Universal PCR Master Mix[10]). Thermal cycling profile used was: 10 min at 95 °C, followed by 50 cycles of 15 s at 95 °C and 1 min at 60 °C. The relative amount of mRNA was calculated using the relative standard curve method (Genex 6.1[13]), and results were expressed as mean fold difference (target / reference genes). Using Normfinder, GAPDH and β-GUS were both selected for normalization (Additional file 8). Molecular investigations were also conducted blinded, in terms of horse 'disease status' and 'challenge' type.

Statistical analyses

Continuous data distributions which were not normally distributed, as assessed by Shapiro-Wilk W test, were log-10 transformed. For hay-related parameters, paired *t* tests (steamed vs. dry) were performed for the bacterial/ mould content. For all horse-related parameters, effects of challenge (steamed vs. dry), time (d + 5 vs. d-2) and disease status (sEA vs. CTL) were investigated by 3-way analysis of variance (ANOVA, General Linear Model) and Tukey-Kramer's post-hoc tests, with age as covariate. Correlations among sEA affected horses were determined by Spearman's correlation coefficient. Absolute values of $R < 0.5$ were arbitrarily not reported. The different analyses were conducted using Prism 7[14] and NCSS12,[15] and values of $P < 0.05$ were considered significant.

Endnotes

[1]Tromelin & Cie, Ploeren, France
[2]Haygain, Lambourn, Berkshire, UK
[3]SCK Inc., Eighty Four, PA, USA
[4]Merck-Millipore, Molsheim, France
[5]Major Science, Saratoga, CA, USA
[6]Charles River Laboratories, Saint-Germain-Nuelles, France
[7]Associates of Cape Cod Inc., East Falmouth, MA, USA
[8]Optomed, Les Ulis, France
[9]Quiagen, Courtabœuf, France
[10]Thermoscientific, Villebon-sur-Yvette, France
[11]Agilent Technologies, Les Ulis, France
[12]Life Technologies, Saint-Aubin, France
[13]bioMMC, Freising, Germany
[14]GraphPad, La Jolla, CA, USA
[15]NCSS – LLC, Kaysville, UT, USA

Additional files

Additional file 1: CONSORT flow diagram for the clinical trial involving 6 control (CTL) horses and 6 horses with severe equine asthma (sEA). (PDF 46 kb)

Additional file 2: Microbiological content in hay ($n = 10$), before and after steaming: a) bacterial content; b) mould content. *** significantly different (*P < 0.001),* based on paired t test. (TIF 917 kb)

Additional file 3: Cytology of bronchoalveolar lavage fluid (BALF), before and after the initiation of each challenge. sEA, severe equine asthma; CTL control; d-2, 2 days before challenge; d + 5, 5 days after challenge. * overall significant difference between groups (sEA vs. CTL horses); # overall significant difference between time points (d + 5 vs. d-2), based on ANOVA investigations. (DOCX 20 kb)

Additional file 4: Relative mRNA expression of cytokines in bronchoalveolar lavage fluid (BALF), before and after the initiation of each challenge: a) interleukin (IL)-2; b) IL-5; c) IL-13; d) TGF-β; e) IL-6; f) IL-8; g) Interferon (IFN)-γ. sEA, severe equine asthma; CTL, control; d-2, 2 days before challenge; d + 5, 5 days after challenge. (TIF 2119 kb)

Additional file 5: Correlations (95% confidence interval) between relative mRNA expression of cytokines and clinical/cytological parameters, before and after the initiation of each challenge. IL, interleukin; (95% CI); ns, non-significant and/or absolute value of R < 0.5. (DOCX 21 kb)

Additional file 6: CONSORT check-list for the clinical trial involving 6 control (CTL) horses and 6 horses with severe equine asthma (sEA). (PDF 134 kb)

Additional file 7: Clinical scoring system for respiratory conditions, adapted from Tesarowski et al. [32]. (DOCX 18 kb)

Additional file 8: Nucleotide sequences of equine-specific primers used in real-time PCR assays. (DOCX 22 kb)

Abbreviations
ACTB: Actin; BALF: Bronchoalveolar lavage fluid; cDNA: Complementary deoxyribonucleic acid; CFUs: Colony forming units; CTL: Control; GAPDH: Glycéraldéhyde-3-phosphate dehydrogenase; IFN: Interferon; IL: Interleukin; mEA: Mild equine asthma; mRNA: Ribonucleic acid messenger; OGA: Oxytetracycline-glucose-yeast extract agar; PCA: Plate count agar; qPCR: Quantitative polymerase chain reaction; RIN: RNA Integrity number; sEA: Severe equine asthma; TGF: Transforming growth factor; Th: T-helper; TNF: Tumor necrosis factor; β-Gus: β-glucuronidase

Acknowledgements
The authors wish to thank the horse's owners, as well as institutional staff (LABÉO, Oniris) for their kind collaboration.

Funding
Funding for this study was provided by Haygain, LABÉO and Oniris. The funders had no role in the design of the study and collection, analysis, and interpretation of data and in writing the manuscript.

Authors, contributions
MO contributed to data collection and study execution, data analysis/interpretation, and preparation of the manuscript. EH contributed to data collection, analysis and interpretation. AC contributed to study design, data collection and study execution. CBM contributed to study design, data collection and study execution. MPT contributed to data collection and study execution. MMC contributed to study design and preparation of the manuscript. LC contributed to study design, data collection and preparation of the manuscript. SP contributed to data analysis and interpretation. RP contributed to data interpretation and preparation of the manuscript. MD contributed to study execution and preparation of the manuscript. EAR contributed to study design, data interpretation, and preparation of the manuscript. All authors provided final approval of the manuscript.

Consent for publication
Not applicable.

Competing interests
MMC is Scientific Consultant for Haygain. The authors declare that they have no competing interests.

Author details
[1]LABÉO Frank Duncombe, Caen, France. [2]Normandie Université, UniCaen, BIOTARGEN, Caen, France. [3]LUNAM Université, Oniris, NP3, Nantes, France. [4]Royal Agricultural University, Cirencester, UK. [5]Purdue University, College of Veterinary Medicine, West Lafayette, IN, USA.

References
1. Pirie RS, Couëtil LL, Robinson NE, Lavoie J-P. Equine asthma: an appropriate, translational and comprehendible terminology? Equine Vet J. 2016;48:403–5.
2. Pirie RS. Recurrent airway obstruction: a review. Equine Vet J. 2014;46:276–88.
3. Couëtil LL, Cardwell JM, Gerber V, Lavoie J-P, Léguillette R, Richard EA. Inflammatory airway disease of horses - revised consensus statement. J Vet Intern Med. 2016;30:503–15.
4. Debrue M, Hamilton E, Joubert P, Lajoie-Kadoch S, Lavoie J-P. Chronic exacerbation of equine heaves is associated with an increased expression of interleukin-17 mRNA in bronchoalveolar lavage cells. Vet Immunol Immunopathol. 2005;105:25–31.
5. Ainsworth DM, Wagner B, Erb HN, Young JC, Retallick DE. Effects of in vitro exposure to hay dust on expression of interleukin-17, −23, −8, and -1beta and chemokine (C-X-C motif) ligand 2 by pulmonary mononuclear cells isolated from horses chronically affected with recurrent airway disease. Am J Vet Res. 2007;68:1361–9.
6. Henríquez C, Perez B, Morales N, Sarmiento J, Carrasco C, Morán G, et al. Participation of T regulatory cells in equine recurrent airway obstruction. Vet Immunol Immunopathol. 2014;158:128–34.
7. Ramseyer A, Gaillard C, Burger D, Straub R, Jost U, Boog C, et al. Effects of genetic and environmental factors on chronic lower airway disease in horses. J Vet Intern Med. 2007;21:149–56.
8. McGorum BC, Dixon PM, Halliwell RE. Responses of horses affected with chronic obstructive pulmonary disease to inhalation challenges with mould antigens. Equine Vet J. 1993;25:261–7.
9. Pirie RS, Collie DDS, Dixon PM, McGorum BC. Inhaled endotoxin and organic dust particulates have synergistic proinflammatory effects in equine heaves (organic dust-induced asthma). Clin Exp Allergy. 2003;33:676–83.
10. Jackson CA, Berney C, Jefcoat AM, Robinson NE. Environment and prednisone interactions in the treatment of recurrent airway obstruction (heaves). Equine Vet J. 2000;32:432–8.
11. Leclere M, Lefebvre-Lavoie J, Beauchamp G, Lavoie J-P. Efficacy of oral prednisolone and dexamethasone in horses with recurrent airway obstruction in the presence of continuous antigen exposure: prednisolone in RAO. Equine Vet J. 2010;42:316–21.
12. Cesarini C, Hamilton E, Picandet V, Lavoie JP. Theophylline does not potentiate the effects of a low dose of dexamethasone in horses with recurrent airway obstruction. Equine Vet J. 2006;38:570–3.
13. Clements JM, Pirie RS. Respirable dust concentrations in equine stables. Part 1: validation of equipment and effect of various management systems. Res Vet Sci. 2007;83:256–62.
14. Whittaker AG, Hughes KJ, Parkin TDH, Love S. Concentrations of dust and endotoxin in equine stabling. Vet Rec. 2009;165:293–5.
15. Clements JM, Pirie RS. Respirable dust concentrations in equine stables. Part 2: the benefits of soaking hay and optimising the environment in a neighbouring stable. Res Vet Sci. 2007;83:263–8.
16. Moore-Colyer MJS, Taylor JLE, James R. The effect of steaming and soaking on the respirable particle, bacteria, mould, and nutrient content in hay for horses. J Equine Vet Sci. 2016;39:62–8.
17. Moore-Colyer MJS, Lumbis K, Longland A, Harris P. The effect of five different wetting treatments on the nutrient content and microbial concentration in hay for horses. PLoS One. 2014;9:e114079.
18. Gerber V, Lindberg A, Berney C, Robinson NE. Airway mucus in recurrent airway obstruction--short-term response to environmental challenge. J Vet Intern Med. 2004;18:92–7.
19. Beeler-Marfisi J, Clark ME, Wen X, Sears W, Huber L, Ackerley C, et al. Experimental induction of recurrent airway obstruction with inhaled fungal spores, lipopolysaccharide, and silica microspheres in horses. Am J Vet Res. 2010;71:682–9.
20. Berndt A, Derksen FJ, Edward Robinson N. Endotoxin concentrations within the breathing zone of horses are higher in stables than on pasture. Vet J. 2010;183:54–7.
21. Ivester KM, Couëtil LL, Moore GE, Zimmerman NJ, Raskin RE. Environmental exposures and airway inflammation in young thoroughbred horses. J Vet Intern Med. 2014;28:918–24.

22. Ivester KM, Smith K, Moore GE, Zimmerman NJ, Couëtil LL. Variability in particulate concentrations in a horse training barn over time. Equine Vet J Suppl. 2012;43:51–6.
23. Ferreira MAR, Matheson MC, Duffy DL, Marks GB, Hui J, Le Souëf P, et al. Identification of IL6R and chromosome 11q13.5 as risk loci for asthma. Lancet. 2011;378:1006–14.
24. Ullah MA, Revez JA, Loh Z, Simpson J, Zhang V, Bain L, et al. Allergen-induced IL-6 trans-signaling activates γδ T cells to promote type 2 and type 17 airway inflammation. J Allergy Clin Immunol. 2015;136:1065–73.
25. Cordeau M-E, Joubert P, Dewachi O, Hamid Q, Lavoie J-P. IL-4, IL-5 and IFN-gamma mRNA expression in pulmonary lymphocytes in equine heaves. Vet Immunol Immunopathol. 2004;97:87–96.
26. Laan TT, Bull S, Pirie R, Fink-Gremmels J. The role of alveolar macrophages in the pathogenesis of recurrent airway obstruction in horses. J Vet Intern Med. 2006;20:167–74.
27. Perkins GA, Viel L, Wagner B, Hoffman A, Erb HN, Ainsworth DM. Histamine bronchoprovocation does not affect bronchoalveolar lavage fluid cytology, gene expression and protein concentrations of IL-4, IL-8 and IFN-gamma. Vet Immunol Immunopathol. 2008;126:230–5.
28. Richard EA, Depecker M, Defontis M, Leleu C, Fortier G, Pitel P-H, et al. Cytokine concentrations in bronchoalveolar lavage fluid from horses with neutrophilic inflammatory airway disease. J Vet Intern Med. 2014; 28:1838–44.
29. Holcombe SJ, Jackson C, Gerber V, Jefcoat A, Berney C, Eberhardt S, et al. Stabling is associated with airway inflammation in young Arabian horses. Equine Vet J. 2001;33:244–9.
30. Moher D, Hopewell S, Schulz KF, Montori V, Gøtzsche PC, Devereaux PJ, et al. CONSORT 2010 explanation and elaboration: updated guidelines for reporting parallel group randomised trials. BMJ. 2010;340:c869.
31. Schulz KF, Altman DG, Moher D, CONSORT Group. CONSORT 2010 statement: updated guidelines for reporting parallel group randomised trials. PLoS Med. 2010;7:e1000251.
32. Tesarowski DB, Viel L, McDonell WN. Pulmonary function measurements during repeated environmental challenge of horses with recurrent airway obstruction (heaves). Am J Vet Res. 1996;57:1214–9.
33. Gerber V, Straub R, Marti E, Hauptman J, Herholz C, King M, et al. Endoscopic scoring of mucus quantity and quality: observer and horse variance and relationship to inflammation, mucus viscoelasticity and volume. Equine Vet J. 2004;36:576–82.
34. Depecker M, Richard EA, Pitel P-H, Fortier G, Leleu C, Courouсé-Malblanc A. Bronchoalveolar lavage fluid in Standardbred racehorses: influence of unilateral/bilateral profiles and cut-off values on lower airway disease diagnosis. Vet J. 2014;199:150–6.
35. Orard M, Depecker M, Hue E, Pitel P-H, Courouсé-Malblanc A, Richard EA. Influence of bronchoalveolar lavage volume on cytological profiles and subsequent diagnosis of inflammatory airway disease in horses. Vet J. 2016; 207:193–5.

19

High intensity, short duration pulling in heavy horses: physiological effects of competition and rapid weight change

Persephone Greco-Otto, Shannon Massie, Erin Shields, Marie-France Roy, Edmond Pajor and Renaud Léguillette*

Abstract

Background: The Heavy Horse Pull is a competition where teams of two horses pull an increasingly heavy sled for a short distance. Similar to human wrestlers, some horses may undergo rapid weight change in order to enter a lower weight category. The objectives were to study the physiological effects of this practice as well as of the pulling competition in draft horses.

Results: Fifty horses were divided into light-, middle- and heavyweight categories based on their arrival weights and competed 1–3 days after. Body weight was measured upon arrival and pre-competition. Blood was sampled for chemistry and high sensitivity cardiac troponin T (hscTnT) at arrival, pre- and post-competition in 34, 26 and 20 horses, respectively. Body weight increased significantly between arrival and pre-competition for light (7.2% (Median: 62.8Kg (41.7–77.0)) and middle (8.6% (Median: 80.5Kg (62.7–90.9)) weight categories. Change in body weight was correlated ($r = 0.69$, $p = 0.002$) with competition ranking for middleweights. The ratios of weight pulled to team body weight were 2.7 (1.9–2.8), 2.6 (2.5–2.6) and 2.4 (2.2–2.5) for the lightweights, middleweights and heavyweights, respectively. Blood chemistry indicated hemoconcentration on arrival in the middleweight and lightweight horses. Hemoconcentration was not seen on arrival in some horses with marked rapid weight change. Overall, no chemistry parameter changed between pre- and post-competition. The hscTnT stayed within normal range post-competition.

Conclusions: While horses arrived to the event with indications of hemoconcentration, they appeared to have sufficient time to rehydrate prior to competition, and the effects of the competition were reversible within 3 h.

Keywords: Draft, Equine, Rapid weight loss, Cardiac troponin, Electrolytes, Serum chemistry

Background

The Heavy Horse Pull is a competition that showcases horses' strength and anaerobic power. Teams of two draft horses pull a weighted sled over 14 ft at increasing load until a maximum is reached. Similar to many human sports, horses compete within a specified weight division and undergo mandatory weigh-ins to ensure equal and fair competition. In wrestling, human athletes attempt to gain what is believed to be a competitive advantage by weighing in at the top of a lower weight division and commonly drop 3–4 kg in the week prior to competition [1]. Weight changes in human athletes are primarily attributed to total body water loss and often exceed 2% of body weight [2]. This rapid weight loss (RWL) is achieved by severely restricting fluid and caloric intake, using laxatives and increasing perspiration [3]. Some heavy horses may also undergo similar RWL practices, commonly referred to as "shrinkage", but unlike human wrestlers, they have 1 to 3 days after weigh-in to rehydrate and regain weight prior to competition. This is a key difference, as these horses undergo rapid weight changes (weight loss followed by weight gain), rather than simply rapid weight loss. Though not documented in the scientific literature, shrinkage is common enough that some pulling competitions explicitly state that excessive shrinking is grounds for disqualification. While RWL in humans has negative physiological effects on the renal, muscular and cardiac systems [4, 5], the effects of severe short term changes in weight are unknown in horses.

* Correspondence: rleguill@ucalgary.ca
Department of Veterinary Clinical and Diagnostic Sciences, Faculty of Veterinary Medicine, University of Calgary, Calgary, AB T2N 4N1, Canada

Additionally, the physiological response to short term high intensity resistance pulling in heavy horses is unknown. Previous work examined the physiological effects of sustained pulling in Draft horses [6, 7], however the workload efforts, physiological demand and metabolic stress of the Heavy Horse Pull are drastically different since it is at a much higher intensity, but for a much shorter duration. The effects of a high intensity short duration exercise on the myocardium are unknown in horses but have been shown to induce a leakage of cardiac troponin in human athletes [8]. In addition, we reported that high sensitivity cardiac troponin (hscTnT) can be increased in racehorses with upper airway obstruction while racing [9]. This may be due to myocardium damage or increased permeability of myocardial membranes or release of cardiac troponin through vesicles [10–12]. It has been documented that 35% of large horse breeds competing in hitch and pulling classes have recurrent laryngeal neuropathy [13], which can result in a drastic reduction in cross-sectional area of the upper airway. Consequently, we hypothesized that hscTnT increases in draft horses competing in pulling events.

The aim of the study was to assess the effect of competition, including "shrinkage", on the physiology of draft horses. We hypothesized that rapid weight changes happen in the lightweight and middleweight categories, which affects performance and results in hemoconcentration and electrolytes imbalances. Additionally, we hypothesized that competition itself would effect plasma homeostasis and induce subclinical myocardial damage. The specific objectives of the study were therefore: 1) To quantify the extent and prevalence of rapid weight changes in this competition and its effect on physiology and performance; and 2) To asses the physiological effects of the Heavy Horse Pull competition on blood chemistry, electrolytes, and hscTnT.

Methods

Heavy Horse Pull competition

The study took place during the official Heavy Horse Pull competition at the 2015 Calgary Stampede. For logistical reasons, Calgary Stampede divides teams into three equal weight categories based on entry weight (lightweight: <1451Kg, middleweight: 1452-1587Kg, heavyweight: >1587Kg). Horses are weighed on arrival (day 1). Lightweights compete on day 2, middleweights on day 3 and heavyweights on day 4, as per Calgary Stampede regulations.

Competition results including rank, maximal weight and distance pulled were collected and analyzed for all horses that entered the competition. Additionally, historical data (over the last 13 years) of the Calgary Stampede heavy horses pulling competition maximal weight pulled results for each weight category were available for discussion.

Horses

Body weight, competition results, horses' age, hauling distance, last feeding and last water prior to arrival was available from the organizers for all 52 horses participating in the event. Out of the 52 horses competing, 35 draft horses (n = 18 teams) were voluntarily enrolled in the study for blood data collection for which owners completed a consent form. This study was approved by the University of Calgary Veterinary Sciences Animal Care Committee.

Physical exam

All horses underwent and passed the Calgary Stampede official "Fitness to Compete" veterinary check, which included a lameness exam, cardiac auscultation, checking for upper airway noise, and heart rate recovery.

Body weight measurements

To quantify the extent and prevalence of rapid weight change (specific objective 1), all horses (n = 52) were weighed on arrival and prior to competition. Indeed, the weight gained between arrival and pre-competition is assumed to be indicative of the weight lost during the "shrinkage" process done prior to arrival. This is because "shrinkage" is believed to create a competitive advantage, where owners want the horses to weigh in at lower-than-normal body weights, but induce rapid weight change (gain) to return to a higher body weight prior to competition. Although documenting the normal body weight on farm would have allowed using it as a reference, it was not part of the specific objectives of the study and it was not practical to do as horses came from across North America.

All horses (n = 52) were weighed between 6 am and 7 am on arrival (day 1) and were assigned to a weight category on that day as per official Calgary Stampede rules and regulations. All horses, except for one pair (n = 50 total), were again weighed on the morning prior to competition (day 2, 3 and 4 for lightweight, middleweight and heavyweight, respectively) for the purpose of the study, though this had no effect on weight division designation. Horses were not weighed following competition, since it was outside the scope of the study to document "shrinkage." In addition, it was not practical, as horses had to leave the premises following competition. The scale was calibrated 41 days prior to the study.

Blood sampling

Venous blood samples were drawn in 7 mL lithium heparin tubes at 3 time points: On arrival (day 1), on the morning of the competition (pre-competition, day 2 for lightweights, day 3 for middleweights and day 4 for heavyweights) and 3 h after the competition (post-competition). Samples were immediately centrifuged (10 min at 2000 x g) and plasma was immediately frozen on site at −20 °C, then at -80 °C until they underwent chemistry,[1] electrolyte[1] (commercial veterinary laboratory) and hscTnT analysis[2,3,4] (commercial human hospital laboratory) within the next month. Chemistry and electrolytes analysis included total protein, albumin, globulins, urea, creatinine, calculated osmolarity (equation: 2 * (Na + K)) + (BUN/2.8) + (Glucose/18)), sodium, chloride, potassium, creatinine kinase (CK), aspartate aminotransferase (AST), alanine aminotransferase (ALT), glucose, total bilirubin. The plasma analysis results were grouped as total protein, albumin, creatinine and urea and calculated osmolarity to study hemoconcentration. Sodium, chloride and potassium were grouped to study specifically electrolytes data. The CK and AST were described together to study muscle damage. The cTnT was used as a specific indicator of myocardial damage. Lastly, glucose, ALT and total bilirubin were reported as other chemistry parameters. Out of the 35 horses for which consent was obtained for blood collection, 34 were sampled on arrival (1 horse too difficult to sample on arrival), 26 were sampled pre- and 20 were sampled post-competition (samples missing due to horses being withdrawn from the study, owner compliance or logistical reasons).

Statistical analysis

Body weight difference between arrival and pre-competition was tested using a paired t-test for all horses (n = 50) and a Wilcoxon matched-pairs signed rank test for within-each category (light, middle and heavy) comparison. Differences between the 3 weight categories in maximum weight pulled and weight ratios was tested using a Kruskal Wallis test with a Dunn's post hoc test for multiple comparisons.

Differences in blood chemistry parameters and electrolytes between arrival, pre-competition and post-competition were analyzed using a repeated ANOVA, followed by a Tukey post hoc test (data from all horses together) or a Kruskal Wallis test (for changes within each weight category), with a Dunn's post hoc test for multiple comparisons. The exception was for the lightweight category where only arrival and pre-competition samples were studied for differences in blood parameters using a Wilcoxon signed rank test because only 3 horses were sampled post-competition and this group was not included in the analysis. Association between weight change and final rank as well as between chemistry parameters from arrival samples were examined using a Pearson Correlation (data from all horses together) or a Spearman Correlation (for horses within each weight category). Data is presented as median and interquartile ranges to accommodate non-normal distribution of data (similar format was applied to the data involving all of the horses for consistency).

Results

Horses

The information provided by the owners to the event's staff indicated that horses were 9 years old (IQR: 8–10), were hauled a median distance of 451Km (IQR: 100–800)) and were fed 10 h (IQR: 2–11)) prior to weigh-in. No horses were disqualified based on the "Fitness to Compete" veterinary exam.

Body weight changes

Arrival (day 1) and pre-competition (day 2, 3 or 4 depending on division) weight was recorded for 50 out of 52 horses competing in the Heavy Horse Pull competition (1 team of 2 horses in the lightweight division missed pre-competition weighing).

Overall for all horses, body weight increased significantly between the arrival (median: 779.0Kg (735.3–885.8)) and pre-competition (median: 844.8Kg (807.3–909.2)) weigh-in ($p < 0.0001$) (Fig. 1).

When looking at specific weight divisions, body weight increased by 7.2% (median: 62.8Kg (41.7–77.0)) ($p < 0.0001$) between arrival and pre-competition (day 2) for horses competing in the lightweight division (n = 16; 8 teams) (Fig. 1). Based on the competition weigh-in thresholds, 6 of the 8 lightweight teams would have qualified for the middleweight division when using the pre-competition weights. Similarly, body weight increased by 8.6% (median: 80.5Kg (62.7–90.9)) ($p < 0.0001$) between arrival and pre-competition (day 3) for horses competing in the middleweight division (n = 16; 8 teams) (Fig. 1). As a result, 7 of the 8 teams exceeded the middleweight division and would have qualified for the heavyweight division. Weight change was not significant in the heavyweight division (n = 18; 9 teams) (p = 0.053) (Fig. 1).

Weight and ratio of weight pulled

The maximal weight pulled for each team is presented in Fig. 2. Ranking is determined by maximum weight and distance pulled (if total distance of 14 ft is not completed). For this reason, there are multiple teams that pulled the same maximal weight, though for different distances. The maximum weight pulled during the competition was 5216Kg by a heavyweight team, though this was not significantly greater than the maximal weight pulled by the winning middleweight or lightweight teams.

Additionally, the middleweights pulled a greater ratio of weight (weight pulled: team weight) than the heavyweights (median: 2.6 (2.5–2.6); 2.4 (2.2–2.5) respectively) (p = 0.01) (Fig. 2). There was no difference in weight pulled: team weight ratio between the lightweights (median: 2.7 (1.9–2.8)) and middleweights or lightweights and heavyweights.

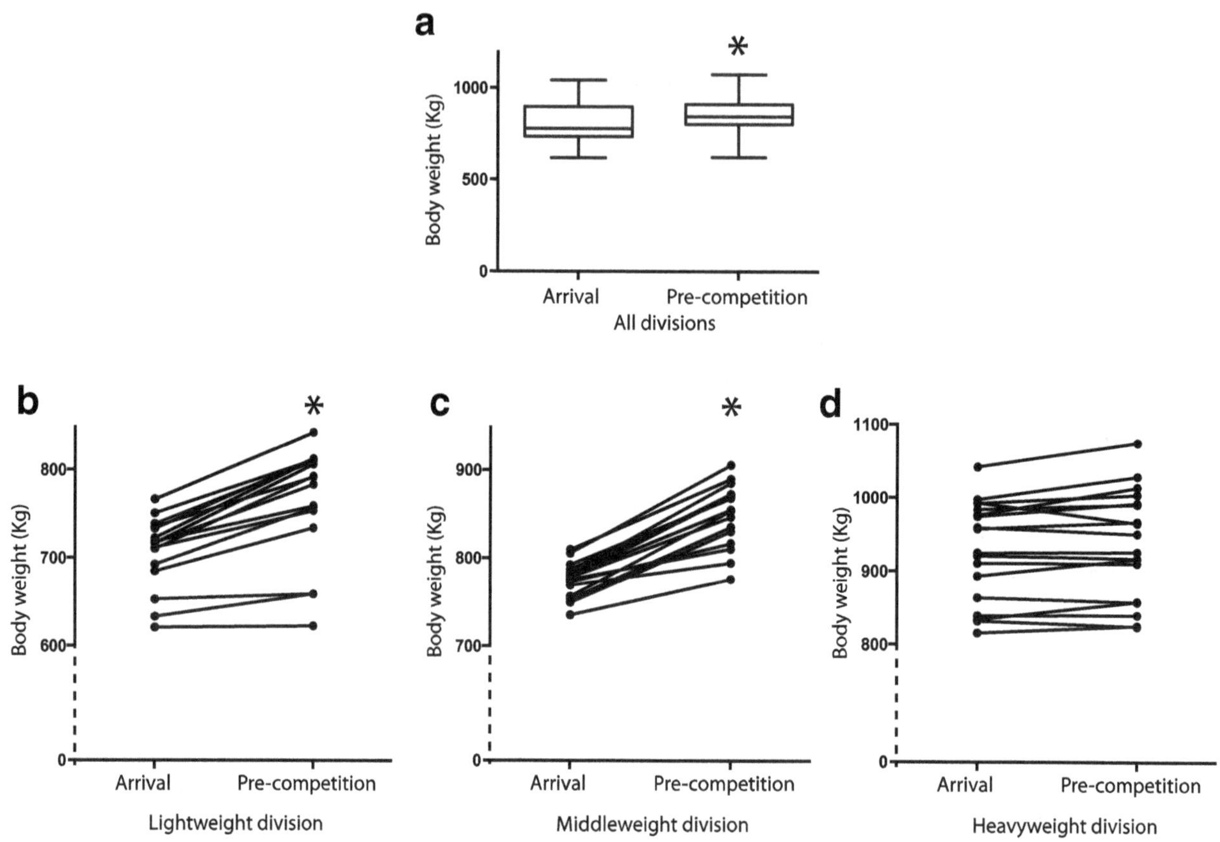

Fig. 1 Body weight change between arrival and pre-competition in draft horses participating in the Heavy Horse Pull competition at the Calgary Stampede. **a** Body weight (in Kg) measured at arrival and pre-competition in all 50 horses participating in the event. **b** Body weight change in the 16 horses from the lightweight division between arrival and pre-competition. **c** Body weight change in the 16 horses from the middleweight division between arrival and pre-competition. **d** Body weight change in the 18 horses from the heavyweight division between arrival and pre-competition. * indicates significantly different from arrival

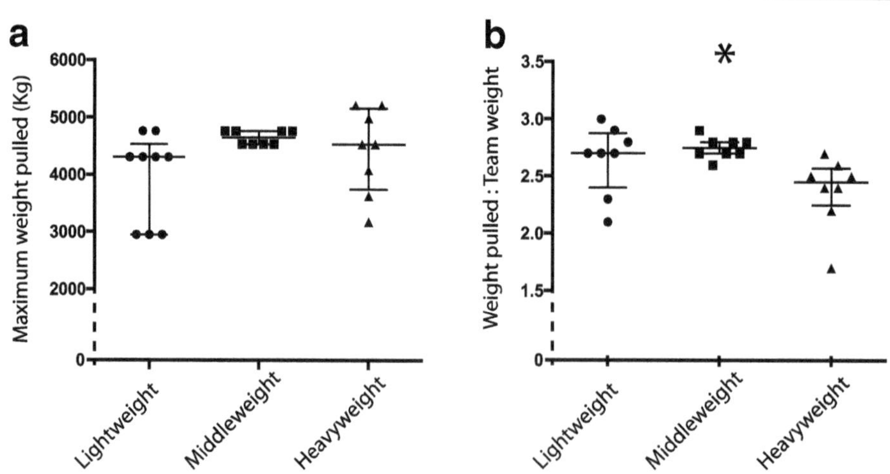

Fig. 2 Maximum weight pulled and weight ratios: **a** Maximum weight pulled (in Kg) by 24 draft horse teams (48 horses total – 1 team was disqualified before reaching maximum weight). Horses are divided based on weight division. **b** Ratio of weight pulled to team weight (Kg) for 24 draft horse teams (48 horses total – 1 team was disqualified before reaching maximum weight). Horses are treated as teams (pairs) with combined total body weights. * indicates significantly different from heavyweights

Weight change vs. competition rank

A strong negative correlation ($r = -0.69$, $p = 0.002$) was found in the middleweight horses between weight change and rank when horses were individually analyzed (Fig. 3). A higher rank is reflected with a lower placing (i.e. 1st place) therefore resulting in a negative correlation where the more weight change the better the competition result. Such correlation was not found for the lightweight and heavyweight divisions.

Plasma sample analysis

Plasma samples were collected upon arrival from all horses volunteering for the study ($n = 35$, minus 1 horse that was too difficult to sample on arrival: lightweight $n = 8$, middleweight $n = 12$, heavyweight $n = 14$). Eight horses (23%) were not sampled at further time points in the study because owners were not present or withdrew from the study. Therefore 26 (74%) pre-competition samples were collected on days 2 to 4 (lightweight $n = 7$, middleweight n = 8, heavyweight $n = 11$). Twenty (57%) post-competition samples were obtained (lightweights n = 3, middleweights n = 8, heavyweights $n = 9$) as some teams had to leave the premises prior to sampling. Median and interquartile range for all plasma parameters at arrival, pre- and post-competition are provided in Table 1 for all horses that participated in the study. Correlations between plasma parameters for all horses are provided in Table 2. Within weight categories, correlations were only found in the lightweight division.

No differences were found between pre- and post-competition for any of the blood parameters analyzed.

Total protein, albumin, creatinine, urea and calculated osmolarity

Overall, total protein was significantly greater at arrival (median: 76.5 g/L (71.3–81.3)) than at pre- (median: 70.0 g/L (68.3–72.8)) or post-competition (median: 70.5 g/L (66.0–74.0)) ($p < 0.001$) (Table 1). On arrival, 26 horses (76%) had a total protein value above 70 g/L, with a maximal value of 92 g/L observed in one horse. Analyzing the change in total protein between pre- and post-competition, we found that out of the 19 horses for which both a pre- and post-competition sample was available, 9/19 horses had a decrease in total protein after competition, whereas 10/19 horses had an increase in total protein (overall change in total protein pre- vs post-competition: Median: 0 g/L (−3.5, 3.5)). The changes in total protein were not significant when horses were split by weight categories.

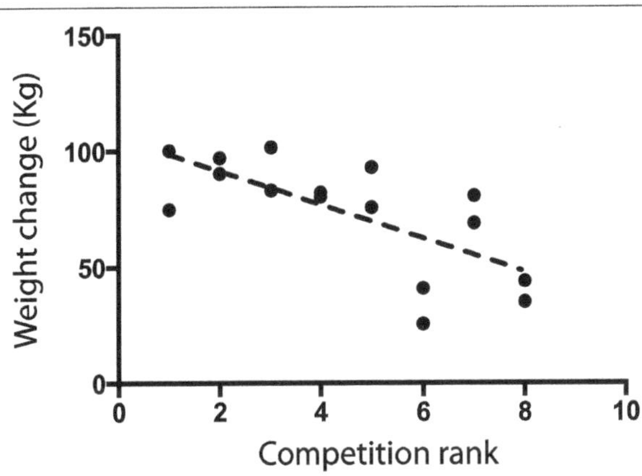

Fig. 3 Correlation between weight change (between arrival and pre-competition, in Kg) and rank for 16 horses competing in the middleweight division. A lower rank is indicative of a better final placing

Similarly to total protein, albumin was overall significantly greater at arrival (32.5 g/L (31.0–36.0)) than at the pre- (29.5 g/L (28.0–31.0)) or post-competition (30.0 g/L (28.0–32.0), respectively) time points ($p < 0.001$). Analysis of the data by weight categories showed that albumin decreased significantly between arrival (median: 37.5 g/L (32.5–39.0); (32.0 g/L (32.0–34.0), respectively) and pre-competition (median: 31.5 g/L (27.8–33.5); 28.0 g/L (26.5–30.0), respectively) for the middle and heavyweight horses ($p = 0.02$ and $p = 0.003$ respectively).

Creatinine was overall significantly greater on arrival (median: 121.0 mmol/L (102.8–144.0)) than at pre- (median: 105.5 mmol/L (92.5–111.75)) and post-competition (median: 111.0 mmol/L (89.8–120.3)) time points ($p = 0.001$ for both). Similarly, creatinine was greater on arrival than at pre-competition for the lightweight and middleweight divisions ($p = 0.015$ and $p = 0.005$ respectively) (Table 1). Five horses (15%) had elevated creatinine levels (Normal range: 70-159 mmol/L) on arrival, reaching a maximum of 235 mmol/L in one horse.

Urea overall significantly decreased from arrival (median: 5.9 mmol/L (5.2–6.9)) to pre- (median: 4.6 mmol/L (4.2–5.7)) and post-competition (median: 4.8 mmol/L (4.2–5.7)) ($p < 0.001$ for both). Urea was greater on arrival (median: 6.6 mmol/L (6.4–6.9); 6.7 mmol/L (5.9–10.5), respectively) than pre-competition (median: 5.8 mmol/L (5.6–6.5); 4.2 mmol/L (3.7–5.0), respectively) for the lightweights and middleweights ($p = 0.047$, $p = 0.004$, respectively). Four horses (12%) had elevated urea levels (Normal laboratory range: 1.8–8.9 mmol/L) on arrival, reaching a maximum of 15.4 mmol/L.

As expected, there was a strong correlation between plasma total protein, albumin, globulin, creatinine and urea (Table 2).

Calculated osmolarity was overall greater on arrival (median: 267.0 mmol/Kg (258.3–278.5)) than pre- (median: 256.0 mmol/Kg (245.3–262.8) and post-competition (median: 250.5 mmol/Kg (241.5–259.5)) ($p < 0.001$). It decreased significantly in the middleweights between arrival (median: 281.0 mmol/Kg (256.5–295.0)) and post-competition (median: 242.0 mmol/Kg (241.0–247.5)) ($p = 0.006$) as well as

Table 1 Plasma chemistry, electrolytes and high sensitivity cardiac troponin in heavy horse pulling competition: Samples on arrival (day 1), on the morning of competition (day 2, 3 or 4, depending on weight category), and 3 h after competition (number of horses indicated for each time point). The first column is based on all horses, with the other columns divided based on weight category. Median (Interquartile Range) shown

	All			Lightweight			Middleweight			Heavyweight		
	Arrival	Pre	Post	Arrival	Pre	Post	Arrival	Pre	Post	Arrival	Pre	Post
N =	34	26	20	8	7	3	12	8	8	14	11	9
Total protein (g/L)	76.5 (71.3–81.3)	70.0 [a] (68.3–72.8) ($p < 0.001$)	70.5 [a] (66.0–74.0) ($p < 0.001$)	76.0 (72.0–80.3)	71.0 (69.5–72.5)	71.0 (69.5–73.5)	78.5 (70.8–90.0)	71.0 (70.0–72.8)	71.0 (68.0–74.3)	75.0 (69.0–79.0)	68.0 (62.0–72.0)	67.0 (66.0–73.0)
Albumin (g/L)	32.5 (31.0–36.0)	29.5 [a] (28.0–31.0) ($p < 0.001$)	30.0 [a] (28.0–32.0) ($p < 0.001$)	31.5 (30.0–32.5)	29.0 [a] (29.0–30.0) ($p = 0.02$)	30.0 (29.0–31.0)	37.5 (32.5–39.0)	31.5 [a] (27.8–33.5) ($p = 0.003$)	30.0 (29.0–34.3)	32.0 (32.0–34.0)	28.0 [a] (26.5–30.0) ($p = 0.003$)	30.0 (26.0–32.0)
Globulin (g/L)	43.0 (39.3–46.8)	41.0 (39.0–43.0)	40.5 (37.0–42.0)	46.0 (42.5–47.8)	42.0 (40.0–43.0)	41.0 (40.5–42.5)	41.5 (39.8–51.0)	41.5 (38.8–43.5)	40.5 (39.0–41.3)	42.5 (39.0–45.0)	40.0 (37.0–43.0)	38.0 (37.0–42.0)
Creatinine (mmol/L)	121.0 (102.8–144.0)	105.5 [a] (92.5–111.75) ($p = 0.001$)	111.0 [a] (89.8–120.3) ($p = 0.001$)	121.0 (113.0–155.0)	111.0 [a] (105.0–112.0) ($p = 0.015$)	115.0 (113.0–118.0)	124.5 (118.0–179.3)	106.0 [a] (96.0–110.0) ($p = 0.005$)	107.0 (88.5–120.0)	109.5 (98.5–129.8)	94.0 (90.5–117.0)	100.0 (90.0–121.0)
Urea (mmol/L)	5.9 (5.2–6.9)	4.6 [a] (4.2–5.7) ($p < 0.001$)	4.8 [a] (4.2–5.7) ($p < 0.001$)	6.6 (6.4–6.9)	5.8 [a] (5.6–6.5) ($p = 0.047$)	5.5 (5.2–6.5)	6.7 (5.9–10.5)	4.2 [a] (3.7–5.0) ($p = 0.004$)	4.0 (3.4–5.2)	5.1 (4.9–5.7)	4.6 (4.5–4.9)	5.4 (4.4–5.6)
Osmolarity (mmol/Kg)	267.0 (258.3–278.5)	256.0 [a] (245.3–262.8) ($p < 0.001$)	250.5 [a] (241.5–259.5) ($p < 0.001$)	267.5 (257.8–274.8)	261.0 (259.5–263.5)	258.0 (254.5–263.5)	281.0 (256.5–295.0)	257.5 (239.5–263.3)	242.0 [a] (241.0–247.5) ($p = 0.006$)	267.0 (264.3–267.8)	247.0 [a] (238.0–256.0) ($p = 0.013$)	250.0 (243.0–265.0)
Sodium (mmol/L)	135.0 (128.5–138.8)	129.5 [a] (123.3–131.0) ($p < 0.001$)	125.5 [a] (122.0–131.5) ($p < 0.001$)	134.0 (129.3–137.0)	130.0 (130.0–132.0)	131.0 (129.0–133.0)	140.0 (127.5–144.0)	129.0 (120.5–131.8)	123.0 [a] (121.8–126.0) ($p = 0.02$)	134.0 (133.0–135.0)	125.0 [a] (119.5–129.5) ($p = 0.02$)	125.0 (122.0–133.0)
Chloride (mmol/L)	99.0 (96.0–103.0)	95.0 [a] (86.0–98.0) ($p = 0.004$)	92.0 [a] (82.8–96.0) ($p = 0.004$)	98.0 (90.0–102.0)	96.0 (93.0–97.0)	91.0 (86.0–95.0)	102.0 (95.5–105.3)	92.5 (83.0–99.5)	91.0 [a] (82.3–94.3) ($p = 0.01$)	98.0 (97.0–101.0)	94.0 (89.0–98.0)	93.0 (88.0–101.0)
Potassium (mmol/L)	3.4 (3.2–3.7)	3.3 (2.8–3.7)	2.9 [a] (2.4–3.4) ($p = 0.034$)	3.45 (3.2–3.7)	3.6 (3.1–3.7)	2.3 (2.1–2.6)	3.3 (3.2–3.5)	3.3 (2.9–4)	2.8 [a] (2.2–2.8) ($p = 0.01$)	3.3 (3.1–3.6)	3.2 (2.5–3.5)	3.3 (3.1–3.5)
CK (IU/L)	175.5 (150.3–253.0)	174.0 (127.8–325.3)	225.5 (142.0–887.5) [a] ($p = 0.04$)	214.0 (189.0–313.8)	215.0 (169.5–622.5)	294.0 (230.0–704.0)	175.0 (160.8–259.0)	143.5 (113.3–504.0)	209.0 (147.5–753.5)	167.0 (147.3–213.8)	178.0 (115.5–293.5)	231.0 (142.0–4544.0)
ALT (IU/L)	7.0 (6.0–15.0)	6.5 (5.3–14.0)	9.5 (6.8–23.5)	6.0 (5.8–6.5)	7.0 (6.0–9.5)	7.5 (7.3–7.8)	11.5 (6.5–21.5)	14.0 (9.0–22.0)	14.5 (10.0–23.5)	7.0 (6.0–9.0)	5.0 (3.5–6.5)	6.0 (5.0–13.0)
cTnT (ng/L)	2.9 (2.9–6.0)	2.9 (2.9–5.5)	4.0 (2.9–10.0)	2.9 (2.9–5.1)	2.9 (2.9–11.5)	15 (8.9–16.5)	4.0 (2.9–7.0)	2.9 (2.9–5.7)	3.5 (2.9–9.5)	2.9 (2.9–3.8)	2.9 (2.9–5.0)	4.0 (2.9–8.0)
Glucose (mmol/L)	5.9 (5.4–6.6)	5.4 [a] (5.0–5.6) ($p = 0.026$)	5.5 (5.1–5.8)	5.8 (5.1–6.1)	5.4 (5.2–5.7)	5.3 (5.2–5.4)	6.4 (5.9–7.2)	5.4 [a] (5.2–5.8) ($p = 0.047$)	5.8 (5.4–6.4)	5.8 (5.3–6.1)	5.0 [a] (4.8–5.5) ($p = 0.044$)	5.5 (5.0–5.7)
T. bilirubin (μmol/L)	26.4 (19.9–31.3)	17.7 [a] (14.9–21.8) ($p = 0.01$)	17.8 (16.3–24.8)	25.0 (16.4–30.0)	15.0 [a] (12.9–18.8) ($p = 0.01$)	19.3 (18.3–23.6)	48.3 (28.7–62.3)	18.7 [a] (17.2–37.4) ($p = 0.02$)	18.4 (16.3–32.1)	21.8 (19.3–25.9)	17.5 (15.3–21.2)	17.3 (13.1–21.1)

[a] **significantly different from arrival.** *CK* Creatinine Kinase, *hscTnT* High sensitivity cardiac troponin T

Table 2 Significant correlations between plasma chemistry parameters for horses sampled at the Heavy Horse Pull ($n = 34$) on arrival (day 1). Correlation is organized in descending order with the associated p-value

Blood parameter	Correlation coefficient	P
Globulin/Total protein	0.959	< 0.001
Creatinine/Urea	0.945	< 0.001
Total bilirubin/Urea	0.942	< 0.001
ALT/AST	0.93	< 0.001
Albumin/Sodium	0.917	< 0.001
Total bilirubin/Creatinine	0.905	< 0.001
Albumin/Total protein	0.896	< 0.001
ALT/CK	0.882	< 0.001
Total protein/Sodium	0.874	< 0.001
Total protein/Urea	0.839	< 0.001
Albumin/Urea	0.826	< 0.001
Glucose/Urea	0.819	< 0.001
Albumin/Total bilirubin	0.814	< 0.001
Glucose/Total bilirubin	0.808	< 0.001
Glucose/Total protein	0.788	< 0.001
Glucose/Creatinine	0.777	< 0.001
Glucose/Albumin	0.767	< 0.001
Total protein/Creatinine	0.759	< 0.001
Globulin/Urea	0.758	< 0.001
Sodium/Urea	0.753	< 0.001

between arrival (median: 267.0 mmol/Kg (264.3–267.8)) and pre-competition (median: 247.0 mmol/Kg (238.0–256.0)) in the heavyweights ($p = 0.013$).

Altogether, the increased values of total proteins, albumin, creatinine, urea and calculated osmolarity indicate that these horses were overall hemoconcentrated on arrival. However, the plasma chemistries of the heavyweight horses did not indicate hemoconcentration (except for higher albumin on arrival than pre-competition) after analysis by weight categories.

Electrolytes

Overall, sodium, chloride and potassium decreased after arrival. Sodium and chloride were significantly greater on arrival (median: 135.0 mmol/L (128.5–138.8); 99.0 mmol/L (96.0–103.0, respectively) than at both pre- (median: 129.5 mmol/L (123.3–131.0); 95.0 mmol/L (86.0–98.0), respectively) and post-competition (median: 125.5 mmol/L (122.0–131.5); 92.0 mmol/L (82.8–96.0), respectively) ($p < 0.001$, $p = 0.004$, respectively) (Table 1), and potassium was greater on arrival (median: 3.4 mmol/L (3.2–3.7)) than post-competition (median: 2.9 mmol/L (2.4–3.4)) ($p = 0.034$). Sodium, chloride and potassium decreased significantly between arrival (median: 140.0 mmol/L (127.5–131.8); 102.0 mmol/L (95.5–105.3); 3.3 mmol/L (3.2–3.5), respectively) and post-competition (median: 123.0 mmol/L (120.5–131.8); 91.0 mmol/L (82.3–94.3); 2.8 mmol/L (2.2–2.8), respectively) for the middleweight horses ($p = 0.02$, $p = 0.01$ and $p = 0.01$ respectively), while only sodium showed a decrease between arrival (median: 134.0 mmol/L (133.0–135.0)) and pre-competition (median: 125.0 mmol/L (119.5–129.5)) in the heavyweights ($p = 0.02$). None of the 3 electrolytes showed any change over time in the lightweight horses.

Arrival samples indicated that 7 (21%) and 4 (12%) of the 34 horses had greater than normal sodium and chloride levels, respectively. The highest chloride and sodium levels on arrival were 112.0 mmol/L and 148.0 mmol/L respectively, in a lightweight horse.

Plasma sodium was strongly correlated to total protein, albumin, and urea when all horses were included in the analysis (Table 2). Plasma chloride was strongly correlated to total protein ($r = 0.92$, $p = 0.003$), globulin ($r = 0.93$, $p = 0.001$) and sodium ($r = 0.80$, $p = 0.02$) only in the lightweight horses.

Muscle enzymes

Overall there was a significant increase in CK between arrival (median: 175.5 IU/L (150.3–253.0)) and post-competition (median: 225.5 IU/L (142.0–887.5)) ($p = 0.04$), though this was not observed within the individual weight categories. Eleven horses had elevated AST (laboratory range: 180-570 IU/L) and/or CK values (laboratory range: 110-700 IU/L) prior to competition (10 horses (30%) at arrival, 9 (35%) at pre-competition). Eight horses (40%) had elevated AST and/or CK post-competition, only one of which was not elevated pre-competition.

There was as strong correlation between AST and ALT, as well as between CK and ALT (Table 2).

Cardiac troponin hscTnT

High sensitivity cTnT stayed within normal range for all horses and the trend to increase after competition was not significant (Table 1).

Other chemistry parameters

Plasma glucose was greater on arrival (median: 5.9 mmol/L (5.4–6.6)) than pre-competition (median: 5.4 mmol/L (5.0–5.6)) overall ($p = 0.026$) as well as for the middleweight (median: 6.4 mmol/L (5.9–7.2); 5.4 mmol/L (5.2–5.8), respectively) ($p = 0.047$) and heavyweight (median: 5.8 mmol/L (5.3–6.1); 5.0 mmol/L (4.8–5.5), respectively) ($p = 0.044$) categories (Table 1).

Glucose was strongly correlated with creatinine, urea, total protein, albumin and globulin (Table 2).

Plasma total bilirubin decreased overall between arrival (median: 26.4 μmol/L (19.9–31.3)) and pre-competition (median: 17.7 μmol/L (14.9–21.8)) ($p = 0.01$), which was also observed for the lightweights (median: 25.0 μmol/L

(16.4–30.0); 15.0 μmol/L (12.9–18.8), respectively) and middleweights (median: 48.3 μmol/L (28.7–62.3); 18.7 μmol/L (17.2–37.4), respectively) (p = 0.01, p = 0.02, respectively).

Total bilirubin was strongly correlated to creatinine, urea, albumin and glucose (Table 2).

Discussion

Our study describes the physiological demands of the Heavy Horse Pull, a unique high-intensity, short duration discipline, where horses pull more than 2.5 times their weight for a distance of 14 ft. This is also the first descriptive analysis of "shrinkage" or rapid weight change in horses, with up to an average change in weight of 8.6%. However, this weight change did not seem to affect performance of the horses, likely because they had 34 to 82 h to recover prior to competition.

Weight change and hemoconcentration

While some human athletes subject themselves to RWL to "make weight" in an attempt to gain a competitive edge, evidence supporting this claim of enhanced performance is disputed. It has been shown that in humans even a 2% change in body weight negatively affects aerobic and endurance performance [2]. It is believed that weight loss through dehydration affects sprint exercises less than endurance events [4, 14], and there is debate as to whether mild dehydration may actually improve performance in sprint and power sports in humans [15]. Although laboratory tests have shown reduced human athletic capacity following 2% weight loss, up to a 4% weight loss has not been shown to affect performance in field tests [16, 17].

There is, however, an important difference in rapid weight change between human athletes and draft horses entering pulling competitions: whereas human athletes compete at their lower-than-normal weight, heavy horses have a period of time regain significant weight before competing. Therefore, although horses may arrive to the event in a dehydrated state, we found that they compete in a euhydrated state. Indeed, in the present study, no horse had plasma creatinine or urea values above normal range at the pre-competition time point, and the calculated osmolarity, creatinine, urea and total protein values decreased significantly between arrival and pre-competition (Table 1). The rapid weight change may therefore have less of an effect on the performance and physiological parameters of these horses than on human athletes.

Work previously conducted in a different type of pulling event in Europe (light horses pulling for 1.3 min) where horses compete in a dehydrated and unfed state found that regardless of weight category, dehydrated horses had increased total protein, albumin, creatinine, sodium and urea [18]. Interestingly in the present study, not all horses that experienced weight loss were hemoconcentrated on arrival. This indicates that while most horses lost weight via a loss of intravascular fluid, some horses instead lost gastrointestinal content, possibly due to feed restriction or laxative use.

Lightweight category horses had the least amount of time to recover between arrival and competition (~34 h) compared to middleweights (~58 h) and heavyweights (~82 h). Based on this minimum period of 34 h, it does not appear that number of days before competition had a significant effect on pre-competition volemic status. Indeed, no horse had increased creatinine or urea at pre-competition, indicating that these horses were able to adequately rehydrate during the 34-h period.

Mild to moderate hemoconcentration (elevated total protein) was observed in 11 horses post-competition, which is a normal response following maximal exercise.

Weight change and overall rank

The strong negative correlation (r = 0.69, p = 0.002) found between the weight change and overall ranking in middleweight horses (Fig. 3) indicates that the more weight the horse gained (indicative more intensive rapid weight change), the better they placed. However, it may also be that the best teams are also the ones that practice shrinkage. A study conducted on work oxen found that weight loss had no effect on pulling performance, however this was achieved through long-term diet restrictions with adequate water [19]. In the present study, horses that showed severe hemoconcentration did rehydrate quickly, and this rapid weight change did not impair performance (Fig. 3). Additionally, in spite of having the least amount of time (34 h) to replenish any weight loss, the lightweight horses pulled the greatest weight relative to their bodyweight, indicating that the rapid weight change is unlikely to have an effect on pulling performance as long as the horses have at least 34 h to recover.

Further research is required to determine if there is a physiological relationship between weight loss and rank at pulling competitions.

Percentage of weight pulled

Draft capacity is often represented in terms of horsepower (the rate at which work is performed) with horses having been selected for their greater capacity and speed than oxen or cattle, indicating their superior horsepower [20]. Horses working in teams will have a greater cumulative draft capacity, however each individual horses' draft capacity will be reduced by up to 7.5% for two horses when compared to a single animal effort [21].

Previously, research has focused on sustained pulling capacity of horses for farming where they pull 10–12% of their body weight [20]. In comparison, we found that these horses could pull over 2.5 times their body weight, though it was over a very short duration.

The competitors perceive that heavier horses have an advantage in the pulling competitions. In that sense, there was a trend in the present study to have a greater maximum weight pulled by the heavyweight teams. Combined data from this study and the historical results available from the Calgary Stampede pulling competitions over the previous 13 years, however, indicate that the maximum weight pulled does not differ between different weight classes. This suggests that the weight of the horses is not the most determining factor for the maximum pulling weight capacity of the teams during competition. It has been reported that small horses are stronger relative to their body weight compared to larger horses [22], with ponies able to pull 66% of the weight that was pulled by horses and 116% of that pulled by cattle [23]. Similarly, we found that lightweight horses pulled the greatest amount of weight relative to body mass (median: 275% (272–286)), which is greater than what a previous study reported on Valencian horses [18]. The Valencian horses described by Munoz et al., pulled 2–2.5 times their bodyweight for 1.3 min during competitions which is also much shorter than the draft horses pulling competition described in the present study,

Plasma electrolytes and other chemistry parameters

There were many differences in plasma parameter levels between arrival and pre- or post-competition, as discussed below; however, no differences were found between pre- and post- competition. These post-competition values indicate that the duration of the event was simply too short to induce significant changes in the variables measured, or that the horses were able to recover from the competition within 3 h. Indeed, a different study found that recovery from pulling exercise happens quickly with a return of blood parameters to baseline levels within 15 to 30 min [18].

On arrival, plasma glucose was significantly greater than at pre-competition and there was a strong correlation between glucose and creatinine, urea, total protein, albumin and globulin. Altogether, these results are likely explained by the stress of shipping (some teams were shipped for longer than 17 h) combined with hemoconcentration.

Sodium and chloride significantly decreased between arrival and pre-competition and then post-competition. It is interesting to note that 9/34 horses on arrival were hyponatremic. The reason for this is unknown, but it is possibly due to sodium losses through the colon. In spite of these 9 horses being hyponatremic, the data shows overall greater plasma sodium levels on arrival than pre-competition. The higher overall plasma sodium and chloride levels on arrival were likely related to hemoconcentration due to shipping and rapid weight change practices. Similarly, a previous study found an increase in plasma sodium and chloride in dehydrated pulling horses compared to euhydrated controls, and found a similar correlation as we did between plasma sodium and urea [18].

In the study from Munoz et al. a pulling exercise induced a short duration increase in sodium and chloride that then decreased back to resting levels within 15 min in euhydrated horses [18]. In the present study however, we actually observed a trend for plasma sodium and chloride to decrease post-competition. This is probably because our post-competition samples were taken 3 h after exercise, when plasma sodium and chloride values were at a steady state and not affected by exercised-induced electrolyte shifts.

Surprisingly, plasma potassium decreased significantly between arrival and post-competition (Table 1). Potassium is usually related to hay intake – it is difficult to explain this finding in the context of RWL, where we would have expected lower potassium values on arrival due to feed withdrawal, and an increase in plasma potassium with time. A confounding factor may be hemoconcentration on arrival.

We found an increase in CK between arrival and post-competition, likely due to the effect of shipping, as CK takes a few hours to peak after muscle damage is initiated. In addition, 7/ 20 horses had increased CK values post-competition (median: 225.5 IU/L (142.0–887.5)). Since these samples were taken 3 h after the competition, we estimate that this is a good indication of the true CK peak values after the pulling event. The CK values noted were under 5000 IU/L for all except for 2 horses (8784 IU/L and 16,605 IU/L). This altogether with the fact that CK values did not increase significantly between pre- and post-competition, shows that the pulling event did not have an effect on the muscle metabolism of these draft horses. There were no significant changes in AST values, however AST peaks later than CK and a longer post-competition period would be required to observe this peak. Total bilirubin decreased significantly overall between arrival and pre-competition, which may be explained by a decreased feed intake right before and during shipping.

In the present study we found a trend for hscTnT to increase post-competition that was not statistically significant. This indicates that there is no myocardial damage induced by the high intensity short duration pulling exercise in draft horses.

Conclusions

Our study showed that horses competing in the Heavy Horse Pull undergo significant weight changes, most marked in the middleweight category. Although we found that horses arrived to the event with some indications of hemoconcentration, the minimum 34 h delay before the competition allowed the horses to recover well from the effects of shipping and rapid weight change. We did not find any effect of the pulling competition on the chemistry parameters, indicating that these events are well tolerated and only induce reversible, short-term stress on the metabolism of the horses.

Endnotes

[1]AU680, Beckman Coulter Inc., Mississauga, ON.
[2]Troponin T hs, Roche Diagnostics, Indianapolis, IN.
[3]Cobas-e601, Roche Diagnostics, Indianapolis, IN.
[4]Calgary Lab Services, Calgary, AB.

Abbreviations

ALT: Alanine aminotransferase; AST: Aspartate aminotransferase; CK: Creatine kinase; cTnT: Cardiac troponin; hscTnT: High-sensitivity cardiac troponin; RWL: Rapid weight loss

Acknowledgements

The authors thank the organizers of the Calgary Stampede and the owners for participating in this study. Thank-you to Rhianna Malcolm, Claire Poulain and Mei Steinnman for their help with data collection.

Funding

This study was supported by an internal University of Calgary start-up fund awarded to EP.

Authors' contributions

PGO, SM, ES, MFR, EP, and RL participated in study design. PGO, SM and ES collected the samples. PGO, MFR, and RL performed statistical analysis. PGO drafted the manuscript with help from SM, ES, MFR, EP, and RL. All authors read and approved the final manuscript.

Authors information

PGO: Bsc – PhD student.
SM: BScKin, CEP, MSc.
ES: HBSc., DC, DVM, Resident ACVSMR (Sports Medicine and Rehabilitation) – MSc.
MFR: PhD, DVM, Dipl. ACVIM.
EP: BSc, MSc, PhD – Anderson-Chisholm Chair in Animal Care and Welfare, Professor UCVM.
RL: MSc., PhD, DMV, Dipl. ACVIM, Dipl. ACVSMR (Sports Medicine and Rehabilitation) – Associate Professor UCVM.

Consent for publication

Not applicable.

Competing interests

The authors declare that they have no competing interests.

References

1. Rankin JW. Weight loss and gain in athletes. Curr Sport. Med Rep. 2002;1:208–13.
2. Bartok C, Schoeller DA, Sullivan JC, Clark RR, Landry GL. Hydration testing in collegiate wrestlers undergoing hypertonic dehydration. Med Sci Sports Exerc. 2004;36:510–7.
3. James LJ, Shirreffs SM. Fluid and electrolyte balance during 24-hour fluid and/or energy restriction. Int J Sport Nutr Exerc Metab. 2013;23:545–53.
4. Yoshida T, Takanishi T, Nakai S, Yorimoto A, Morimoto T. The critical level of water deficit causing a decrease in human exercise performance: a practical field study. Eur J Appl Physiol. 2002;87:529–34.
5. Judelson DA, Maresh CM, Anderson JM, Armstrong LE, Casa DJ, Kraemer WJ, et al. Hydration and muscular performance: does fluid balance affect strength, power and high-intensity endurance? Sports Med. 2007;37:907–21.
6. Perez R, Recabarren SE, Valdes P, Hetz E. Biochemical and physiological parameters and estimated work output in draught horses pulling loads for long periods. Vet Res Commun. 1992;16:231–46.
7. Pérez R, Recabarren SE, Mora G, Jara C, Quijada G, Hetz E. Cardiorespiratory parameters in draught horses before and after short term draught work pulling loads. J Vet Med Ser A. 1992;39:215–22.
8. Shave R, Baggish A, George K, Wood M, Scharhag J, Whyte G, et al. Exercise-induced cardiac Troponin elevation. J Am Coll Cardiol. 2010;56:169–76.
9. Shields E, Seiden-Long I, Massie S, Passante S, Leguillette R. Analytical validation and establishment of reference intervals for a 'high-sensitivity' cardiac troponin-T assay in horses. BMC Vet Res. 2016;12:104.
10. Shave R, Baggish A, George K, Wood M, Scharhag J, Whyte G, et al. Exercise-induced cardiac troponin elevation: evidence, mechanisms, and implications. J Am Coll Cardiol. 2010;56:169–76.
11. Hessel MHM, Michielsen ECHJ, Atsma DE, Schalij MJ, van der Valk EJM, Bax WH, et al. Release kinetics of intact and degraded troponin I and T after irreversible cell damage. Exp Mol Pathol. 2008;85:90–5.
12. Hessel MHM, Atsma DE, van der Valk EJM, Bax WH, Schalij MJ, van der Laarse A. Release of cardiac troponin I from viable cardiomyocytes is mediated by integrin stimulation. Eur J Phys. 2008;455:979–86.
13. Brakenhoff JE, Holcombe SJ, Hauptman JOEG, Smith HK, Nickels FA, Caron JP, et al. The prevalence of laryngeal disease in a large population of competition draft horses. Vet Surg. 2006:579–83.
14. Webster S, Rutt R, Weltman A. Physiological effects of a weight loss regimen practiced by college wrestlers. Med Sci Sports Exerc. 1990;22:229–34.
15. Viitasalo JT, Kyröläinen H, Bosco C, Alen M. Effects of rapid weight reduction on force production and vertical jumping height. Int J Sports Med. 1987;8:281–5.
16. Cheuvront SN, Carter R III, Sawka MN. Fluid balance and endurance exercise performance. Curr Sport Med Rep. 2003;2:202–8.
17. Goulet EDB. Effect of exercise-induced dehydration on endurance performance: evaluating the impact of exercise protocols on outcomes using a meta-analytic procedure. Br J Sports Med. 2013;47:679–86.
18. Muñoz A, Riber C, Trigo P, Castejón FM, Lucas RG, Palacio J. The effects of hypertonic dehydration changes on renal function and arginine vasopressin in the horse during pulling exercises. Vet J. 2011;189:83–8.
19. Astatke A, Reed JD, Butterworth MH. Effect of diet restriction on work performance and weight loss of local zebu and Friesian X Boran crossbred oxen. ILCA Bull. 1986;23:11–4.
20. Goe MR, McDowell RE. Animal traction: guidelines for utilization. Cornell Int Agric Mimeogr. 1980;81
21. Centre d'études et d'expérimentation du machinisme agricole tropical. Employment of Draught Animals in Agriculture. 1972.
22. Back W, Clayton HM. Equine locomotion: Elsevier Health Sciences; 2013.
23. Hesse HJ. Working ability and food requirements of small horses compared with large horses and cattle. Anim Breed. 1956;24:160–3.

Deletion of the ORF2 gene of the neuropathogenic equine herpesvirus type 1 strain Ab4 reduces virulence while maintaining strong immunogenicity

Christiane L. Schnabel[1], Christine L. Wimer[1], Gillian Perkins[2], Susanna Babasyan[1], Heather Freer[1], Christina Watts[1], Alicia Rollins[1], Nikolaus Osterrieder[3] and Bettina Wagner[1*]

Abstract

Background: Equine herpesvirus type 1 (EHV-1) induces respiratory infection, abortion, and neurologic disease with significant impact. Virulence factors contributing to infection and immune evasion are of particular interest. A potential virulence factor of the neuropathogenic EHV-1 strain Ab4 is ORF2.

This study on 24 Icelandic horses, 2 to 4 years of age, describes the infection with EHV-1 Ab4, or its deletion mutant devoid of ORF2 (Ab4ΔORF2) compared to non-infected controls (each group $n = 8$). The horses' clinical presentation, virus shedding, viremia, antibody and cellular immune responses were monitored over 260 days after experimental infection.

Results: Infection with Ab4ΔORF2 reduced fever and minimized nasal virus shedding after infection compared to the parent virus strain Ab4, while Ab4ΔORF2 established viremia similar to Ab4. Concurrently with virus shedding, intranasal cytokine and interferon α (IFN-α) production increased in the Ab4 group, while horses infected with Ab4ΔORF2 expressed less IFN-α.

The antibody response to EHV-1 was evaluated by a bead-based multiplex assay and was similar in both infected groups, Ab4 and Ab4ΔORF2. EHV-1 specific immunoglobulin (Ig) G1 was induced 8 days after infection (d8 pi) with a peak on d10–12 pi. EHV-1 specific IgG4/7 increased starting on d10 pi, and remained elevated in serum until the end of the study. The intranasal antibody response to EHV-1 was dominated by the same IgG isotypes and remained elevated in both infected groups until d130 pi. In contrast to the distinct antibody response, no induction of EHV-1 specific T-cells was detectable by flow cytometry after ex vivo re-stimulation of peripheral blood mononuclear cells (PBMC) with EHV-1 in any group. The cellular immune response was characterized by increased secretion of IFN-γ and interleukin10 in response to ex vivo re-stimulation of PBMC with EHV-1. This response was present during the time of viremia (d5–10 pi) and was similar in both infected groups, Ab4 and Ab4ΔORF2.

Conclusions: ORF2 is a virulence factor of EHV-1 Ab4 with impact on pyrexia and virus shedding from the nasal mucosa. In contrast, ORF2 does not influence viremia. The immunogenicity of the Ab4ΔORF2 and parent Ab4 viruses are identical.

Keywords: Horse, EHV-1, ORF2, Virulence factor, Immunoglobulin, Mucosal immune response

* Correspondence: bw73@cornell.edu
[1]Department of Population Medicine and Diagnostic Sciences, College of Veterinary Medicine, Cornell University, Ithaca, NY 14853, USA
Full list of author information is available at the end of the article

Background

Equine herpesvirus type 1 (EHV-1), an alphaherpesvirus, frequently induces clinical disease in horses and other equids. Clinical manifestations include upper respiratory tract disease with pyrexia as well as late-term abortions, or neurologic disease (equine herpesvirus myeloencephalopathy, EHM) [1–4]. EHV-1 is transmitted from horse to horse during close contact via respiratory secretions. The virus initially infects the epithelium of the upper respiratory tract. Subsequently, it spreads through the underlying connective tissue to the regional lymphoid tissues, and next establishes cell-associated viremia in leukocytes [5–8]. Viremia is a prerequisite for the infection of endothelial cells by EHV-1 and induction of vasculitis in the pregnant uterus or central nervous system. These events can lead to the severe manifestations of EHV-1, abortions or EHM, respectively [1, 3, 5, 9–11]. Furthermore, EHV-1 establishes latency. Latent EHV-1 is believed to reside in the trigeminal ganglia and in lymphoid tissues of the respiratory tract [12–16].

Latency and immune evasion are two important characteristics of EHV-1 preventing EHV-1 elimination by the immune system of the horse. Latently infected horses serve as a reservoir of the virus. EHV-1 can be reactivated with or without signs of clinical disease in the reservoir horse [17]. Lack of vaccination and incomplete protection after vaccination provide sufficient susceptible hosts within the population for EHV-1 to spread periodically after reactivation from latency or from newly infected horses [4, 17]. The prevalence of EHV-1 is high with detection in 54–88% of horses post mortem [14, 18, 19]. Outbreaks of EHV-1 associated clinical disease occur in variable frequencies but the severity of EHV-1 manifestations seems to be increasing [4, 14, 20]. Consequently, EHV-1 has a significant impact on animal health and the equine economy worldwide and EHM has been classified as an emerging disease in the USA [20, 21]. Management practices and biosecurity measures are applied to contain EHM outbreaks. Many horses are regularly vaccinated in order to prevent infection and disease. However, the use of inactivated or attenuated live virus vaccines has not been sufficient to completely protect from EHV-1 infection and outbreaks [22, 23]. Protective immune responses after vaccination with available vaccines and after natural infection in horses are transient and re-infection is possible between 4 and 8 weeks post vaccination or 6–18 months post infection of adult horses [22, 24–27].

Recent research has focused on the identification of EHV-1 virulence factors such as the mutation of the DNA polymerase gene (ORF30) at nucleotide position 2554, which has been associated with the manifestation of EHM and the establishment of latency after EHV-1 infection. Strains of the genotype G2554 are thus classified as neuropathogenic [2, 28–31]. However, this classification rather points to an increased risk of the G2554 strains causing EHM. During neurological outbreaks between 3 and 45% of the horses developed EHM [32–34] while non-neuropathogenic strains can also cause neurologic disease [2]. The identification and better characterization of virulence factors underlying the pathogenicity, immune modulation, and establishment of latency by EHV-1 can enable targeted approaches to develop a vaccine providing advanced protection from the virus.

In vitro infection of equine peripheral blood mononuclear cells (PBMC) with the non-neuropathogenic EHV-1 strain RacL11 reduced the down-regulation of MHC class I expression [35], and increased interleukin10 (IL-10) secretion [36] and chemokine expression [37] compared to infection with the neuropathogenic strain Ab4. These findings point to differences of EHV-1 strains in modulating the host immune response, which may also be relevant in vivo. Potential virulence factors of the Ab4 strain are the ORF1 and ORF2 gene products. ORF1 and ORF2 genes are absent in RacL11, the RacL11-derived modified-live vaccine strain RacH [38], as well as in the apathogenic strain KyA [39, 40]. Hence, the ORF1 and ORF2 genes could encode for immunomodulatory proteins leading to differences in virulence or pathogenicity. The ORF1 gene product pUL56 of Ab4 is responsible for MHC class I down-regulation and seems to be involved in the suppression of cytokine expression and chemokine secretion in vitro [35, 41]. The ORF2 gene is related to ORF1, but is less well characterized. The ORF2 gene product was classified as a membrane protein due to its predicted hydrophobic profile [40]. The deletion of ORF1 and ORF2 genes from EHV-1 Ab4 significantly reduced pyrexia duration and viral shedding compared to the parent Ab4 virus in experimentally infected ponies [42]. This effect could be attributed to either gene or the combination of ORF1 and ORF2.

Here, we performed an experimental infection in horses using a single ORF2 gene deletion mutant of the EHV-1 strain Ab4, Ab4ΔORF2 [35], in comparison to the parent Ab4 virus. The goals of the approach were to identify ORF2 as a potential virulence factor, to characterize the effects of ORF2 on EHV-1 infection and immune responses in horses with known EHV-1 infection and immunity background.

Methods

Horses

Twenty-four horses from the Cornell University herd of Icelandic horses with known EHV-1 status were enrolled in this study [43, 44]. All horses were offspring of one stallion, were born at Cornell University, and kept at an isolated facility as a group from birth. They had no contact with other horses in the USA prior to and for the duration of this study. All horses were previously experimentally infected with the EHV-1 strain NY03 after weaning at 7 months of age [44, and unpublished data]. By the time of the present study, the horses were 2–4 years of age and their EHV-1 specific immunity had waned to values typically observed in EHV-1 susceptible horses. EHV-1 specific protective immunity is short-lasting and believed to be maintained for 6–9 months after a single experimental infection [27]. The horses were vaccinated annually against rabies, tetanus, West Nile virus, Eastern and Western Encephalitis virus. They were also dewormed twice a year. Prior to the EHV-1 infection described here, the horses were kept on pasture and were clinically healthy. Grass hay was fed to the horses *ad libitum*. All horses survived and were kept for research purposes at Cornell University after the study.

Virus preparation

Viruses for experimental infection were EHV-1 Ab4, a neuropathogenic strain isolated from a quadriplegic mare [9, 28, 45] and its ORF2 gene deletion mutant, Ab4Δ ORF2, produced by two-step Red-mediated recombination of a recombinant BAC Ab4 as previously described in detail [35]. The viruses were propagated in rabbit kidney cells (RK13) in MEM medium supplemented with 0.292 g/l L-glutamine, 1 mM sodium pyruvate, 100 U/ml Penicillin, 100 μg/ml Streptomycin, 50 μg/ml gentamycin, (all Thermo Fisher Scientific Waltham, MA, USA), and 10% FCS (Atlanta biological, Flowery Branch, GA, USA). Virus titers were determined in RK13 cells as previously described [22, 37].

The identity of each virus preparation was confirmed by conventional PCR on 2 μg of extracted viral DNA, using primers flanking the ORF1 and ORF2 gene region of the EHV-1 strain Ab4: forward primer – 5'-AACA ACCCTGGGCTCTTTA -3′ and reverse primer – 5'-G ATTCGCACCTCATCTCCAC -3′. The resulting PCR products had a distinct size of 2043 bp for Ab4 and of 1446 bp for Ab4ΔORF2. The deletion of ORF2 in Ab4Δ ORF2 was furthermore confirmed by sequencing of the PCR product at the Biotechnology Core Facility of Cornell University. After infection, the titer of each virus preparation was confirmed by titration on a plaque assay as described below.

Experimental EHV-1 infection

For experimental EHV-1 infection horses were assigned to three groups of eight horses each with four mares and four geldings per group. One group of horses served as non-infected controls (control group) and had a median age of 2 years (range 2–3 years). Horses in a second group were infected with the neuropathogenic EHV-1 strain Ab4 (Ab4 group) and had a median age of 2.5 years (range 2–3 years). The third group was infected with the Ab4ΔORF2 deletion mutant virus (Ab4ΔORF2 group) and had a median age of 2.5 years (range 2–4 years).

One day prior to EHV-1 infection the horses were moved into the isolation barns with individual box stalls and allowed to acclimate. The stalls did not allow the horses to have direct nose-to-nose contact. The non-infected control group was housed in a separate barn and always handled prior to the other groups. The two infected groups were housed in a barn with two separate sections, one for each group, divided by a barrier. Airflow between sections was not possible. Each section had a separate entry with an area for donning personal protective equipment including disposable coveralls, boots, hats, and gloves. Biosecurity precautions were taken and people changed personal protective equipment upon entering and exiting each of the sections to prevent the spread of viruses between the three groups. Within each barn section, the barn had a center hallway with the same airspace and horses were handled in each section as one group. No other specific care was taken to prevent spread of virus from horse-to-horse within each group by animal handlers except for changing gloves after taking nasal swab samples from each horse.

Baseline serum and nasopharyngeal secretion (NS) samples were taken the day before EHV-1 infection (d-1). Baseline physical examination measurements were taken on d-1 and again immediately before EHV-1 infection on d0. Then, Ab4 group horses were infected intranasally with $1 \, x \, 10^7$ plaque-forming units (PFU) of EHV-1 strain Ab4 in 4 ml of saline with a mucosal atomizer device (Wolfe Tory Medical, Salt Lake City, UT). Horses in the Ab4ΔORF2 group received $1x10^7$ PFU of the Ab4ΔORF2 virus in 4 ml saline intranasally. Horses in the control group received 4 ml saline without any virus using the mucosal atomizer device.

Clinical examination

Rectal temperatures were recorded on d-1, twice daily from d0 until d10 post infection (pi) and then daily on days 11 to 14 pi. Fever was defined as body temperatures exceeding 101.5 °F (38.6 °C). Clinical scores were recorded daily between d-1 and d14 pi by veterinarians according to the grade of depression (0–3), reduced appetite (0–2), nasal discharge (0–6), eye discharge (0–3), mandibular lymph node swelling (0–3) and ataxia (0–5). To determine ataxia, neurologic examinations were performed as previously described [46]. The gait was evaluated by walking the horses individually in the aisle, including turns to both sides. A summarized clinical score for each horse and day was calculated as the sum of the scores (possible range 0–22). Due to the housing arrangement examiners were aware of the identity of the control group, but blinded to the identification of the Ab4 or Ab4ΔORF2 groups. The control group was always worked with first.

Sample collection and processing

The horses were assigned randomized ID numbers, which did not reveal the group affiliation to the laboratory personnel. Samples were processed based on ID numbers and the group affiliation remained blinded until data collection and assay evaluation was completed.

NS were acquired on d-1, and d1-d9 pi using two polyester tipped applicators (Puritan Medical Products Company, Gullford, Maine, USA) swabbed on the nasal mucosa of one nostril for 5 s. Swabs were immediately put into 1 ml of sterile phosphate buffered saline (PBS) in a polystyrene tube. The swabs (in PBS) were transported to the laboratory, maintained at 4 °C and processed within 2 hours after sampling. For virus isolation, NS samples were not further processed. For the analysis of intranasal cytokines and antibodies, NS samples were spun at 1000×g at 4 °C for 5 min leaving the swabs in the collection tube. The diluted NS surrounding the swabs was collected into a 1.5 ml centrifuge tube and the cleared fluid supernatant was stored at − 20 °C until analysis.

Blood samples were collected on d-8, d-1, d1 to d14, d24, d60, d100, d130, d170, d220, and d260 pi by jugular venipuncture with a vacutainer system (20G Monoject Covidien, Medtronic Minneapolis, MN, USA) into glass tubes without anticoagulant or with sodium heparin (both BD, Franklin Lakes, NJ, USA). Serum and heparinized blood samples were processed as described previously [43, 44].

Within 3 h after blood collection PBMC were isolated by density gradient centrifugation (Ficoll-Paque Plus, GE Healthcare, Piscataway, NJ, USA) and re-suspended in cell culture media (DMEM supplemented with 1% (*v*/v) non-essential amino acids, 2 mM L-glutamine, 50 μM 2-mercaptoethanol, 50 μg/ml Gentamicin, 100 U/ml penicillin, 100 μg/ml streptomycin, all from all Thermo Fisher Scientific Waltham, MA, USA and 10% FCS, Atlanta biological, Flowery Branch, GA, USA) at 6×10^6 cells/ml for the following experiments. For PCR detection of viremia, 1×10^7 PBMC were washed twice in PBS, dry cell pellets were snap frozen in liquid nitrogen, and stored at − 80 °C until PCR was performed.

Serum samples were stored in aliquots at − 20 °C until analysis.

Virus isolation

To determine nasal virus shedding virus isolation was performed as plaque assays as previously described [22]. Briefly, vortexed NS were titrated on confluent RK13 cells. Virus penetration into the cells was allowed during an incubation for 2-4 h at 37 °C before supernatants were aspirated and an overlay with 0.5% Methylcellulose (Sigma Aldrich, St. Louis, MO, USA) in cell culture medium (Gibco MEM medium, supplemented with 0.292 g/l L-glutamine, 1 mM sodium pyruvate, 50 μg/ml Gentamicin, 300 U/ml Penicillin, 300 μg/ml Streptomycin, 0.75 μg/ml Amphotericin B, all from Thermo Fisher Scientific and 10% inactivated FCS, Atlanta biological) was performed. After 5 days of incubation, plaques were counted after fixation and staining in crystal violet staining solution (PBS containing 4% *v*/v Paraformaldehyde, 1% *v*/*w* Methanol, 0.05% *w*/*v* Crystal Violet, all Sigma Aldrich). Viral titers were expressed as PFU per ml NS.

EHV-1 PCR

Cell associated viremia was evaluated by real-time PCR targeting the gB gene of EHV-1 performed exactly as previously described [44, 47]. A total of 1×10^7 PBMC was used for DNA extraction per horse and time point. The PCR was performed at the Animal Health Diagnostic Center at Cornell University.

EHV-1 multiplex assay

EHV-1 specific antibodies in serum and NS samples were determined using a fluorescent bead-based EHV-1 multiplex assay. The assay was previously described in detail [43] and has been slightly modified for this approach: Instead of coupling viral glycoproteins directly to the beads a monoclonal anti-equine IL-4 antibody (clone 25, [48]) was coupled to all three beads numbered 33, 35 and 36 (Luminex Corp., Austin, TX, USA). Bead 33 was then incubated with IL-4/EHV-1 glycoprotein B (gB), bead 35 with IL-4/EHV-1 gC, and bead 36 with IL-4/EHV-1 gD. All three IL-4/EHV-1 glycoproteins were expressed as described previously [43]. The EHV-1 gB, gC and gD coated beads were then multiplexed, and incubated with diluted serum (1:400) or undiluted NS samples, followed by the respective detection antibodies as described [43]. Total EHV-1 specific immunoglobulin (Ig) was detected by biotinylated goat anti-horse IgG (H + L) antibody (Jackson Immunoresearch Laboratories, WestGrove, PA, USA). Ig isotype detection was performed by biotinylated monoclonal antibodies specific for IgG1 (CVS45) and IgG4/7 (CVS39) [both [49]], IgG1/3 (clone 159–4), IgG3/5 (clone 586), IgG6 (clone 267) [all three [50]], and IgA (BVS2) [51]. Data were reported as median fluorescent intensities (MFI).

Ex vivo re-stimulation of PBMC with EHV-1

EHV-1 re-stimulation of PBMC was performed as previously described in detail [36, 44, 52]. In brief, PBMC were re-stimulated ex vivo with EHV-1 strain Ab4 at a multiplicity of infection of 1 for 48 h. As controls culture in medium alone or stimulation with Phorbol12-myristate13-acetate (PMA; 25 ng/ml) and ionomycin (1 μM; both Sigma Aldrich) were included. Supernatants were collected for the analysis of secreted cytokines. In assays for intracellular staining of cytokines and flow cytometric analysis, protein secretion was blocked by Brefeldin

A (10 μg/ml; Sigma Aldrich) added for the last 24 h of incubation, before the cells were fixed.

Multiplex assay detection of cytokine secretion

Equine cytokines were quantified in PBMC supernatants, serum and NS samples using a fluorescent bead-based multiplex cytokine assay as previously described [53]. Interferon (IFN)-α, IL-4, and IL-10 were reported in pg/ml and IFN-γ, and IL-17 were reported as U/ml. Furthermore, soluble cluster of differentiation 14 (sCD14), an inflammatory marker, was determined in serum and NS samples by a separate bead-based assay as previously described in detail [54] and was reported in ng/ml. All samples were measured undiluted except for the sCD14 analysis in serum. The latter samples were diluted at 1:200.

EHV-1-specific T-cell detection by flow cytometry

Flow cytometric analysis of EHV-1 specific cells was performed as previously described [43, 44, 52]. In brief, after EHV-1 re-stimulation PBMC were fixed, permeabilized, and triple stained for CD4, and CD8 on the cell surface and intracellular IFN-γ production or intracellular IL-10, IL-17A, and IL-4, respectively. For each sample 100,000 events were analyzed in a FACS Canto II flow cytometer (BD Biosciences, San Diego, CA). The evaluation of the data was performed using FlowJo version 10.2 (FlowJO LLC, Ashland, OR, USA). A small lymphocyte gate was set by morphology and the proportions of IFN-γ positive lymphocytes after re-stimulation, compared to medium controls were assessed as previously described [52]. The average intracellular cytokine detection in PMA/ionomycin stimulated PBMC (positive controls) was 14.7% IFN-γ positive, 2.2% IL-4 positive, 2.2% IL-10 positive, and 0.1% IL-17 positive lymphocytes.

Statistical analysis

The data sets of this study were not normally distributed according to D'Agostino and Pearson normality tests. All data sets were analyzed by repeated measures ANOVA with Tukey's Post-hoc test to identify group differences for each time point analyzed. *P*-values < 0.05 were considered significant. Correlation of peak virus shedding and peak nasal cytokine concentrations were analyzed by two-tailed Spearman rank correlation. The statistical analysis was performed using GraphPad Prism software version 6 or higher (GraphPad Software Inc., La Jolla, CA, USA).

Results

Clinical signs after EHV-1 infection

Horses in both infected groups, Ab4 and Ab4ΔORF2, displayed clinical signs of mild upper respiratory tract disease as well as fever, while horses in the control group did not (Fig. 1a and b). Horses in the Ab4 group developed an initial fever peak from d1.5 to d2.5 pi, which was significantly higher than the control group ($p < 0.0001$). The initial fever peak was less pronounced in the Ab4ΔORF2 group. Although Ab4ΔORF2 horses had increased body temperatures compared to the control group on d1.5 ($p < 0.001$), d2 and d2.5 pi (both $p < 0.0001$), the fever in the Ab4ΔORF2 group was lower than in the Ab4 group on d2 ($p < 0.001$) and d2.5 pi ($p < 0.01$). Afterwards, body temperatures in both infected groups were significantly increased compared to the control group at several time points until d5 pi (Fig. 1a).

Horses in the control group had low clinical scores between 0 and 5 (median 3) resulting from mild nasal or ocular discharge while stabled. In both infected groups, nasal discharge and enlarged submandibular lymph nodes were the most prevalent clinical signs of disease. Clinical scores in the Ab4 and Ab4ΔORF2 groups were similar over the course of the study and higher than in the controls on days 2 to 7 pi (Fig. 1b). Mild signs of ataxia (score 1) were seen in one horse each in the infected groups. These were noted in the Ab4 group on days 9 and 10 pi and in the Ab4ΔORF2 group on days 5, 6 and 9 pi, respectively. These symptoms resolved completely in both horses by d10 pi.

Viral shedding and viremia after EHV-1 infection

Virus was isolated from the NS samples of horses in the infected groups between d1to d6 pi and peaked on d2 pi (Fig. 1c). Viral shedding on d2 pi was reduced in Ab4ΔORF2 infected horses compared to those in the Ab4 group ($p < 0.0001$). Although viral shedding was detected in horses of the Ab4ΔORF2 group, their NS virus amounts were low and not different from the control group throughout the study. No virus was detected in NS of the control group.

Cell-associated viremia was detected by PCR. Viral DNA was detectable in PBMC of both infected groups and significantly elevated compared to the control group between days 4 to 8 pi ($p < 0.01$, Fig. 1d). On d8 pi, higher amounts of viral DNA were detected in PBMC of the Ab4ΔORF2 group than in those of the Ab4 group ($p < 0.01$) and on d10 pi viral DNA was still elevated in this group compared to the control group ($p < 0.01$). Viremia was not detected in the control group.

Intranasal cytokine production in response to EHV-1 infection

Within the first days after intranasal infection with Ab4 or Ab4ΔORF2 cytokines were detected in the NS. As the first cytokine, IFN-α was detected and peaked in both infected groups at d2 pi, (Fig. 2a) which corresponds with the time of maximum nasal virus shedding (Fig. 1c). The intranasal IFN-α concentration of the Ab4 group exceeded that of the Ab4ΔORF2 group on d2 pi ($p < 0.001$) and it remained significantly higher than in the control group on d3 pi (*p*

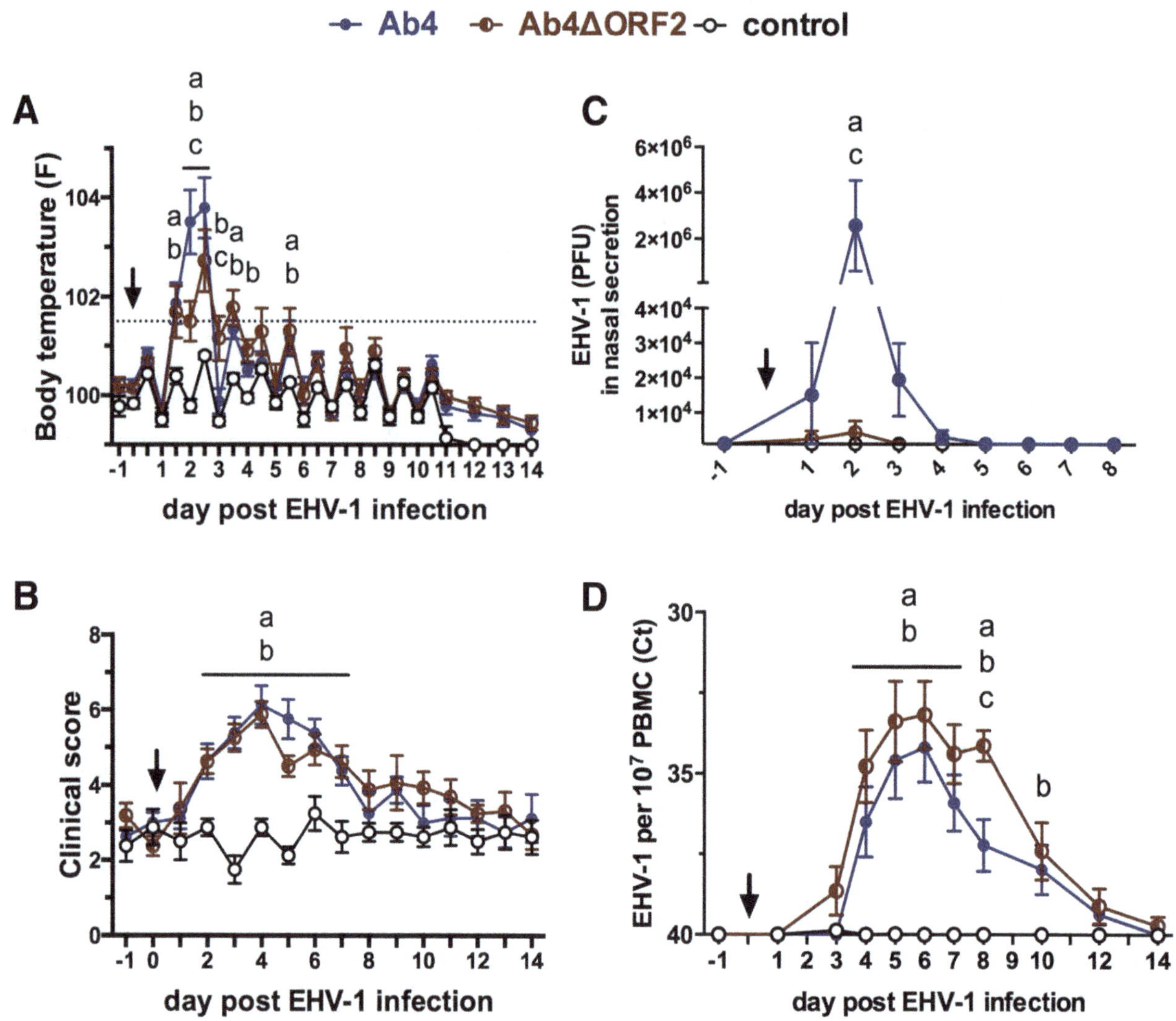

Fig. 1 Clinical findings and virus detection after experimental infection with the EHV-1 strain Ab4 or its deletion mutant Ab4ΔORF2. Three groups of horses ($n = 8$/group) were either not infected (control), infected with the neuropathogenic EHV-1 strain Ab4 (Ab4) or infected with its ORF2 deletion mutant (Ab4ΔORF2) on day 0 (arrow). Clinical signs were monitored and virus detection was performed before (day − 1) and after infection (day 1 to 14). Body temperature (**a**); clinical score calculated as the sum of numerical scores for nasal discharge, ocular discharge, lymph node enlargement, ataxia, depression and reduced appetite ranging from 0 to 22 (**b**); viral shedding expressed as plaque forming units (PFU/ml) detected by virus isolation in nasopharyngeal secretions (**c**); viremia determined in 1×10^7 PBMC by real time PCR and shown as Ct values for the gB gene (**d**) were analyzed; Mean and standard errors are plotted for each group. Dotted horizontal lines represent a cutoff of fever at 101.5 °F (**a**) and EHV-1 detection at a Ct 38 (D). Significant differences between groups are marked: **a** = Ab4 vs. control, **b** = Ab4ΔORF2 vs. control, **c** = Ab4 vs. Ab4ΔORF2

< 0.001). IFN-α concentrations declined to undetectable values by d4 pi. Intranasal IFN-α was not detected in the control group.

The inflammatory protein sCD14 increased in NS of both infected groups starting on d2 pi to peak on d3 pi, and remained elevated compared to the control group until d5 pi (Fig. 2b). In Ab4ΔORF2 infected horses sCD14 was increased on d2 pi in comparison to the control and Ab4 groups (both $p < 0.001$), while the peak sCD14 concentration on d3 pi was higher in Ab4 infected than in Ab4ΔORF2 infected horses ($p < 0.05$).

Nasal IFN-γ increased as a sharp peak on d3 pi in the Ab4 and Ab4ΔORF2 groups while it remained undetectable in the control group. Differences in IFN-γ values between the Ab4 and Ab4ΔORF2 infected groups were not observed (Fig. 2c). At d4 pi IL-10 concentrations peaked in NS of both infected groups compared to the control group ($p > 0.0001$) and declined gradually to baseline values by d6 pi in the Ab4 or d7 pi in the Ab4ΔORF2 group. Differences in IL-10 values between the Ab4 and Ab4ΔORF2 infected groups were not observed (Fig. 2d). Intranasal IL-4 and IL-17 were overall

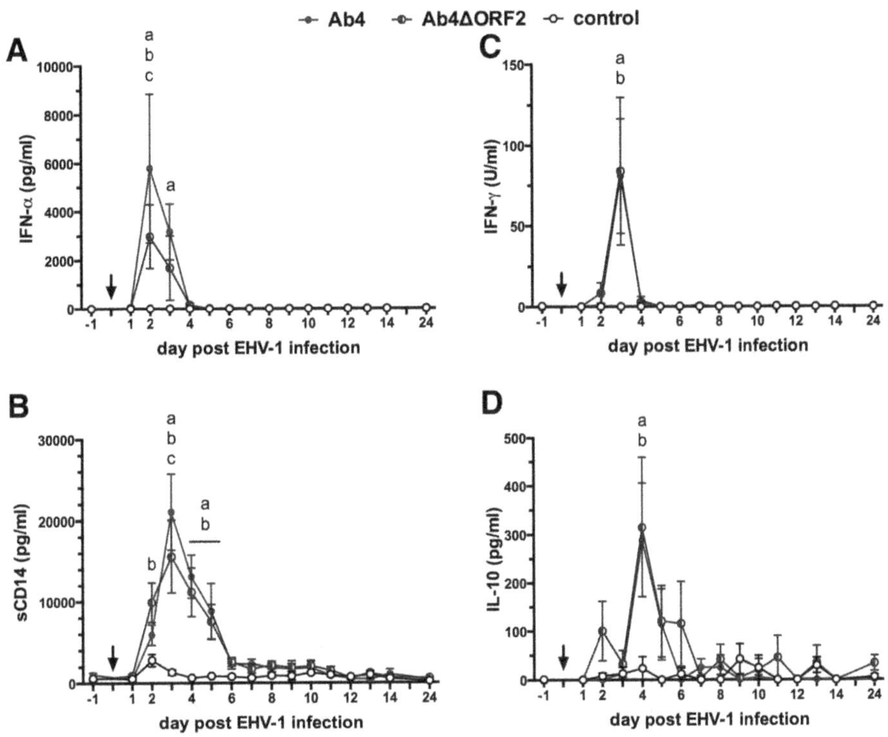

Fig. 2 Intranasal cytokine secretion after infection with EHV-1 strain Ab4 or its deletion mutant Ab4ΔORF2. Three groups of horses ($n = 8$/group) were either not infected (control), infected with the neuropathogenic EHV-1 strain Ab4 (Ab4) or infected with its ORF2 deletion mutant (Ab4**Δ**ORF2) on day 0 (arrow). Before (day − 1) and after (day 1–24) experimental infection IFN-α (**a**), sCD14 (**b**), IFN-γ (**c**), and IL-10 (**d**) were quantified in nasopharyngeal secretions by fluorescent bead-based assays. Mean and standard errors are plotted for each group. Significant differences between groups are marked: **a** = Ab4 vs. control, **b** = Ab4**Δ**ORF2 vs. control, **c** = Ab4 vs. Ab4**Δ**ORF2

low or not detectable and similar between all three groups (data not shown).

The maximum values of virus shedding on d2 pi positively correlated with the peak values of nasal IFN- α and sCD14 (Table 1).

Antibody response to infection

Antibodies specific for EHV-1 gB, gC, and gD were determined before and following infection in NS and serum. The antibody responses to the three EHV-1 antigens were slightly different in magnitude (gB = gD << gC) but followed a similar overall pattern. Thus, representative results of EHV-1 gC-specific antibodies are presented here. Total EHV-1 gC-specific Ig in NS and serum were low

Table 1 Spearman rank correlations of peak nasal cytokines and sCD14 with maximum virus shedding on day 2 pi

day pi	IFN-α d2 pi	sCD14 d3 pi	IFN-γ d3 pi	IL-10 d4 pi
r	0.8066	0.7866	0.6442	0.4860
95% CI[a]	0.5894 to 0.9150	0.5526 to 0.9056	0.3140 to 0.8354	0.09026 to 0.7492
P value	< 0.0001	< 0.0001	0.0007	0.0160

[a]*CI* confidence interval

before infection (d-8, d-1) in all horses and EHV-1 specific antibody induction was not detected in the control group throughout the study (Fig. 3).

Intranasal antibody response to infection

Infection with either virus, Ab4 or Ab4ΔORF2, induced EHV-1 gC-specific intranasal antibodies following a wave-like pattern, characterized by several peaks on days 3–4, 10, 24–60, and 130 pi (Fig. 3a). The highest magnitude of the anti-gC antibody response was observed at d24 pi (Ab4ΔORF2 group) or d60 pi (Ab4 group). The increase of total anti-gC antibodies was significantly higher in both infected groups compared to the control group from days 8 to 130 pi, and in the Ab4 group also on days 4 and 7 pi. After d170 pi, nasal EHV-1 specific antibodies in both infected groups returned to low values until the end of the study period on d260 pi, which were not significantly different from the control group. Intranasal gC-specific antibodies were higher in the Ab4ΔORF2 group than in the Ab4 group on d13 pi ($p < 0.01$) and d24 pi ($p < 0.05$), while the Ab4 group exceeded the Ab4ΔORF2 group on d60 pi ($p < 0.05$) (Fig. 3a).

The initial intranasal antibody increase on d3-4pi was composed of low amounts of different gC-specific IgG

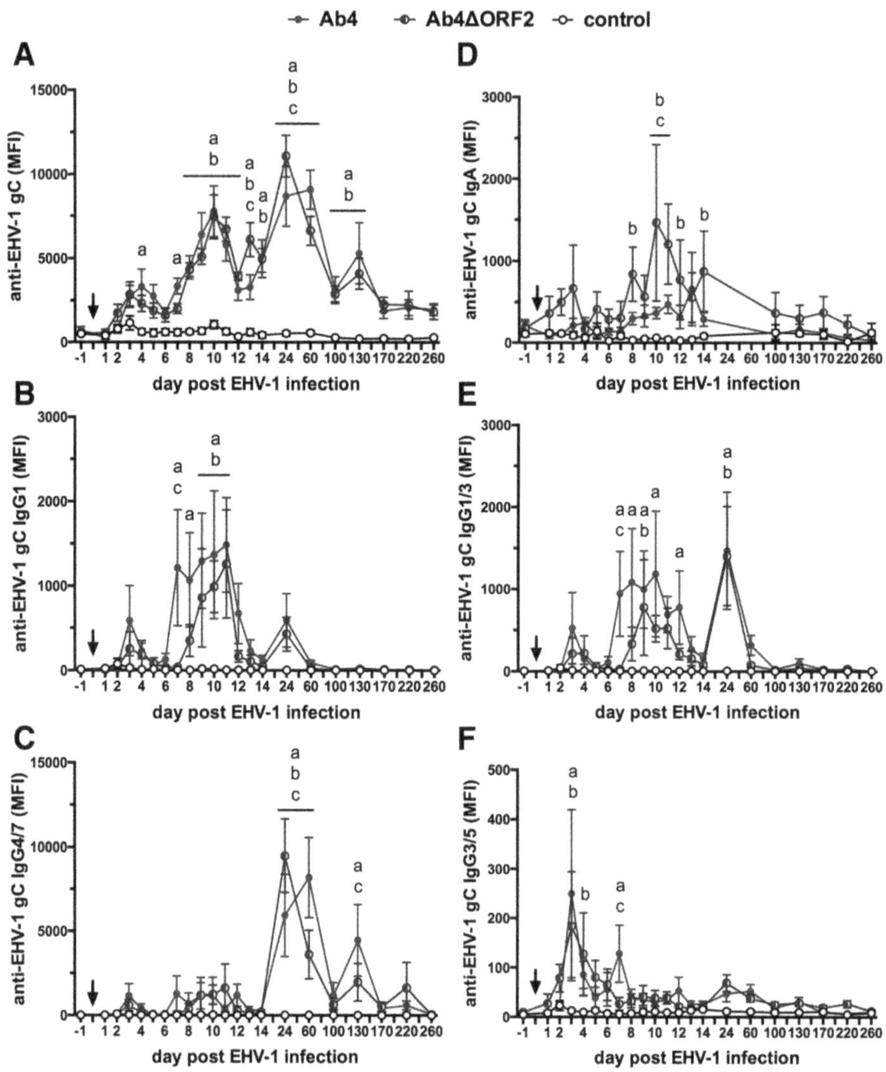

Fig. 3 Anti-EHV-1 gC antibodies in nasal secretions after infection with EHV-1 strain Ab4 or its deletion mutant Ab4**Δ**ORF2. Three groups of horses ($n = 8$/group) were either not infected (control), infected with the neuropathogenic EHV-1 strain Ab4 (Ab4) or infected with its ORF2 deletion mutant (Ab4**Δ**ORF2) on day 0 (arrow). Before (day − 1) and after (day 1–260) experimental infection EHV-1 gC specific total Ig (**a**), IgG1 (**b**), IgG4/7 (**c**), IgA (**d**), IgG1/3 (**e**), and IgG3/5 (**f**) were quantified in nasopharyngeal secretions by fluorescent bead-based multiplex assays and expressed as median fluorescent intensities (MFI). Note that Y-axes scales differ depending on isotype. Mean and standard errors are plotted for each group. Significant differences between groups are marked: **a** = Ab4 vs. control, **b** = Ab4**Δ**ORF2 vs. control, **c** = Ab4 vs. Ab4**Δ**ORF2

isotypes, and in the Ab4ΔORF2 group also some IgA (Fig. 3b-f). Afterwards, the intranasal anti-gC total antibody peaks (Fig. 3a) were each dominated by different isotypes. The second anti-gC peak on day 10 pi corresponded to an increase of primarily IgG1 in both infected groups (Fig. 3b). IgG1 was induced slightly earlier (d7, $p < 0.001$) in the Ab4 than in the Ab4 ΔORF2 group (d8). Similarly, the third anti-gC antibody peak on days 24 (Ab4ΔORF2) and 60 pi (Ab4), respectively, and the fourth peak on d130 pi were mainly composed of IgG4/7 (Fig. 3c). Anti-gC IgG4/7 antibodies almost mimicked the total anti-gC response shown in Fig. 3a from d24 pi on. This included the higher IgG4/7 in the AbΔORF2 compared to the Ab4 group on d24 pi ($p < 0.01$), the lower intranasal IgG4/7 in the AbΔORF2 group on d60 pi ($p < 0.0001$), and on d130 pi ($p < 0.05$) compared to the Ab4 group.

Notably, intranasal gC-specific IgA after infecting horses with the Ab4 virus was not different from the control horses at any time after infection. In contrast, gC-specific IgA was increased in the Ab4ΔORF2 group compared to the control group on days 8, 10 to 12 and 14 pi. It was also higher than in the Ab4 group on d10 and d11 pi (Fig. 3d). Overall the intranasal EHV-1 specific IgA response in the Ab4ΔORF2 group appeared to be of low magnitude and short duration.

EHV-1 gC-specific IgG1/3 induction mimicked IgG1 antibodies until d14 pi (Fig. 3e). IgG3/5 antibodies were overall low including the early peak on d3pi (Fig. 3f). This supports that the IgG1/3 antibody response until d14 pi was mainly composed of IgG1. On d24 pi, an increase in IgG1/3 antibodies was observed in both infected groups ($p < 0.0001$). This increase was higher than the corresponding IgG1 response in Fig. 3b and likely results from a mixture of anti-gC IgG1 and IgG3 on d24 pi.

EHV-1 specific IgG6 in nasal secretion was low for all groups throughout the study and no group differences were observed (data not shown).

Serum antibody response to EHV-1 infection

Infection with either Ab4 or Ab4ΔORF2 resulted in the induction of EHV-1 gC-specific Ig in serum which was first increased on d8 pi compared to the control group ($p < 0.01$). Anti-gC antibodies peaked on d24 pi, slowly declined until d170 pi, and then remained constant in both infected groups for the remainder of the study (Fig. 4a) with p-values< 0.0001 between days 10 to

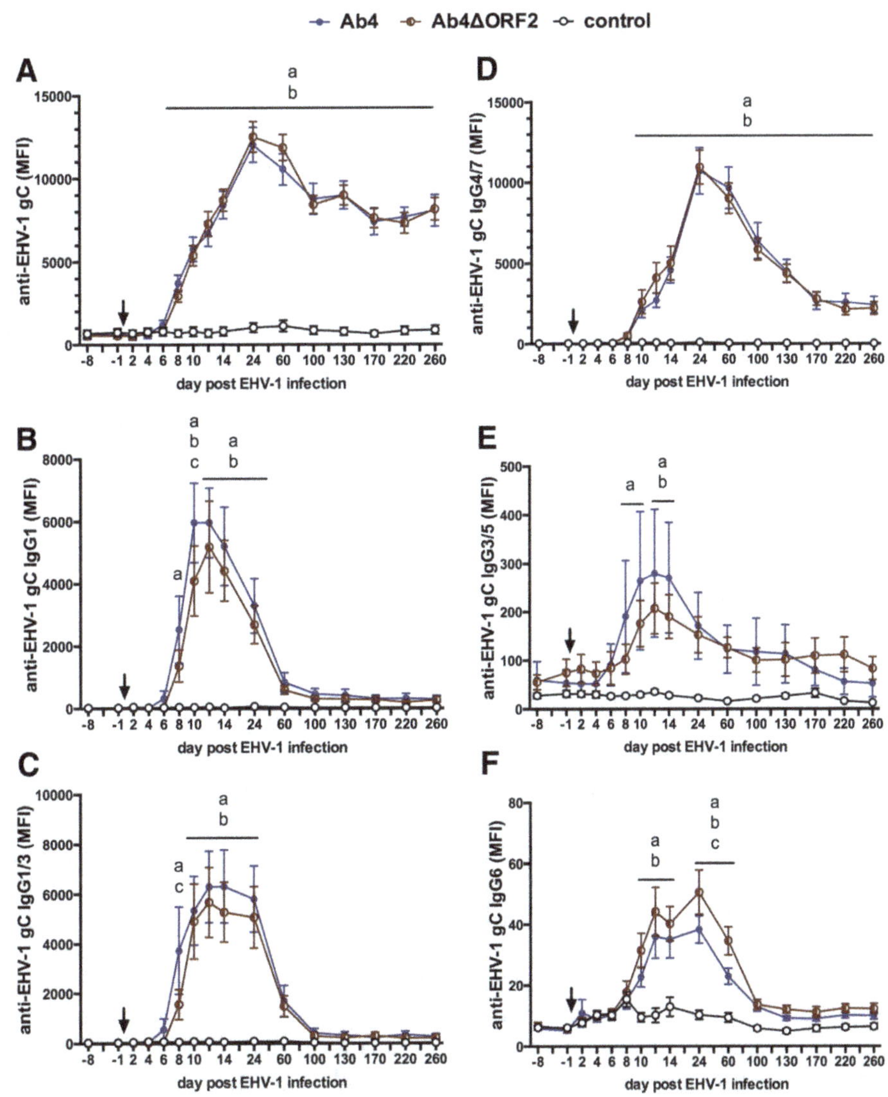

Fig. 4 Anti-EHV-1 gC antibodies in serum after EHV-1 infection. Three groups of horses ($n = 8$/group) were either not infected (control), infected with the neuropathogenic EHV-1 strain Ab4 (Ab4) or infected with its ORF2 deletion mutant (Ab4ΔORF2) on day 0 (arrow). Before (day − 1) and after (day 1–260). EHV-1 gC specific total Ig (**a**), IgG1 (**b**), IgG1/3 (**c**), IgG4/7 (**d**), IgG3/5 (**e**) and IgG6 (**f**) were quantified in serum by fluorescent bead-based multiplex assays and expressed as median fluorescent intensities (MFI). Note that Y-axes scales differ depending on isotype. Mean and standard errors are plotted for each group. Significant differences between groups are marked: **a** = Ab4 vs. control, **b** = Ab4ΔORF2 vs. control, **c** = Ab4 vs. Ab4ΔORF2

260 pi for both infected groups in comparison to the control group. Total gC-specific Ig was similar between the Ab4 or Ab4ΔORF2 groups for the duration of the study and until d260 pi.

In both infected groups, Ab4 and Ab4ΔORF2, IgG1 (Fig. 4b) and IgG1/3 isotypes (Fig. 4c) were detectable early after infection. They peaked on d10 or d12 pi and declined by d60 pi to baseline values. In the Ab4 group, IgG1 and IgG1/3 induction was slightly earlier than in the Ab4ΔORF2 group (d8 vs. d10) and reached higher IgG1 values on d10 pi ($p < 0.05$).

Anti-gC IgG4/7 antibodies were first detectable on d10 pi in both infected groups and peaked on d24 pi. IgG4/7 primarily contributed to the long-term EHV-1 specific antibody response with both infected groups exceeding the antibody values of the control group from d10 until d260 pi (p-values between $p < 0.0001$ and $p < 0.05$) (Fig. 2d). Differences in the IgG4/7 response of the Ab4 and Ab4ΔORF2 groups were not observed.

EHV-1 specific IgG3/5 was weakly induced and elevated in comparison to the control group in the Ab4 group on days 8 to 14 pi ($p < 0.05$ to $p < 0.001$), and in the Ab4ΔORF2 group on d12 and d14 pi (both $p < 0.05$) (Fig. 4e). IgG6 was present in low quantities, which were increased compared to the control group in the Ab4 and Ab4ΔORF2 group on days 10–60 pi ($p < 0.05$). On days 24 and 60 pi the IgG6 antibodies in the Ab4ΔORF2 group exceeded those in the Ab4 group (both $p < 0.05$) (Fig. 4f). EHV-1-specific IgA was not detected in serum at any time point (data not shown).

Cellular immune response to EHV-1

Cellular immune responses of all groups were analyzed by ex vivo re-stimulation of PBMC with the EHV-1 strain Ab4. Between 5 and 10 days pi, IFN-γ secretion was elevated in horses of both the Ab4 group (days 5, 6, 8 pi, $p < 0.05$) and the Ab4ΔORF2group (days 6, 10 pi, $p < 0.05$) (Fig. 5a) compared to the control group. The IL-10 secretion displayed a similar biphasic response with the IL-10 peak on d5 pi slightly preceding the maximal IFN-γ response on d6pi. Both infected groups had greater IL-10 secretion from re-stimulated PBMC on days 5 and 6 pi ($p < 0.05$), and IL-10 was again elevated at d8 pi in the Ab4 group ($p < 0.01$) while the Ab4ΔORF2 group had a non-significant trend at d8 pi (Fig. 5b) compared to the control group. At later time points (d60-d260 pi) induction of cytokine secretion from PBMC in response to ex vivo re-stimulation was not observed for any group. Significant IL-4 and IL-17 secretion was not induced at any time (data not shown). Secretion of IFN-α was induced by the in vitro infection of PBMC at all time points, but there was no difference between the three groups of horses during the study (data not shown).

In addition, EHV-1 specific T-cells were analyzed by flow cytometry for intracellular IFN-γ, IL-4, IL-10 and IL-17 production. IFN-γ production by lymphocytes in PBMC were overall low and not different between the three groups for the duration of the study (Fig. 5c). IL-4, IL-10 or IL-17 were not induced in lymphocytes after ex vivo re-stimulation with EHV-1 (data not shown).

Cytokine responses in serum

Cytokine measurements in serum were overall similar between the control and the infected groups with a few exceptions. IFN-α was increased in serum early after infection on days 2 and 4 pi in the Ab4ΔORF2 group compared to the control group ($p < 0.05$, Additional file 1: Figure S1A). In the Ab4 group there was a non-significant trend of increased serum IFN-α on d2 pi. It remained at a similar level to uninfected controls for the remainder of the measurements in both infected groups. Serum sCD14 was elevated in the Ab4 group compared to the control group at d3 pi ($p < 0.01$). In addition, sCD14 was higher in the control group compared to the Ab4ΔORF2 group at d13 pi ($p < 0.05$) but was increased in the Ab4ΔORF2 group compared to both, Ab4 and the controls at d24 pi, while it was still significantly higher in Ab4 than in controls at that day ($p < 0.05$, Additional file 1: Figure S1B). The levels of serum IFN-γ did not differ between the three groups at any point during the experiment (Additional file 1: Figure S1C). IL-4 and IL-17 concentrations were overall low in serum and without any differences between the three groups (data not shown).

Discussion

An experimental infection with Ab4ΔORF2 deletion mutant virus in comparison to the parental neuropathogenic Ab4 virus was performed in horses to characterize the effects of the ORF2 gene product on EHV-1 infection and host immunity. Clinical signs, nasal shedding, and viremia induced by both viruses were evaluated to identify differences in virulence. Host immunity was analyzed locally and systemically summarizing the influence of both viruses on innate and adaptive cellular immunity and antibody induction. Overall, the infection of the horses with the parent Ab4 strain in the present study induced similar clinical signs, virus shedding, and viremia as previously described for EHV-1 infections of susceptible hosts [14, 42, 55]. Most importantly, the deletion of ORF2 reduced the virulence of the neuropathogenic EHV-1 Ab4 virus. This was evident by clearly reduced magnitude of the initial fever and significantly lower viral shedding in horses infected with the Ab4 ΔORF2 deletion mutant virus. The reduced virulence observed here for Ab4ΔORF2 was comparable to the

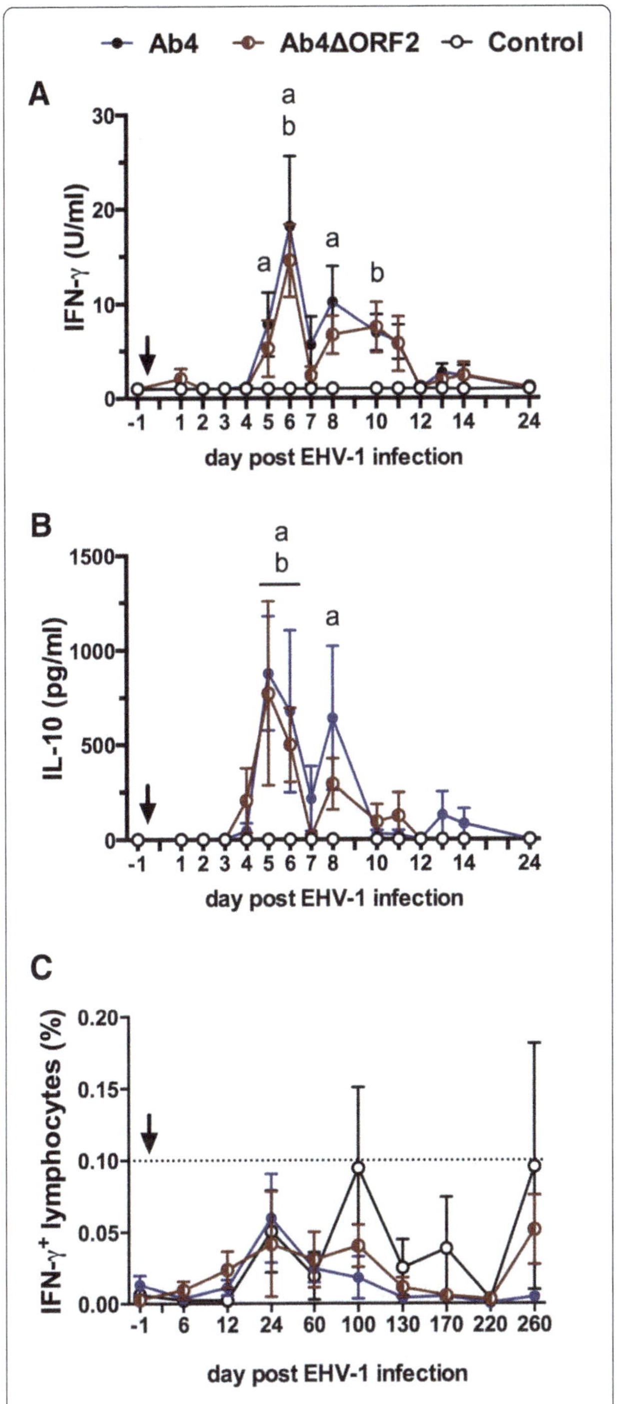

Fig. 5 Cellular immune responses to infection in PBMC. Three groups of horses ($n = 8$/group) were either not infected (control), infected with the neuropathogenic EHV-1 strain Ab4 (Ab4) or infected with its ORF2 deletion mutant (Ab4ΔORF2) on day 0 (arrow). PBMC were isolated before (day − 1) and after infection (day 1–24) and re-stimulated ex vivo for 48 h with EHV-1 (strain Ab4). Cytokine production (**a** and **b**) was analyzed in supernatants by a fluorescent bead-based multiplex assay. All values are cell culture medium control corrected. Mean and standard errors of secreted IFN-γ (**a**) and IL-10 (**b**) are shown. EHV-1 stimulated PBMC were also fixed, stained for intracellular IFN-γ and analyzed by flow cytometry. Total EHV-1 specific IFN-γ producing lymphocytes are displayed (**c**). Values have been corrected by the respective medium control of each horse. The dotted horizontal line (**c**) represents a cutoff of 0.1% IFN-γ + lymphocytes. PBMC controls kept in medium alone typically result in values below this cutoff value. Significant differences between groups are marked: **a** = Ab4 vs. control, **b** = Ab4ΔORF2 vs. control, **c** = Ab4 vs. Ab4ΔORF2

shorter duration of pyrexia, decreased magnitude and duration of virus shedding but unaffected viremia after infection of ponies with Ab4ΔORF1/2 compared to Ab4 in an earlier approach [42]. Differences in the magnitude of the fever induced by Ab4 infection may be based on individual differences between the ponies used by Soboll et al. [42] and the Icelandic horses used in the present study. Importantly, the reduction of virus shedding after deleting the ORF2 gene from the Ab4 virus versus using an Ab mutant deprived of ORF1 and ORF2 in the previous study [42] should be directly compared: Soboll et al. quantified EHV-1 DNA by PCR, while we used a plaque assay for virus isolation from nasal secretion, which measures infectious virus and thus correlates more directly with viral shedding and the ability of the infected horse to infect other horses.

The virulence factor ORF2 impacted the infection of the upper respiratory tract and local innate immune response to EHV-1 infection. In this study, we provided a comprehensive evaluation of intranasal cytokine and antibody secretion to longitudinally describe local innate and adaptive host immune responses during EHV-1 infection and potential differences induced by the ORF2 gene product. The onset of the local innate immune response against Ab4 was observed during virus shedding as determined by isolation of infectious virus from nasal discharge on days 2–4 pi. Intranasal innate immunity was characterized by sequential increases of the cytokines IFN-α (peak on d2pi), IFN-γ (peak on d3pi), and IL-10 (peak on d4pi) followed by a quick decline of all three cytokines. The nasal secretion of bioactive IFN was correlated with the time of EHV-1 shedding in a prior experimental infection study by Edington [56]. Here, we identified that high IFN-α in nasal secretion positively correlates with EHV-1 shedding in the Ab4 infected horses. In comparison, Ab4ΔORF2 infection induced low viral shedding combined with decreased IFN-α secretion. It has been demonstrated earlier, that equine IFN-α detected by the mAb pair used for quantification here, is also bioactive [57]. This suggests that intranasal IFN-α serves as an early danger signal during EHV-1 infection and, as previously pointed out by Randall [58], likely supports the induction of an antiviral state in the infected mucosal tissues. Notably, local IFN-γ and IL-10 induction was similar in both infected groups, Ab4ΔORF2 and Ab4, indicating that the ORF2 gene product does not influence these two immune regulatory cytokines.

Besides the short-term and pointed IFN-α, IFN-γ, and IL-10 secretion, elevated sCD14 concentrations were locally induced by EHV-1 between days 2–5 pi, while the horses were shedding virus. Peak intranasal sCD14 concentrations were slightly reduced in Ab4ΔORF2 infected horses supporting a possible direct or indirect influence of the ORF2 gene on intranasal sCD14 secretion. Lipopolysaccharide (LPS) binding sCD14 is produced by exocytosis and shedding of CD14 from monocyte or macrophage cell surfaces [59–61] and has a neutralizing, anti-inflammatory role for protection against LPS-induced cell death [62, 63]. The exact mechanisms of sCD14 induction after EHV-1 infection still needs to be unraveled in future approaches. However, EHV-1 was described to infect monocytes in vitro and in vivo [7, 64, 65] and the nasal sCD14 increase could thus result from a stress response of EHV-1 infected macrophages of the upper respiratory tract or reflect responses related to phagocytosis of virus and infected cells.

Overall, these findings point towards a role of ORF2 in the lytic virus replication cycle in the nasopharyngeal epithelia, which supported the release of infectious virions and increased the local viral load and nasal shedding. Nevertheless, the transmission of EHV-1 to mononuclear cells resulting in cell-associated viremia [7, 66] appears to be independent of ORF2. Here, viremia in the Ab4ΔORF2 and Ab4 groups was similar. Additionally, in vitro replication of Ab4ΔORF2 or Ab4ΔORF1/2 in RK13 cells and equine dermal cells (NBL-6) was not impaired compared to Ab4 [42]. Thus, the impact of ORF2 on nasal virus replication can only be shown after in vivo infection of the mucosal epithelial tissue including an intact local innate immune response.

In contrast to the clear reduction of virulence and intranasal IFN-α and sCD14 secretion, the immunogenicity of EHV-1 was not influenced by the deletion of the ORF2 gene from Ab4, with the only exception of a slightly earlier onset of IgG1 antibody responses in serum and during the second intranasal IgG1 peak in Ab4 infected horses. Local EHV-1 specific antibodies were detectable intranasally within 3–4 days after infection at low values. At this time, antibody responses were not yet detectable in serum. This very early nasal Ig secretion was similarly composed of different IgG isotypes and seems to be derived from local cells, such as *lamina propria* memory B-cells or those located in the regional lymph nodes. It should again be pointed out that all horses in this study were infected with EHV-1 about 1.5 to 2.5 years prior to the EHV-1 infection performed here. This confirmed the transient nature of protective immunity to EHV-1 described earlier [3, 27]. Although our horses did not mount a rapid and sufficiently high immune response to be protected from the EHV-1 infection performed here, they likely still had EHV-1 specific memory B-cells in their lymphatic tissues. Binding of viral antigens may have stimulated these memory B-cells to quickly secrete EHV-1 specific antibodies in low, but detectable quantities 3–4 days after infection.

Interestingly, this initial local IgG response waned quickly and was followed by peaks of higher local antibody responses that were dominated by IgG1 between d8–12 pi and IgG4/7 after d14 pi. Our findings clearly indicate that mucosal immune responses against the EHV-1strain Ab4 are dominated by IgG antibodies. Intranasal EHV-1 specific IgG antibodies are secreted in waves for several months post infection. The reason for the wave-like local antibody pattern is not yet clear. It requires further evaluation to identify if they could reflect local subclinical EHV-1 re-activation stages or other mechanisms. In contrast, the nasal EHV-1 specific IgA response after Ab4 infection was of overall low magnitude with slightly higher values for some horses that were infected with Ab4ΔORF2 during d8–14 pi. EHV-1 specific IgA was not detectable at later time points supporting that IgA is neither a major nor a long-lasting antibody during the mucosal EHV-1 specific immune response. This finding is contradictory to Breathnach [67], who found significant induction of nasal EHV-1 specific IgA together with IgG isotypes 2 weeks after primary infection with the neuropathogenic EHV-1 strain Army 183. Both, Breathnach [67] and our analysis here were based on the same monoclonal IgA antibody, BVS2, but used different assays for antibody detection. Future research could analyze if the observed difference in the EHV-1 specific IgA response are related to viral strain differences or if they have other reasons.

Robust systemic EHV-1 specific antibody responses were found in serum by d8 pi and were still detectable at high values by 9 months after infection with Ab4 or Ab4ΔORF2. Similar to nasal secretions, IgG1 was the dominating isotype of the early systemic response to EHV-1 infection, while IgG4/7 maintained the long-term response for more than 9 months. Similar serum antibody kinetics and IgG isotypes were previously reported after experimental EHV-1 infection with different EHV-1 strains including Ab4 and NY03 [42, 44]. This report exceeds the longitudinal observation period of previous articles of monitoring the immune response for weeks [67, 68] to 2–3 months [42, 69] after EHV-1 infection.

The glycoproteins gC and gD of EHV-1 are entry receptors of EHV-1 and highly immunogenic [70, 71]. In horses, gC and gD specific serum Ig and IgG4/7 highly correlate with EHV-1 serum neutralization titers [43]. Here, EHV-1 gC and gD specific antibodies were measured as representative markers for local and systemic EHV-1 specific immune responses with anti-gD responses closely resembling those of anti-gC. Equine IgG1 and IgG4/7 antibodies expressed effector functions such as strong complement activation and a high affinity to bind to IgG Fc-receptors in vitro [72]. EHV-1 specific IgG1 and IgG4/7 were thus assumed to have neutralizing activity and mediate protection against EHV-1 infection [22, 52]. Furthermore, IgG1 and IgG4/7 have been associated with a Th1 dominated B-cell response against EHV-1 [43].

In contrast to the robust antibody induction, an EHV-1 specific T-cell response could not be detected after infection with Ab4 or Ab4ΔORF2. Similarly, only weak T-cell responses were observed in former studies after experimental infection with EHV-1 Ab4 or NY03 [42, 44, 69]. However, we and others demonstrated increased EHV-1 specific cytotoxic T-cells frequencies or IFN-γ producing T-cells during viremia in older horses [13, 73], a few weeks after infection [74–76], or in horses that experienced an EHM outbreak and several vaccinations afterwards [52]. This suggests that EHV-1 specific T-cell activation is not consistently observed after infection, can be a slow process, and may require several immune recognition and activation events with EHV-1 or an EHV vaccine to develop substantial EHV-1 specific T-cell immunity. In the present study, a detectable cellular response was limited to EHV-1 re-stimulation ex vivo, occurred during viremia, and was represented by increased secretion of IL-10 and IFN-γ from PBMC. Likely, the transient stimulations of cytokine secretion from PBMC resulted from an innate response to the viral infection of circulating immune cells. It is believed that EHV-1 down-regulates cellular immunity and thereby allows the establishment of cell-associated viremia, which is a prerequisite for infection of endothelial cells prior to developing EHM or abortions [27, 66]. Current modified-live vaccines containing deletions of ORF2 and other genes [38, 40], similar to Ab4ΔORF2, fail to induce T-cell immunity and thus do not prevent viremia [22, 23, 52]. The EHV-1 genes responsible for the down-regulation of T-cell immunity still need to be identified to achieve robust cellular host immunity against EHV-1.

Conclusions

The ORF2 gene of the EHV-1 strain Ab4 is a virulence factor which contributes to fever and viral shedding but does not affect viremia or adaptive host immunity against the virus (Graphical abstract). Infection with EHV-1 Ab4 and its ORF2 deletion mutant induces high local and systemic antibody responses dominated by early IgG1 and long-lasting IgG4/7 isotypes. Local EHV-1 specific IgA antibodies are only a minor component of the mucosal immune response. Antibody responses dominate EHV-1 immunity while T-cell immunity is overall low.

Additional file

Additional file 1: Figure S1. Cytokines in serum after infection with EHV-1 strain Ab4 or its deletion mutant Ab4ΔORF2. Horses ($n = 8$/group) were infected with one of two EHV-1 strains (Ab4) or Ab4ΔORF2 at day 0 or kept as uninfected controls. Serum was sampled at several times before (days – 8, – 1) and after (day 1- day 24) infection, cytokines and the inflammatory marker sCD14 were evaluated with fluorescent bead-based assays. Mean and standard errors for IFN-α (A), sCD14 (B), and IFN-γ (C) in the serum are displayed. Significant differences between groups are marked: a = Ab4 vs. control, b = Ab4ΔORF2 vs. control, c = Ab4 vs. Ab4ΔORF2. (JPG 332 kb)

Abbreviations

Ab4ΔORF2: Deletion mutant of Ab4 devoid of open reading frame 2; CI: Confidence interval; d pi: Days post infection; EHM: Herpesvirus myeloencephalopathy; EHV-1: Equine herpesvirus type 1; gB/C/D: Envelope glycoprotein B/C/D; IFN: Interferon; Ig: Immunoglobulin; IL: Interleukin; LPS: Lipopolysaccharide; MFI: Median fluorescent intensities; NS: Nasopharyngeal secretion; ORF: Open reading frame; PBMC: Peripheral blood mononuclear cells; PBS: Phosphate buffered saline; PFU: Plaque-forming units; PMA: Phorbol12-myristate13-acetate; RK13: Rabbit kidney 13 cells; sCD14: Soluble cluster of differentiation 14

Acknowledgements

The authors would like to thank Fahad Raza, Franziska Kaiser, Karynn Kilts and Adam Alejandro for their help with sample collection and processing; Laura Goodman and Amy Glaser at the Animal Health Diagnostic Center at Cornell for performing the EHV-1 PCR on PBMC; Kevin Yager, Larry Carlisle, and Brooke Burke for excellent horse care and barn management; Rob Felt, Christine Bellezza, Debra Dwyer, and the IACUC committee at Cornell University for their input and recommendation; and USDA/APHIS for their support and help to establish an EHV-1-free herd at Cornell University and supervision during import quarantine.

Funding

The experimental EHV-1 infection study described in this manuscript was performed with funding from the Agriculture and Food Research Initiative Competitive Grant no. 2015-67015-23091 'The effect of ORF1 and ORF2 gene expression on Innate and Adaptive Immunity and Protection Against Equine Herpes Virus Type 1 (EHV-1)' supported by the USDA National Institute of Food and Agriculture. Reagent development for horse Ig isotype and cytokine monoclonal antibodies was supported by Agriculture and Food Research Initiative Competitive Grants no. 2005-01812 'The US Veterinary Immune Reagent Network' and no. 2015-67015-23072 'Equine Immune Reagents: Development of monoclonal antibodies to improve the analysis of immunity in horses' also supported by the USDA National Institute of Food and Agriculture. The horses used for this project were obtained through funding provided by the Harry M. Zweig Memorial Fund for Equine Research at Cornell University.

Authors' contributions

BW and GP designed the study. NO constructed and provided the ORF2 deletion mutant virus. CLS, GP, and BW performed the experimental infection study and sample acquisition. Cytokine, antibody and cellular assays were performed by CLS, SB, HF, CW, CLW and AR. CLS and BW performed the data analyses. CLS and BW drafted the manuscript. All authors read and approved the final version.

work also followed the Guide for Care and Use of Animals in Agricultural Research and Teaching. All efforts were made to minimize suffering of the animals, for example by sedation of nervous or excited horses before sampling. At the end of this experimental study, all horses were kept at the facility at Cornell University as research horses.

Consent for publication
Not applicable.

Competing interests
The authors declare that they have no competing interests with the content of this article.

Author details
[1]Department of Population Medicine and Diagnostic Sciences, College of Veterinary Medicine, Cornell University, Ithaca, NY 14853, USA. [2]Department of Clinical Sciences, College of Veterinary Medicine, Cornell University, Ithaca, NY 14853, USA. [3]Institut für Virologie, Freie Universität Berlin, Philippstrasse 13, 10115 Berlin, Germany.

References
1. Borchers K, Thein R, Sterner-Kock A. Pathogenesis of equine herpesvirus-associated neurological disease: a revised explanation. Equine Vet J. 2006;38: 283–7.
2. Perkins GA, Goodman LB, Tsujimura K, Van de Walle GR, Kim SG, Dubovi EJ, et al. Investigation of the prevalence of neurologic equine herpes virus type 1 (EHV-1) in a 23-year retrospective analysis (1984-2007). Vet Microbiol. 2009; 139:375–8.
3. Pusterla N, David Wilson W, Madigan JE, Ferraro GL. Equine herpesvirus-1 myeloencephalopathy: a review of recent developments. Vet J. 2009;180: 279–89.
4. Lunn DP, Davis-Poynter N, Flaminio MJBF, Horohov DW, Osterrieder K, Pusterla N, et al. Equine Herpesvirus-1 Consensus Statement. J Vet Intern Med. 2009;23:450–61.
5. Patel JR, Edington N, Mumford JA. Variation in cellular tropism between isolates of equine herpesvirus-1 in foals. Arch Virol. 1982;74:41–51.
6. Kydd JH, Smith KC, Hannant D, Livesay GJ, Mumford JA. Distribution of equid herpesvirus-1 (EHV-1) in the respiratory tract of ponies: implications for vaccination strategies. Equine Vet J. 1994;26:466–9.
7. Kydd JH, Smith KC, Hannant D, Livesay GJ, Mumford JA. Distribution of equid herpesvirus-1 (EHV-1) in respiratory tract associated lymphoid tissue: implications for cellular immunity. Equine Vet J. 1994;26:470–3.
8. Vandekerckhove AP, Glorieux S, Gryspeerdt AC, Steukers L, Van Doorsselaere J, Osterrieder N, et al. Equine alphaherpesviruses (EHV-1 and EHV-4) differ in their efficiency to infect mononuclear cells during early steps of infection in nasal mucosal explants. Vet Microbiol. 2011;152:21–8.
9. Edington N, Bridges CG, Patel JR. Endothelial cell infection and thrombosis in paralysis caused by equid herpesvirus-1: equine stroke. Arch Virol. 1986; 90:111–24.
10. Edington N, Smyth B, Griffiths L. The role of endothelial cell infection in the endometrium, placenta and foetus of equid herpesvirus 1 (EHV-1) abortions. J Comp Pathol. 1991;104:379–87.
11. Smith KC, Mumford JA, Lakhani K. A comparison of equid herpesvirus-1 (EHV-1) vascular lesions in the early versus late pregnant equine uterus. J Comp Pathol. 1996;114:231–47.
12. Slater JD, Borchers K, Thackray AM, Field HJ. The trigeminal ganglion is a location for equine herpesvirus 1 latency and reactivation in the horse. J Gen Virol. 1994;75:2007–16.
13. Allen GP. Risk factors for development of neurologic disease after experimental exposure to equine herpesvirus-1 in horses. Am J Vet Res. 2008;69:1595–600.
14. Allen GP. Antemortem detection of latent infection with neuropathogenic strains of equine herpesvirus-1 in horses. Am J Vet Res. 2006;67:1401–5.
15. Pusterla N, Mapes S, Wilson WD. Prevalence of equine herpesvirus type 1 in trigeminal ganglia and submandibular lymph nodes of equids examined postmortem. Vet Rec. 2010;167:376–9.
16. Pusterla N, Mapes S, David WW. Prevalence of latent alpha-herpesviruses in thoroughbred racing horses. Vet J. 2012;193:579–82.
17. Edington N, Bridges CG, Huckle A. Experimental reactivation of equid herpesvirus 1 (EHV 1) following the administration of corticosteroids. Equine Vet J. 1985;17:369–72.
18. Edington N, Welch HM, Griffiths L. The prevalence of latent equid herpesviruses in the tissues of 40 abattoir horses. Equine Vet J. 1994;26:140–2.
19. Taouji S, Collobert C, Gicquel B, Sailleau C, Brisseau N, Moussu C, et al. Detection and isolation of equine herpesviruses 1 and 4 from horses in Normandy: an autopsy study of tissue distribution in relation to vaccination status. J Vet Med B Infect Dis Vet Public Health. 2002;49:394–9.
20. USDA APHIS. Equine herpesvirus Myeloencephalopathy: a potentially emerging disease. Vet. Serv. Info Sheet. 2007. https://www.aphis.usda.gov/animal_health/emergingissues/downloads/ehv1final.pdf. Accessed 11 Aug 2018.
21. Patel JR, Heldens J. Equine herpesviruses 1 (EHV-1) and 4 (EHV-4) – epidemiology, disease and immunoprophylaxis: a brief review. Vet J. 2005; 170:14–23.
22. Goodman L, Wagner B, Flaminio M, Sussman K, Metzger S, Holland R, et al. Comparison of the efficacy of inactivated combination and modified-live virus vaccines against challenge infection with neuropathogenic equine herpesvirus type 1 (EHV-1). Vaccine. 2006;24:3636–45.
23. Goehring LS, Wagner B, Bigbie R, Hussey SB, Rao S, Morley PS, et al. Control of EHV-1 viremia and nasal shedding by commercial vaccines. Vaccine. 2010;28:5203–11.
24. Kydd JH, Hannant D, Mumford JA. Residence and recruitment of leucocytes to the equine lung after EHV-1 infection. Vet Immunol Immunopathol. 1996; 52:15–26.
25. Heldens JG, Hannant D, Cullinane AA, Prendergast MJ, Mumford JA, Nelly M, et al. Clinical and virological evaluation of the efficacy of an inactivated EHV1 and EHV4 whole virus vaccine (Duvaxyn EHV1,4). Vaccination/challenge experiments in foals and pregnant mares. Vaccine. 2001;19:4307–17.
26. Breathnach CC, Yeargan MR, Timoney JF, Allen GP. Detection of equine herpesvirus-specific effector and memory cytotoxic immunity in the equine upper respiratory tract. Vet Immunol Immunopathol. 2006;111:117–25.
27. Kydd JH, Townsend HGG, Hannant D. The equine immune response to equine herpesvirus-1: the virus and its vaccines. Vet Immunol Immunopathol. 2006;111:15–30.
28. Nugent J, Birch-Machin I, Smith KC, Mumford JA, Swann Z, Newton JR, et al. Analysis of equid herpesvirus 1 strain variation reveals a point mutation of the DNA polymerase strongly associated with Neuropathogenic versus Nonneuropathogenic disease outbreaks. J Virol. 2006;80:4047–60.
29. Goodman LB, Loregian A, Perkins GA, Nugent J, Buckles EL, Mercorelli B, et al. A point mutation in a herpesvirus polymerase determines Neuropathogenicity. PLoS Pathog. 2007;3:e160.
30. Van de Walle G, Goupil R, Wishon C, Damiani A, Perkins G, Osterrieder N. A single nucleotide polymorphism in a herpesvirus DNA polymerase is sufficient to cause lethal neurological disease. J Infect Dis. 2009;200:20–5.
31. Allen GP, Breathnach CC. Quantification by real-time PCR of the magnitude and duration of leucocyte-associated viraemia in horses infected with neuropathogenic vs. non-neuropathogenic strains of EHV- 1. Equine Vet J. 2006;38:252–7.
32. Henninger RW, Reed SM, Saville WJ, Allen GP, Hass GF, Kohn CW, et al. Outbreak of neurologic disease caused by equine herpesvirus-1 at a university equestrian center. J Vet Intern Med. 2007;21:157–65.
33. Gryspeerdt A, Vandekerckhove A, Van Doorsselaere J, Van de Walle G, Nauwynck H. Description of an unusually large outbreak of nervous system disorders caused by equine herpesvirus 1 (EHV1) in 2009 in Belgium. Vlaams Diergeneeskd Tijdschr. 2011;80:147–53.
34. Barbić L, Lojkić I, Stevanović V, Bedeković T, Starešina V, Lemo N, et al. Two outbreaks of neuropathogenic equine herpesvirus type 1 with breed-dependent clinical signs. Vet Rec. 2012;170:227.
35. Ma G, Feineis S, Osterrieder N, Van de Walle GR. Identification and characterization of equine herpesvirus type 1 pUL56 and its role in virus-induced downregulation of major histocompatibility complex class I. J Virol. 2012;86:3554–63.
36. Wagner B, Wimer C, Freer H, Osterrieder N, Erb HN. Infection of peripheral blood mononuclear cells with neuropathogenic equine herpesvirus type-1 strain Ab4 reveals intact interferon-α induction and induces suppression of anti-inflammatory interleukin-10 responses in comparison to other viral strains. Vet Immunol Immunopathol. 2011;143:116–24.

37. Wimer CL, Damiani A, Osterrieder N, Wagner B. Equine herpesvirus type-1 modulates CCL2, CCL3, CCL5, CXCL9, and CXCL10 chemokine expression. Vet Immunol Immunopathol. 2011;140:266–74.
38. Hübert PH, Birkenmaier S, Rziha HJ, Osterrieder N. Alterations in the equine herpesvirus type-1 (EHV-1) strain RacH during attenuation. Zentralblatt vet. Reihe B J Vet Med Ser B. 1996;43:1–14.
39. Yalamanchili RR, Raengsakulrach B, O'Callaghan DJ. Equine herpesvirus 1 sequence near the left terminus codes for two open reading frames. Virus Res. 1991;18:109–16.
40. Telford EA, Watson MS, McBride K, Davison AJ. The DNA sequence of equine herpesvirus-1. Virology. 1992;189:304–16.
41. Soboll Hussey G, Ashton LV, Quintana AM, Van de Walle GR, Osterrieder N, Lunn DP. Equine herpesvirus type 1 pUL56 modulates innate responses of airway epithelial cells. Virology. 2014;464–465:76–86.
42. Soboll Hussey G, Hussey SB, Wagner B, Horohov DW, Van de Walle GR, Osterrieder N, et al. Evaluation of immune responses following infection of ponies with an EHV-1 ORF1/2 deletion mutant. Vet Res. 2011;42:23.
43. Wagner B, Goodman LB, Babasyan S, Freer H, Torsteinsdóttir S, Svansson V, et al. Antibody and cellular immune responses of naïve mares to repeated vaccination with an inactivated equine herpesvirus vaccine. Vaccine. 2015; 33:5588–97.
44. Wagner B, Perkins G, Babasyan S, Freer H, Keggan A, Goodman LB, et al. Neonatal Immunization with a Single IL-4/Antigen Dose Induces Increased Antibody Responses after Challenge Infection with Equine Herpesvirus Type 1 (EHV-1) at Weanling Age. Murthy AK, editor. PLOS ONE. 2017;12:e0169072.
45. Crowhurst FA, Dickinson G, Burrows R. An outbreak of paresis in mares and geldings associated with equid herpesvirus 1. Vet Rec. 1981;109:527–8.
46. Furr M, Reed S. Equine Neurology: Wiley; 2008. Available from: https://books.google.de/books?id=atRmlbfxu5UC
47. Elia G, Decaro N, Martella V, Campolo M, Desario C, Lorusso E, et al. Detection of equine herpesvirus type 1 by real time PCR. J Virol Methods. 2006;133:70–5.
48. Wagner B, Hillegas JM, Babasyan S. Monoclonal antibodies to equine CD23 identify the low-affinity receptor for IgE on subpopulations of IgM+ and IgG1+ B-cells in horses. Vet Immunol Immunopathol. 2012;146:125–34.
49. Lunn DP, Holmes MA, Antczak DF, Agerwal N, Baker J, Bendali-Ahcene S, et al. Report of the second equine leucocyte antigen workshop, squaw valley, California, July 1995. Vet Immunol Immunopathol. 1998;62:101–43.
50. Keggan A, Freer H, Rollins A, Wagner B. Production of seven monoclonal equine immunoglobulins isotyped by multiplex analysis. Vet Immunol Immunopathol. 2013;153:187–93.
51. Lunn DP, Holmes MA, Schram B, Duffus WP. Monoclonal antibodies specific for equine IgG sub-isotypes including an antibody which recognizes B lymphocytes. Vet Immunol Immunopathol. 1995;47:239–51.
52. Goodman LB, Wimer C, Dubovi EJ, Gold C, Wagner B. Immunological correlates of vaccination and infection for equine herpesvirus 1. Clin Vaccine Immunol. 2012;19:235–41.
53. Wagner B, Freer H. Development of a bead-based multiplex assay for simultaneous quantification of cytokines in horses. Vet Immunol Immunopathol. 2009;127:242–8.
54. Wagner B, Ainsworth DM, Freer H. Analysis of soluble CD14 and its use as a biomarker in neonatal foals with septicemia and horses with recurrent airway obstruction. Vet Immunol Immunopathol. 2013;155:124–8.
55. Brosnahan MM, Damiani A, van de Walle G, Erb H, Perkins GA, Osterrieder N. The effect of siRNA treatment on experimental equine herpesvirus type 1 (EHV-1) infection in horses. Virus Res. 2010;147:176–81.
56. Edington N, Bridges CG, Griffiths L. Equine interferons following exposure to equid herpesvirus-1 or −4. J Interf Res. 1989;9:389–92.
57. Wagner B, Hillegas JM, Flaminio MJ, Wattrang E. Monoclonal antibodies to equine interferon-alpha (IFN-alpha): new tools to neutralize IFN-activity and to detect secreted IFN-alpha. Vet Immunol Immunopathol. 2008;125(3–4): 315–25.
58. Randall RE, Goodbourn S. Interferons and viruses: an interplay between induction, signalling, antiviral responses and virus countermeasures. J Gen Virol. 2008;89:1–47.
59. Bazil V, Horejsí V, Baudys M, Kristofová H, Strominger JL, Kostka W, et al. Biochemical characterization of a soluble form of the 53-kDa monocyte surface antigen. Eur J Immunol. 1986;16:1583–9.
60. Landmann R, Fisscher AE, Obrecht JP. Interferon-gamma and interleukin-4 down-regulate soluble CD14 release in human monocytes and macrophages. J Leukoc Biol. 1992;52:323–30.
61. Labeta MO, Durieux J-J, Fernandez N, Herrmann R, Ferrara P. Release from a human monocyte-like cell line of two different soluble forms of the lipopolysaccharide receptor, CD14. Eur J Immunol. 1993;23: 2144–51.
62. Schütt C, Schilling T, Grunwald U, Schönfeld W, Krüger C. Endotoxin-neutralizing capacity of soluble CD14. Res Immunol. 1992;143:71–8.
63. Haziot A, Rong GW, Lin XY, Silver J, Goyert SM. Recombinant soluble CD14 prevents mortality in mice treated with endotoxin (lipopolysaccharide). J Immunol. 1995;154:6529.
64. Wilsterman S, Soboll-Hussey G, Lunn DP, Ashton LV, Callan RJ, Hussey SB, et al. Equine herpesvirus-1 infected peripheral blood mononuclear cell subpopulations during viremia. Vet Microbiol. 2011;149:40–7.
65. Baghi HB, Nauwynck HJ. Impact of equine herpesvirus type 1 (EHV-1) infection on the migration of monocytic cells through equine nasal mucosa. Comp Immunol Microbiol Infect Dis. 2014;37:321–9.
66. Osterrieder N, Van de Walle GR. Pathogenic potential of equine alphaherpesviruses: the importance of the mononuclear cell compartment in disease outcome. Vet Microbiol. 2010;143:21–8.
67. Breathnach CC, Yeargan MR, Sheoran AS, Allen GP. The mucosal humoral immune response of the horse to infective challenge and vaccination with equine herpesvirus-1 antigens. Equine Vet J. 2001;33:651–7.
68. Coombs DK, Patton T, Kohler AK, Soboll G, Breathnach C, Townsend HGG, et al. Cytokine responses to EHV-1 infection in immune and non-immune ponies. Vet Immunol Immunopathol. 2006;111:109–16.
69. Paillot R, Daly JM, Juillard V, Minke JM, Hannant D, Kydd JH. Equine interferon gamma synthesis in lymphocytes after in vivo infection and in vitro stimulation with EHV-1. Vaccine. 2005;23:4541–51.
70. Packiarajah P, Walker C, Gilkerson JR, Whalley JM, Love DN. Immune responses and protective efficacy of recombinant baculovirus expressed glycoproteins of equine herpesvirus 1 (EHV-1) gB gC and gD alone or in combinations in BALB/c mice. Vet Microbiol. 1998;61:261–78.
71. Tewari D, Nair SV, De Ungria MC, Lawrence CL, Hayden M, Love DN, Field HJ, Whalley JM. Immunization with glycoprotein C of equine herpesvirus-1 is associated with accelerated virus clearance in a murine model. Arch Virol. 1995;140:789–97.
72. Lewis MJ, Wagner B, Woof JM. The different effector function capabilities of the seven equine IgG subclasses have implications for vaccine strategies. Mol Immunol. 2008;45(3):818–27.
73. Breathnach CC, Soboll G, Suresh M, Lunn DP. Equine herpesvirus-1 infection induces IFN-γ production by equine T lymphocyte subsets. Vet Immunol Immunopathol. 2005;103:207–15.
74. Allen G, Yeargan M, Costa LR, Cross R. Major histocompatibility complex class I-restricted cytotoxic T-lymphocyte responses in horses infected with equine herpesvirus 1. J Virol. 1995;69:606–12.
75. Kydd J, Wattrang E, Hannant D. Pre-infection frequencies of equine herpesvirus-1 specific, cytotoxic T lymphocytes correlate with protection against abortion following experimental infection of pregnant mares. Vet Immunol Immunopathol. 2003;96:207–17.
76. O'Neill T, Kydd JH, Allen GP, Wattrang E, Mumford JA, Hannant D. Determination of equid herpesvirus 1-specific, CD8+, cytotoxic T lymphocyte precursor frequencies in ponies. Vet Immunol Immunopathol. 1999;70:43–54.

21

Effects of orally administered galacto-oligosaccharides on immunological parameters in foals

Johannes Cornelis Vendrig[1*], Luc Edgar Coffeng[2] and Johanna Fink-Gremmels[1]

Abstract

Background: In the first phase of life, in which the immune system is primed and the bacterial colonization of epithelial surfaces takes place, foals are highly susceptible to bacterial infections. Next to strategies to optimize maternally acquired immunity in individual foals, current research explores other options to modulate immune responses in foals. During the past decades, oligosaccharide supplements were developed to mimic beneficial properties of the oligosaccharides, which are present in colostrum and milk. In human infants and laboratory animal species, dietary supplementation with galacto-oligosaccharides (GOS) has been shown to result in prebiotic and immunomodulating effects, with long-term beneficial consequences for both defensive and allergic immune responses. As yet, no studies are published concerning the *in vivo* effects of GOS in horses. The current study was designed as a pilot study to investigate the effects of an orally applied, commercially available GOS product in a group of pony foals. The treatment and the control group consisted of six and four foals, respectively. Foals were treated during the first four weeks of life and subsequently followed up for another ten weeks.

Results: In peripheral blood mononuclear cells (PBMCs) derived from GOS-treated foals at day 28, a standardized lipopolysaccharide challenge resulted in significantly lower relative mRNA expression levels of the pro-inflammatory cytokines interferon-γ and interleukin-6 compared with PBMCs of control foals. In the 98-day period of investigation, no significant effects of the GOS supplement were observed on clinical and blood parameters for immunity and general health in these foals.

Conclusions: Based on these first results, we can conclude that this dose regimen of GOS was well accepted by the foals and did not result in any detectable undesirable side effects. More clinical trials are required to confirm the attenuating effects of GOS treatment on equine pro-inflammatory immune responses and to implement this into practice.

Keywords: Horse, Foal, Oligosaccharides, PBMC, GOS, Immunomodulation, Cytokines, Bayesian Hierarchical linear regression

Background

With birth, the foal's immune system is subjected to a range of environmental challenges. Bacterial colonization of epithelial surfaces is one of the major events in early life determining immune responses in later phases of life [1]. In addition to the basic concept of protection by maternal antibodies present in colostrum, recently more interest has arisen for the influence of other colostral constituents, such as oligosaccharides. In human infants and experimental animals, dietary supplements containing commercially produced galacto-oligosaccharides (GOS) have been proven to elicit prebiotic effects [2-4] and to be beneficial for health in several ways [5], for instance by enhancing defensive immune responses [6-8] and lowering the incidence of infections [9,10]. Still, the evidence supporting the use of such oligosaccharide supplements is not conclusive, as other studies have reported only temporary or non-significant effects of similar supplements on infection and immunity [11-13].

* Correspondence: J.C.Vendrig@uu.nl
[1]Veterinary Pharmacology, Pharmacotherapy and Toxicology, Institute for Risk Assessment Sciences, Faculty of Veterinary Medicine, Utrecht University, P.O. box 80152, 3508 TD Utrecht, The Netherlands
Full list of author information is available at the end of the article

A limited amount of research into the effects of oligosaccharides in horses has been conducted so far. Prebiotic properties of short-chain fructo-oligosaccharides in horses have been confirmed [14,15], but to our knowledge no studies into *in vivo* effects of GOS or other oligosaccharide supplements in horses or foals have been published. Our previous *in vitro* studies with equine peripheral blood mononuclear cells (PBMCs) revealed immunomodulatory properties of both equine colostral carbohydrates and several commercially available oligosaccharide products, including GOS [16,17].

The present study was designed as a pilot study to investigate the *in vivo* effects of a commercially available GOS product in young foals. Next to assessing the safety of the chosen dose regimen of GOS and its effects on immunity and general health, we compared the responses to a standardized lipopolysaccharide (LPS) challenge in *ex vivo* PBMCs after 4 weeks of treatment.

Methods

Foals

Twelve warmblood pony foals (crossbreed New Forest* Arabian) were included in the study, all born at a horse dairy farm in The Netherlands, where the experiment was carried out. All mares and foals were housed together as a group under identical and stable conditions. Foals were born by natural delivery within a period of ten weeks and were allocated to the treatment group and the control group at random. In total, six foals were supplemented with GOS and four foals were included in the control group (two foals were excluded during the course of the study: see results section). Foals were naturally nursed by the mares and were also free to eat roughage (hay, grass, straw) as soon as they were ready for it. All experimental procedures were approved by the committee of ethical considerations in animal experiments of Utrecht University (DEC Utrecht, Permit Number: 2012.III.05.053).

Dietary supplementation

Foals in the treatment group were orally supplemented with GOS for 28 days, starting at the day of birth. The applied GOS product (Vivinal GOS syrup, Friesland-Campina Domo, Zwolle, The Netherlands) consisted of approximately 45% GOS, 16% lactose, 14% glucose, and 25% water. The product contained short chain GOS, which are oligomers (degree of polymerization 2–6) constructed from lactose [18]. An amount of 15 g GOS syrup was supplemented twice daily. Foals in the control group were orally supplemented with 2.4 g lactose and 2.1 g glucose (twice daily for 28 days), resembling the amounts of glucose and lactose that the GOS treated foals received through the GOS syrup. Both the GOS syrup and the control treatments were administered directly into the mouth of the foals (with a syringe).

Sampling and output parameters

At day 0, 1, 7, 14, 21, 28, 42, 56, 70, 84, and 98, approximately 14 mL of blood was collected by jugular venipuncture directly into sterile blood collection tubes; one 10 mL serum tube and one 4 mL spray-coated EDTA tube (BD Vacutainer Systems, Plymouth, United Kingdom). At all time points, samples were sent to the University Veterinary Diagnostic Laboratory in Utrecht to determine red and white blood cell parameters (including hematocrit, leukocyte count, and leukocyte differentiation) and the total protein concentrations including a protein electrophoresis (albumin and differentiation of globulins). In addition, aliquots of the serum samples were stored at −80°C to perform several ELISAs. Serum concentrations of the immunoglobulin subtypes IgG(a), IgG(b), IgG(T), IgM and IgA were quantified, using commercial ELISA kits according to the manufacturer's instructions (Bethyl Laboratories Inc., Montgomery, AL, USA). Mare colostrum was sampled within 12 hours postpartum to investigate the concentrations of immunoglobulin subtypes by means of the same ELISA kits (Bethyl Laboratories Inc., Montgomery, AL, USA).

PBMC experiments

At day 28, the last day of GOS application, PBMCs were isolated from each foal according to previously described methods [16]. PBMCs were resuspended in RPMI 1640 Medium (Lonza, Basel, Switzerland) containing 2 mM glutamine (Lonza, Basel, Switzerland), 100 IU/mL penicillin (Lonza, Basel, Switzerland), 100 µg/mL streptomycin (Lonza, Basel, Switzerland) and 10% horse serum. Horse serum was prepared by collecting full blood, allowing it to clot for 45 minutes, and then collecting the serum following centrifugation. The serum for all experiments was prepared at once by collection of blood from one pony (not enrolled in the study) from the same herd.

PBMCs were seeded in 24 well plates at a density of $4*10^6$ cells/mL medium/well. Subsequently, the plates were incubated for 2 hours at 37°C and 5% CO_2. The plates were then centrifuged for 10 minutes at 400× *g* before refreshing the medium without removing PBMCs. The experiments were started by replacing the medium with medium containing 0 or 1 µg/mL LPS (*Escherichia coli* O111:B4, Sigma-Aldrich, St. Louis, MO, USA). After 4 hours of incubation, supernatants were collected for ELISA and stored at −80°C; for qPCR, PBMCs were lysed using RNA lysis buffer (Promega, Madison, WI, USA) and stored at −80°C. All individual incubations were performed in triplicate for each foal.

Protein levels of tumor necrosis factor-α (TNF-α), interferon-γ (IFN-γ) and interleukin-10 (IL-10) were measured by means of ELISA on the cell culture supernatants, using Duoset® ELISA Development System for equine TNF-α, equine IFN-γ, and equine IL-10 (R&D Systems, Minneapolis, MN, USA). Standard operating procedures of the manufacturer were followed, applying all required buffers and solutions in the form provided by the manufacturer (R&D Systems, Minneapolis, MN, USA). The lower limits of detection of the ELISAs were 15.6 pg/mL, 62.5 pg/mL, and 156.3 pg/mL for TNF-α, IFN-γ, and IL-10, respectively.

RNA was isolated from PBMCs using SV Total RNA isolation system according to the manufacturer's instructions (Promega, Madison, WI, USA). Isolated fractions were dissolved in 50 μL RNAse free water and stored at −80°C. Quality and quantity of RNA was determined spectrophotometrically (Nanodrop). cDNA was generated using iScript™ cDNA Synthesis Kit (Biorad, Hercules, CA, USA) according to the manufacturer's protocol. For reverse transcriptase reaction, 1000 ng RNA was applied per sample. Expression of mRNA was assessed by real-time PCR using a Biorad iQ5 Multicolor Real-time PCR detection system and iQ™ SYBR® Green Supermix (Biorad, Hercules, CA, USA). Specific primer pairs were designed and tested for efficiency and accuracy, after having checked their specificity using the NCBI-BLASTN search program. Primer pairs were synthesized commercially (Eurogentec Nederland B.V., Maastricht, The Netherlands). For this study, mRNA expression of IFN-γ, IL-4, IL-6, IL-10, IL-13, IL-17, transforming growth factor-β1 (TGF-β1), TNF-α, β-actin, and glyceraldehyde 3-phosphate dehydrogenase (GAPDH) was determined using the following primer pairs:

IFN-γ: F 5′-GATCTGAAGGTCCAGCGCAA-3′ R 5′-TCCGGCCTCGAAATGGATTC-3′;
IL-4: F 5′-GCCCGAAGAACACAGATGGA-3′ R 5′-CAGTACAGCAGGTCCCGTTT-3′;
IL-6: F 5′-TGGCTGAAGAACACAACAACT-3′ R 5′-GAATGCCCATGAACTACAACA-3′;
IL-10: F 5′-GAGAACCACGGCCCAGACATCAAG-3′ R 5′-GACAGCGCCGCAGCCTCACT-3′;
IL-13: F 5′-AGCAGTCATTGCTCTCGCTT-3′ R 5′-TGGGTGATGTTGACCAGCTC-3′;
IL-17: F 5′-GCTGAGTCTGGTGGCTATCG-3′ R 5′-TTCTTGTCCCCAGTGTTCGG-3′;
TGF-β1: F 5′-TGTCCACCTGCAAGACCATC-3′ R 5′-CCGCAACTTGGACAGGATCT-3′;
TNF-α: F 5′-TCCAGACGGTGCTTGTGC-3′ R 5′-GGCCAGAGGGTTGATTGACT-3′;
β-actin: F 5′-CAAGGCCAACCGCGAGAAGA TGAC-3′ R 5′-GCCAGAGGCGTACAGGGACAG CA-3′;
GAPDH: F 5′-TGGCATGGCCTTCCGTGTCC-3′ R 5′-GCCCTCCGATGCCTGCTTCAC-3′.

Statistical analysis

Data were analyzed in a Bayesian framework. This means that we considered the data as fixed (which it is once observed) and parameters as random variables because they are unknown (in a frequentist framework, data are considered random and parameters are fixed). In other words, our inferences are conditioned on the observed data, and not on the distribution of test statistics across a range of unobserved repeated samples. Related to this, the Bayesian context facilitates a common-sense interpretation of uncertainty in parameter estimates [19]. For example, a posterior 95% credible interval of 1–10 means that the true value of the parameter lies between one and ten with 95% probability (conditional on the chosen model). Model selection can be done based on the deviance-based information criterion (and several other criteria), which can even be used to compare hierarchical models. Also, a Bayesian framework provides more robust parameter estimates, as such estimates are exact (we need not rely on asymptotic theory as we would in a frequentist framework) and we do not have to be concerned about multiple testing. These last two points are especially relevant to the current study (small sample size, many outcome parameters).

Data on blood parameters (day 28 separately, and the entire period from day 0–98) as well as PBMC data (day 28 only) were analyzed by means of Bayesian linear regression. Similar to previous analyses [17], PBMC responses were allowed to vary between horses in general (random intercept), and with regard to incubation with LPS (random slope). To stabilize the variance, all blood and PBMC data were log-transformed, except for hematocrit data, which were analyzed on the unit scale. For the analysis of the blood data over the entire period, time was entered into the model as a continuous variable. To account for the sometimes non-linear association between time and blood data, time was transformed by means of fractional polynomials, such that the statistical model best fitted the data. To minimize bias in blood data due to variable uptake of colostral globulins, the first weeks of life were not included in the analysis for β-2 and γ globulins (up to day 42), IgA and IgM (up to day 28), IgG(a) (up to day 42), and IgG(b) and IgG(T) (up to day 56). The selection of these periods was based on visual inspection of the data, and was made such that at worst, estimates of the difference between the control and GOS group would be conservative.

For each data type, the best fitting fractional polynomials were determined in R (version 2.15.3; [20]), using the package *mfp* (version 1.4.9; [21]), not yet accounting for variation between horses. Final models, including random intercepts and fractional polynomials, were analyzed in JAGS, a program for analysis of Bayesian models using Markov Chain Monte Carlo simulation (version 3.3.0; [22]). Simulations in JAGS were performed using

R packages *rjags* (version 3–10; [23]) and *R2jags* (version 0.03-08; [24]). Posterior distributions were estimated based on uninformative prior distributions (normal distributions with mean 0 and standard deviation 100 for parameter means; inverse gamma distributions with mean 1 and variance 10,000 for variance of measurement error; uniform distributions with range 0 to 100 for standard deviation of random intercepts). Differences between control and GOS groups were stated significant, based on 95% Bayesian credible intervals, which were defined as the 2.5% and 97.5% percentiles of the posterior distributions. Posterior distributions were simulated by means of four Markov chains, each consisting of 10,000 Monte Carlo samples. The first 5,000 samples were discarded for burn-in, allowing the model to converge. Model convergence was assessed by means of Gelman and Rubin's convergence diagnostic, the potential scale reduction factor [25].

qPCR data validation

Variation of mRNA expression was excluded as a confounding factor, as no significant differences in either β-actin or GAPDH expression were detected between PBMCs from GOS-treated foals and foals from the control group, or between the blank incubations and the incubations with LPS.

In addition, we analyzed the data with a correction for GAPDH, according to the method described by Livak and Schmittgen [26]. In our case, normalization of data (based on housekeeping genes) did not change point estimates for differences between incubation types. Furthermore, normalization did not reduce the variation in the data (as should be expected in case of confounding due to variation in total mRNA levels), but rather increased it. This indicated that the error due to variation in mRNA expression, if any, was negligible compared to basic measurement error in the data. Based on this knowledge and the fact that housekeeping genes for equine PBMCs have not yet been validated, we decided to present the data in this manuscript without any corrections.

Results

Course of the study

During the 98-day period of investigation, no effects of the treatment on the apparent clinical health parameters were observed, either in the GOS-treated foals or in the control group. The treatments were well accepted by the foals and no undesirable side effects (including diarrhea) were encountered.

Two foals in the control group were excluded from the study; one foal was stillborn, and another foal was not treated on the first two days of life due to colic. Therefore, the results comprise the data of six GOS-treated foals and four foals from the control group.

Blood parameters

Table 1 represents the comparison of the blood parameters between GOS-treated and control foals during the entire period of investigation. None of the blood parameters differed significantly between the two groups of foals. In Figure 1, a quantification of blood parameters is given for all foals at each time point for the entire period of investigation. Table 2 illustrates the comparison of the blood parameters between the two groups of foals at day 28 (at the moment of PBMC isolation). At day 28, the blood concentration of IgG(a) was found to be significantly higher in the group of GOS-treated foals compared to control group. Apart from this, no significant differences were observed between the two groups at day 28.

An additional file is provided to illustrate the data in more detail for the individual foals in both groups (see [Additional file 1]).

Table 1 Blood parameters: comparison between GOS-treated and control foals throughout the 98 days of the experiment

	Difference between treatment and control group including 95% Bayesian credible intervals[1]		
	Median	Lower bound	Upper bound
Leukocytes	0.88	0.66	1.15
Lymphocytes	0.89	0.66	1.19
Mature granulocytes	0.89	0.62	1.28
Total protein[2]	1.03	0.94	1.13
Albumin (absolute values)	1.05	0.96	1.15
α-1 globulins (absolute values)	1.09	0.87	1.36
α-2 globulins (absolute values)	0.94	0.84	1.04
β-1 globulins (absolute values)	1.16	0.72	1.97
β-2 globulins (absolute values)	1.05	0.74	1.54
γ globulins (absolute values)	1.10	0.83	1.44
Albumin (% of total protein)	1.01	0.94	1.09
α-1 globulins (% of total protein)	1.05	0.83	1.36
α-2 globulins (% of total protein)	0.91	0.81	1.02
β-1 globulins (% of total protein)	1.09	0.74	1.61
β-2 globulins (% of total protein)	1.01	0.71	1.44
γ globulins (% of total protein)	1.07	0.87	1.30
IgA	1.02	0.66	1.55
IgM	1.20	0.72	1.99
IgG(a)	1.13	0.91	1.42
IgG(b)	1.77	0.66	4.99
IgG(T)	1.34	0.74	2.38

[1]Relative differences are stated (significant if ≠ 1). For the hematocrit, the absolute difference was 0.00 (interval ranging from −0.04 to 0.05). [2]The protein spectrum (albumin and different globulins) are compared both as absolute values (g/L) and as a percentage of the total protein concentration.

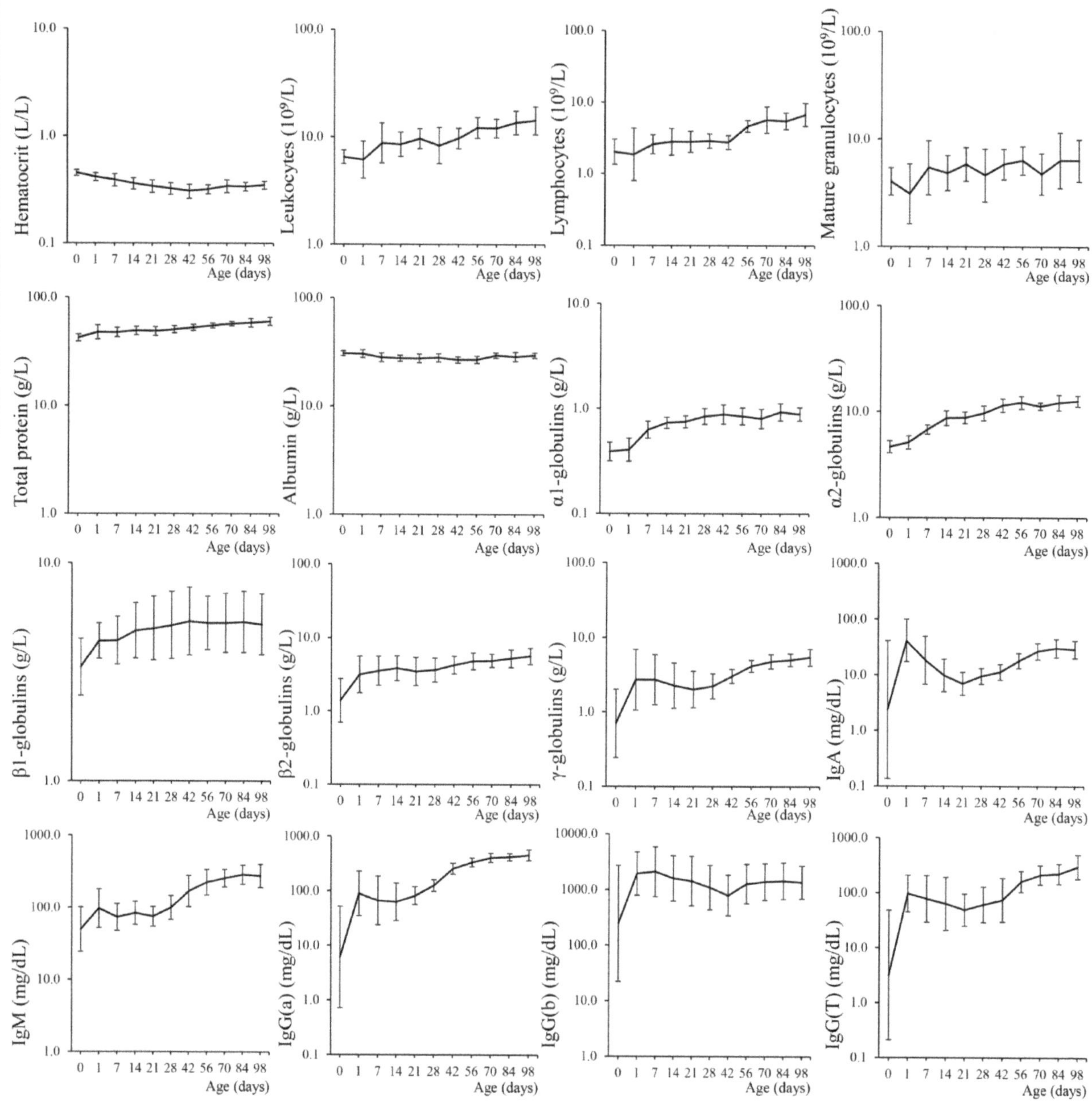

Figure 1 Blood parameters. Mean values and standard deviations for the investigated blood parameters at each time point for all foals included in the study.

Colostral and serum immunoglobulins

The measured concentrations of immunoglobulin subtypes in the colostral samples of the individual mares are added to the immunoglobulin data of the corresponding foals in the provided additional file (see [Additional file 1]). No significant differences were observed with regard to concentrations of the measured immunoglobulin subtypes in the mares' colostrum between the two groups. The colostral immunoglobulin levels for all mares exceeded the minimal quality standards for equine colostrum (for instance 3000 mg/dL for IgG [27]). Moreover, the colostrum of the dams of foals with relatively low serum globulin concentrations during the first weeks did not contain lower amounts of immunoglobulins relative to the colostrum of dams belonging to foals with high serum globulin concentrations.

The passive transfer of immunity at day 1 was within the expected range, as all foals reached serum IgG concentrations well above 800 mg/dL, except for one foal in the control group (i.e., 294 mg/dL 24 hours postpartum). In the analysis of endogenously produced immunoglobulins, no significant differences were found in the entire group of foals and the serum of the aforementioned foal reached comparable immunoglobulin concentrations as

Table 2 Blood parameters: comparison between GOS-treated and control foals at day 28 (at the moment of PBMC isolation)

	Difference between treatment and control group including 95% Bayesian credible intervals[1]		
	Median	Lower bound	Upper bound
Leukocytes	0.85	0.47	1.57
Lymphocytes	0.83	0.60	1.15
Mature granulocytes	0.83	0.34	2.02
Total protein[2]	1.03	0.92	1.16
Albumin (absolute values)	0.99	0.87	1.14
α-1 globulins (absolute values)	1.01	0.77	1.33
α-2 globulins (absolute values)	1.06	0.82	1.36
β-1 globulins (absolute values)	1.18	0.68	2.02
β-2 globulins (absolute values)	1.14	0.63	2.01
γ globulins (absolute values)	1.11	0.61	2.02
Albumin (% of total protein)	0.96	0.87	1.08
α-1 globulins (% of total protein)	0.98	0.71	1.37
α-2 globulins (% of total protein)	1.03	0.81	1.29
β-1 globulins (% of total protein)	1.15	0.70	1.88
β-2 globulins (% of total protein)	1.10	0.62	1.95
γ globulins (% of total protein)	1.07	0.64	1.81
IgA	1.41	0.92	2.18
IgM	1.15	0.62	2.08
IgG(a) *	**1.43**	**1.10**	**1.83**
IgG(b)	2.14	0.58	7.99
IgG(T)	1.70	0.56	5.00

[1]Relative differences are stated (significant if ≠ 1, marked with asterisk). For the hematocrit, the absolute difference was −0.01 (interval ranging from −0.07 to 0.06). [2]The protein spectrum (albumin and different globulins) are compared both as absolute values (g/L) and as a percentage of the total protein concentration.

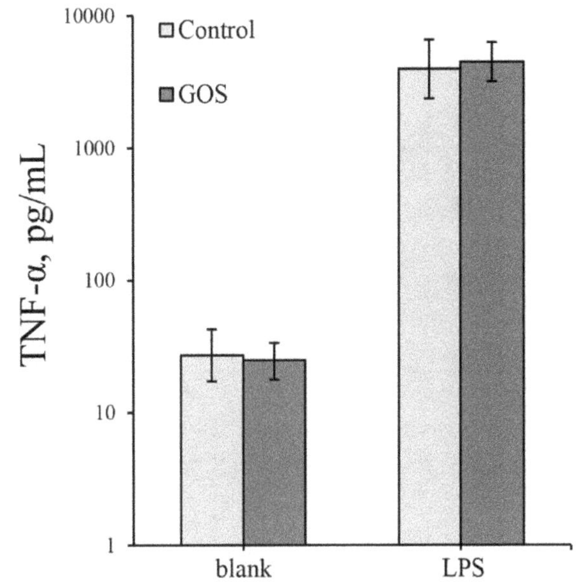

Figure 2 TNF-α production. Mean supernatant concentrations of TNF-α (in pg/mL) including 95% Bayesian credible intervals for unchallenged (blank) and LPS-challenged PBMCs derived from foals treated with either GOS or glucose/lactose (control).

well (in the period >42 days of age, as can be observed in the graphs of [Additional file 1]).

PBMC experiments

Figure 2 illustrates supernatant concentrations of TNF-α for unchallenged and LPS-challenged PBMCs. No significant difference in TNF-α production was observed between the two groups. The data for supernatant concentrations of IL-10 and IFN-γ were mostly below the detection limit of the applied assay. Hence, analysis of these data was not possible.

Relative cytokine expression levels after LPS stimulation in PBMCs are presented in Figure 3. In both groups, *ex vivo* LPS stimulation resulted in a significant up-regulation of mRNA expression for all investigated cytokines, except IL-4 and TGF-β1. IL-4 expression was not significantly influenced by the LPS challenge in neither of the groups, and the expression of TGF-β1 was significantly down-regulated in both groups. For IFN-γ and IL-6, the relative mRNA expression levels after LPS challenge were significantly lower in PBMCs derived from GOS-treated foals compared with the control group (80% and 40% reduction for IFN-γ and IL-6, respectively). No other significant differences were detected between the two groups.

Discussion

In this pilot study, we found that GOS was well accepted and tolerated by newborn foals, causing no observable negative side effects. Furthermore, we did not find any significant differences between GOS-treated and control foals with regard to the investigated blood parameters. The serum globulin contents varied highly during the first weeks of life, most likely due to differences in the uptake of maternal globulins by individual foals. The measured globulin concentrations of the colostrum samples indicate that this variation was not caused by insufficient quality of the mares' colostrum. Despite the variation in maternally acquired immunoglobulin levels, all foals eventually reached comparable and sufficient levels of immunoglobulins during the experimental period, through endogenous production (in the period >42 days of age). This active immunity of the foal itself becomes pivotal to prevent pathogens from causing disease, when maternal immunity fades [28].

At the moment of PBMC isolation, no significant differences were observed among the blood parameters of

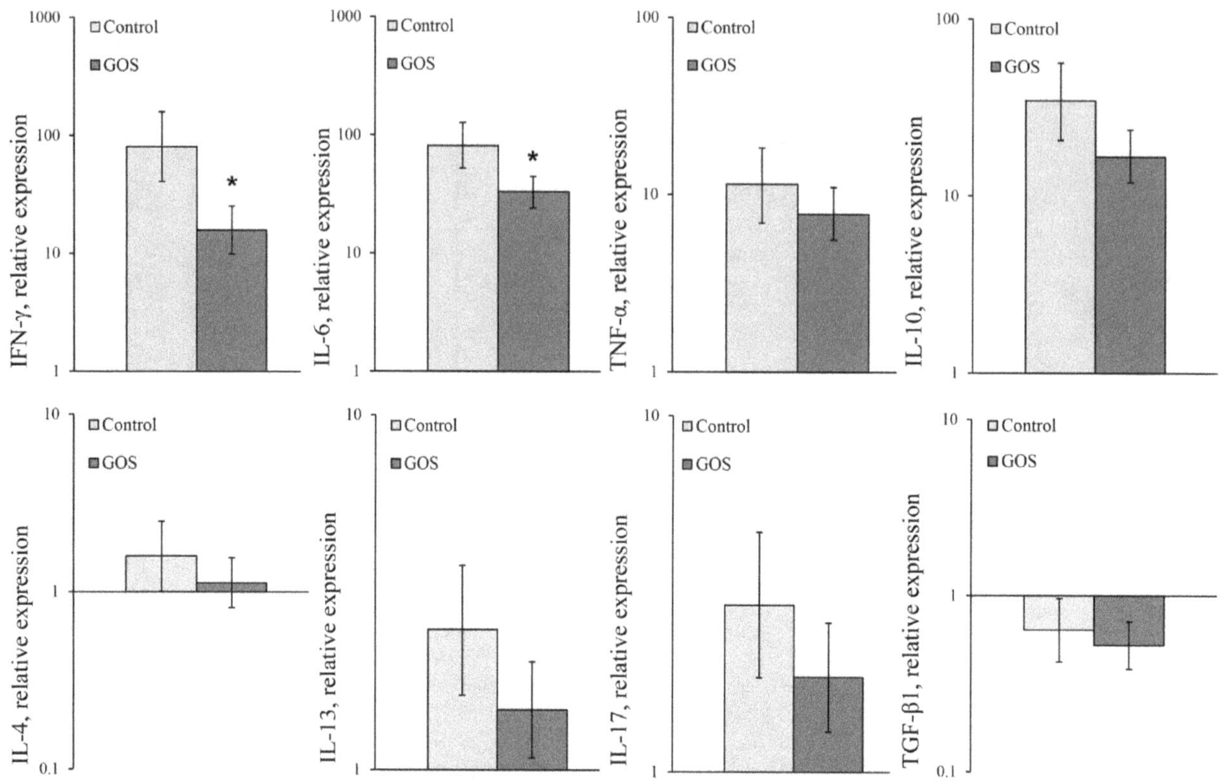

Figure 3 Cytokine mRNA expression levels. Mean relative cytokine mRNA expression levels including 95% Bayesian credible intervals in LPS-challenged PBMCs, relative to blank controls. Significant differences between PBMCs derived from foals treated with GOS and glucose/lactose (control) are indicated with an asterisk (*).

the two groups, apart from the serum concentration of IgG(a), which was significantly higher in the group of GOS-treated foals compared to the control group (see Table 2). This difference can be attributed to the particularly low serum IgG(a) concentration of the one foal with failure of passive transfer. One may be concerned about a possible influence of the serum IgG(a) concentration on the mRNA expression of cytokines in the foals' PBMCs following LPS stimulation. If this were the case, one would expect particularly high mRNA expression rates for IFN-γ and IL-6 in the PBMCs of foals with relatively low serum IgG(a) concentrations. However, such a pattern was not present in our data; in contrast, the data showed relatively low mRNA expression levels of IFN-γ and IL-6 for the PBMCs of foals with relatively low IgG(a) concentrations. Therefore, we conclude that the differences in the PBMC experiments were probably not caused by differences in serum IgG(a) concentrations at day 28.

Our results show that the LPS-induced mRNA expression levels of IFN-γ and IL-6, which are both related to type 1 T helper cell (Th1) responses, were significantly lower in PBMCs derived from GOS-treated foals compared with the control group. However, the LPS-induced production of TNF-α in PBMCs did not differ between the two groups; similarly, there was no significant difference in mRNA expression of TNF-α. Recently, anti-inflammatory effects of oligosaccharide supplements containing GOS have been described in preterm human infants as well, though these effects were found to be transient [12]. Therefore, the PBMC data from our pilot study in foals call for future studies with PBMC experiments at multiple time points during the treatment period.

Several studies have reported measurable immunomodulatory effects of oligosaccharides through direct interaction with Toll-like receptors (TLRs) [29-31]. Moreover, transfer of oligosaccharides across the epithelial barrier was proven by Eiwegger et al.[32], suggesting that direct contact between orally supplied oligosaccharides and the cells of the immune system is possible. Taking these findings into account, we hypothesize that oral supplementation of GOS in the present study led to long-term *in vivo* interaction of PBMCs with TLRs, eventually resulting in a measurable endotoxin tolerance and less responsive PBMCs. This hypothesis is in line with our data from a previous study, in which we demonstrated direct (short-term) immunomodulatory effects of GOS on equine PBMCs *ex vivo*; co-incubation of equine PBMCs with GOS enhanced the LPS-induced cytokine responses [16].

Moreover, recently TLR-4 activation by GOS was demonstrated in several cell types [33,34]. To investigate this further, future *in vitro* experiments with repeated or long-term exposure to oligosaccharides are desirable. However, the limited viability of primary equine cells and the lack of a functional equine immortal cell line make it difficult to perform reliable experiments over a longer time frame.

Young foals have previously been shown to display lower expression levels of Th1 related cytokines, including IFN-γ and IL-6, compared with older individuals [35-37]. Immature lymphocyte responses in neonates, with a bias towards Th2 responses, are thought to play a role in the increased susceptibility to infections in early life. Therefore, immunomodulation in young individuals is generally focused on the enhancement of defensive cytokine responses instead of reducing them [38]. On the other hand, a modulated immune response to bacteria that colonize epithelial surfaces during the first period of life, including the intestines, is a prerequisite to establish bacterial colonization and concurrently maintain homeostasis [39]. Exaggerated immune responses to bacteria in the phase of colonization could influence the composition of the microbiota and even may cause tissue damage and decreased epithelial barrier function, possibly leading to bacterial infections and sepsis. If indeed GOS treatment in foals results in a lower responsiveness of gut-associated lymphocytes and dendritic cells to LPS (or other challenges), this could be an interesting finding with regard to the eventual introduction of oligosaccharide supplements in practice. Depending on the clinical context, next to disease prevention through enhancing defensive immune responses, the suppression of exaggerated cytokine responses to bacterial compounds could prevent pathology in early life, particularly in the gastrointestinal tract. On the other hand, very pronounced suppression of immune responses by GOS is not desirable as it could increase the susceptibility to infections. This question should be addressed in forthcoming *in vivo* experiments that include a pathogen challenge of treated foals. More research is required to further investigate the long-term effects of GOS, other oligosaccharides, and oligosaccharide mixtures, and to eventually optimize the use of oligosaccharide supplements in different clinical settings.

In addition, beneficial effects of oligosaccharide supplements on allergic immune responses have been reported in various mammalian species [40-45]. Recently, a Cochrane review was published on this subject, in which these significant beneficial effects are stated as well, together with the limitations of these studies and the need for more conclusive evidence [46]. The reported beneficial effects of oligosaccharide supplements in other species suggest another possible indication for the use of oligosaccharides in horses, with the aim to reduce the long-term incidence and severity of relevant immune-mediated inflammatory diseases, such as recurrent airway obstruction, inflammatory airway disease, and insect hypersensitivity (summer eczema). Further investigations into this topic are warranted.

Conclusions

In conclusion, the results from this pilot study indicate that the chosen dose regimen of GOS was well accepted by the foals, and that no undesirable side effects were encountered. At the same time, no differences in the investigated hematological parameters, including serum immunoglobulins, could be detected between GOS-treated foals and the control group. GOS treatment appeared to reduce the pro-inflammatory responses in PBMCs after an *ex vivo* LPS challenge. With this knowledge, additional experiments with the GOS preparation can be performed in larger groups of foals, including the application of higher dosages and longer periods of treatment. Moreover, a longer follow up of GOS-treated foals may reveal long-term beneficial effects on the incidence and severity of immune-mediated inflammatory diseases, in line with published studies in other mammalian species.

Abbreviations

GAPDH: Glyceraldehyde 3-phosphate dehydrogenase; GOS: Galacto-oligosaccharides; IFN: Interferon; Ig: Immunoglobulin; IL: Interleukin; LPS: Lipopolysaccharide; PBMC: Peripheral blood mononuclear cell; TGF: Transforming growth factor; Th: T helper cell; TLR: Toll- like receptor; TNF: Tumor necrosis factor.

Competing interests

The authors declare that they have no competing interests.

Authors' contributions

Conceived and designed the study: JFG, JCV. Collected materials and performed experiments: JCV. Analyzed the data: JCV, LEC. Wrote the manuscript: JCV. Reviewed and revised the manuscript: JFG, JCV, LEC. All authors read and approved the final manuscript.

Acknowledgements

The authors thank the owners of the participating studfarm for their cooperation and Danone/Nutricia Research (Utrecht, The Netherlands) for kindly donating the oligo-, mono-, and disaccharide fractions, which were applied in this study.

Author details

[1]Veterinary Pharmacology, Pharmacotherapy and Toxicology, Institute for Risk Assessment Sciences, Faculty of Veterinary Medicine, Utrecht University, P.O. box 80152, 3508 TD Utrecht, The Netherlands. [2]Department of Public Health, Erasmus MC University Medical Center Rotterdam, P.O. box 3000, 2040 CA Rotterdam, The Netherlands.

References

1. Martin R, Nauta AJ, Ben Amor K, Knippels LM, Knol J, Garssen J: **Early life: gut microbiota and immune development in infancy.** *Benef Microbes* 2010, **1**(4):367–382.
2. Davis LM, Martinez I, Walter J, Hutkins R: **A dose dependent impact of prebiotic galactooligosaccharides on the intestinal microbiota of healthy adults.** *Int J Food Microbiol* 2010, **144**(2):285–292.
3. Fanaro S, Marten B, Bagna R, Vigi V, Fabris C, Pena-Quintana L, Arguelles F, Scholz-Ahrens KE, Sawatzki G, Zelenka R, Schrezenmeir J, de Vrese M, Bertino E: **Galacto-oligosaccharides are bifidogenic and safe at weaning: a double-blind randomized multicenter study.** *J Pediatr Gastroenterol Nutr* 2009, **48**(1):82–88.
4. Ben XM, Li J, Feng ZT, Shi SY, Lu YD, Chen R, Zhou XY: **Low level of galacto-oligosaccharide in infant formula stimulates growth of intestinal Bifidobacteria and Lactobacilli.** *World J Gastroenterol* 2008, **14**(42):6564–6568.
5. Sangwan V, Tomar SK, Singh RR, Singh AK, Ali B: **Galactooligosaccharides: novel components of designer foods.** *J Food Sci* 2011, **76**(4):R103–11.
6. Gopalakrishnan A, Clinthorne JF, Rondini EA, McCaskey SJ, Gurzell EA, Langohr IM, Gardner EM, Fenton JI: **Supplementation with galacto-oligosaccharides increases the percentage of NK cells and reduces colitis severity in Smad3-deficient mice.** *J Nutr* 2012, **142**(7):1336–1342.
7. Vos AP, Haarman M, van Ginkel JW, Knol J, Garssen J, Stahl B, Boehm G, M'Rabet L: **Dietary supplementation of neutral and acidic oligosaccharides enhances Th1-dependent vaccination responses in mice.** *Pediatr Allergy Immunol* 2007, **18**(4):304–312.
8. Schijf MA, Kruijsen D, Bastiaans J, Coenjaerts FE, Garssen J, van Bleek GM, Van't Land B: **Specific dietary oligosaccharides increase Th1 responses in a mouse respiratory syncytial virus infection model.** *J Virol* 2012, **86**(21):11472–11482.
9. Arslanoglu S, Moro GE, Boehm G: **Early supplementation of prebiotic oligosaccharides protects formula-fed infants against infections during the first 6 months of life.** *J Nutr* 2007, **137**(11):2420–2424.
10. Chatchatee P, Lee WS, Carrilho E, Kosuwon P, Simakachorn N, Yavuz Y, Schouten B, Graaff PL, Szajewska H: **Effects of growing-up milk supplemented with prebiotics and LCPUFAs on infections in young children.** *J Pediatr Gastroenterol Nutr* 2014, **58**(4):428–437.
11. Niele N, van Zwol A, Westerbeek EA, Lafeber HN, van Elburg RM: **Effect of non-human neutral and acidic oligosaccharides on allergic and infectious diseases in preterm infants.** *Eur J Pediatr* 2013, **172**(3):317–323.
12. van den Berg JP, van Zwieteren N, Westerbeek EA, Garssen J, van Elburg RM: **Neonatal modulation of serum cytokine profiles by a specific mixture of anti-inflammatory neutral and acidic oligosaccharides in preterm infants.** *Cytokine* 2013, **64**(1):188–195.
13. van den Berg JP, Westerbeek EA, van der Klis FR, Berbers GA, Lafeber HN, van Elburg RM: **Neutral and acidic oligosaccharides supplementation does not increase the vaccine antibody response in preterm infants in a randomized clinical trial.** *PLoS One* 2013, **8**(8):e70904.
14. Respondek F, Goachet AG, Julliand V: **Effects of dietary short-chain fructooligosaccharides on the intestinal microflora of horses subjected to a sudden change in diet.** *J Anim Sci* 2008, **86**(2):316–323.
15. Berg EL, Fu CJ, Porter JH, Kerley MS: **Fructooligosaccharide supplementation in the yearling horse: effects on fecal pH, microbial content, and volatile fatty acid concentrations.** *J Anim Sci* 2005, **83**(7):1549–1553.
16. Vendrig JC, Coffeng LE, Fink-Gremmels J: **In vitro evaluation of defined oligosaccharide fractions in an equine model of inflammation.** *BMC Vet Res* 2013, **9**:147.
17. Vendrig JC, Coffeng LE, Fink-Gremmels J: **Equine colostral carbohydrates reduce lipopolysaccharide-induced inflammatory responses in equine peripheral blood mononuclear cells.** *Equine Vet J Suppl* 2012, **44**(Suppl 43):68–72.
18. Rijnierse A, Jeurink PV, van Esch BC, Garssen J, Knippels LM: **Food-derived oligosaccharides exhibit pharmaceutical properties.** *Eur J Pharmacol* 2011, **668**(Suppl 1):S117–23.
19. Gelman A, Carlin JB, Stern HS, Dunson DB, Vehtari A, Rubin DB: *Bayesian Data Analysis: 3rd ed.* CRC Press; 2014.
20. R Development Core Team: *R: A language and environment for statistical computing.* Vienna, Austria: R Foundation for Statistical Computing; 2011.
21. Amber G, Banner A: 2010 [http://CRAN.R-project.org/package=mfp]
22. Plummer M: 2012 [http://mcmc-jags.sourceforge.net]
23. Plummer M: 2011 [http://CRAN.R-project.org/package=rjags]
24. Su Y, Yajima M: 2011 [http://CRAN.R-project.org/package=R2jags]
25. Gelman A, Rubin DB: **Inference from iterative simulation using multiple sequences.** *Statistical Sci* 1992, **7**(4):457–511.
26. Livak KJ, Schmittgen TD: **Analysis of relative gene expression data using real-time quantitative PCR and the 2(−Delta Delta C(T)) Method.** *Methods* 2001, **25**(4):402–408.
27. Reed SM, Bayly WM, Sellon DC: *Equine Internal Medicine.* 3rd edition. USA: Elsevier; 2010. ISBN 978-1-4160-5670-6.
28. Giguere S, Polkes AC: **Immunologic disorders in neonatal foals.** *Vet Clin North Am Equine Pract* 2005, **21**(2):241–72. v.
29. Termeer C, Benedix F, Sleeman J, Fieber C, Voith U, Ahrens T, Miyake K, Freudenberg M, Galanos C, Simon JC: **Oligosaccharides of Hyaluronan activate dendritic cells via toll-like receptor 4.** *J Exp Med* 2002, **195**(1):99–111.
30. Campo GM, Avenoso A, D'Ascola A, Prestipino V, Scuruchi M, Nastasi G, Calatroni A, Campo S: **Hyaluronan differently modulates TLR-4 and the inflammatory response in mouse chondrocytes.** *Biofactors* 2012, **38**(1):69–76.
31. Tsai CC, Lin CR, Tsai HY, Chen CJ, Li WT, Yu HM, Ke YY, Hsieh WY, Chang CY, Wu CY, Chen ST, Wong CH: **The immunologically active oligosaccharides isolated from wheatgrass modulate monocytes via Toll-like receptor-2 signaling.** *J Biol Chem* 2013, **288**(24):17689–17697.
32. Eiwegger T, Stahl B, Haidl P, Schmitt J, Boehm G, Dehlink E, Urbanek R, Szepfalusi Z: **Prebiotic oligosaccharides: in vitro evidence for gastrointestinal epithelial transfer and immunomodulatory properties.** *Pediatr Allergy Immunol* 2010, **21**(8):1179–1188.
33. Capitan-Canadas F, Ortega-Gonzalez M, Guadix E, Zarzuelo A, Suarez MD, de Medina FS, Martinez-Augustin O: **Prebiotic oligosaccharides directly modulate proinflammatory cytokine production in monocytes via activation of TLR4.** *Mol Nutr Food Res* 2014, **58**(5):1098–1110.
34. Ortega-Gonzalez M, Ocon B, Romero-Calvo I, Anzola A, Guadix E, Zarzuelo A, Suarez MD, Sanchez de Medina F, Martinez-Augustin O: **Nondigestible oligosaccharides exert nonprebiotic effects on intestinal epithelial cells enhancing the immune response via activation of TLR4-NFkappaB.** *Mol Nutr Food Res* 2014, **58**(2):384–393.
35. Liu T, Nerren J, Liu M, Martens R, Cohen N: **Basal and stimulus-induced cytokine expression is selectively impaired in peripheral blood mononuclear cells of newborn foals.** *Vaccine* 2009, **27**(5):674–683.
36. Merant C, Breathnach CC, Kohler K, Rashid C, Van Meter P, Horohov DW: **Young foal and adult horse monocyte-derived dendritic cells differ by their degree of phenotypic maturity.** *Vet Immunol Immunopathol* 2009, **131**(1–2):1–8.
37. Breathnach CC, Sturgill-Wright T, Stiltner JL, Adams AA, Lunn DP, Horohov DW: **Foals are interferon gamma-deficient at birth.** *Vet Immunol Immunopathol* 2006, **112**(3–4):199–209.
38. Diesner SC, Forster-Waldl E, Olivera A, Pollak A, Jensen-Jarolim E, Untersmayr E: **Perspectives on immunomodulation early in life.** *Pediatr Allergy Immunol* 2012, **23**(3):210–223.
39. Walker WA: **Initial intestinal colonization in the human infant and immune homeostasis.** *Ann Nutr Metab* 2013, **63**(Suppl 2):8–15.
40. van Hoffen E, Ruiter B, Faber J, M'Rabet L, Knol EF, Stahl B, Arslanoglu S, Moro G, Boehm G, Garssen J: **A specific mixture of short-chain galacto-oligosaccharides and long-chain fructo-oligosaccharides induces a beneficial immunoglobulin profile in infants at high risk for allergy.** *Allergy* 2009, **64**(3):484–487.
41. Yasuda A, Inoue K, Sanbongi C, Yanagisawa R, Ichinose T, Tanaka M, Yoshikawa T, Takano H: **Dietary supplementation with fructooligosaccharides attenuates allergic peritonitis in mice.** *Biochem Biophys Res Commun* 2012, **422**(4):546–550.
42. Moro G, Arslanoglu S, Stahl B, Jelinek J, Wahn U, Boehm G: **A mixture of prebiotic oligosaccharides reduces the incidence of atopic dermatitis during the first six months of age.** *Arch Dis Child* 2006, **91**(10):814–819.
43. Vos AP, van Esch BC, Stahl B, M'Rabet L, Folkerts G, Nijkamp FP, Garssen J: **Dietary supplementation with specific oligosaccharide mixtures decreases parameters of allergic asthma in mice.** *Int Immunopharmacol* 2007, **7**(12):1582–1587.

44. Arslanoglu S, Moro GE, Schmitt J, Tandoi L, Rizzardi S, Boehm G: **Early dietary intervention with a mixture of prebiotic oligosaccharides reduces the incidence of allergic manifestations and infections during the first two years of life.** *J Nutr* 2008, **138**(6):1091–1095.
45. Sagar S, Morgan ME, Chen S, Vos AP, Garssen J, van Bergenhenegouwen J, Boon L, Georgiou NA, Kraneveld AD, Folkerts G: **Bifidobacterium breve and Lactobacillus rhamnosus treatment is as effective as budesonide at reducing inflammation in a murine model for chronic asthma.** *Respir Res* 2014, **15**:46.
46. Osborn DA, Sinn JK: **Prebiotics in infants for prevention of allergy.** *Cochrane Database Syst Rev* 2013, **3**, CD006474.

Immune response of healthy horses to DNA constructs formulated with a cationic lipid transfection reagent

Christiane L. Schnabel[1*], P. Steinig[1], M. Koy[2], H.-J. Schuberth[2], C. Juhls[3,4], D. Oswald[3,4], B. Wittig[4], S. Willenbrock[5], H. Murua Escobar[5,6], C. Pfarrer[7], B. Wagner[8], P. Jaehnig[9], A. Moritz[10], K. Feige[1] and J.-M. V. Cavalleri[1]

Abstract

Background: Deoxyribonucleic acid (DNA) vaccines are used for experimental immunotherapy of equine melanoma. The injection of complexed linear DNA encoding interleukin (IL)-12/IL-18 induced partial tumour remission in a clinical study including 27 grey horses. To date, the detailed mechanism of the anti-tumour effect of this treatment is unknown.

Results: In the present study, the clinical and cellular responses of 24 healthy horses were monitored over 72 h after simultaneous intradermal and intramuscular application of equine IL-12/IL-18 DNA (complexed with a transfection reagent) or comparative substances (transfection reagent only, nonsense DNA, nonsense DNA depleted of CG). Although the strongest effect was observed in horses treated with expressing DNA, horses in all groups treated with DNA showed systemic responses. In these horses treated with DNA, rectal temperatures were elevated after treatment and serum amyloid A increased. Total leukocyte and neutrophil counts increased, while lymphocyte numbers decreased. The secretion of tumour necrosis factor alpha (TNFα) and interferon gamma (IFNγ) from peripheral mononuclear blood cells *ex vivo* increased after treatments with DNA, while IL-10 secretion decreased. Horses treated with DNA had significantly higher myeloid cell numbers and chemokine (C-X-C motif) ligand (CXCL)-10 expression in skin samples at the intradermal injection sites compared to horses treated with transfection reagent only, suggesting an inflammatory response to DNA treatment.

In horses treated with expressing DNA, however, local CXCL-10 expression was highest and immunohistochemistry revealed more intradermal IL-12-positive cells when compared to the other treatment groups.

In contrast to non-grey horses, grey horses showed fewer effects of DNA treatments on blood lymphocyte counts, TNFα secretion and myeloid cell infiltration in the dermis.

Conclusion: Treatment with complexed linear DNA constructs induced an inflammatory response independent of the coding sequence and of CG motif content. Expressing IL-12/IL-18 DNA locally induces expression of the downstream mediator CXCL-10.

The grey horses included appeared to display an attenuated immune response to DNA treatment, although grey horses bearing melanoma responded to this treatment with moderate tumour remission in a preceding study. Whether the different immunological reactivity compared to other horses may contributes to the melanoma susceptibility of grey horses remains to be elucidated.

Keywords: Equine melanoma, Grey horse, MIDGE vector, Cytokines, CpG, IL-12, IL-18, Transfection reagent, DNA vaccine, Cationic lipid

* Correspondence: Christiane.Schnabel@tiho-hannover.de
[1]University of Veterinary Medicine Hannover, Clinic for Horses, Buenteweg 9, 30559 Hannover, Germany
Full list of author information is available at the end of the article

Background

Melanoma is one of the most common equine cutaneous neoplasms [1–3]. Prevalence is up to 80 % in grey horses older than 15 years, while horses of other colours are rarely affected by this disease [4, 5]. To date, there is no satisfactory therapeutic approach available in advanced cases of grey horse melanoma [1, 4, 6]. One experimental *in vivo* approach is immunotherapy with melanoma antigens and/or immune modulating cytokines encoded by deoxyribonucleic acid (DNA) vectors taking advantage of systemic effects on metastases [7–9]. Interleukin (IL)-12 and IL-18 have been employed as they synergistically stimulate cytotoxic T-cells and natural killer cells [10–12], which are typically involved in anti-tumour immune responses. The two cytokines improve antigen presentation [13] and form a link between innate and adoptive immunity [14, 15]. Furthermore, anti-angiogenic properties have been described which could contribute to anti-tumour effects [16, 17].

A moderate decrease in the tumour volume of melanomas was observed by Mählmann et al. [18] during a study period of 120 days after immunotherapy of 27 grey horses with mixed linear DNA vectors (minimalistic immunologic defined gene expression (MIDGE)-Th1) encoding equine IL-12 and IL-18. These DNA vectors were formulated with the transfection reagent SAINT-18 and administered simultaneously intramuscularly (i.m.) and peritumourally intradermally (i.d.).

MIDGE-Th1 vectors are minimalistic linear double-stranded DNA molecules lacking plasmid backbone sequences. The vectors are covalently closed with single-strand hairpin loops at both ends. They contain the expression cassette only, i.e. a promoter, the coding sequence of interest and a polyadenylation site [19, 20]. One of the ends is covalently bound to a nuclear localisation signal peptide, triggering an improved humoral and cellular response of a T_H1 phenotype [21, 22]. *In vivo* transfection is established and can be facilitated by the formulation of the DNA vectors with cationic lipids, such as SAINT-18, to form complexes with these molecules [23, 24].

Signs of a systemic immune response, i.e. the development of fever 12 h after administration of MIDGE-Th1 formulated with SAINT-18 and the size reduction of metastases which had not been treated locally, were observed in the study of Mählmann et al. [18]. Local immunological responses were indicated by signs of acute inflammation (swelling, reddening, etc.) and depigmentation of the skin at the site of injection. The exact mechanisms of this anti-tumour therapy are still unknown.

Effects of DNA vectors are usually explained by their transgene products [9, 19, 23, 25], by immunologic effects caused by CG motifs randomly contained in the vector constructs which activate toll-like receptor (TLR-) 9 pathways [26–28], by reactions triggered by interaction with cytosolic receptors for dsDNA [29–33], or by combinations of these effects.

The mechanisms of the immunotherapeutic effects of MIDGE-Th1 encoding equine IL-12 and IL-18 demonstrated by Mählmann et al. [18] in grey horses affected with melanoma need to be elucidated in order to improve the directed clinical use of anti-tumour treatments. Therefore, the aim of this study was the characterisation of the immune response to the treatment by investigation of various candidate immune parameters on the systemic and local level in healthy horses. Furthermore, potential immunologically active components of the therapeutic were analysed for their contribution to the immune response. This was conducted comparatively in four treatment groups, representing effects by transfection reagent only, transgene products, CG motifs or DNA independent of its sequence.

Methods

Ethical statement

All procedures were carried out according to the ethical guidelines of the law on animal welfare (Tierschutzgesetz) approved by the "Niedersächsisches Landesamt für Verbraucherschutz und Lebensmittelsicherheit" in the animal experiment No. 33.9-42502-04-11/0399. Informed consent was obtained from all animal owners.

Study design

A prospective, randomised, double-blinded study was performed in 24 horses assigned randomly to four groups of six horses each (A–D) by the criteria of colour, age and breed (Table 1).

Animals

Clinically healthy horses (6 mares, 15 geldings and 3 stallions) aged between 2 and 21 years (mean 10.6 years) with a body weight of 425–680 kg (mean 572 kg) were included in the study. There were six Thoroughbred (ThB) type horses (two Arabians, two Arabian-mix and two English ThBs) and 18 Warmblood (WBl) type horses (nine Hanoverian WBls, one Hessian WBl, one Polish WBl, two Pura Raza Españolas (PRE), one PRE-mix, one Standardbred, one Oldenburg WBl, and one Westfalian WBl; Table 1). One horse of treatment group A had a history of insect bite hypersensitivity and one horse of each of the treatment groups A, B and C had a history of chronic obstructive bronchitis/bronchiolitis, but all horses were asymptomatic throughout the study period. No systemic and potentially immunomodifying treatments were administered in the two weeks preceding the experiments.

The animals were kept in stables of the Clinic for Horses, University of Veterinary Medicine, Hannover, Foundation,

Table 1 Distributions of horses within treatment groups

Treatment group	Treatment	Mean age (years)	Mean weight (kg)	Mares (n)	Geldings (n)	Stallions (n)	WBl (n)	ThB (n)	Grey (n)	Non-grey (n)
A	SAINT18	11.1	561	2	3	1	4	2	2	4
B	SAINT18+ eqIL12 + eqIL18	10.8	589	2	3	1	5	1	2	4
C	SAINT18+ eqIL12-ATG + eqIL18-ATG	10.1	548	0	5	1	4	2	2	4
D	SAINT18+ eqIL12-ATG-CG + eqIL18-ATG-CG	11.3	591	2	4	0	5	1	2	4

IL interleukin, *–ATG* nonsense DNA, *–ATC-CG* nonsense DNA depleted of CG, *WBl* warmblood, *ThB* thoroughbred

housed in standard single boxes on straw or wood shavings under a natural light–dark cycle of German summer (15–16.3 h of light, sunrise between 05:12 and 05:44, light from large windows or adjacent paddocks). The horses were fed hay and concentrates twice a day (at 07:00 and 18:00), according to their body weight, and had access to water ad libitum. Horses had access to an outdoor 20 × 60 m sand area once a day, in the late afternoon or early evening, with a minimum of 2 h rest prior to examination and sampling.

The horses were allowed to acclimatise for at least 2 days before starting the experiment and were trained by classical and operant conditioning for blood sampling to minimise stress during blood collection. Horses stayed in the clinic for 8 days (t-96 – t72). Examinations were performed and samples were acquired at the horses' home stables at day 11 (t264) after treatment (Fig. 1).

Test items and groups

Four horses at a time were kept in the clinic and each was treated with one of the four different treatments, A–D. Injection solutions were provided in blinded tubes in a volume of 1 ml buffered with phosphate-buffered saline (PBS). Treatment letter codes were kept at the DNA vector manufacturing site and opened only after all study data had been acquired and evaluated.

Group A received only the transfection reagent (SAINT-18, Synvolux Therapeutics B.V., Groningen, Netherlands; containing 6 nmol/ml 1-methyl-4-(cis-9-dioleyl) methylpyridinium-chloride).

Group B received SAINT-18 and linear DNA vectors (MIDGE-Th1, eqIL12 and IL-1beta receptor antagonist protein (ILRAP)-eqIL18) encoding equine IL-12 [NM_001082511.1; NM_001082516.1] and IL-18 [NM_001082512.1] fused to the coding sequence of the IL-1beta receptor antagonist protein (ILRAP) signal peptide.

Group C received SAINT-18 and non-expressing MIDGE-Th1 vector of equine IL-18 with point mutations in all ATG sequences to delete potential start codons (nonsense DNA; eqIL18-ATG). These vectors had 1.02 times the number of total CG sequences, thus, potential CG motifs, as those given in the dose of group B.

Group D received SAINT-18 and nonsense DNA, similar to group C, but with inverted CG motifs (eqIL18-ATG-CG).

DNA vectors

The construction and synthesis of MIDGE-Th1 vectors was performed by MOLOGEN AG (Berlin, Germany), analogous to the method described by Schirmbeck et al. [21]. Briefly, the expression cassettes containing the cytomegalo virus immediate-early enhancer/promoter, a chimeric intron, the gene sequence (eqIL12; eqIL18; eqIL18-ATG or eqIL18-ATG-CG) and the SV40 late protein polyadenylation site were inserted into the plasmid pMCV1.4. The coding sequence for the ILRAP signal peptide was fused to the eqIL18 coding sequence in all eqIL18 MIDGE vectors. A digestion with the restriction endonuclease Eco31-I (MBI Fermentas, Vilnius, Lithuania) was performed to set the expression cassette free. The open ends of the expression cassette were sealed with loop-forming oligodeoxyribonucleotides, one of them linked to a peptide nuclear localisation sequence (a peptide with the amino acid sequence PKKKRKVEDPYC) [21]. Unbound DNA fragments were degraded with T7 DNA polymerase (MBI Fermentas, Vilnius, Lithuania) followed by purification of MIDGE-Th1 vectors.

Formulation of DNA vectors or phosphate-buffered saline with SAINT-18

The transfection reagent SAINT-18 (0.5 ml dissolved in water) was vortexed for 1 min and then mixed manually with 2× PBS (Biochrom AG, Berlin, Germany), or the DNA was dissolved in 2× PBS, obtaining the test item at a volume of 1 ml. Lipid-DNA complexes were allowed to form at room temperature (rt) for approximately 10 min prior to injection, achieving a mixture of 1 ml in 1× PBS. MIDGE-Th1/SAINT-18 complexes in groups B, C and D were formed at a ratio of 1 mg DNA to 0.75 μmol SAINT-18 and the DNA concentration was 0.4 mg/ml 1× PBS.

Treatment

All time points (t) in the following are reported as h before or after treatment (t-48 to t264; Fig. 1).

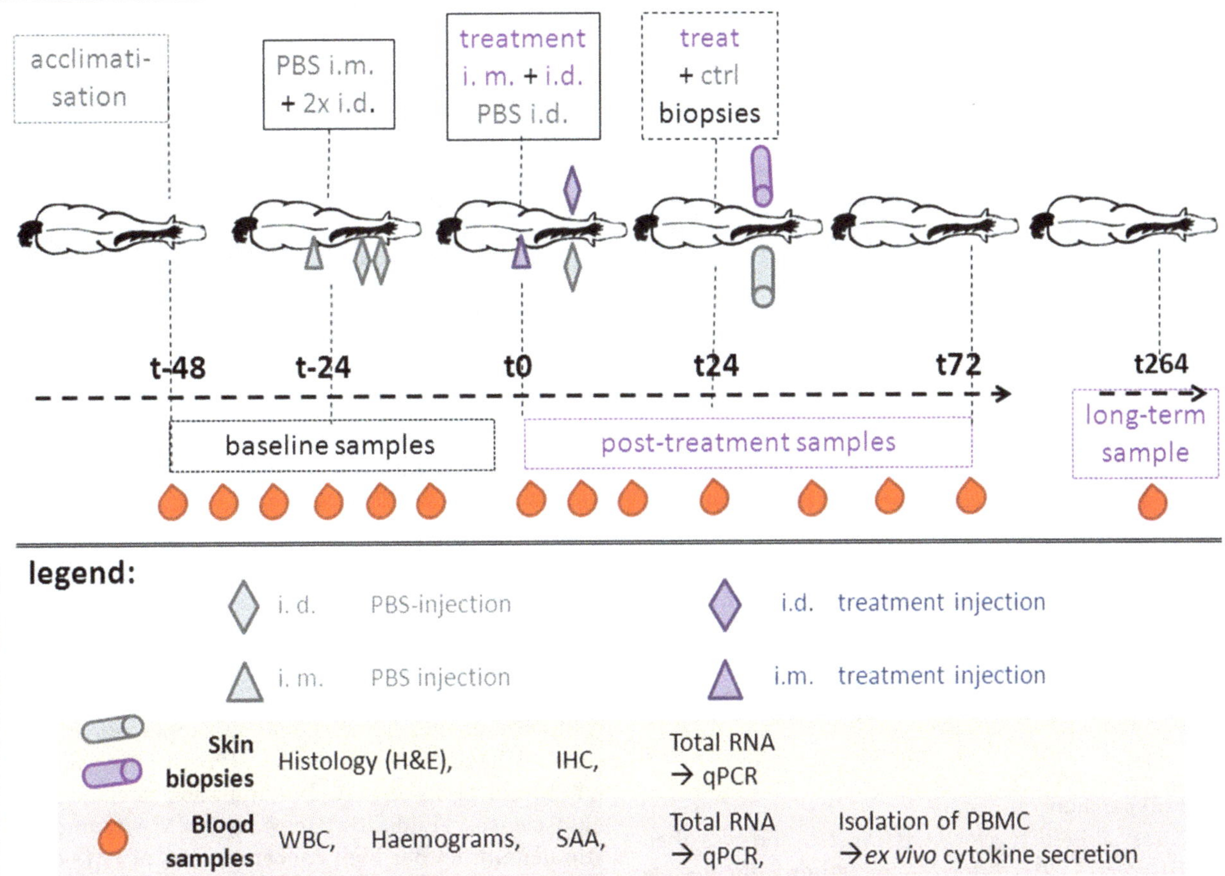

Fig. 1 Procedure Test procedure illustrated in course of time. The horses were left to acclimatise for at least three days. At t-24, the horses were injected with PBS (grey symbols) i.m. (0.5 ml) and i.d. (2 × 0.5 ml). Baseline samples (blood) as internal controls for systemic parameters were acquired from t-48 – t0. At t0, horses were injected with treatments A – D (purple symbols) i.m. (0.5 ml) and i.d. (0.5 ml) and contralaterally with PBS (grey symbol, 0.5 ml). From t6 – t72, post-treatment samples (blood) of systemic parameters were acquired. At t24, skin biopsies were acquired of treatment (purple) and PBS control (grey) sites. Eleven days post-treatment (t264), one long-term sample was acquired at the home stable of each horse. General examinations were performed at all sampling times. Blood samples were used to determine WBC, haemograms, SAA, cytokine mRNA and *ex vivo* cytokine secretion by PBMC. Skin samples were used to perform histological examinations, IHC of IL-12, IL-18 and calprotectin, and qPCR of cytokine and chemokine mRNA

The test item dose of 1 ml was split. One half (0.5 ml) was injected into the pectoralis muscle. The other 0.5 ml was injected i.d. into the middle third of the neck under subcutaneous local anaesthesia with 1 ml of lidocaine (Lidocainhydrochlorid 2 %, Bela-Pharm, Vechta, Germany) after aseptic preparation of the i.d. injection site with chlorhexidine (Hibiscrub, tk pharma trade, Hasbergen, Germany). The i.d. injection site (*treat*) was marked.

In order to evaluate local effects related to the application procedure, but unrelated to the test items at the time of treatment (t0), the contralateral side of the neck was treated with 0.5 ml of PBS i.d. (*ctrl*) after the same preparation and local anaesthesia as the *treat* site.

Clipping and shaving of i.d. injection sites was performed at t-36 to allow local irritation to resolve before injections (t0) and biopsy sampling (t24).

Twenty-four hours prior to treatment (t-24), the horses were injected with PBS in the same manner, but contralaterally (0.5 ml i.m. and 1 ml i.d. split into two injections of 0.5 ml each, injected at least 5 cm distant from each other and 20 cm from the injection sites of t0; Fig. 1). This injection of PBS was performed in order to evaluate the systemic effects of the injection procedure unrelated to the test item.

Examinations

The horses underwent a general clinical examination 4 times a day between t-48 and t48 and twice a day during the rest of their stay.

The skin at the injection sites was also examined clinically at these time points and digital photographs were taken. Changes were described in the categories oedema, pain, heat, depigmentation and exudate by a non-linear scale (0–3 representing absent – high-grade, respectively). Scores were summarised as the sums of all categories in a single clinical skin score.

Blood samples were drawn at 09:00, 15:00 and 21:00 from t-24–t24, and at 09:00 and 21:00 from t-48– -24 and from t24–t72. One general examination, clinical scoring of the injection site and blood sampling were performed on each horse at t264.

Blood sampling

Blood samples were drawn from the jugular vein after disinfection on the surface area with ethanol, by use of a vacutainer system (Vacuette, greiner bio-one, Frickenhausen, Germany) with a 20 G single-use cannula. Blood was collected in ethylenediaminetetraacetate (EDTA)-coated tubes for routine clinical laboratory measurements, in clot-activator-coated tubes for serum, in heparinised (sodium-heparin) tubes for the determination of SAA, and in PAXgene blood tubes (BD, Heidelberg, Germany) for the isolation of peripheral blood mononuclear cells (PBMC) and for the conservation of total messenger ribonucleic acid (mRNA).

Serum preparation

Blood was allowed to clot at rt for 2 h and was then centrifuged at 1430 × g for 6 min. Serum without clots was stored in aliquots at 4 °C for a maximum of 48 h until further analysis.

Routine clinical laboratory measurements

Analysis by routine clinical laboratory measurements included total plasma protein (TPP), haematocrit (Hct), white blood cell counts (WBC) and differential haemograms, measured by a manual refractometer (TPP), a Sysmex kx-21 N (Sysmex Deutschland GmbH, Norderstedt, Germany) (Hct, WBC) and an ADVIA 120 (Siemens Healthcare Diagnostics GmbH, Eschborn, Germany) (haemograms), respectively. Due to the availability of laboratory devices, differential haemograms were obtained after storage of EDTA-blood at rt for a maximum of 36 h. Absolute leukocyte subset (neutrophils, lymphocytes, monocytes) counts were calculated from percentages of the ADVIA measurement and total WBC measured immediately after sampling by Sysmex kx-21 N.

Serum amyloid A determination

Serum amyloid A was determined by an immunoturbidimetric latex agglutination test (LZ Test Eiken SAA, Eiken Chemical Co. Ltd., Tokyo, Japan). Limits of detection were 5–300 μg/ml. This assay for human serum amyloid A (SAA) had been evaluated for horses [34].

Isolation of peripheral blood mononuclear cells

The PBMC were isolated from heparinised blood by density gradient separation. Briefly, after sedimentation at rt for 1 h, leukocyte-rich plasma was layered onto LSM 1077 (density gradient solution, PAA, Pasching, Austria) and centrifuged (1000 × g, rt, for 30 min). Interphase PBMC were harvested and washed three times in PBS (500/250/150 × g, rt, 10 min). Cells were counted using the Cellometer Auto T4 cell-counting system (Nexcelom Bioscience, Massachusetts, USA).

Cell culture

A total of 2×10^6 PBMC per well were seeded in sterile cell culture 12-well plates and incubated for 12 h in a humidified atmosphere at 37 °C (5 % CO_2 in air) in 1 ml culture medium [(Roswell Park Memorial Institute: RPMI, Biochrom AG, Berlin, Germany) supplemented with 10 % heat-inactivated foetal calf serum (FCS; PAA Laboratories GmbH, Pasching, Austria) and penicillin 100 U/ml, streptomycin 0.1 mg/ml (PAA)] (medium only), supplemented with 1 μg/ml lipopolysaccharide (LPS; #L2755, Sigma-Aldrich, Munich, Germany) (LPS-stimulated), or in medium supplemented with phorbol 12-myristate 13-acetate (PMA; 50 ng/ml) and ionomycin (1.34 μM) (Cell stimulation cocktail 500×, eBioscience, Frankfurt, Germany) (PMA/ionomycin-stimulated). Rather high concentrations of PMA/ionomycin were chosen after preliminary experiments (data not shown) to obtain positive controls of cytokine secretion for each individual.

After incubation, cell-free supernatants were obtained and stored at −80 °C until further analysis. Thawing was performed at 37 °C immediately prior to the cytokine determinations.

Cells in medium only were used to evaluate spontaneous cytokine release. Lipopolysaccharide stimulation was used to evaluate TLR4-response [35] and PMA/ionomycin stimulation to assess cytokine induction by non-specific stimulation [36–38] as positive controls.

Determination of equine cytokines in cell culture supernatants

Tumour necrosis factor alpha was measured in duplicates by a sandwich ELISA for equine TNFα (Duo Set DY 1814, RnD, Wiesbaden, Germany), performed according to the manufacturer's protocol with the exception that coating was carried out at 4 °C overnight, as described previously [39]. Absorption was measured using a Synergy 2 instrument (BioTek, Bad Friedrichshall, Germany) and data was analysed by Gene 5 1.11 software (BioTek). The lower and upper limits of detection of the assay were 31.2–2000 pg/ml. Dilutions of standards and supernatant samples (if necessary due to exceeding upper detection limit) were made with PBS containing 1 % bovine serum albumin (BSA; # P3688, Sigma-Aldrich).

Two samples (one value from group A at t6; one value from group C at t24) were excluded from further analysis as the differences measured between TNFα duplicates were excessive.

Interferon alpha, IFNγ, IL-4, IL-10 and IL-17 were measured using a bead-based multiplex assay based on equine-specific monoclonal antibodies on a Luminex 100 System (Luminex, Austin, TX, USA), as validated previously [40]. Limits of detection were as follows: IFNα (12–30,000 pg/ml), IFNγ (10–5000 U/ml), IL-4 (40–80,000 pg/ml), IL-10 (15–35,000 pg/ml) and IL-17 (10–10,000 U/ml).

Examination of messenger ribonucleic acid

Preparation of messenger ribonucleic acid from blood samples

Ribonucleic acid was isolated from whole blood in PAXgene blood RNA tubes with the PAXgene blood RNA Kit (Qiagen GmbH, Hilden, Germany). Isolation was performed according to the manufacturer's instruction. The RNA concentration of the resulting solution was measured by automated electrophoresis (Experion System, Bio-Rad Laboratories GmbH, Munich, Germany) using the Experion RNA StdSens Starter Kit (Bio-Rad Laboratories GmbH), according to the manufacturer's instructions.

Preparation of messenger ribonucleic acid of skin samples

Punch biopsies of 4 mm diameter were transferred into 300 μl RLT buffer (Qiagen GmbH) and homogenised with TissueLyser II (30 Hz, four times for 5 min each, Qiagen GmbH). Subsequently, the RNA was extracted using the RNeasy Fibrous Tissue Mini Kit (Qiagen GmbH), according to the manufacturer's instructions. The resulting RNA solution was used for analysis by quantitative PCR (qPCR).

Transcription into cDNA

In order to perform the qPCR, 100 ng RNA diluted to a final volume of 10 μl with DNase/RNase-free water was transcribed into cDNA. SuperScriptII RT (Invitrogen, Karlsruhe, Germany) was used in combination with RNaseOUT Recombinant Ribonuclease Inhibitor (Invitrogen), according to the manufacturer's instructions.

The resulting RNA solutions were stored at −80 °C and the cDNA solutions at −20 °C.

Standard series for qPCR

Target-specific primers were designed for conventional and qPCR using the National Centre for Biotechnology Information primer blast in observance of the Equus caballus genome, and were produced by Eurofins MWG Operon, Ebersberg (Table 2). In order to perform the real-time PCR based on SYBR green, standard dilutions were produced for absolute quantification of the cDNA copy numbers.

Ribonucleic acid was eluted from equine liver, uterus and PBMC by standard procedures using the RNeasy Plus Mini Kit (Qiagen GmbH). The RNA was reverse transcribed into cDNA, as described previously.

A conventional PCR was performed with target-specific primer and Taq DNA Polymerase (5 U/ μl; Invitrogen). The reaction mixture had a final volume of 20 μl, consisting of 2 μl of 10× reaction mix, 0.4 μl of ROTI-MIX PCR 3 (pH 7; Carl Roth GmbH, Karlsruhe, Germany), 0.6 μl of magnesium chloride (50 mM; Invitrogen), 0.2 μl Taq DNA Polymerase (5 U/μl; Invitrogen), 1.5 μl of forward and 1.5 μl of reverse primer (5 pmol/μl), 12.8 μl DNase/RNase-free water (Sigma-Aldrich, Steinheim, Germany) and 1 μl of the cDNA. All samples were incubated at 95 °C for 10 min followed by 40 cycles of 30 s at 95 °C, 30 s at 56 °C and 45 s at 72 °C. Finally, the mixture was incubated at 72 °C for 10 min and stored at −20 °C.

All samples were analysed on 2.5 % agarose gel with Gel Loading Dye Blue (0.08 μl/ml; New England Biolabs GmbH, Frankfurt am Main, Germany) by electrophoresis. The rather high agarose concentration was chosen due to the best separation, as determined in preliminary experiments (data not shown). When the expected size was reached, the product was isolated from the gel band by the QIAEX II Gel Extraction Kit (Qiagen GmbH), according to the manufacturer's instructions.

One Shot TOP10 Chemically Competent *E. coli* (Invitrogen) was transformed with the target sequences isolated from the gel bands using the pCR 2.1 TOPO TA Cloning Kit (Invitrogen). The *E. coli* solution was transferred to LB medium (32 g LB agar powder (Lennox; Carl Roth GmbH) in 1 l *Aqua tridest*) breeding plates containing ampicillin (Sigma-Aldrich), 5-Brom-4-chlor-3-indoxyl-β-D-galactopyranosid (Invitrogen) and Isopro pyl-β-D-thiogalactopyranosid (Invitrogen). The *E. coli* were cultured for at least 24 h at 37 °C. Afterwards, colonies were transferred into 5 ml liquid LB medium (20 g LB agar (Lennox; Carl Roth GmbH) in 1 l A. tridest.) containing 50 μl ampicillin, and cultured for 16 h at 37 °C and 370 rpm. Subsequently, the plasmids were isolated from transformed *E. coli* by the PureLink Quick Plasmid Miniprep Kit (Invitrogen). The plasmids were sequenced by Sequence Laboratories Göttingen GmbH (Göttingen, Germany) to monitor the success of the transformation. Properly transformed plasmids were linearised using the restriction enzyme ScaI (Thermo-Scientific, Schwerte, Germany).

Table 2 qPCR settings

Cytokine	Accession number	Amplicon size (bp)	Forward primer (5'->3')	Forward primer volume (µl)	Reverse primer (5'->3')	Reverse primer volume (µl)	Concentration of primers (pmol/µl)
IL12p35	NM_001082511.1	76	GCTGACAGCCATTGACAAGCT	1.5	TTCAAGGGAGGGCTTTTGTG	4.5	0.5
IL12p40	NM_001082516.1	76	TGCTGTTCACAAGCTCAAGTATGA	1.5	GGGTGGGTCTGGTTTGATGA	1.5	0.5
IL18	NM_001082512.1	124	TGCTGGACCAGTAGAAGACA	1.5	AGGTTCAAGCCTGCCAAAGT	1.5	5
IFNγ	NM_001081949.1	417	GCTGTGTGCGATTTTGGGTT	1.5	CTCAGGTTAGCTTTGGGCGA	4.5	5
CXCL10	NM_001114940.1	153	GACTCTGAGTGGAACTCAAGGAAT	1.5	GTGGCAATGATCTCAACACG	4.5	5

The concentrations of the resulting solutions were measured by BioPhotometer (Eppendorf, Hamburg, Germany) and the copy number per µl was calculated. Finally, solutions with a known concentration of copy numbers were diluted and used as standard series in the qPCR in duplicate.

qPCR

Real-time SYBR Green PCR was performed on a StepO nePlus Real-Time PCR System (Applied Biosystems, Darmstadt, Germany) with MicroAmp Fast Optical 96-Well Reaction Plates, 0.1 ml (Applied Biosystems) and MicroAmp Optical Adhesive Film (Applied Biosystems). A real-time PCR reaction mixture was used with 12.5 µl SYBR green (Applied Biosystems), forward and reverse primers (Table 2) and the addition of DNase/RNase-free water to achieve a final volume of 25 µl. A volume of 1 µl of sample cDNA solution was added. In order to quantify the amount of copy numbers, the standard dilution series produced were used for comparison (10^2–10^6 copies/µl). All measurements were performed in duplicate. The samples were denatured for 10 min at 95 °C, followed by 40 cycles of 15 s at 95 °C and 60 s at 60 °C. A DNA melting curve analysis was carried out to ensure the production of a single PCR product.

Skin sampling

Four skin samples were taken 24 h after treatment under local anaesthesia after aseptic preparation of the skin at a distance of 1 cm from each injection site. This was the closest distance possible to achieve four equal biopsy samples and to still be able to close the sites afterwards without a high risk of scar formations. Skin biopsy samples were obtained using 8 mm (for histology) and 4 mm (for qPCR) diameter biopsy punches (Stiefel, Munich, Germany). Biopsy sites were closed aseptically by routine surgical closure.

Punch biopsies for qPCR were snap frozen in 1.5 ml RNAlater (Ambion, Carlsbad, USA) in liquid nitrogen and stored at −80 °C until further analysis.

Biopsies for histological examinations were fixed in 4 % neutral buffered formalin [41] for 24 h and then cut into two halves perpendicular to the surface.

Subsequently, formalin-fixed specimens were rinsed in slowly running tap-water for 6 h. After this, specimens were blinded again and embedded in paraffin for storage at rt until further analysis.

Histology

Sections of the paraffin-embedded tissues were cut (each 3 µm), mounted on glass slides and dried at 60 °C overnight.

Haematoxylin and eosin (H&E) stainings were prepared of each specimen for a general histopathological examination. One half of each specimen was chosen by the criteria of lowest artefacts, presence of all layers of the skin and best plane of cutting (exact sagittal slices preferred) for further evaluation.

Evaluation

Histopathological alterations were assessed according to a semi-quantitative score of inflammation (Table 3) separately in each layer of the skin [epidermis (Ep); dermis, papillary layer (*Dpap*) including adnexa; dermis, reticular layer (*Dret*); subcutis]. Inflammatory cell patterns were documented and individual cell types were ranked (0 to 3) according to their proportion of the cell infiltrate.

Table 3 Histological scores

Score	Epithelium	Dermis
0	No abnormalities	No leukocytes
1	One small ulcer / a few suspect areas with subepithelial infiltration of leukocytes	A few leukocytes, usually perivascular
2	A few ulcers, but predominantly epithelium without alterations	Some leukocytes, usually perivascular mononuclear cells
3	Some ulcers	Many leukocytes, countable
4	Frequent ulcers, intact epithelium between ulcers	Many leukocytes, uncountable due to overlapping or high-density masking cell edges
5	Many ulcers, no epithelium without alterations	Many leukocytes, uncountable tissue structure masked

Descriptions of histological scores for evaluations of epithelium and dermal layers (papillary and reticular) in skin samples stained with H&E

Immunohistochemistry

Immunohistochemistry (IHC) was performed on slices of the half of the formalin-fixed paraffin-embedded skin samples chosen. Macrophages and neutrophilic granulocytes were detected by staining of calprotectin, which is expressed by these cells [42]. Equine IL-12 and IL-18 were detected by cross-reactive monoclonal antibodies (mAbs), as described previously [43].

Slices of 3 μm were cut and dried on salined glass slides (Histobond, Marienfeld, Lauda-Königshofen, Germany) at 60 °C overnight. The sections were deparaffinised in xylene and rehydrated in a series of alcohols of descending grades. Endogenous peroxidase was blocked in 0.6 % hydrogen peroxide in 80 % ethanol at rt for 30 min. Sections were rinsed 3 times in PBS at rt for 5 min each.

All the following incubation steps were performed in a moist chamber. Pretreatment for antigen retrieval was performed with MAC 387 for optimum results (Table 4). The sections were incubated with proteinase K (#P2308, 7.0–14.0 U/mg, Sigma Aldrich) diluted in PBS at rt for 30 min. The sections were then rinsed in distilled water twice at rt for 2 min and once in PBS at rt for 5 min. The sections were incubated with heat-inactivated normal goat serum (NGS) diluted 1:5 in PBS for 20 min at rt to block unspecific protein binding.

The NGS was decanted and the sections were covered with primary antibodies (Table 4) diluted in PBS with 1 % BSA and incubated at 4 °C overnight. Negative controls were incubated with PBS/BSA only. On the following day, sections were rinsed 3 times in PBS for 5 min at rt (negative controls were handled separately).

The sections were then incubated with biotinylated secondary antibodies diluted in PBS at rt for 45 min, followed by rinsing in PBS and signal amplification with avidin-biotin complex (vector laboratories, Burlingame, Canada), according to the manufacturer's instructions for interleukins, or a ready-to-use kit (IHC Kit, DCS Immunoline, Hamburg, Germany) was employed, according to the manufacturer's instructions, for calprotectin as a secondary antibody and signal amplification (Table 4).

After rinsing the sections 3 times in PBS for 5 min, visualisation was performed with the chromogen, 3-amino-9-ethylcarbazole (AEC; Peroxidase-Substrat-Kit AEC, Biologo, Kronshagen, Germany), which was applied according to the manufacturer's instructions. After incubation for 10 min at rt, the slides were rinsed in PBS for 5 min and in slowly running tap-water for 10 min.

Sections were counterstained in Delafield's haematoxylin for 2 s and rinsed in running tap-water for 10 min to facilitate identification of specific tissue components.

Slides were mounted with Kaiser's glycerol gelatine (Merck, Darmstadt, Germany) and cover-slips and left to dry at rt.

Sections were viewed with a Zeiss Axioskop (Carl Zeiss Jena GmbH, Jena, Germany) and images were digitally captured using an Olympus DP Soft Camera (Olympus Deutschland GmbH, Hamburg, Germany).

Distinct red staining of cells was interpreted as a positive reaction of the primary antibodies given that negative controls showed no such staining. Negative controls were run in each batch, and isotype controls and positive controls in other tissues had been performed when establishing the IHC settings used.

Evaluation of immunohistochemistry-stained specimens

Cells stained positive for the respective targets in IHC were separately evaluated in the different layers of the skin (*Ep, Dpap, Dret*). Since only a few specimens contained sufficient amounts of subcutis, this layer was not assessed further.

Five fields of view (FOV, 0.1435 mm^2) with a 20,000 × magnification were chosen randomly in *Dpap* and *Dret*, and positively stained cells were counted in images of these by means of the manual tag function of the Image Pro programme (Media Cybernetics, Inc., Rockville, MD, USA). Epithelia were evaluated descriptively.

Statistical analysis

Statistical analysis was performed with SAS Analytics Pro (SAS Institute Inc., Cary, NC, USA) version 9.3 or higher. P-values < 0.05 were considered significant.

Cytokine data were log transformed due to log-normal distribution of the values for statistical comparisons. Stimulation ratios (times release) were calculated for each cytokine as cytokine $_{LPS}$/cytokine $_{medium}$ and cytokine $_{PMA/ionomycin}$/cytokine $_{medium}$.

Determination of baselines as internal controls for systemic parameters

Analysis of variance (ANOVA) was employed with time-of-day as a fixed factor and horses as random factors considering the interaction of time-of-day and horses for the analysis of the influence of sampling times on all systemic parameters measured and calculated before treatment.

For parameters influenced by sampling time, baselines were calculated separately for each sampling time (09:00, 15:00, 21:00, 03:00) as means of all values measured at the respective time before treatment. For parameters independent of sampling time (cytokines in PBMC supernatants), baselines were calculated as means over all measurements before treatment.

All measurements were evaluated in relation to individual baselines. This decision was confirmed by an

Table 4 Protocols in immunohistochemistry

Target	Antibody	Clone, immuno-globulin subclass	Source	Catalogue no.	Pretreatment for antigen retrieval	Dilution final concentration	Secondary antibody, dilution	Signal amplification	Tissue for positive control	Isotype control
Cal-protectin	Macrophage/ MAC 387	MAC 387, mouse IgG1	DCS I mmunoline, Hamburg, Germany	MI657C01	Proteinase K 5 μg/ml, in PBS, 30 min	1:400 0.1 μg/ml	IHC Kit MouseLink, HRP Label (DCS Immunoline) enhancer	IHC Kit MouseLink, HRP Label (DCS Immunoline) polymer	Tonsil	Mouse IgG1 (Dako, Hamburg, Germany)
IL-12	Mouse anti-bovine IL-12	CC301, mouse IgG2a	AbD Serotec, Puchheim, Germany	MCA1782	None	1:100 10 μg/ml	Anti-mouse-biotin (vector laboratories, Burlingame, Canada) 1:200	Vectastain Elite ABC Kit (vector laboratories)	Colon	Mouse IgG2a (AbD Serotec)
IL-18	Mouse anti-pig IL-18	5-C-5, mouse IgG1	AbD Serotec	MCA2094	None	1:1000 1 μg/ml	Anti-mouse-biotin (vector laboratories) 1:200	Vectastain Elite ABC Kit (vector laboratories)	Colon	Mouse IgG1 (Dako)

analysis of the influence of baseline values on measurements after treatment in an ANOVA with respect to interactions of treatment and baseline, which showed significant influences of the baseline measurements.

Influence of treatment on systemic parameters

The influence of the treatments on systemic parameters in relation to calculated baseline measurements was analysed by univariate (uv) and multivariate (mv) ANOVA over all measurements post-treatment. If influences were significant in both models, they were considered relevant.

Questionable parameters of treatment effect, judged by graphic evaluation and ANOVA results, were analysed in detail for measurements at t12 and t24, SAA as a long-term indicator, for all sampling times. The influences of single treatments were analysed by paired t-tests of time-of-day matched baseline values compared to values at t12 and t24. Comparison of treatment effects of A–D at t12 and t24 was performed by estimated pairwise group differences with corresponding p-values and 95 % confidence intervals derived by analysis of covariance (ANCOVA) methods with baseline as covariate (*t*-test, baseline adjusted), not adjusted for multiplicity.

Influence of treatment on local parameters

The Wilcoxon signed-rank test was employed for clinical and histological scores to compare treatment and control sample for each treatment and parameter.

The Kruskal-Wallis test was used to detect overall differences between treatments employing differences between *treat* and *ctrl* site for individual horses and Wilcoxon signed-rank test was employed to analyse differences from 0 or comparisons of single treatments.

Data were log transformed for immunohistochemistry parameters, except for IL-12/IL-18 ratios, and ANOVA was performed with a Tukey post hoc test to determine differences between treatments and controls and between different treatments.

Determination of responders

Parameters statistically significantly affected by treatments (differences to baseline, t-tests) were used to determine responders herein. Thresholds and response periods discriminating responders from non-responders were defined by graphic evaluation of courses of the measurements in each parameter. Horses were regarded as responders if their values exceeded the thresholds in at least three parameters. Responders and parameters with responses exceeding thresholds were counted for each group.

Influence of treatment on messenger ribonucleic acid expression

The difference of copy numbers of mRNA in *treat* (in blood t12) and *ctrl* samples (in blood t0) was calculated for the analysis of mRNA expression in blood and skin samples. These differences were analysed by Wilcoxon signed-rank test.

Influences of the horse factors: age, sex, type and colour

Horses of groups which had shown no difference by treatment on respective parameters were analysed together for these parameters. The influences of age were analysed by uv ANOVA. Sex, type and colour influences were analysed by unpaired t-tests.

Results and discussion

Changes of systemic parameters measured were induced by DNA containing treatments (B, C, D) and occurred within 24 h after injection for all parameters measured, except for SAA, an acute phase protein, which was used as a long-term indicator demonstrating effects by 72 h after injection.

In summary, horses showed elevated rectal temperatures (RT) and increased WBC, with the increase mainly attributable to elevated granulocyte levels, after treatment with DNA complexed with SAINT-18 (B, C, D). These effects were interpreted as signs of a mild systemic inflammatory reaction [44, 45].

Clinical findings

Treatment with SAINT-18 and MIDGE-Th1 vectors was well tolerated in all horses. Clinical parameters were within normal ranges after treatments, except for elevated RT exceeding 38 °C in seven horses. This matches the findings described for this treatment in horses bearing melanoma [18]. Overall, short-term safety of the treatment can be assumed.

In comparison to individual time-of-day matched baselines, the RTs of horses in groups B–D were elevated between 12 and 18 h after treatments. This difference reached statistical significance in group B (*t*-test, $p = 0.0467$). However, these elevations of RTs were not significantly different between different treatments (ANCOVA; Fig. 2a).

Rectal temperature increases or development of fever (RT > 38.5 °C) in the healthy horses included were far less frequently observed and tended to last for a shorter time compared to the previous study by Mählmann et al. [18] of horses affected by melanoma. However, since injection of MIDGE-Th1 complexed with SAINT-18 coding for luciferase in five healthy horses had also led to fever in that study, this difference cannot be easily explained by the mere presence or absence of melanoma. Further differences between the studies were the different site of the i.d. injection (peri-tumorally versus neck) and use of local anaesthetics at these sites in the present study. Based on the present data, the authors cannot exclude that the use of subcutaneous lidocaine especially may have inhibited the initial local inflammation at the i.d. injection site and the

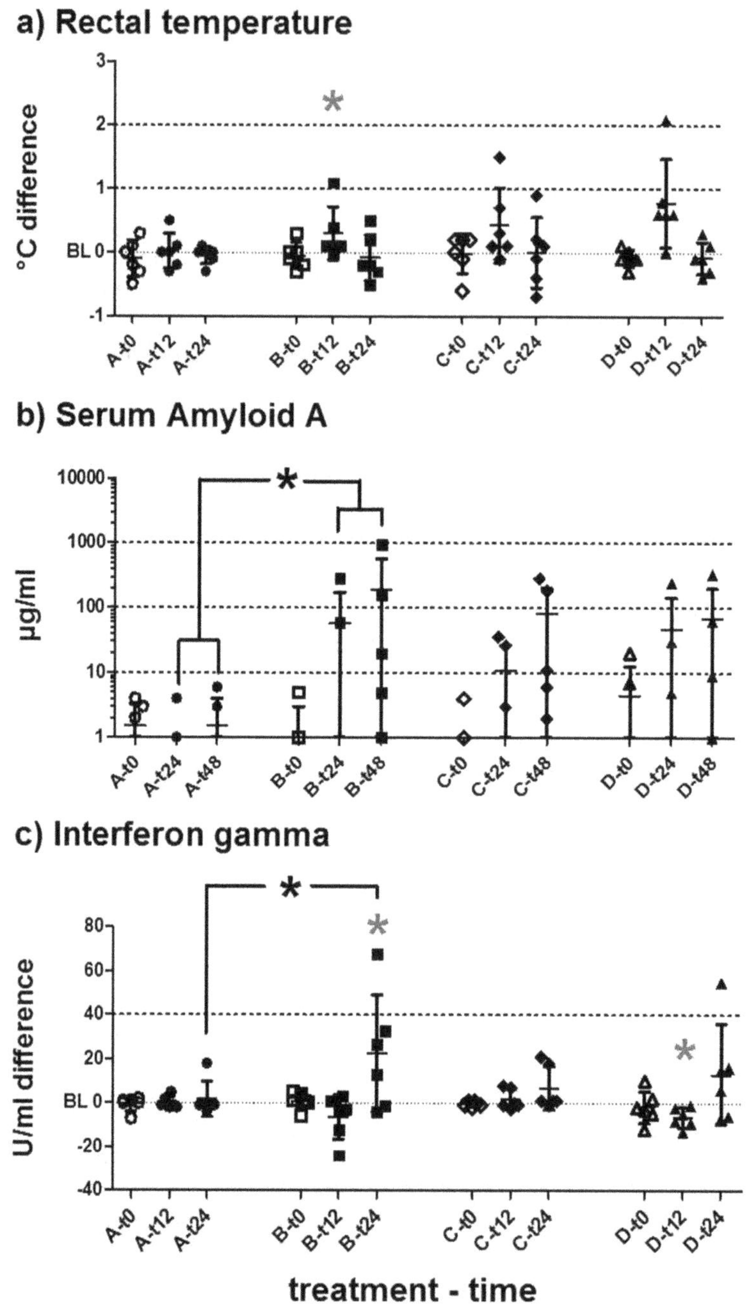

Fig. 2 Responses to treatments. **a** Rectal temperature differences to individual time-of-day matched baselines (BL), (**b**) Serum Amyloid A (SAA, absolute concentrations) and (**c**) Interferon gamma (IFNγ) differences to individual baselines in PBMC supernatants (medium only) are plotted in histograms for t0 and two measurements post-treatment. Datasets are marked as (group)-(hours post-treatment) at the X-axis. Horizontal bars represent mean and SD. Grey asterisks (*) represent significant differences from baseline in the respective dataset. Asterisks (*) with brackets (┌ ┌) represent significantly different comparisons. Group B showed values significantly different from baseline in rectal temperatures at t12 and in IFNγ at t24. Horses of this group, furthermore, differed significantly from group A in SAA measurements and IFNγ post-treatment

following increase of RT. Other parameters of potential influence, such as distributions of ages, sexes, breeds and the seasons of treatments, were not statistically significantly different between the previous and the present study. Hence, the reason for this variance between studies remains to be elucidated.

Blood counts and haemograms

All haematologic values measured remained within physiological ranges during all observations, with a tendency towards signs of an acute systemic inflammatory response [45], as follows: WBC increased in comparison to individual time-of-day matched baselines in horses of groups B, C and D between 12 and 36 h after treatment. Treatment effects in group B differed statistically significantly from all other treatments (uv and mv ANOVA, $p < 0.05$). For single comparisons, treatment effects on WBC induced by B and D at t24 were significantly higher than in A (ANCOVA, $p = 0.0494$; 0.0227; Fig. 3a).

Neutrophil numbers increased after all treatments, similar to the WBC effects. The overall effect of treatment on neutrophil numbers was significant (uv and mv ANOVA, $p < 0.05$). However, comparisons of neutrophil numbers to individual baselines showed statistically significant differences 24 h after treatment in group B (t-test, $p = 0.0406$)

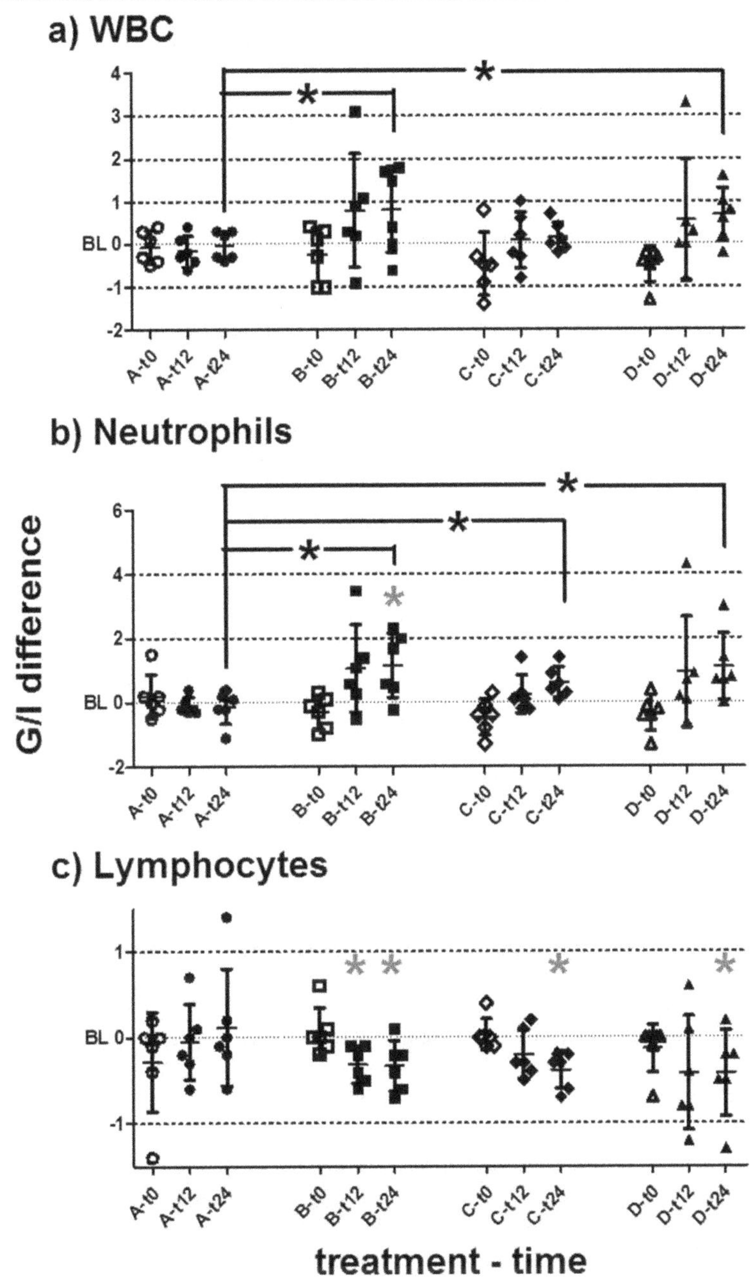

Fig. 3 Leucocyte counts. Leucocyte quantities in peripheral blood measured by automated haematology systems are plotted as differences to individual time-of-day matched baselines (BL) for t0, t12 and t24. Datasets are marked as (group)-(hours post-treatment) at the X-axes. Horizontal bars represent mean and SD. Grey asterisks (*) represent significant differences from baseline in the respective dataset. Asterisks (*) with brackets (┌ ┌) represent significantly different comparisons. **a** Increases of WBC induced by B and D at t24 were significantly higher than in A. **b** The increase in neutrophils was significantly different from baseline in B at t24. Group A showed significantly less treatment effects than B, C and D at t24. **c** In comparison to individual baselines, lymphocyte numbers decreased significantly after treatment B at t12 and t24, and at t24 in C and D

only. Group A showed statistically significantly fewer treatment effects than B, C or D (ANCOVA, $p = 0.0167$, 0.0497 and 0.0184, respectively; Fig. 3b).

Lymphocyte numbers decreased after treatments B, C and D. In comparison to individual baselines, lymphocyte numbers decreased significantly after treatment B at t12 and t24 (*t*-test, $p = 0.0399$ and 0.0111, respectively), and after treatments C and D (*t*-test, $p = 0.0005$ and 0.0276, respectively) only at t24 (Fig. 3c).

The decrease of lymphocyte numbers after the treatments can be explained in the context of an acute systemic inflammatory state of the horses treated with DNA, which may occasionally include lymphopenia, as seen after endotoxin challenge [46]. Decrease in lymphocytes and increase in neutrophils has been demonstrated in mice after systemic administration of complexed plasmid DNA paralleling the present findings in horses [47]. Lymphocyte decrease may be due to extravasation following endothelial activation, as indicated by endothelial swelling and increased perivascular infiltration of lymphocytes in histologic sections of skin samples at locally treated sites in the present study.

Serum Amyloid A

The horses included usually showed physiological levels of SAA below the lower limit of detection of 5 μg/ml before treatment. Levels of SAA after treatment were highly variable between individual horses of the same treatment group. Despite not reaching statistical significance, SAA in some horses in groups B–D clearly increased 24 to 72 h after treatment. Group B showed statistically significantly higher values after treatment compared to group A (ANOVA uv $p = 0.0176$; mv $p = 0.0197$; Fig. 2b).

All horses had SAA levels below 7 μg/ml at t264, except for one horse (horse # H), which had shown no increase by t72, but had a history of infectious diseases in the herd of its home stable to which it returned at t96.

The increase of SAA indicates an acute phase response, for which it is a sensitive marker in the horse [48]. This again suggests a systemic inflammatory reaction to the DNA treatment in individual horses. Most horses in which SAA increased displayed the rise at t24, but maximums were usually reached at t48 or t72. Serum Amyloid A is known to rise 6 to 12 h after surgery or experimental inflammation and to peak after 48 or even 72 h [34, 49, 50]. This matches the present findings, but may also be due to prolonged response or secondary mechanisms in response to treatments with MIDGE-Th1 vectors, which are detectable long-term after application [51]. Furthermore, biopsy sampling at t24 may have contributed to the acute phase response of the horses. The reaction affecting SAA, however, seems to resolve in a short time, as measurements at t264 no longer displayed increased values.

Cytokine messenger ribonucleic acid in blood samples

Cytokine expression in peripheral blood samples, determined by qPCR, was not significantly altered between controls (t0) and treatment (t12) in any treatment group or between different treatments. Interferon γ transcripts could not be detected at all in peripheral blood (Additional file 1: Table S1). Insufficient sensitivity of the qPCR assay for *IFNγ* may be assumed, as its absence is contrary to the detection of IFNγ protein. Analysis of mRNA in blood at t12 had been chosen as the horses in the previous study [18] had developed fever 12 to 18 h post-treatment and, thus, systemic effects on mRNA around these time points were expected to be noticed as well. The examination of more time points would be warranted in future studies to track the dynamics of cytokine expressions and to identify later changes.

Equine cytokines in cell culture supernatants

Cytokines were usually detectable by enzyme-linked immunosorbent assay (ELISA) or bead-based assay in supernatants of *ex vivo*-cultured PBMC (with and without stimuli) and displayed great interindividual variances. Interferon-α was hardly detectable, even after stimulation, and was, thus, excluded from further analysis (Additional file 2: Table S2).

There were no treatment effects detected in individual concentrations and alterations of IL-4 and IL-17 in supernatants of cells cultured without stimuli compared to individual baselines.

Stimulation ratios (e.g. $IFN\gamma_{\text{PMA-ionomycin}}/IFN\gamma_{\text{medium}}$) showed high interindividual variances in all cytokines, but no treatment effects were observed.

Tumour necrosis factor alpha (TNFα, in medium only) increased in single horses of all treatment groups compared to individual baselines. *Ex vivo* LPS stimulation of TNFα secretion was mild (mean stimulation ratio = 3.717 times secretion). Changes post-treatment were usually similar in medium and LPS settings. The increase of TNFα after treatments was statistically significant in groups B, C and D. Treatment effects in groups C and D were higher than in A (details given in Fig. 4).

Within 24 h after treatment, levels of IFNγ increased (without *ex vivo* stimuli) only in group B to a mean value statistically significant from group A. Four out of six horses in group B displayed an increase of IFNγ (Fig. 1c). Lipopolysaccharide stimulation of PBMC *ex vivo* resulted in only mild induction of IFNγ (mean stimulation ratio = 2.041 times secretion). Changes after treatments were similar to those in medium settings, but did not reach statistical significance.

Interleukin-10 in medium settings decreased at t6 after treatment B and at t12 after all other treatments. In general, LPS mildly induced IL-10 secretion *ex vivo* (mean stimulation ratio = 2.821 times secretion). The stimulated

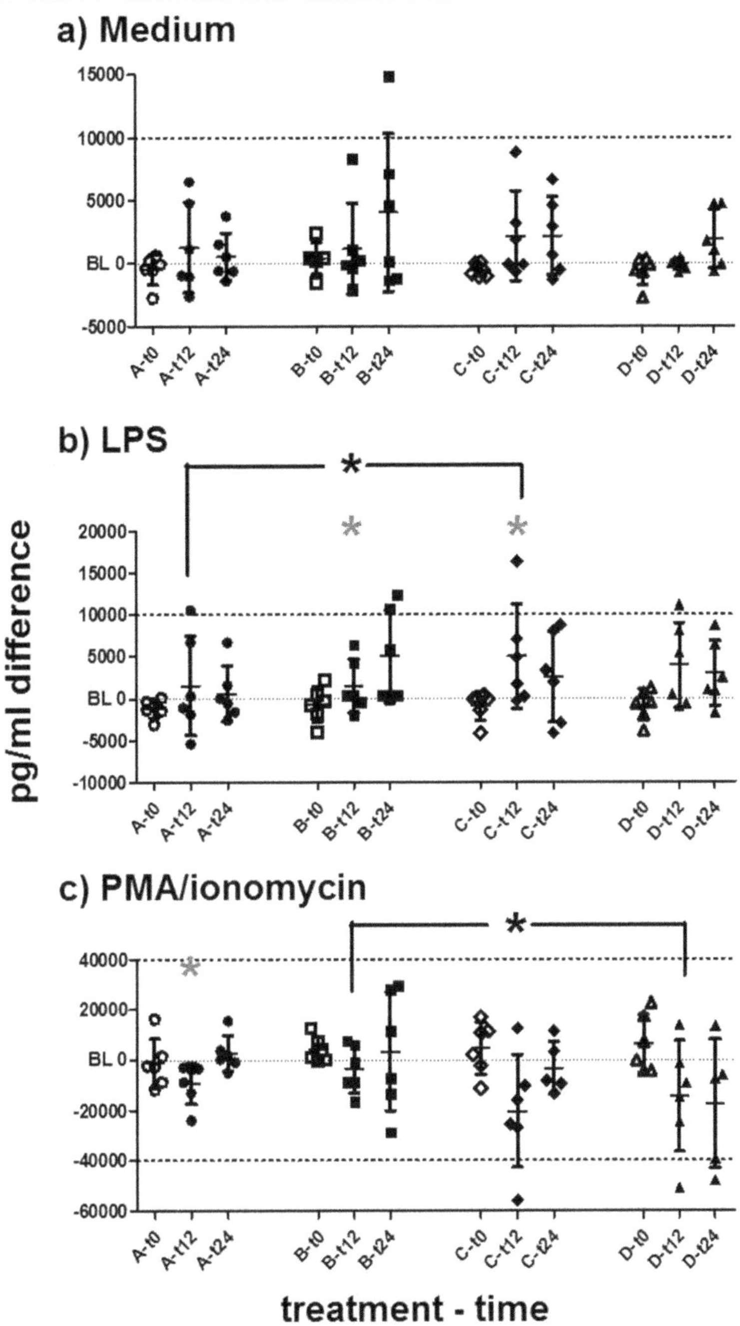

Fig. 4 Tumour necrosis factor alpha. Tumour necrosis factor alpha differences to individual baselines in PBMC supernatants measured by ELISA are plotted for releases (**a**) in medium only, (**b**) after LPS stimulation and (**c**) after PMA/ionomycin stimulation for t0, t12 and t24. Datasets are marked as (group)-(hours post-treatment) at the X-axes. Horizontal bars represent mean and SD. Grey asterisks (*) represent significant differences from baseline in the respective dataset. Asterisks (*) with brackets (┌ ┌) represent significantly different comparisons. The increase of TNFα could be statistically noticed in B (t12, medium and LPS), in C (t12, LPS) and in D (t24, medium and LPS). Treatment effects after LPS stimulation at t12 in C or D were higher than in A. Treatments containing DNA (B – D) induced higher TNFα secretion than transfection reagent alone (A)

IL-10 secretion in PMA and ionomycin settings decreased at t12 in groups B, C and D (Fig. 5).

Detection of cytokine effects proved challenging, as the variance of *ex vivo* cytokine release was high even before treatments. This variance in immune parameters is not unexpected in outbred species such as the horse [52, 53]. However, in comparison to individual baselines, increases of TNFα and IFNγ proteins were systemically induced by treatment with MIDGE-Th1/SAINT-18 (B, C and D), while IL-10 synthesis tended to decrease. These

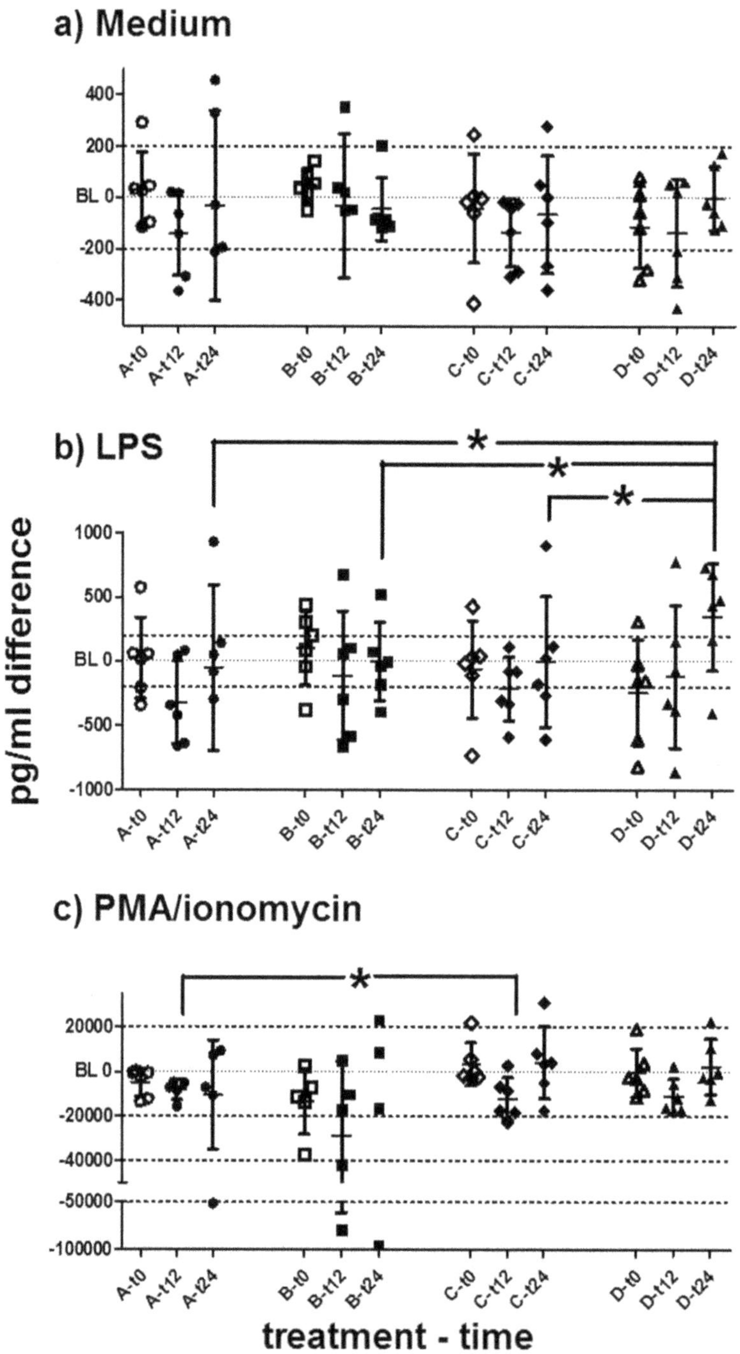

Fig. 5 Interleukin 10. Interleukin 10 differences to individual baselines in PBMC supernatants measured by a bead-based assay are plotted for releases (**a**) in medium only, (**b**) after LPS stimulation and (**c**) after PMA/ionomycin stimulation. Data presented at t0, t12 and t24. Datasets are marked as (group)-(hours post-treatment) at the X-axes. Horizontal bars represent mean and SD. Asterisks (*) with brackets (┌ ┌) represent significantly different comparisons. Interleukin 10 decreased after all treatments. Treatment effects after LPS stimulation (b) in group D at t24 (increase) differed significantly from those in A, B and C. After PMA and ionomycin stimulation, treatment effects in C (decrease) differed significantly from those in **a** (near baseline) at t12. The greatest interindividual variances were seen in group **b**

changes after each treatment containing DNA indicate a bias towards a pro-inflammatory immune state [54–58]. It was intended to confirm this at the mRNA level of whole blood leukocytes. However, the qPCR used here was possibly not sensitive enough to detect low numbers of mRNA copies, which may, nevertheless, have been repeatedly translated to detectable amounts of cytokine proteins.

Systemic effects of DNA treatment

According to the evaluations of systemic parameters in the present study (RT, haemograms, SAA, cytokines in PBMC supernatants), simultaneous i.m. and i.d. treatment with DNA complexed with cationic lipid provokes a systemic immune reaction in horses in accordance with previous reports on inflammation induced by the combination of DNA and cationic transfection reagent in mice [59, 60]. The inflammatory response herein was shown to be independent of transgene expression or CG motif content of the DNA injected, as differences between groups B and D were usually not statistically significant. It could, therefore, be hypothesised that this stimulation of the immune system may be responsible for parts of the antimetastatic effects demonstrated by Mählmann et al. [18] due to subtle modifications of the immune system induced by this antigen-unspecific modulation. However, plasmids containing nonsense DNA alone were not effective in melanoma therapy in previous studies in horses [7, 8], indicating that not just any DNA can be assumed to be effective and complexation with a cationic lipid might be required.

Although most of the recent literature on DNA effects focuses on the immunological effects of CG motifs [26, 61–63], *in vivo* application of complexed DNA herein induced systemic and local effects independent of the CG motif content. It should be mentioned that the CG motif contents of the vectors have been estimated on the basis of counting CG without analysis of the flanking sequences. A detailed analysis was not possible as information on the exact sequences of stimulatory motifs or their allocation to classes are only known for a few oligodeoxynucleotides in the horse [53, 62, 64] and have yet not been completely recognised. In comparison to plasmids, which often carry CG motifs in the backbone, MIDGE vectors only contain CG motifs in their expression cassettes [20, 65]. According to the rather low CG motif content in the MIDGE-Th1 vectors utilised and the absence of statistically significant differences of treatment effects between DNA containing CG and depleted of CG, the authors conclude that signalling via TLR-9 receptors is probably not the primary mechanism of immunostimulatory action of *in vivo* applied complexed MIDGE-Th1 vectors in horses.

Non-nuclear DNA, independent of CG motif and TLR signalling, stimulates innate immune responses, such as pro-inflammatory cytokine production via different pathways, as described more recently [30–33]. The signalling cascades employed are induced by intracellular double-stranded DNA and usually involve cGAS (cyclic GMP-AMP synthase) and STING (stimulator of IFN genes), AIM2 (absent in melanoma 2) and inflammasome activation or ribonucleic acid (RNA) polymerase III and RIG-I (retinoic acid-inducible gene), leading to pro-inflammatory and antiviral immune responses [29, 31, 32]. To the best of the authors' knowledge, there are no reports of these mechanisms in horses. However, due to their high phylogenetical conservation, they are very likely to exist in horses as well. Thus, although the causative molecular mechanism of the systemic and local immunostimulatory effect independent of the CG motif content of the DNA herein cannot be identified based on the present data, the stimulation of the pathways of the innate immune system by complexed DNA reaching cytosolic compartments described seems likely.

Responder classification in systemic effects of treatments

The parameters included for responder classification were RT, SAA, neutrophil and lymphocyte counts, TNFα release in response to LPS stimulation and IFNγ release from unstimulated cells (medium only). White blood cell counts, although influenced by treatments, were not included, as this parameter is dependent on neutrophil and lymphocyte counts which were already being considered. Response periods up to t24 were usually chosen, except for SAA (until t72; Table 5). A classification into responders and non-responders was not performed for local parameters evaluated in skin samples because it was not possible to define threshold values by visual inspection due to the lack of graphical dichotomy of the values measured.

Responders were found in all groups. There were no noteworthy changes of SAA, neutrophil counts or IFNγ in group A. In groups B–D, there were more responses than in A, but no clear differences between types of DNA. Interestingly, not a single grey horse was classified as a responder after treatment with complexed DNA (B, C or D; Table 5).

While some horses displayed systemic effects following DNA application (usually in RT, haematological parameters, acute phase proteins and cytokine secretion), others showed no effects at all. Similar to findings in melanoma patients, responders and non-responders to DNA treatment seem to exist in healthy horses. In accordance with single parameters of systemic evaluations, significant differences between expressing (B) and non-expressing (C) or CG motif-free non-expressing (D) DNA could not be found by the responder classification.

Since no grey horse was classified as a responder, the authors cannot conclude reasonably on the predictive value of the parameters, thresholds and response periods chosen for the responder classification or on anti-tumour effects in grey horses bearing melanomas.

Evaluation of local treatment effects in clinical and histological examinations

The skin was unaffected and clinical scores were usually classified as grade 0 before treatment. Treatment (A–D injected i.d. locally treated skin samples: *treat*) and control

Table 5 Responders in systemic parameters

Treatment group / horses			A)	# A	# E	# I	# N	# R	# W	B)	# B	# F	# K	# S	# O	# X	C)	# C	# G	# L	# P	# U	# Y	D)	# D	# H	# M	# Q	# V	# Z
Age (years) (groups: mean)			11.1	21	4	11	8	13	9	10.6	5	17	19	7	5	10	10.3	2	8	11	8	20	11	10.9	8	8	10	14	17	8
Sex				fe	fe	mc	mc	mc	mi		fe	mc	mc	fe	mc	mi		mc	mc	mc	mc	mc	mi		fe	fe	mc	mc	mc	mc
Type				ThB	WBl	WBl	WBl	WBl	ThB		ThB	WBl	WBl	WBl	WBl	WBl		ThB	WBl	WBl	WBl	WBl	ThB		ThB	WBl	WBl	WBl	WBl	WBl
Colour				g	g	o	o	o	o		g	o	o	o	o	g		g	o	g	o	o	o		o	g	o	o	g	o
Para-meter	Thre-shold	Period (h)																												
SAA (µg/ml)	10	72	0	–	–	–	–	–	–	3	–	–	+	+	+	–	3	–	–	+	–	+	+	2	+	–	–	–	–	+
RT (°C)[a]	0.5	24	3	+	+	–	–	+	–	3	–	–	+	+	+	–	3	+	–	–	–	+	+	5	+	+	+	+	–	+
Neu (G/l)[a]	1	24	0	–	–	–	–	–	–	3	+	–	–	+	+	–	2	–	–	–	–	+	+	2	+	–	–	–	–	+
Lymph (G/l)[a]	-0.4	24	1	+	–	–	–	–	–	4	–	–	+	+	+	+	2	–	–	–	–	+	+	5	+	+	+	+	–	+
TNFα (pg/ml)[b, LPS]	5000	24	2	+	–	+	–	–	–	3	–	–	+	+	+	–	3	–	–	+	–	+	+	4	+	–	+	+	–	+
IFNγ (U/ml)[b, med]	20	24	0	–	–	–	–	–	–	3	+	–	+	–	–	+	1	–	–	–	–	–	+	2	+	–	–	–	–	+
Responder			1	+	–	–	–	–	–	3	–	–	+	+	+	–	2	–	–	–	–	+	+	4	+	–	+	+	–	+
Responses/group parameters with response			6	3	1	1	0	1	0	19	2	0	5	5	5	2	17	1	0	2	0	5	6	20	6	1	3	3	0	6

Numbers of horses that display values of ≥ threshold given in each cell of group columns; response present (+, threshold reached) or absent (–, threshold not reached) given in each cell of individual horses (IDs)
fe female, mare, *mc* male castrated, gelding, *mi* male intact, stallion, *Wbl* Warmblood, *ThB* thoroughbred, *g* grey, *o* other (non-grey), *WBC* white blood cell counts, *Neu* neutrophil counts, *Lymph* lymphocyte counts, *med* medium settings, *LPS* LPS settings, *responder* (response + in min. 3 parameters), *response in groups* at least two horses +
[a]differences to individual time-of-day matched baselines
[b]differences to individual baselines over all times of day

(PBS injected i.d. control skin samples: *ctrl*) sites showed mild oedema (grade 1–2) after treatments. Other alterations were very rare (painfulness: $n = 2$ in *treat* and *ctrl*; redness $n = 2$ in *treat* and *ctrl*; depigmentation = 2 in *ctrl* and *treat*). Clinical scores were not statistically different between control and treatment sites or between different treatments.

The evaluation of skin biopsies stained with H&E revealed ulceration of the epithelia (Additional file 3a–c) and perivascular mixed-cell dermatitis with some additional infiltrating leukocytes in a diffuse pattern, especially in the *Dret*. Inflammatory cells were predominantly of lymphoid origin. Macrophages appeared perivascularly in subepithelial positions proximate to most ulcers and infrequently in diffuse patterns. Neutrophilic granulocytes were randomly seen intravascularly and sometimes found perivascularly and abundantly in a diffuse pattern in higher grade inflammation in *Dret* (Additional files 3a, c and 4a–c).

Scores of inflammation did not differ significantly between treatments and controls or between different treatments in any layer.

Shaving of the skin was performed to optimise the cutting of histological slices of biopsy samples after fixation, as hairs often cause disruption of slices and artefacts in microscopic views. An early time point (t-72) was chosen for shaving to facilitate gross recovery before treatment. Shaving and scrubbing alone led to ulcerative inflammation of the epithelium visible in histologic slides, as shown in six additional healthy horses which underwent shaving and scrubbing without further treatment (Additional file 5). This preparation of the skin may have hidden treatment effects on epithelia, but not on deeper skin layers where the main alterations in response to treatments A–D were expected. However, shaving immediately prior to taking biopsies might have been better. Nevertheless, since the effect of DNA was noted mainly in the dermis, this aspect of the study design may not be of relevance for interpretation of the data.

Local anaesthesia was performed at the i.d. injection sites due to ethical reasons, to facilitate secure intradermal application without complication by defensive actions of the horses and to avoid the need for sedation, as this could have influenced parameters characterizing the systemic immune response. The volume applied is likely to have contributed to the oedema observed. It is, furthermore, possible that the application of local anaesthetics at the i.d. injection sites influenced the immune response to the treatments applied. Local anaesthetics are known to have anti-inflammatory properties [66] and could, thus, have inhibited the inflammatory response. The lidocaine used was applied subcutaneously. Its anaesthetic action is thought to last a maximum of three hours after subcutaneous infiltration [67], allowing the assumption that the majority of the substance should then be cleared from the injection site. MIDGE-Th1 DNA applied intradermally has been described to stay in the dermis long-term, thus, the authors assume that the potential anti-inflammatory effect of lidocaine did not mask the effects of the treatments completely. It still cannot be excluded that local anaesthesia partially influenced the immune response to DNA/SAINT-18.

Immunohistochemistry results in the skin

Calprotectin stained by MAC387

The *strata spinosum, granulosum* and *lucidum*, and hairs' epithelial sheaths of the stratified squamous epithelium in all specimens were generally immunopositive for calprotectin. Ulcers in the epithelium usually did not stain, except for single infiltrated cells or debris (Additional file 6a, c). Calprotectin positive cells in the dermis were frequent in perivascular locations, but also occurred infrequently in other localisations in a diffuse pattern (Additional files 6b–d and 7a, c). Calprotectin, detected by MAC 387, is a marker for myeloid cells [68] and for epithelial stress [69]. The immunohistochemical staining pattern observed in the present skin samples corresponded well with neutrophilic granulocytes and macrophages identified by H&E staining.

Overall, *treat* specimens contained more calprotectin-positive cells than *ctrls* in both layers. For single comparisons, this was significant in the *Dret* in A (Aa) and B (Bb). The *ctrl* samples of B, C and D contained more calprotectin-positive cells than *ctrl* samples of A without reaching significance. In the *Dret*, the *treat* samples of B contained statistically significantly more calprotectin-positive cells than the *treat* samples of A (details given in Fig. 6a, b).

Myeloid cell infiltration reveals that inflammation was induced in both the *treat* and *ctrl* samples. Thus, an acute inflammatory response was induced locally by i.d. injections in general, and by the transfection reagent, SAINT-18, which induced an influx of leukocytes and expression of the cytokines IL-12 and IL-18 (see below). The addition of DNA tended to enhance the inflammatory response, without reaching statistical significance by means of inflammation scores and IHC evaluation. This may be due to the overlapping of the systemic effects causing increased tissue reactivity and effects of the local stimulus by, for example, the pressure of the injection demonstrated in *ctrl* sites.

The treatment schedule closely resembled that of the previous study by Mählmann et al. [18]. The i.m. and i.d. administered portions of the treatments were carried out simultaneously. Therefore, it is not possible to distinguish their contribution to the systemic effects. However, the impact of the route of administration on systemic effects is an interesting aspect that warrants investigation in future studies, considering the routes used and, for

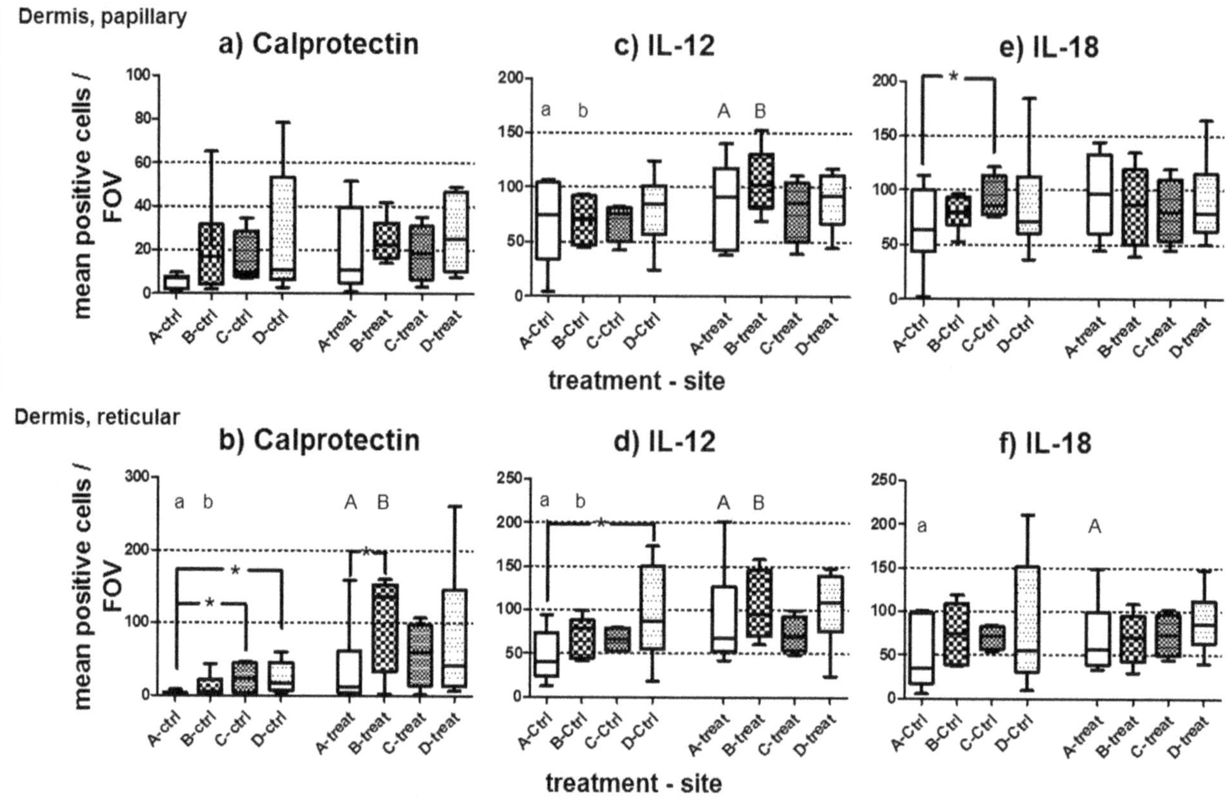

Fig. 6 Immunohistochemistry results. Mean positive cells per FOV are plotted for the papillary dermis (*Dpap*, top) and the reticular dermis (*Dret*, bottom) for each treatment (A – D) and site (*Ctrl*: control; *treat*: local treatment) for calprotectin (**a**, **b**), Interleukin (IL)12 (**c**, **d**) and IL-18 (**e**, **f**) determined by immunohistochemistry. Median, quartiles, minimum and maximum plotted for each dataset. Asterisks (*) with brackets (┌ ┌) and same letters (Aa, Bb) represent significantly different comparisons. *Treat* samples overall contained significantly more calprotectin-positive cells and IL-12 positive cells than *ctrls* in the *Dpap* (a), *and Dret* (b). For single comparisons, this was significant in *Dret* (b) in treatment groups A (Aa) and B (Bb). Control samples of A had significantly fewer calprotectin-, IL-18- and IL-12-positive cells than those of other treatment groups. *Treat* samples of B contained significantly more calprotectin-positive cells in *Dret* than those of A (*)

example, transdermal application methods used for DNA vaccines [70, 71].

Local expression of IL-12 and IL-18 proteins in skin samples after treatment

The IL-12 and IL-18 proteins were stained by monoclonal antibodies in IHC for the investigation of transgene expression.

In general, IL-12 and IL-18 were present in the same tissues and cell types in skin samples of the sites treated and of healthy control animals: squamous epithelium, hairs, glands (sebaceous and apocrine), fibrocytes, endothelia (unstained in some bigger vessels), pericytes, muscle cells, nerves (in parts) and leukocytes (Additional files 8, 9, 10, 11, 12 and 13). However, intensity varied, and some cell types (e.g. inflammatory cells) were present more frequently in samples after treatment, resulting in a theoretically higher amount of locally available IL-12 and IL-18.

The *treat* samples contained more IL-12 positive cells than the *ctrls*. This was statistically significant for single comparisons in treatments A and B in both layers, *Dpap* and *Dret*. Furthermore, the *Dret ctrls* contained significantly fewer IL-12-positive cells in A than the *Dret ctrls* in D. The *treat* samples did not differ statistically significantly between different treatments in the absolute numbers of IL-12-positive cells in any layer (details given in Fig. 6c, d).

There was no statistically significant overall difference in the IL-18-positive cells in the *Dpap* between *treat* and *ctrl*. The *Dpap ctrls* contained statistically significantly fewer IL-18-positive cells in A than in C. The *treat* samples in *Dret* contained more IL-18-positive cells overall than the *ctrls*. This was statistically significant in A. The *treat* samples did not differ statistically significantly between different groups in the numbers of IL-18-positive cells (details given in Fig. 6e, f).

Cytokine and chemokine mRNA in skin biopsies

For further investigation of *in vivo* expression of recombinant *IL-12* and *IL-18*, IL-12 and IL-18 mRNA were measured in skin biopsies by SYBR green qPCR. Furthermore, in order to confirm these and their biologic activity, in addition to the interleukins, the downstream mediator typically induced by IL-12, IFNγ [7] was analysed, as well as a chemokine strongly induced by the latter, CXCL-10 [68] (Additional file 1: Table S1).

The detection of IL-12 expression by qPCR was hampered by the interference of MIDGE- Th1 DNA in the (*treat*) samples, as MIDGE-Th1 vectors present at the site of injection could not be digested completely prior to reverse transcription of mRNA into cDNA (complementary DNA), and PCR primers could not be designed to discriminate between equine recombinant *IL-12* transcripts expressed by MIDGE-Th1 vectors and endogenous *IL-12* transcripts. Consequently, measurement of *IL-12* by qPCR always resulted in positive results and discrimination from false-positive results was not possible.

Copy number differences between *treat* and *ctrl* samples of *IL-18* were lowest in group A, which varied statistically significantly from B to D (Fig. 7a).

Copy number differences of *CXCL-10* between *treat* and *ctrl* of individual horses were statistically significantly lower in group A compared to the other groups. Group B, furthermore, showed statistically significantly higher differences of *CXCL-10* mRNA copy numbers between *ctrl* and *treat* than the other groups treated with complexed DNA (C or D) (Fig. 7b).

Similar to the blood samples, *IFNγ* mRNA/cDNA was not detected at all. For IHC, unfortunately, no antibody was available to detect IFNγ protein in comparison. Again, insufficient sensitivity of the qPCR assay for *IFNγ* mRNA/cDNA detection cannot be excluded, as the result on *IFNγ* mRNA levels is contrary to the significant detection of *CXCL-10*.

Transgene expression

In vitro transgene expression after transfection of mammalian cells with MIDGE-Th1 eqIL12 and eqIL18 was proven on the mRNA level [18] and *in vivo* transfection of MIDGE-Th1 vectors was generally confirmed in other species, e.g. in rats, on the protein level as well [72].

Although expression of recombinant IL-12 and IL-18 in group B could not be verified directly by detection of *IL-12* and *IL-18* transcripts, the mRNA of *CXCL-10*, a downstream mediator of IL-12 and IFNγ [73, 74], was significantly elevated in skin samples treated with expressing MIDGE-Th1 (group B, *treat*). As it has been shown that effects on downstream mediators are amplified due to enhancing loops [74], *CXCL-10* mRNA could be detected even if recombinant IL-12 and IL-18, and IFNγ induced by these, are not detectably increased. As CXCL-10 has been shown to be produced after intratumoural injection of IL-12 plasmids in human melanoma [75], subsequent to IFNγ after IL-12 treatment in mice [74] and after transfection of B16 melanoma with IL-18, also in mice [76], it is likely that CXCL-10 is a relevant anti-tumour mediator in melanoma immunotherapy with IL-12/IL-18 DNA also in horses.

Treatment with DNA complexed with SAINT-18 did not lead to vast amounts of cytokines being released by PBMC or expressed by blood leukocytes. The *IL-12* and *IL-18* expression levels were not increased in blood cells

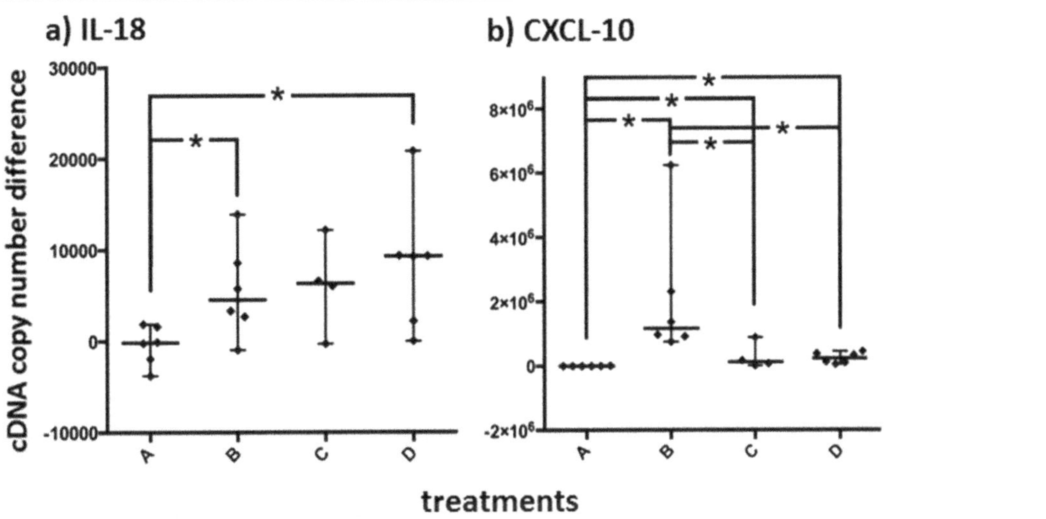

Fig. 7 Treatment effects on messenger ribonucleic acid expression in the skin. The *treat-ctrl* differences of copy numbers of IL-18 (**a**) and CXCL-10 (**b**) measured by qPCR in skin samples are shown in histograms. Horizontal bars represent medians and ranges. Asterisks (*) with brackets (┌ ┐) represent significantly different comparisons. The expressions of IL-18 increased by local treatment in comparison to *ctrl*s in groups B – D. The expression of CXCL-10 in skin biopsies of the *treat* site was significantly higher overall than in the *ctrl* samples in all treatment groups. The *treat-ctrl* difference (b) of copy numbers examined was significantly lower in A than in the other treatment groups. Group B, furthermore, displayed significantly higher *treat-ctrl* differences of CXCL-10 copy numbers than C or D

after treatments and IL-12 protein could not be detected by a bead-based assay (validated in horses previously [77]) in PBMC supernatants, even after stimulation as evaluated in samples of eight horses of groups A–D, including four responders (data not shown). It can be concluded that circulating leukocytes and tissues influencing these were not transfected to a great extent by expressing DNA vectors, as recombinant *IL-12* and *IL-18* were not statistically significantly elevated in post-treatment blood samples of B and only a moderate increase in the production of IFNγ protein was detected as an induced downstream cytokine of IL-12 and IL-18 [14–16].

However, local treatment with DNA expressing IL-12 and IL-18 (B) induced an increase in IL-12-positive cells in the dermis in comparison to PBS controls. This could be due to local transfection of cells or to induction of endogenous IL-12. This cannot be discriminated herein by means of IHC.

Influences of horse factors on treatment effects

The authors noted great interindividual variances in treatment effects on most parameters. The following possible influencing factors were evaluated to elucidate the origin of these variances: age, sex (mares vs. geldings; two stallions were excluded from analysis due to limited number), type (breed) and colour of coat.

As treatment differences were usually observed between treatment with (groups B, C and D) and without DNA (group A), horses of groups B, C and D were combined for the analysis of influences on treatment effects.

Mares showed higher increases in WBC (*t*-test, $p = 0.0068$) and neutrophils (*t*-test, $p = 0.0282$), and higher TNFα responses (medium settings; *t*-test, $p = 0.0172$) than geldings (Additional file 14). This is in accordance with the finding of higher plasma levels of TNFα in healthy mares [78] and the authors' finding of a rather pro-inflammatory tendency of mares compared to geldings when analysing baseline measurements prior to treatments [79].

Thoroughbred type horses showed higher TNFα responses (medium settings; *t*-test, $p = 0.0240$) than WBl type horses (Additional file 14). The breed has previously been shown to influence the cytokine response in TNFα to *in vivo* stimuli [80], but this has not yet been investigated for DNA treatment. The allocation of different breeds to the types of WBl and ThB in the present study may be arbitrary to some degree and does not necessarily represent

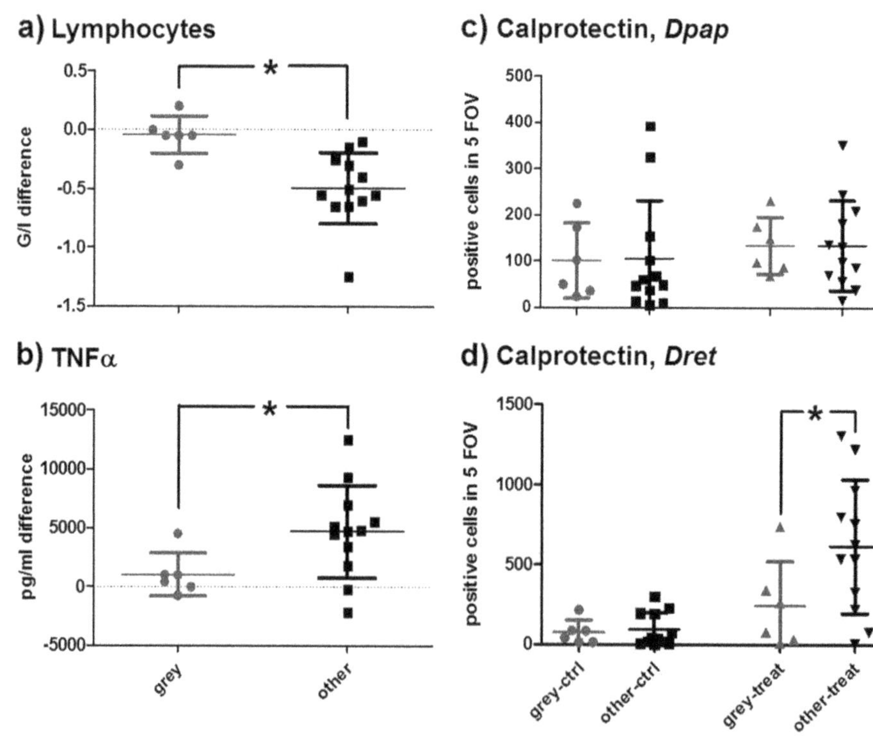

Fig. 8 Influence of colour. The results of horses treated with DNA (groups B – D) are summarized. Differences of (**a**) lymphocytes and (**b**) TNFα release after LPS stimulation to individual baselines calculated at t12 and t24 are plotted in histograms for grey horses (grey) and horses of other colours (other). Calprotectin-positive cells in five fields of view (FOV) are plotted (**c**) for the papillary dermis (*Dpap*), and (**d**) the reticular dermis (*Dret*) in histograms for PBS *ctrl* and *treat* sites. Horizontal bars represent mean and SD. Asterisks (*) with brackets (┐ ┐) represent significantly different comparisons. Lymphocyte decreases (a) to individual time-of-day matched baselines were significantly less in grey than in other horses. The TNFα increases to individual baselines in PBMC supernatants were significantly lower in grey than in other horses. Significantly fewer calprotectin-positive cells were found in the *Dret* (b) of *treat* sites of grey horses than in samples of non-grey (other) horses

biological dichotomy. Thus, this limitation should be considered for the judgement of its influence.

Sex and type are known to influence immunological parameters [80–84] and to find such effects herein was not unexpected. As the treatment groups of horses were balanced with respect to these horse parameters, bias of the interpretation of the results concerning treatment effects is not likely.

In addition, there was a relation between the coat colour of the horses and their responses to treatment with DNA. Grey horses showed statistically significantly fewer lymphocyte decreases than horses of other colours (*t*-test, $p = 0.0037$) and fewer increases of *ex vivo* secreted TNFα in response to stimulation with LPS (*t*-test, $p = 0.0470$; Fig. 8). Statistically significantly fewer myeloid (calprotectin-, MAC-387-positive) cells were found (*t*-test, $p = 0.0413$; Fig. 8) in the *Dret* of *treat* samples of grey horses than of non-grey horses, resulting in statistically significantly lower *treat-ctrl* differences (*t*-test, $p = 0.0379$).

Furthermore, none of the grey horses included was classified as a responder to DNA treatment with regard to systemic parameters. Therefore, the acute immune reaction of grey horses to DNA treatment seems to be milder than that of non-grey horses as defined by the parameters included in the present report. Some differences between grey and non-grey horses in immunological parameters reported previously, such as different associations of microsatellites and single nucleotide polymorphisms with immune responses to Equine Herpes Virus vaccination [85], match the findings of different immune reactivity reported herein. The milder response of grey horses to DNA complexed with transfection reagent may require stronger stimulation in DNA vaccination, as inflammation enhances DNA uptake and antigen processing [86].

It might even be speculated whether this different acute immunological response contributes to melanoma development in grey horses, as genetic bases of grey coat colour are proposed to have an influence on other organ systems, including cell cycle regulation and immune functions [87–89], which may affect tumour development and immune escape. This is speculative based on the present data of healthy horses, but certainly warrants further investigation.

Conclusions

Treatment with DNA complexed with the transfection reagent SAINT-18 is immunostimulatory in healthy horses, independent of transgene expression and CG motif content. Grey horses and horses of other colours differ in their systemic and local acute immune reaction to treatment with linear DNA vectors complexed with a cationic lipid. Grey horses seem to be non-responders with respect to non-specific systemic effects of DNA. It cannot be excluded that this characteristic of grey horses may be related to the development of melanoma. Further research elucidating this issue is warranted.

Additional files

Additional file 1: Table S1. Cytokine cDNA copy numbers (qPCR). Equine cytokine expression measured with absolute quantification by qPCR after transferring mRNA into cDNA. Medians of copy numbers given per µl; t0: before treatment; t12: 12 h after treatment; *ctrl*: local PBS control sample; *treat*: locally treated (A–D) sample; n.d. = not detectable (<100 cDNA copies/µl).2

Additional file 2: Table S2. *Ex vivo* secreted cytokines. Equine cytokines in PBMC supernatants after 12 h of cell culture: mean concentration (STD); BL: Baseline (mean t-24–t0); t12: 12 h post-treatment; t24: 24 h post-treatment; Detection limits: IFNα (12–30,000 pg/ml), TNFα (31.2–2000 pg/ml), IFNγ (10–5000 U/ml), IL-4 (40–80,000 pg/ml), IL-10 (15–35,000 pg/ml), and IL-17 (10–10,000 U/ml).

Additional file 3: Histology of epithelia and papillary dermis. Illustration of findings in representative skin samples (H&E staining). Evaluation was performed for single layers: epithelium (Ep), papillary dermis (*Dpap*), reticular dermis (*Dret*). a) Overview of Ep with two ulcers (arrows) and areas of subepithelial infiltration. Note beginning of ulceration in two additional localisations (dashed arrows). b) Detail of Ep with ulceration (magnification of frame in A). Note cell debris in ulcer (arrow) and subepithelial infiltration of leukocytes (arrowhead) in *Dpap*.c) Inflammation in *Dpap* with adnexa. Distinct infiltration of leukocytes in perivascular localisations (asterisks), while only a few leukocytes are present in a diffuse distribution pattern in other areas.

Additional file 4: Histology of the reticular dermis. Illustration of findings in representative skin samples (H&E staining) in *Dret*. a) Overview of *Dret* with haemorrhage (arrows). b) Detail of *Dret* with haemorrhage (magnification of A). Note haemorrhage (arrows) and massive perivascular infiltration of leukocytes (asterisks). c) Detail of inflammation in *Dret*. Distinct infiltration of leukocytes in perivascular (asterisks) and intravascular (arrowheads) localisation, while only a few leukocytes are present in a diffuse distribution pattern in other areas.

Additional file 5: Evaluation of shaving and scrubbing effects on skin irritation. Description of an additional experiment to evaluate the impact of shaving and scrubbing on skin alterations.

Additional file 6: Immunohistochemistry for calprotectin. Immunohistochemical localisation of calprotectin (red) in representative skin samples (counterstained with haematoxylin). a) Overview of Ep and Dermis with low grade inflammation. Calprotectin-positive cells are present in *Dpap* (arrows). In addition, *Ep* and hairs were immunopositive in parts. b) Overview of *Dret* with haemorrhage (arrows). Some leukocytes (asterisks) near and within haemorrhage stained positive for calprotectin (red). c) Epithelial Ulcer (arrow). Subepithelial leukocytes frequently stained calprotectin-positive (red). In addition, parts of the *Ep* (*Str. spinosum and Str. granulosum*) are positive for calprotectin. d) *Dpap* with adnexa. Infiltrating calprotectin-positive (red) leukocytes in perivascular localisation indicate a distinct inflammation. Hairs (H) and excretory ducts of apocrine glands (G) were negative.

Additional file 7: Detail of calprotectin immunohistochemistry (continued). Immunohistochemical localisation of calprotectin (red) in representative skin samples (counterstained with haematoxylin), a) *Dret* with perivascular inflammation around larger vessels. Detail of large artery (A) and vein (V), which are surrounded by multiple calprotectin-positive (red) leukocytes. b) *Dret* – Isotype control. Similar localisation as a) with large artery (A) and smaller veins (V), where a perivascular infiltration (asterisks) is visible, but red staining is absent (negative). c) Perineural leukocyte infiltration in *Dret*. Detail of nerve (N) and vessels; note the distinct perivascular and perineural infiltration with calprotectin-positive leukocytes.

Additional file 8: Immunohistochemistry for Interleukin 12. Immunostaining for IL-12 (red) illustrated in representative skin samples (counterstaining with haematoxylin). a) Overview of Ep and dermis in inflamed skin. *Ep*, hairs (H) and sebaceous glands (G) stained immunopositive for IL-12 (red). b) Detail of Ep and *Dpap*. The *strata granulosum, spinosum* and *basale* of the stratified squamous epithelium (Ep) showed a cytoplasmic red staining for IL-12. Sebaceous glands (G) and hairs (H) usually stained positive for IL-12. *Musculi arrectores pilorum* (Mm) were also positive for IL-12. In addition, infiltrating leukocytes were frequently positive for IL-12 (arrows). c) Epithelial ulcers. Ulcers (arrows) were unstained in otherwise IL-12-positive stained squamous epithelium. Parts of the fibrocytes (asterisks) in *Dpap* also stained positive for IL-12. d) Isotype control. No immunopositive staining is visible in a similar localisation as in c).

Additional file 9: Immunohistochemistry for Interleukin 12 in papillary dermis. Red immunoreactions for IL-12 are shown in representative skin samples with haematoxylin counterstaining. a) Detail of *Dpap* with adnexa. Epithelia of various kinds were usually positive for IL-12, e.g. cortex and epithelial root sheath of hairs (H), and glands and their excretory ducts (asterisks). Please note the patchy staining pattern of the excretory ducts. Endothelia stained positive (arrows) or negative (dashed arrows) for IL-12. Additionally, *Mm. arrectores pilorum* (Mm) stained positive for IL-12. Fibrocytes usually appeared negative for IL-12, but some perinuclear immunopositive staining of fusiform cells in the connective tissue could be noted (circles). b) Detail of *Dpap* illustrating appearance of apocrine glands. Apocrine glands were positive for IL-12 (asterisks), but showed a patchy staining. Epithelial components of hairs (H) were immunopositive, while fibrocytes in this detail were negative for IL-12.c) *Dpap* – detail of subepithelial inflammation. Infiltrating leukocytes can be found perivascularly and are dispersed diffusely in the connective tissue. They frequently show a red perinuclear and cytoplasmic immunostaining for IL-12 (arrows). *Mm. arrectores pilorum* (Mm) and endothelia (dashed arrows) stained positive for IL-12, while fibrocytes were usually negative for IL-12. Epithelium (Ep) and a gland (G) are indicated at the edges of the image (top right and bottom left, respectively).

Additional file 10: Immunohistochemistry for Interleukin 12 in reticular dermis. Immunostaining for IL-12 (red) in representative skin samples (counterstaining with haematoxylin). a) Large artery and nerve in *Dret*. Walls and endothelia (dashed arrows) of a large artery (A) and small blood vessels stained positive for IL-12, as did the nerve (N). In addition, infiltrated leukocytes (arrows) were positive for IL-12. Fibrocytes and extracellular matrix were usually negative. b) *Dret* – detail with perivascular inflammation. Leukocytic perivascular infiltration of high degree proximate to artery (A) and vein (V). In addition, vessel walls and endothelia (arrows) infiltrated cells (asterisks) are positive for IL-12. Fibrocytes and extracellular matrix are negative apart from a weak background staining. c) Isotype control *Dret* with artery (A). All tissue components are negative in detail of *Dret*.

Additional file 11: Immunohistochemistry for Interleukin 18. Illustration of red IL-18 immunoreaction in representative skin samples (counterstained with haematoxylin). a) Overview of Ep and dermis in mildly inflamed skin. *Ep* (except for ulcers, arrows), hairs (H) and glands (G) stained positive for IL-18. b) Isotype control – overview of Ep and dermis. No immunopositive staining is visible in a similar localisation as in a) in the papillary layer. c) Detail of Ep with ulcer (arrow) and *Dpap* with medium grade leukocyte infiltration. All epithelial tissues [*stratum granulosum, spinosum* and *basale* of the stratified squamous epithelium (Ep), cortex and epithelial root sheath of hairs (arrowheads), sebaceous glands (G)] showed a cytoplasmic immunoreaction for IL-18, while ulcers (arrow) were negative for IL-18. Infiltrating leukocytes (arrowheads) were frequently positive for IL-18. The IL-18 staining of fibrocytes and endothelia (dashed arrows) varied from positive to negative. d) Detail of Ep and *Dpap*, isotype control. A corresponding section to c) did not show any reaction for IL-18. Symbols: stratified squamous epithelium (Ep) with an ulcer (arrow), hairs (cross-section, H), sebaceous glands (G), endothelia (dashed arrows) and leukocyte infiltration (arrowheads). e) Detail of *Dpap* with vessels and excretory ducts of apocrine glands (G). Blood vessel walls and endothelia (dashed arrows) of a larger artery (A) and smaller vessels stained positive for IL-18 (dashed arrows) usually appeared with immunopositive *Lamina media* and endothelia (dashed arrows). Excretory ducts of apocrine glands (G) were positive for IL-18. Fibrocytes and extracellular matrix were usually negative. f) Detail of adnexa in *Dpap*. The epithelial root sheath of a hair (H) and *Mm. arrectores pilorum* (Mm) always stained immunopositive for IL-18, while apocrine glands (G) stained positive, but with some patchy appearance. Fibrocytes and extracellular matrix were usually negative.

Additional file 12: Immunohistochemistry for Interleukin 18 (continued). Immunostaining for IL-18 (red) in representative skin samples (counterstaining with haematoxylin). a) *Dret* – detail with perivascular inflammation. Leukocytic perivascular infiltration is visible proximate to artery (A) and vein (V). Vessel walls and endothelia (dashed arrows), as well as infiltrated cells (arrows) are positive for IL-18. Fibrocytes and extracellular matrix are negative, apart from a weak background staining. b) Cross-sectioned nerve (N) in subcutis. Most parts of the nerve (N) stained immunopositive. In addition, adjacent capillary endothelia were positive for IL-18 (dashed arrows). c) Detail of infiltrated cells in *Dpap*. Infiltrating subepithelial immune cells were usually positive for IL-18 (arrowheads), as well as capillary endothelia (dashed arrows). Positive stratified squamous epithelium (Ep) and negative basis of an ulcer (arrow) are visible at the top edge of the detail.

Additional file 13: Staining characteristics of IL-12 and IL-18 in IHC. Detailed description of IL-12 and IL-18 stainings of skin biopsies.

Additional file 14: Influence of sex and type on systemic parameters. Differences to individual baselines of a) WBC, b) neutrophils and c, d) TNFα release (in medium only) of horses treated with DNA (groups B–D) calculated at t12 and t24 are plotted in histograms for mares and geldings (a–c) or Thoroughbreds (ThB) and Warmbloods (WBl) (d). Horizontal bars represent mean and SD. Asterisks (*) with brackets (┌┐) represent significantly different comparisons. The WBC, neutrophil and TNFα increases to individual baselines after treatments with SAINT-18 formulated DNA were significantly higher in mares than in geldings. Increases of TNFα releases were significantly higher in ThB than in WBl.

Abbreviations

#: Horse identification (letters); AIM2: Absent in melanoma 2; ANCOVA: Analysis of covariance; ANOVA: Analysis of variance; BSA: Bovine serum albumin; cDNA: Complementary DNA; cGAS: Cyclic GMP-AMP synthase; *ctrl*: Control skin samples, locally treated with PBS; CXCL: Chemokine (C-X-C motif) ligand; DNA: Deoxyribonucleic acid; *Dpap*: Papillary dermis; *Dret*: Reticular dermis; *E. coli*: *Escherichia coli*; EDTA: Ethylenediaminetetraacetate; ELISA: Enzyme-linked immunosorbent assay; FOV: Fields of view; H&E: Haematoxylin and eosin; Hct: Haematocrit; i.d.: Intradermal; i.m.: Intramuscular; IFN: Interferon; IHC: Immunohistochemistry; IL: Interleukin; ILRAP: IL-1beta receptor antagonist protein; LB: Luria-Bertani medium; LPS: Lipopolysaccharide; mAb: Monoclonal antibody; MIDGE: Minimalistic immunologic defined gene expression; mRNA: Messenger ribonucleic acid; mv: Multivariate; NGS: Normal goat serum; PBMC: Peripheral blood mononuclear cells; PBS: Phosphate buffered saline; PMA: Phorbol 12-myristate 13-acetate; qPCR: Quantitative PCR; RIG-I: Retinoic acid-inducible gene; RNA: Ribonucleic acid; rpm: Rounds per minute; RPMI: Roswell Park Memorial Institute; RT: Rectal temperature; rt: Room temperature; SAA: Serum amyloid A; SD: Standard deviation; STING: Stimulator of IFN genes; t(hours): Time post-treatment; t-(hours): Time pretreatment; t0: Time immediately prior to treatment; ThB: Thoroughbred; TLR: Toll-like receptor; TNF: Tumour necrosis factor; TPP: Total plasma protein; *treat*: Locally treated skin samples; uv: Univariate; WBC: White blood cell counts; WBl: Warm blood.

Competing interests

DO and CJ are employees of MOLOGEN AG. MOLOGEN AG owns a patent for the MIDGE-Th1 vector (PCT/DE02/03798P74). These affiliations do not alter the authors' adherence to the policies of Biomed Central Veterinary Research on sharing data and materials. BWi consulted and received funding from MOLOGEN AG.

Authors' contributions

CLS, HJS, KF and JMVC designed the concept of the study and created the manuscript. BWi, CJ and DO designed the treatment constructs, determined the application details and contributed to quantitative PCR assays. CLS, PS, MK, HME, SW, BWa, CP and AM contributed essentially to the development of analysis methods used herein. CLS and PS conducted the experiments of the present study and acquired the laboratory data. PJ performed the statistical analysis. All authors contributed to the critical revision and finalisation of the manuscript. All authors read and approved the final manuscript.

Acknowledgements

The authors thank Dr Kerstin Kapp for her valuable advice concerning CG motifs and their effects, Dirk Menzel for the technical support in haematological observations, and Marion Gähle and Doris Walter for excellent technical assistance in histology and immunohistochemistry.

Sources of funding

Christiane Schnabel is funded by the Friedrich-Ebert-Stiftung (Bonn, Germany).

Author details

[1]University of Veterinary Medicine Hannover, Clinic for Horses, Buenteweg 9, 30559 Hannover, Germany. [2]University of Veterinary Medicine Hannover, Immunology Unit, Bischofsholer Damm 15, 30173 Hannover, Germany. [3]Mologen AG, Fabeckstrasse 30, 14195 Berlin, Germany. [4]Foundation Institute Molecular Biology and Bioinformatics, Freie Universitaet Berlin, Berlin, Germany. [5]University of Veterinary Medicine Hannover, Small Animal Clinic, Buenteweg 9, 30559 Hannover, Germany. [6]Division of Medicine, Clinic III, Haematology, Oncology and Palliative Medicine, University of Rostock, 18057 Rostock, Germany. [7]University of Veterinary Medicine Hannover, Institute of Anatomy, Bischofsholer Damm 15, 30173 Hannover, Germany. [8]Department of Population Medicine and Diagnostic Sciences, College of Veterinary Medicine, Cornell Universit, 240 Farrier Rd, Ithaca, NY 14853, USA. [9]pj statistics, Niedstrasse 16, 12159 Berlin, Germany. [10]Department of Veterinary Medicine, Clinical Sciences, Clinical Pathology and Clinical Pathophysiology, Justus-Liebig-Universitaet, Frankfurter Strasse 126, 35392 Giessen, Germany.

References

1. Cavalleri JMV, Mählmann K, Steinig P, Feige K. Aetiology, clinical presentation and current treatment options of equine malignant melanoma - a review of the literature. Pferdeheilkunde. 2014;30(4):455–60.
2. Cotchin E. A general survey of tumours in the horse. Equine Vet J. 1977;9(1):16–21.
3. Valentine BA. Survey of equine cutaneous neoplasia in the Pacific Northwest. J Vet Diagn Invest. 2006;18(1):123–6.
4. Phillips JC, Lembcke LM. Equine melanocytic tumors. Vet Clin North Am Equine Pract. 2013;29(3):673–87.
5. Mcfadyean J. Equine melanomatosis. J Comp Path Ther. 1933;46:186–204.
6. Jeglum KA. Melanomas. In: Company RWBS, editor. Current therapy in equine medicine. 4th ed. Pennsylvania, USA: W.B. Saunders Company; 1999. p. 399–400.
7. Heinzerling LM, Feige K, Rieder S, Akens MK, Dummer R, Stranzinger G, et al. Tumor regression induced by intratumoral injection of DNA coding for human interleukin 12 into melanoma metastases in gray horses. J Mol Med. 2001;78(12):692–702.
8. Müller JMV, Feige K, Wunderlin P, Hodl A, Meli ML, Seltenhammer M, et al. Double-blind placebo-controlled study with interleukin-18 and interleukin-12-encoding plasmid DNA shows antitumor effect in metastatic melanoma in gray horses. J Immunother. 2011;34(1):58–64.
9. Phillips JC, Lembcke LM, Noltenius CE, Newman SJ, Blackford JT, Grosenbaugh DA, et al. Evaluation of tyrosinase expression in canine and equine melanocytic tumors. Am J Vet Res. 2012;73(2):272–8.
10. Dinarello CA. Interleukin-18. Methods. 1999;19(1):121–32.
11. Brunda MJ, Luistro L, Warrier RR, Wright RB, Hubbard BR, Murphy M, et al. Antitumor and antimetastatic activity of interleukin 12 against murine tumors. J Exp Med. 1993;178(4):1223–30.
12. Mortarini R, Borri A, Tragni G, Bersani I, Vegetti C, Bajetta E, et al. Peripheral burst of tumor-specific cytotoxic T lymphocytes and infiltration of metastatic lesions by memory CD8+ T cells in melanoma patients receiving interleukin 12. Cancer Res. 2000;60(13):3559–68.
13. Colombo MP, Trinchieri G. Interleukin-12 in anti-tumor immunity and immunotherapy. Cytokine Growth Factor Rev. 2002;13(2):155–68.
14. Shizuo A. The role of IL-18 in innate immunity. Curr Opin Immunol. 2000;12(1):59–63.
15. Trinchieri G. Interleukin-12 and the regulation of innate resistance and adaptive immunity. Nat Rev Immunol. 2003;3(2):133–46.
16. Del Vecchio M, Bajetta E, Canova S, Lotze MT, Wesa A, Parmiani G, et al. Interleukin-12: biological properties and clinical application. Clin Cancer Res. 2007;13(16):4677–85.
17. Coughlin CM, Salhany KE, Wysocka M, Aruga E, Kurzawa H, Chang AE, et al. Interleukin-12 and interleukin-18 synergistically induce murine tumor regression which involves inhibition of angiogenesis. J Clin Invest. 1998;101(6):1441–52.
18. Mählmann K, Feige K, Juhls C, Endmann A, Schuberth H-J, Oswald D, et al. Local and systemic effect of transfection-reagent formulated DNA vectors on equine melanoma. BMC Vet Res. 2015. accepted; doi: 10.1186/s12917-015-0422-9.
19. Lopez-Fuertes L, Perez-Jimenez E, Vila-Coro AJ, Sack F, Moreno S, Konig SA, et al. DNA vaccination with linear minimalistic (MIDGE) vectors confers protection against Leishmania major infection in mice. Vaccine. 2002;21(3–4):247–57.
20. Moreno S, López-Fuertes L, Vila-Coro AJ, Sack F, Smith CA, Konig SA, et al. DNA immunisation with minimalistic expression constructs. Vaccine. 2004;22(13–14):1709–16.
21. Schirmbeck R, König-Merediz S, Riedl P, Kwissa M, Sack F, Schroff M, et al. Priming of immune responses to hepatitis B surface antigen with minimal DNA expression constructs modified with a nuclear localization signal peptide. J Mol Med. 2001;79(5–6):343–50.
22. Zheng C, Juhls C, Oswald D, Sack F, Westfehling I, Wittig B, et al. Effect of different nuclear localization sequences on the immune responses induced by a MIDGE vector encoding bovine herpesvirus-1 glycoprotein D. Vaccine. 2006;24(21):4625–9.
23. Endmann A, Baden M, Weisermann E, Kapp K, Schroff M, Kleuss C, et al. Immune response induced by a linear DNA vector: Influence of dose, formulation and route of injection. Vaccine. 2010;28(21):3642–9.
24. Audouy SA, de Leij LF, Hoekstra D, Molema G. In vivo characteristics of cationic liposomes as delivery vectors for gene therapy. Pharm Res. 2002;19(11):1599–605.
25. Heinzerling L, Basch V, Maloy K, Johansen P1, Senti G, Wüthrich B, et al. Critical role for DNA vaccination frequency in induction of antigen-specific cytotoxic responses. Vaccine. 2006;24(9):1389–94.
26. Lopez AM, Hecker R, Mutwiri G, van Drunen Littel-van den Hurk S, Babiuk LA, Townsend HGG. Formulation with CpG ODN enhances antibody responses to an equine influenza virus vaccine. Vet Immunol Immunopathol. 2006;114(1–2):103–10.
27. Hafner M, Zawatzky R, Hirtreiter C, Buurman WA, Echtenacher B, Hehlgans T, et al. Antimetastatic effect of CpG DNA mediated by type I IFN. Cancer Res. 2001;61(14):5523–8.
28. McCluskie M, Weeratna R, Davis H. The role of CpG in DNA vaccines. Springer Semin Immunopathol. 2000;22(1):125–32.
29. Unterholzner L. The interferon response to intracellular DNA: why so many receptors? Immunobiology. 2013;218(11):1312–21.
30. Unterholzner L, Keating SE, Baran M, Horan KA, Jensen SB, Sharma S, et al. IFI16 is an innate immune sensor for intracellular DNA. Nat Immunol. 2010;11(11):997–1004.
31. Hornung V, Ablasser A, Charrel-Dennis M, Bauernfeind F, Horvath G, Caffrey DR, et al. AIM2 recognizes cytosolic dsDNA and forms a caspase-1-activating inflammasome with ASC. Nature. 2009;458(7237):514–8.
32. Hornung V, Hartmann R, Ablasser A, Hopfner KP. OAS proteins and cGAS: unifying concepts in sensing and responding to cytosolic nucleic acids. Nat Rev Immunol. 2014;14(8):521–8.
33. Ishii KJ, Coban C, Kato H, Takahashi K, Torii Y, Takeshita F, et al. A Toll-like receptor-independent antiviral response induced by double-stranded B-form DNA. Nat Immunol. 2006;7(1):40–8.
34. Jacobsen S, Kjelgaard-Hansen M, Hagbard Petersen H, Jensen AL. Evaluation of a commercially available human serum amyloid A (SAA) turbidometric immunoassay for determination of equine SAA concentrations. Vet J. 2006;172(2):315–9.
35. Ahmad-Nejad P, Hacker H, Rutz M, Bauer S, Vabulas RM, Wagner H. Bacterial CpG-DNA and lipopolysaccharides activate Toll-like receptors at distinct cellular compartments. Eur J Immunol. 2002;32(7):1958–68.
36. Barten MJ, Gummert JF, van Gelder T, Shorthouse R, Morris RE. Flow cytometric quantitation of calcium-dependent and -independent mitogen-stimulation of T cell functions in whole blood: inhibition by immunosuppressive drugs in vitro. J Immunol Methods. 2001;253(1–2):95–112.
37. He H, Courtney AN, Wieder E, Sastry KJ. Multicolor flow cytometry analyses of cellular immune response in rhesus macaques. J Vis Exp. 2010. doi:10.3791/1743.
38. Li L, Chi PD, Meng R, Yang BY, Wu CY. Abstract [Correlation of BrdU incorporation with activation and cytokine expression of T cells]. Xi Bao Yu Fen Zi Mian Yi Xue Za Zhi. 2008;24(1):72–5.
39. Lavoie-Lamoureux A, Maghni K, Lavoie J-P. Optimization of a procedure to accurately detect equine TNFalpha in serum samples. Vet Immunol Immunopathol. 2010;138(1–2):118–23.

40. Wagner B, Freer H. Development of a bead-based multiplex assay for simultaneous quantification of cytokines in horses. Vet Immunol Immunopathol. 2009;127(3–4):242–8.
41. Lillie RD, Fullmer HM. Histopathologic technic and practical histochemistry. New York, NY, USA: McGraw-Hill; 1976.
42. Grosche A, Morton AJ, Polyak MMR, Matyjaszek S, Freeman DE. Detection of calprotectin and its correlation to the accumulation of neutrophils within equine large colon during ischaemia and reperfusion. Equine Vet J. 2008;40(4):393–9.
43. Schnabel CL, Wagner S, Wagner B, Duran MC, Babasyan S, Nolte I, et al. Evaluation of the reactivity of commercially available monoclonal antibodies with equine cytokines. Vet Immunol Immunopathol. 2013;156(1–2):1–19.
44. MacKay RJ. Inflammation in horses. Vet Clin North Am Equine Pract. 2000;16(1):15–27.
45. Reed SM, Bayly WM, Sellon DC. Equine internal medicine. St. Louis, MO, USA: Elsevier Health Sciences; 2009.
46. Peiró JR, Barnabé PA, Cadioli FA, Cunha FQ, Lima VMF, Mendonça VH, et al. Effects of lidocaine infusion during experimental endotoxemia in horses. J Vet Intern Med. 2010;24(4):940–8.
47. Tousignant JD, Gates AL, Ingram LA, Johnson CL, Nietupski JB, Cheng SH, et al. Comprehensive analysis of the acute toxicities induced by systemic administration of cationic lipid:plasmid DNA complexes in mice. Hum Gene Ther. 2000;11(18):2493–513.
48. Jacobsen S, Andersen PH. The acute phase protein serum amyloid A (SAA) as a marker of inflammation in horses. Equine Vet Educ. 2007;19(1):38–46.
49. Jacobsen S, Niewold TA, Halling-Thomsen M, Nanni S, Olsen E, Lindegaard C, et al. Serum amyloid A isoforms in serum and synovial fluid in horses with lipopolysaccharide-induced arthritis. Vet Immunol Immunopathol. 2006;110(3–4):325–30.
50. Shanker A, Brooks AD, Jacobsen KM, Wine JW, Wiltrout RH, Yagita H, et al. Antigen presented by tumors in vivo determines the nature of CD8+ T-cell cytotoxicity. Cancer Res. 2009;69(16):6615–23.
51. Endmann A, Oswald D, Riede O, Talman EG, Vos RE, Schroff M, et al. Combination of MIDGE-Th1 DNA vaccines with the cationic lipid SAINT-18: studies on formulation, biodistribution and vector clearance. Vaccine. 2014;32(27):3460–7.
52. Lembcke LM, Kania SA, Blackford JT, Trent DJ, Odoi A, Grosenbaugh DA, et al. Development of immunologic assays to measure response in horses vaccinated with xenogeneic plasmid DNA encoding human tyrosinase. J Equine Vet Sci. 2012;32:607–15.
53. Klier J, May A, Fuchs S, Schillinger U, Plank C, Winter G, et al. Immunostimulation of bronchoalveolar lavage cells from recurrent airway obstruction-affected horses by different CpG-classes bound to gelatin nanoparticles. Vet Immunol Immunopathol. 2011;144(1/2):79–87.
54. Wagner B, Hillegas JM, Brinker DR, Horohov DW, Antczak DF. Characterization of monoclonal antibodies to equine interleukin-10 and detection of T regulatory 1 cells in horses. Vet Immunol Immunopathol. 2008;122(1–2):57–64.
55. Dinarello CA. Proinflammatory cytokines. Chest. 2000;118(2):503–8.
56. Kelso A. Cytokines: principles and prospects. Immunol Cell Biol. 1998;76(4):300–17.
57. Petrovsky N, McNair P, Harrison LC. Diurnal rhythms of pro-inflammatory cytokines: regulation by plasma cortisol and therapeutic implications. Cytokine. 1998;10(4):307–12.
58. Cavaillon JM. Pro- versus anti-inflammatory cytokines: myth or reality. Cell Mol Biol (Noisy-le-Grand). 2001;47(4):695–702.
59. Dow SW, Elmslie RE, Fradkin LG, Liggitt DH, Heath TD, Willson AP, et al. Intravenous cytokine gene delivery by lipid-DNA complexes controls the growth of established lung metastases. Hum Gene Ther. 1999;10(18):2961–72.
60. Dow SW, Fradkin LG, Liggitt DH, Willson AP, Heath TD, Potter TA. Lipid-DNA complexes induce potent activation of innate immune responses and antitumor activity when administered intravenously. J Immunol. 1999;163(3):1552–61.
61. Wattrang E, Berg M, Magnusson M. Immunostimulatory DNA activates production of type I interferons and interleukin-6 in equine peripheral blood mononuclear cells in vitro. Vet Immunol Immunopathol. 2005;107(3–4):265–79.
62. Wattrang E, Palm A-K, Wagner B. Cytokine production and proliferation upon in vitro oligodeoxyribonucleotide stimulation of equine peripheral blood mononuclear cells. Vet Immunol Immunopathol. 2012;146(2):113–24.
63. Leise BS, Yin C, Pettigrew A, Belknap JK. Proinflammatory cytokine responses of cultured equine keratinocytes to bacterial pathogen-associated molecular pattern motifs. Equine Vet J. 2010;42(4):294–303.
64. Bordin AI, Liu M, Nerren JR, Buntain SL, Brake CN, Kogut MH, et al. Neutrophil function of neonatal foals is enhanced in vitro by CpG oligodeoxynucleotide stimulation. Vet Immunol Immunopathol. 2012;145(1–2):290–7.
65. Schakowski F, Gorschluter M, Buttgereit P, Marten A, Lilienfeld-Toal MV, Junghans C, et al. Minimal size MIDGE vectors improve transgene expression in vivo. In Vivo. 2007;21(1):17–23.
66. Caracas HCPM, Maciel JVB, Martins PMRS, de Souza MMG, Maia LC. The use of lidocaine as an anti-inflammatory substance: a systematic review. J Dent. 2009;37(2):93–7.
67. Muir WW, Hubbell JAE. Equine anesthesia: monitoring and emergency therapy. St. Louis, Missouri, USA: Saunders Elsevier; 2008.
68. Coughlin CM, Salhany KE, Gee MS, LaTemple DC, Kotenko S, Ma X, et al. Tumor cell responses to IFNgamma affect tumorigenicity and response to IL-12 therapy and antiangiogenesis. Immunity. 1998;9(1):25–34.
69. Faleiros RR, Nuovo GJ, Belknap JK. Calprotectin in myeloid and epithelial cells of laminae from horses with black walnut extract-induced laminitis. J Vet Intern Med. 2009;23(1):174–81.
70. Phillips JC, Blackford JT, Lembcke LM, Grosenbaugh DA, Leard T. Evaluation of needle-free injection devices for intramuscular vaccination in horses. J Equine Vet Sci. 2011;31(12):738–43.
71. Goubier A, Fuhrmann L, Forest L, Cachet N, Evrad-Blanchard M, Juillard V, et al. Superiority of needle-free transdermal plasmid delivery for the induction of antigen-specific IFNgamma T cell responses in the dog. Vaccine. 2008;26(18):2186–90.
72. Machelska H, Schroff M, Oswald D, Binder W, Sitte N, Mousa SA, et al. Peripheral non-viral MIDGE vector-driven delivery of beta-endorphin in inflammatory pain. Mol Pain. 2009;5:72.
73. Cassatella MA, Gasperini S, Calzetti F, Bertagnin A, Luster AD, McDonald PP. Regulated production of the interferon-γ-inducible protein – 10 (IP-10) chemokine by human neutrophils. Eur J Immunol. 1997;27(1):111–5.
74. Tannenbaum CS, Wicker N, Armstrong D, Tubbs R, Finke J, Bukowski RM, et al. Cytokine and chemokine expression in tumors of mice receiving systemic therapy with IL-12. J Immunol. 1996;156(2):693–9.
75. Heinzerling L, Burg G, Dummer R, Maier T, Oberholzer PA, Schultz J, et al. Intratumoral injection of DNA encoding human interleukin 12 into patients with metastatic melanoma: clinical efficacy. Hum Gene Ther. 2005;16(1):35–48.
76. Nagai H, Hara I, Horikawa T, Oka M, Kamidono S, Ichihashi M. Gene transfer of secreted-type modified interleukin-18 gene to B16F10 belanoma cells suppresses in vivo tumor growth through inhibition of tumor vessel formation. J Investig Dermatol. 2002;119(3):541–8.
77. Durán MC, Willenbrock S, Müller J-MV, Nolte I, Feige K, Murua Escobar H. Establishment and evaluation of a bead-based luminex assay allowing simultaneous quantification of equine IL-12 and IFN gamma. Anticancer Res. 2013;33(4):1325–36.
78. Suagee JK, Corl BA, Crisman MV, Pleasant RS, Thatcher CD, Geor RJ. Relationships between body condition score and plasma inflammatory cytokines, insulin, and lipids in a mixed population of light-breed horses. J Vet Intern Med. 2013;27(1):157–63.
79. Schnabel CL, Steinig P, Schuberth HJ, Koy M, Wagner B, Wittig B, et al. Influences of age and sex on leukocytes of healthy horses and their ex vivo cytokine release. Vet Immunol Immunopathol. 2015;165(1–2):64–74.
80. Wilmink JM, Veenman JN, van den Boom R, Rutten VPMG, Niewold TA, Broekhuisen-Davies JM, et al. Differences in polymorphonucleocyte function and local inflammatory response between horses and ponies. Equine Vet J. 2003;35(6):561–9.
81. Adams AA, Breathnach CC, Katepalli MP, Kohler K, Horohov DW. Advanced age in horses affects divisional history of T cells and inflammatory cytokine production. Mech Ageing Dev. 2008;129(11):656–64.
82. Hansen S, Sun L, Baptiste KE, Fjeldborg J, Horohov DW. Age-related changes in intracellular expression of IFN-gamma and TNF-alpha in equine lymphocytes measured in bronchoalveolar lavage and peripheral blood. Dev Comp Immunol. 2013;39(3):228–33.
83. Katepalli MP, Adams AA, Lear TL, Horohov DW. The effect of age and telomere length on immune function in the horse. Dev Comp Immunol. 2008;32(12):1409–15.
84. Giraldo CE, Lopez C, Alvarez ME, Samudio IJ, Prades M, Carmona JU. Effects of the breed, sex and age on cellular content and growth factor release from equine pure-platelet rich plasma and pure-platelet rich gel. BMC Vet Res. 2013;9:29.

85. Rusek J, Klumplerova M, Molinkova D, Sedlinska M, Dusek L, Muzik J, et al. Genetics of anti-EHV antibody responses in a horse population. Res Vet Sci. 2013;95(1):137–42.
86. Weide B, Garbe C, Rammensee H-G, Pascolo S. Plasmid DNA- and messenger RNA-based anti-cancer vaccination. Immunol Lett. 2008;115(1):33–42.
87. Rosengren Pielberg G, Golovko A, Sundstrom E, Curik I, Lennartsson J, Seltenhammer M, et al. A cis-acting regulatory mutation causes premature hair graying and susceptibility to melanoma in the horse. Nat Genet. 2008;40(8):1004–9.
88. Comfort A. The longevity and mortality of thoroughbred mares. J Gerontol. 1958;13(4):342–50.
89. Mayr B, Niebauer GW, Gebhart W, Hofecker G, Kügl A, Schleger W. Untersuchungen an peripheren Leukozyten melanomtragender und melanomfreier Schimmelpferde verschiedener Altersstufen. Zentralbl Veterinarmed A. 1979;26(5):417–24.

PERMISSIONS

All chapters in this book were first published in VR, by BioMed Central; hereby published with permission under the Creative Commons Attribution License or equivalent. Every chapter published in this book has been scrutinized by our experts. Their significance has been extensively debated. The topics covered herein carry significant findings which will fuel the growth of the discipline. They may even be implemented as practical applications or may be referred to as a beginning point for another development.

The contributors of this book come from diverse backgrounds, making this book a truly international effort. This book will bring forth new frontiers with its revolutionizing research information and detailed analysis of the nascent developments around the world.

We would like to thank all the contributing authors for lending their expertise to make the book truly unique. They have played a crucial role in the development of this book. Without their invaluable contributions this book wouldn't have been possible. They have made vital efforts to compile up to date information on the varied aspects of this subject to make this book a valuable addition to the collection of many professionals and students.

This book was conceptualized with the vision of imparting up-to-date information and advanced data in this field. To ensure the same, a matchless editorial board was set up. Every individual on the board went through rigorous rounds of assessment to prove their worth. After which they invested a large part of their time researching and compiling the most relevant data for our readers.

The editorial board has been involved in producing this book since its inception. They have spent rigorous hours researching and exploring the diverse topics which have resulted in the successful publishing of this book. They have passed on their knowledge of decades through this book. To expedite this challenging task, the publisher supported the team at every step. A small team of assistant editors was also appointed to further simplify the editing procedure and attain best results for the readers.

Apart from the editorial board, the designing team has also invested a significant amount of their time in understanding the subject and creating the most relevant covers. They scrutinized every image to scout for the most suitable representation of the subject and create an appropriate cover for the book.

The publishing team has been an ardent support to the editorial, designing and production team. Their endless efforts to recruit the best for this project, has resulted in the accomplishment of this book. They are a veteran in the field of academics and their pool of knowledge is as vast as their experience in printing. Their expertise and guidance has proved useful at every step. Their uncompromising quality standards have made this book an exceptional effort. Their encouragement from time to time has been an inspiration for everyone.

The publisher and the editorial board hope that this book will prove to be a valuable piece of knowledge for researchers, students, practitioners and scholars across the globe.

LIST OF CONTRIBUTORS

Akihiro Ochi, Takanori Ueno and Yoshinari Katayama
Equine Research Institute, Japan Racing Association, 1400-4 Shiba, Shimotsuke, Tochigi 329-0412, Japan

Tatsuro Hifumi
Laboratory of Veterinary Histopathology, Joint Faculty of Veterinary Medicine, Kagoshima University, Kagoshima 890-0065, Japan

Ann Kristin Barton and Heidrun Gehlen
Equine Clinic, Freie Universitaet Berlin, Oertzenweg 19b, Berlin 10163, Germany

Tarek Shety
Equine Clinic, Freie Universitaet Berlin, Oertzenweg 19b, Berlin 10163, Germany
Animal Medicine Department, Faculty of Veterinary Medicine, Zagazig University, Zagazig, Egypt

Angelika Bondzio and Ralf Einspanier
Institute of Veterinary Biochemistry, Freie Universitaet Berlin, Oertzenweg 19b, Berlin 10163, Germany

Jorge U. Carmona, Diana L. Ríos and Catalina López
Grupo de Investigación Terapia Regenerativa, Departamento de Salud Animal, Universidad de Caldas, Manizales, Colombia

María E. Álvarez
Grupo de Investigación Terapia Regenerativa, Departamento de Salud Animal, Universidad de Caldas, Manizales, Colombia
Grupo de investigación Biosalud, Departamento de Ciencias Básicas para la Salud, Universidad de Caldas, Manizales, Colombia

Jorge E. Pérez
Grupo de investigación Biosalud, Departamento de Ciencias Básicas para la Salud, Universidad de Caldas, Manizales, Colombia

Mabel E. Bohórquez
Grupo de Investigación en Citogenética, Filogenia y Evolución de Poblaciones, Universidad del Tolima, Ibagué, Colombia

D. S. Trachsel
CIRALE-Hippolia, Médecine Sportive, RD 674, F-14430 Goustranville, France
Université Paris-Est, Ecole Nationale Vétérinaire d'Alfort, 7 avenue du Général de Gaulle, F-94704 Maisons-Alfort, France

A. Giraudet, D. Maso and G. Hervé
Université Paris-Est, Ecole Nationale Vétérinaire d'Alfort, 7 avenue du Général de Gaulle, F-94704 Maisons-Alfort, France

C. Robert
Université Paris-Est, Ecole Nationale Vétérinaire d'Alfort, 7 avenue du Général de Gaulle, F-94704 Maisons-Alfort, France
INRA, GABI-UMR1313, 78350 Jouy-en-Josas, France

D. D. Hauri
Office Fédéral de la Statistique, Espace de l'Europe 10, CH-2010 Neuchâtel, Switzerland

E. Barrey
INRA, GABI-UMR1313, 78350 Jouy-en-Josas, France

Anja Ziegler and Eliane Marti
Department of Clinical Research and Veterinary Public Health, Vetsuisse Faculty, University of Bern, Länggassstrasse 124, 3001 Bern, Switzerland

Eman Hamza
Department of Clinical Research and Veterinary Public Health, Vetsuisse Faculty, University of Bern, Länggassstrasse 124, 3001 Bern, Switzerland
Department of Zoonoses, Faculty of Veterinary Medicine, Cairo University, Cairo, Egypt

Helen Everett
Virology Department, Animal and Plant Health Agency-Weybridge, Woodham Lane, Addlestone, Surrey KT15 3NB, UK

Mattia Garbani
Swiss Institute of Allergy and Asthma Research (SIAF), University of Zürich, Davos, Switzerland

Vinzenz Gerber
Swiss Institute of Equine Medicine, University of Bern, Bern, Switzerland

Falko Steinbach
Faculty of Health and Medical Sciences, School of Veterinary Medicine, University of Surrey, Daphne Jackson Road, Guildford GU2 7AL, UK

Tytti M. Niemelä, Riitta-Mari Tulamo and Anna K. Hielm-Björkman
Department of Equine and Small Animal Medicine, Faculty of Veterinary Medicine, University of Helsinki, Helsinki, Finland

Kathrin Buntenkötter, Maren Osmers and Manfred Kietzmann
Institute of Pharmacology, Toxicology and Pharmacy, University of Veterinary Medicine Hannover Foundation, Hannover, Germany

Ina Schenk, Wilhelm Schänzer and Marc Machnik
Institute for Biochemistry, German Sport University, Cologne, Germany

Michael Düe
Sassenberg, Germany

Metha Chanda, Ratchakrit Srikuea, Arthit Chairoungdua and Pawinee Piyachaturawat
Department of Physiology, Faculty of Science, Mahidol University, Rama Rd., Rachatewee, Bangkok 10400, Thailand

Worakij Cherdchutam
Department of Large Animal and Wildlife Clinical Science, Faculty of Veterinary Medicine, Kasetsart University Kamphaeng Saen Campus, Nakornpathom 73140, Thailand

Daniel Gutiérrez-Expósito, Luis M. Ortega-Mora and G. Álvarez-García
SALUVET, Animal Health Department, Faculty of Veterinary Sciences, Complutense University of Madrid, Ciudad Universitaria s/n, 28040 Madrid, Spain

Ignacio García-Bocanegra and Antonio Arenas-Montes
Animal Health Department, Faculty of Veterinary Sciences, University of Cordoba-Agrifood Excellence International Campus (ceiA3), Cordoba, Spain

Daniel K. Howe and Michelle R. Yeargan
Department of Veterinary Science, M.H. Gluck Equine Research Center, University of Kentucky, Lexington, KY 40546-0099, USA

Sally Anne and L. Ness
Department of Clinical Sciences, College of Veterinary Medicine, Cornell University, Ithaca, NY 14853, USA

Tiny Motlatso Hlokwe
Zoonotic Diseases Section, ARC-Onderstepoort Veterinary Institute, Soutpan Rd., Onderstepoort 0110, South Africa
Department of Veterinary Tropical Diseases, Faculty of Veterinary Science, University of Pretoria, Soutpan Rd., Onderstepoort 0110, South Africa

Patrick Page
Department of Companion Animal Clinical Studies, Faculty of Veterinary Science, University of Pretoria, Soutpan Rd., Onderstepoort 0110, South Africa

David Sutton
Department of Companion Animal Clinical Studies, Faculty of Veterinary Science, University of Pretoria, Soutpan Rd., Onderstepoort 0110, South Africa
The Weipers Centre Equine Hospital, School of Veterinary Medicine, University of Glasgow, Glasgow, UK

Anita Luise Michel
Department of Veterinary Tropical Diseases, Faculty of Veterinary Science, University of Pretoria, Soutpan Rd., Onderstepoort 0110, South Africa

Lynn B. Williams and Judith B. Koenig
Department of Clinical Studies, Ontario Veterinary College, University of Guelph, Guelph, Ontario, Canada

Keith A. Russell and Thomas G. Koch
Department of Biomedical Sciences, Ontario Veterinary College, University of Guelph, Guelph, Ontario, Canada

Yuji Takahashi and Toshiyuki Takahashi
Sports Science Division, Equine Research Institute, Japan Racing Association, 1400-4, Shiba, Shimotsuke, Tochigi 329-0412, Japan

Florian Geburek, Moritz Gaus and Peter M. Stadler
Clinic for Horses, University of Veterinary Medicine Hannover, Foundation, Bünteweg 9, 30559 Hannover, Germany

Hans T. M. van Schie
Department of Equine Sciences, Faculty of Veterinary Medicine, Utrecht University, Yalelaan 112, 3584 CM Utrecht, Netherlands

Karl Rohn
Institute for Biometry, Epidemiology and Information Processing, University of Veterinary Medicine Hannover, Foundation, Bünteweg 2, 30559 Hannover, Germany

Sarah Vondran and Ingrid Vervuert
Institute of Animal Nutrition, Nutrition Diseases and Dietetics, Faculty of Veterinary Medicine, University of Leipzig, D-04103 Leipzig, Germany

Monica Venner
Equine Veterinary Clinic, D-38162 Destedt, Germany

Ann Kristin Barton, Anna Pelli and Heidrun Gehlen
Equine Clinic, Freie Universitaet Berlin, Oertzenweg 19b, 10163 Berlin, Germany

Martin Rieger
Research unit microbe-plant interactions, Helmholtz Zentrum Muenchen, Ingolstädter Landstraße 1, 85764 Neuherberg, Germany

E. Shields, S. Massie, S. Passante and R. Leguillette
University of Calgary Faculty of Veterinary Medicine (UCVM), 3330 Hospital Dr. NW, Calgary T2N 4 N1, AB, Canada

I. Seiden-Long
Foothills Medical Centre, University of Calgary Faculty of Medicine and Calgary Lab Services (CLS), Room C618B, 1403-29th St. NW, Calgary T2N 2 T9, AB, Canada

Sava Lazić, Diana Lupulović, Tamas Petrovic and Gospava Lazić
Scientific Veterinary Institute "Novi Sad", Novi Sad, Serbia

Aymeric Hans and Delphine Gaudaire
ANSES, Laboratory for Equine Diseases, Virology Unit, Dozulé, France

Marie Orard, Erika Hue, Marie-Pierre Toquet, Stéphane Pronost, Romain Paillot and Eric A. Richard
LABÉO Frank Duncombe, Caen, France
Normandie Université, UniCaen, BIOTARGEN, Caen, France

Magali Demoor
Normandie Université, UniCaen, BIOTARGEN, Caen, France
Anne Couroucé and Céline Bizon-Mercier
LUNAM Université, Oniris, NP3, Nantes, France

Meriel Moore-Colyer
Royal Agricultural University, Cirencester, UK

Laurent Couëtil
Purdue University, College of Veterinary Medicine, West Lafayette, IN, USA

Persephone Greco-Otto, Shannon Massie, Erin Shields, Marie-France Roy, Edmond Pajor and Renaud Léguillette
Department of Veterinary Clinical and Diagnostic Sciences, Faculty of Veterinary Medicine, University of Calgary, Calgary, AB T2N 4N1, Canada

Christiane L. Schnabel, Christine L. Wimer, Susanna Babasyan, Heather Freer, Christina Watts, Alicia Rollins and Bettina Wagner
Department of Population Medicine and Diagnostic Sciences, College of Veterinary Medicine, Cornell University, Ithaca, NY 14853, USA

Gillian Perkins
Department of Clinical Sciences, College of Veterinary Medicine, Cornell University, Ithaca, NY 14853, USA

Nikolaus Osterrieder
Institut für Virologie, Freie Universität Berlin, Philippstrasse 13, 10115 Berlin, Germany

Index

www.ingramcontent.com/pod-product-compliance
Lightning Source LLC
LaVergne TN
LVHW080728210926
848485LV00003B/534